THE BIG PICTURE
Physiology

Medical Course & Step 1 Review

Second Edition

a LANGE medical book

Jonathan D. Kibble, PhD
Professor of Physiology
Assistant Dean for Students
College of Medicine
University of Central Florida
Orlando, Florida

New York Chicago San Francisco Athens London Madrid
Mexico City Milan New Delhi Seoul Singapore Sydney Toronto

The Big Picture Physiology: Medical Course & Step 1 Review, Second Edition

Copyright © 2020 by McGraw Hill. All rights reserved. Printed in China. Except as permitted under the United States Copyright Act of 1976, no part of this publication may be reproduced or distributed in any form or by any means, or stored in a data base or retrieval system, without the prior written permission of the publisher.

Originally published as *Medical Physiology: The Big Picture,* copyright © 2009 by the McGraw-Hill Companies.

1 2 3 4 5 6 7 8 9   DSS   25 24 23 22 21 20

ISBN 978-1-260-12250-3

MHID 1-260-12250-6

This book was set in Minion Pro by MPS Limited.

The editors were Michael Weitz and Peter J. Boyle.

The production supervisor was Richard Ruzycka.

Production management was provided by Touseen Qadri, MPS Limited.

The designer was Mary McKeon.

This book is printed on acid-free paper.

Library of Congress Cataloging-in-Publication Data

Names: Kibble, Jonathan David, author.

Title: The big picture physiology : medical course & step 1 review / Jonathan D. Kibble.

Other titles: Big picture.

Description: Second edition. | New York : McGraw Hill, [2020] | Preceded by
    The big picture : medical physiology / by Jonathan David Kibble, Colby
    Ray Halsey. 2009. | Includes bibliographical references and index.

Identifiers: LCCN 2020012163 (print) | LCCN 2020012164 (ebook) |
    ISBN 9781260122503 (paperback ; alk. paper) | ISBN 9781260122510 (ebook)

Subjects: MESH: Physiological Phenomena | Outline

Classification: LCC QP34.5 (print) | LCC QP34.5 (ebook) | NLM QT 18.2 |
    DDC 612—dc23

LC record available at https://lccn.loc.gov/2020012163

LC ebook record available at https://lccn.loc.gov/2020012164

DEDICATION

In loving memory of my brother Gary.

Contents

Preface

The goal of this textbook is to help medical students to efficiently learn and review physiology. The text offers a complete yet concise treatment of the major topics in medical physiology. Several design features are included to make the text easy to use.

- High-yield clinical pearls ▼ are integrated throughout to the text; and clinical examples highlight the relevance and application of physiologic concepts.
- *Key concepts* are highlighted using italics, and **basic terms** are shown in bold when first used.
- Full-color figures illustrate essential processes; explanatory figure legends allow figures to be used for review.
- Bullets and numbering are used to break down complex processes.

Study questions and answers are provided at the end of each chapter. A final examination is also provided, which is organized by body system to allow either comprehensive testing or focused review.

Acknowledgments

Particular thanks to my first edition coauthor Colby Halsey and artist Matt Chansky; to the second edition editorial team from McGraw-Hill, especially Touseen Qadri and Kirti Sharma Kaistha; and to the project leader Michael Weitz for his patience and support.

About the Author

Jonathan Kibble is a professor of physiology at the University of Central Florida, College of Medicine in Orlando. He was recognized by the American Physiological Society in 2018 as the Arthur C. Guyton Physiology Educator of the Year and also received the Alpha Omega Alpha, Robert J. Glaser Distinguished Teacher Award in 2015 from the Association of American Medical Colleges. Jon trained in the United Kingdom in the early 1990s and also worked in the Caribbean and Canada before moving to the United States in 2008. Dr. Kibble brings 25 years of experience in teaching medical physiology to write a text that is both accessible and relevant for students of medicine.

General Physiology

CHAPTER 1

Homeostasis

1. Medical physiology is about how the body systems function and how they are controlled.
2. **Homeostasis** is the *maintenance of a stable internal environment* and requires integration of organ system functions (Table 1-1).
3. Negative feedback control.
   a. The stability of the body's internal environment is defined by the maintenance of **physiologic controlled variables** within narrow normal ranges (Table 1-2).
   b. Minimal variation in a controlled variable is explained by the presence of negative feedback control mechanisms.
   c. Negative feedback responses counter deviations of a controlled variable from its normal range; *this is the major control process used to maintain homeostasis.*

Table 1-1. Major Components and Functions of the Body Systems

Body System	Components	Major Function(s)
Cardiovascular	Heart, blood vessels, blood	Transport of materials throughout the body
Digestive	Gastrointestinal tract, liver, pancreas	Assimilation of nutrients; elimination of some wastes
Endocrine	Endocrine glands	Coordination of body functions through release of regulatory molecules
Immune	Thymus, spleen, lymphatic system, white blood cells	Defense against pathogens
Integumentary	Skin	Protection against external environment
Musculoskeletal	Skeletal muscle and bones	Movement and support
Nervous	Brain, spinal cord, peripheral nerves	Coordination of body functions through electrical signals and release of regulatory molecules; cognition
Reproductive	Gonads, penis, vagina, uterus	Procreation
Respiratory	Lungs	Oxygen and carbon dioxide and exchange with external environment
Urinary	Kidneys, bladder	Homeostasis of ion concentrations in internal environment; elimination of wastes

Table 1-2. Some Examples of Physiologic Controlled Variables

Controlled Variable (Arterial Blood Sample)	Typical Set Point Value
Arterial O_2 partial pressure	100 mm Hg
Arterial CO_2 partial pressure	40 mm Hg
Arterial blood pH	7.4
Glucose	90 mg/dL (5 mM)
Core body temperature	98.4°F (37°C)
Serum Na^+	140 mM
Serum K^+	4.0 mM
Serum Ca^{2+}	2.5 mM
Mean arterial blood pressure	90 mm Hg
Glomerular filtration rate	120 mL/min

   d. A negative feedback control system has the following elements (Figure 1-1):

      i. A **set point** value, which is at the center of the normal range and is treated by the control system as the target value.

      ii. **Sensors** that monitor the controlled variable.

      iii. A **comparator,** which interprets input from the sensors to determine when deviations from the set point have occurred. The comparator initiates a counter response.

      iv. **Effectors** are the mechanisms that restore the set point.

   e. Using the control of blood pressure as an example:

      i. The controlled variable is mean arterial blood pressure (MAP).

      ii. The normal set point for MAP is approximately 95 mm Hg.

      iii. Pressure sensors are located in the carotid sinus and relay information to a comparator located in the central nervous system.

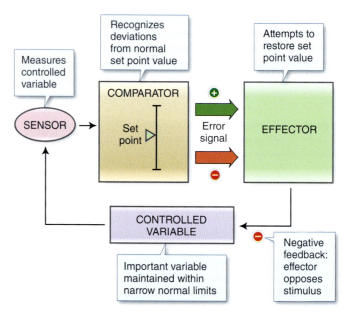

Figure 1-1. Components of a negative feedback control system.

    iv. If MAP suddenly changes, the activity of effectors (e.g., cardiac contractility, vascular tone, and urinary fluid excretion) is altered to restore normal blood pressure.

4. The internal environment.
   a. *The purpose of homeostasis is to provide an optimal fluid environment for cellular function.*
   b. The body fluids are divided into two major functional **compartments:**
      i. **Intracellular fluid (ICF)** is the fluid inside cells.
      ii. **Extracellular fluid (ECF)** is the fluid outside cells, which is subdivided into the **interstitial fluid** and the blood **plasma.**
   c. The concept of an internal environment in the body correlates with the interstitial fluid bathing cells.
   d. There is free exchange of water and small solutes in the ECF between interstitial fluid and plasma across the blood capillaries.
   e. Exchange between interstitial fluid and ICF is highly regulated and occurs across cell membranes.
   f. The volume of **total body water** is approximately 60% of the body weight in men and 50% in women.
      i. About 60% of the total body water is ICF and 40% is ECF (Figure 1-2).

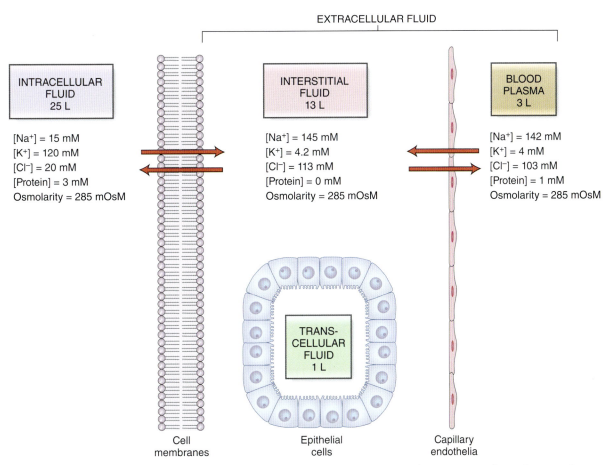

Figure 1-2. Body fluid compartments. Intracellular fluid (ICF) is separated from extracellular fluid (ECF) by cell membranes. ECF is composed of the interstitial fluid bathing cells and the blood plasma within the vascular system. Interstitial fluid is separated from plasma by capillary endothelia. Transcellular fluid is part of the ECF and includes epithelial secretions such as the cerebrospinal and extraocular fluids. ECF has a high [Na$^+$] and a low [K$^+$], whereas the opposite is true of ICF. All compartments have the same osmolarity at steady state.

ii. Approximately 80% of the ECF is interstitial fluid and the remaining 20% is blood plasma.

iii. ECF is high in NaCl and low in K^+, whereas ICF is high in K^+ and low in NaCl.

iv. Interstitial fluid is similar in composition to plasma, except that *interstitial fluid has almost no protein.*

v. Osmolarity is the same in all compartments.

g. ▼ Fluid can move freely from the interstitial to plasma compartments and helps to maintain blood volume during **hemorrhage.**

i. Because approximately 80% of the ECF is interstitial fluid and 20% is blood plasma, a hemorrhaging patient must lose about 5 L of ECF before the plasma volume is decreased by 1 L.

ii. The reverse is also true; to replace 1 L of plasma volume, approximately 5 L of intravascular isotonic saline must be infused. ▼

Membrane Transport Mechanisms

1. The transport of solutes across cell membranes is fundamental to the survival of all cells. Specializations in membrane transport mechanisms often underlie tissue function. For example, voltage-sensitive ion channels account for the ability to generate electrical signals.

2. Cell membranes separate the cytosol from the ECF.

a. Cell membranes are formed from phospholipids that are an effective barrier against the free movement of most water-soluble solutes.

b. Most biologically important substances require a protein-mediated pathway to cross cell membranes.

3. **Solute transport** can be categorized based on the use of cellular energy or the type of transport pathway (Figure 1-3):

a. **Active transport** requires adenosine triphosphate (ATP) hydrolysis.

i. **Primary active transport** occurs via membrane proteins that *directly couple ATP hydrolysis to solute movement.*

ii. **Secondary active transport** couples the transport of two or more solutes together. Energy is used to develop a favorable electrochemical driving force for one solute, which is then used to power the transport of other solutes (e.g., the inwardly directed Na^+ gradient is used to drive glucose uptake from the intestine).

b. **Passive transport** does not require ATP hydrolysis or coupling to another solute.

c. Primary active transporters (Figure 1-4A):

i. **The Na^+/K^+-ATPase** (known as the "sodium pump") is present in all cells and transports $3Na^+$ out of a cell in exchange for $2K^+$, using 1 ATP molecule in each transport cycle. *The action of sodium pumps accounts for high Na^+ concentration in ECF and high K^+ concentration in ICF.*

ii. **Ca^{2+}-ATPases** are located in the plasma membrane and endoplasmic reticulum membrane and function to maintain very low intracellular $[Ca^{2+}]$.

iii. **H^+/K^+-ATPases** pump H^+ out of cells in exchange for K^+ and are present in several epithelia. H^+/K^+-ATPase is responsible for the secretion of acidic gastric juice in the stomach.

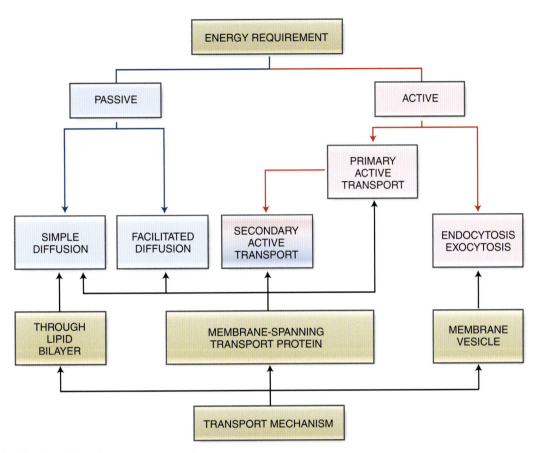

Figure 1-3. Classification of membrane transport systems.

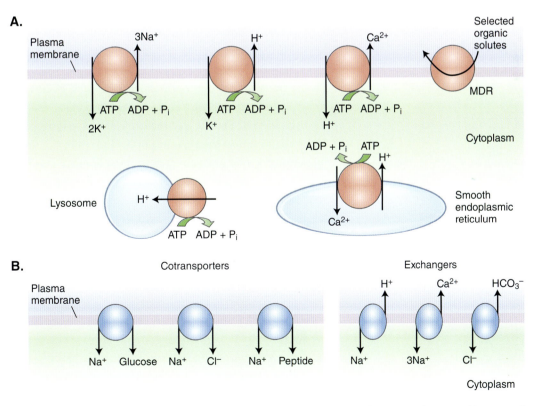

Figure 1-4. Active transport. **A.** Examples of primary active transporters (ATPases) in the plasma membrane and in organelles. **B.** Examples of secondary active transporters; cotransporters transport solutes in the same direction, and exchangers transport solutes in opposite directions. ADP, adenosine diphosphate; ATP, adenosine triphosphate; MDR, multidrug resistance.

    iv. **H⁺-ATPases** are mainly expressed inside cells, including the vacuolar H⁺-ATPase, which acidifies lysosomes; **ATP synthase** is a form of H⁺-ATPase, which operates in reverse to synthesize ATP in mitochondria.

    v. The **multidrug resistance (MDR) transporters** are ATPases that extrude a wide variety of organic molecules from cells. MDRs are physiologically expressed in the liver, kidney, and blood-brain barrier.

      • ▼ The expression of **MDR transporters** (e.g., P-glycoprotein) is one mechanism by which bacteria and cancer cells can become drug resistant. The effectiveness of a drug will be reduced if it is transported out of the target cell by MDR transporters. ▼

d. There are many examples of secondary active transporters (Figure 1-4B):

    i. **Cotransporters (symporters)** couple the movement of two or more solutes in the same direction.

      • Examples of Na⁺-driven cotransporters include Na⁺/glucose uptake in the intestine and diuretic-sensitive Na⁺/K⁺/Cl⁻ and Na⁺/Cl⁻ uptake in the kidney.

      • H⁺/peptide cotransport in the intestine is an example of Na⁺-independent cotransport.

    ii. **Exchangers (antiporters)** couple the movement of two solutes in the opposite direction.

      • Na⁺-driven antiporters include Na⁺/Ca²⁺ and Na⁺/H⁺ exchange, which are important for maintaining low intracellular [Ca²⁺] and [H⁺], respectively.

      • Cl⁻/HCO₃⁻ exchange is an example of an anion exchanger. It is widely expressed, for example, in red blood cells, where it assists in HCO₃⁻ transport into and out of the cell as part of the blood-CO₂ transport system.

e. Passive transport can only occur along a favorable electrochemical gradient.

f. **Simple passive transport** is characterized by a linear relationship between the transport rate and the electrochemical driving force.

g. Pathways for simple passive transport include diffusion through the lipid bilayer or via pores or channels in the membrane (Figure 1-5A).

h. **Fick's law of diffusion** describes the simple diffusion of an uncharged solute (*s*):

$$J_s = -P_s \Delta C_s \hspace{3cm} \textbf{Equation 1-1}$$

    J_s = Net flux per unit area
    P_s = Permeability
    ΔC_s = Concentration difference of *s* across the membrane

i. **Permeability** is a single coefficient relating the driving force for diffusion to net flux.

    i. The membrane permeability to a solute is proportional to the lipid solubility of the solute and inversely proportional to its molecular size.

    ii. *Gases are an example of molecules that are able to move through the lipid bilayer of cell membranes by simple diffusion because they are small and lipid soluble.*

A. Routes available for passive transport

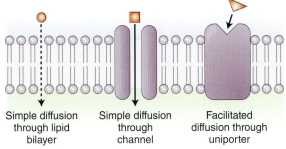

Simple diffusion through lipid bilayer

Simple diffusion through channel

Facilitated diffusion through uniporter

B. Components of ion channels

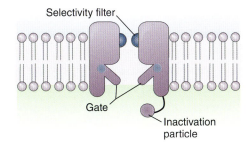

Selectivity filter

Gate

Inactivation particle

C. Kinetics of passive transport

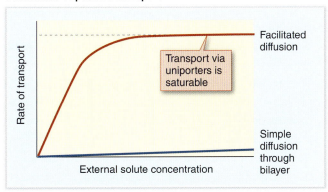

Rate of transport

Facilitated diffusion

Transport via uniporters is saturable

Simple diffusion through bilayer

External solute concentration

Figure 1-5. A. Passive transport pathways. **B.** General components of ion channels components. **C.** Kinetics of passive transport. Note the linear relationship between simple diffusion and flux; facilitated diffusion via uniporters is faster than simple diffusion but is saturable.

j. The passive transport of ions and other small water-soluble molecules across a cell membrane requires transport proteins that span the membrane.

k. **Ion channels** are the most numerous example of passive transporters. Ion channels have the following **general components** (Figure 1-5B):
   i. A **pore region,** through which ions diffuse.
   ii. A **selectivity filter** within the pore, causing the channel to be highly selective for a particular ion (e.g., Na^+ channels).
   iii. A **gating mechanism** that opens and closes the channel; gates may be controlled by membrane voltage (**voltage-gated channels**), chemicals (**ligand-gated channels**), or mechanical forces in the membrane (e.g., **stretch-activated channels**).

l. Passive transport can also occur via **uniporters,** which selectively bind a single solute at one side of the membrane and undergo a conformational change to deliver it to the other side.

       i. Solute transport via uniporters is called **facilitated diffusion** because it is faster than simple diffusion (Figure 1-5C).

       ii. *A characteristic feature of facilitated diffusion is the saturation of the transport rate at high solute concentrations.*

       iii. The **GLUT family** are examples of uniporters for glucose transport that are expressed in many tissues.

   m. *Macromolecules are transported between the ICF and the ECF using membrane-limited vesicles.*

       i. **Endocytosis** is the ingestion of extracellular material to form endocytic vesicles inside a cell. There are three **types of endocytosis:**

- **Pinocytosis** is the ingestion of small particles and ECF that occurs constitutively in most cells.
- **Phagocytosis** is the uptake of large particles (e.g., microorganisms) that occurs in specialized immune cells.
- **Receptor-mediated endocytosis** allows uptake of specific molecules and occurs at specialized areas of membrane called **clathrin-coated pits** (e.g., uptake of cholesterol from low-density lipoproteins).

       ii. **Exocytosis** is export of soluble proteins into the extracellular space by vesicular transport. When vesicles containing proteins fuse with the plasma membrane, the soluble proteins are secreted and the vesicle membrane is incorporated in the plasma membrane. There are two **pathways for exocytosis:**

- The **constitutive pathway** is present in most cells and is used to export extracellular matrix proteins.
- The **regulated pathway** is present in cells that are specialized for the secretion of proteins such as hormones, neurotransmitters, and digestive enzymes. *An increase in the intracellular Ca^{2+} concentration is a key event that triggers regulated exocytosis.*
- ▼ **Lambert-Eaton syndrome** is a neurologic condition resulting from autoantibodies that bind to and block Ca^{2+} channels on the presynaptic motor nerve terminals. By blocking the Ca^{2+} channels, the Ca^{2+}-dependent exocytosis of vesicles filled with acetylcholine (a neurotransmitter needed for muscle contraction) is inhibited, resulting in muscle weakness. ▼

4. **Osmosis.**

   a. *Water transport across a barrier is always passive, driven either by a diffusion gradient or by a hydrostatic pressure gradient.*

   b. Osmosis is water movement that is driven by a **water concentration gradient** across a membrane (Figure 1-6A).

   c. Water concentration is expressed in terms of total solute concentration; the more dilute a solution, the lower its solute concentration and the higher its water concentration.

   d. When two solutions are separated by a **semipermeable membrane** (i.e., one that allows the transport of water but not solutes), *water moves by osmosis away from the more dilute solution.*

   e. *Osmolarity* is an expression of the osmotic strength of a solution and is the ***total solute concentration.***

       i. Osmolarity is the product of the molar solute concentration and the number of particles that the solute dissociates into when dissolved. For example:

A. Osmosis

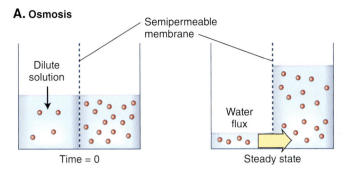

B. Concept of osmotic pressure

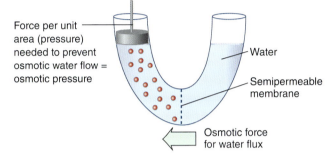

C. Reflection coefficient

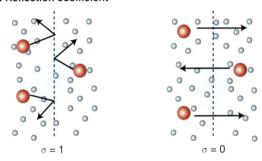

Figure 1-6. Osmosis. **A.** Illustration of osmotic water movement across a semipermeable membrane. **B.** The concept of osmotic pressure. **C.** Reflection coefficients: Solutes that do not permeate the membrane exert all their osmotic pressure ($\sigma = 1$); freely permeable solutes ($\sigma = 0$) do not exert any osmotic pressure.

- 1 mol of glucose dissolved in 1 L of water produces a solution of 1 Osm/L.
- 1 mol of NaCl dissolved in 1 L of water produces a solution of approximately 2 Osm/L.

ii.   Two solutions of the same osmolarity are termed **isosmotic.** A solution with a greater osmolarity than a reference solution is said to be **hyperosmotic,** and a solution of lower osmolarity is described as **hyposmotic.**

iii.   Osmolarity can be converted into units of pressure, which allow osmotic and hydrostatic pressure gradients to be mathematically combined; for example, when considering fluid filtration across capillary walls (see Chapter 4).

iv.   The concept of osmotic pressure (π) is illustrated in Figure 1-6B and is calculated by **van't Hoff law:**

$$\pi = g \times C \times RT \qquad \text{Equation 1-2}$$

g = Number of particles produced when the solute dissociates in solution

C = Molar solute concentration

R = Gas constant

T = Temperature

f. Although blood plasma contains many solutes, a simplified **clinical estimate of plasma osmolarity** can be obtained by considering only the Na^+, glucose, and urea concentrations:

$$P_{Osm} = 2P_{Na} + (P_{glucose} / 18) + (P_{urea} / 2.8) \qquad \textbf{Equation 1-3}$$

P_{Osm} = Plasma osmolarity (mOsm/L)

P_{Na} = Plasma [Na] (mEq/L)

$P_{glucose}$ = Plasma [glucose] (mg/dL)

P_{urea} = Plasma [urea] (mg/dL)

g. A difference between the measured and estimated osmolarity is called an **osmolar gap** and is *caused by the presence of additional solutes in plasma.*

  i. ▼ Patients with **alcohol intoxication** or **ethylene glycol poisoning** will have an increased osmolar gap. ▼

h. The concept of effective osmolarity (tonicity) includes the effect of solute permeation through membranes (Figure 1-6C).

  i. Most biologic membranes are not completely semipermeable.

  ii. *When the membrane is permeated by the solute, the observed osmotic pressure gradient is reduced.*

  iii. The **reflection coefficient (σ)** is the fraction of the measured osmolarity actually applied:

  - $\sigma = 1.0$ for solutes that do not permeate a membrane.
  - $\sigma = 0$ when the membrane is freely permeable to the solute.
  - The effective osmolarity of a solution is calculated as the product of the osmolarity and the reflection coefficient (e.g., *if $\sigma = 0.5$, the effective osmolarity exerted is only 50% of the measured osmolarity*).

  iv. The terms **isotonic, hypotonic, and hypertonic** are used to describe the effective osmolarity of a solution relative to a cell:

  - An **isotonic solution** has the same effective osmolarity as the cell and causes *no net water movement.*
  - A **hypotonic solution** has a smaller effective osmolarity and *causes cells to swell.*
  - A **hypertonic solution** has a larger effective osmolarity and *causes cells to shrink.*

  v. ▼ *At steady state the ECF is isotonic with respect to the ICF because water moves freely across most cell membranes. When the steady state is temporarily disrupted, water moves until ICF and ECF tonicity again becomes equal. For example, if a patient is intravenously infused with a* **hypotonic saline solution,** *the ECF tonicity is initially decreased and some water moves into the ICF by osmosis (i.e., cells swell).* ▼

Membrane Potentials

1. All living cells have a membrane potential difference in which the cytoplasm is negative with respect to the ECF (Figure 1-7A).

A. Resting membrane potential

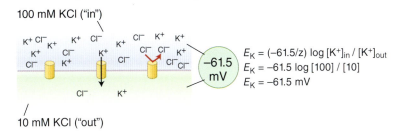

B. Diffusion potentials and Nernst equation

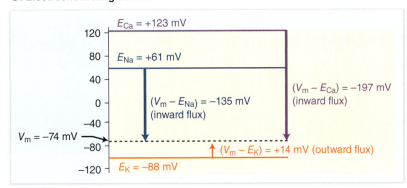

100 mM KCl ("in")

$E_K = (-61.5/z) \log [K^+]_{in} / [K^+]_{out}$
$E_K = -61.5 \log [100] / [10]$
$E_K = -61.5$ mV

10 mM KCl ("out")

C. Electrochemical gradients

$E_{Ca} = +123$ mV

$E_{Na} = +61$ mV

$(V_m - E_{Ca}) = -197$ mV (inward flux)

$(V_m - E_{Na}) = -135$ mV (inward flux)

$V_m = -74$ mV

$(V_m - E_K) = +14$ mV (outward flux)

$E_K = -88$ mV

Figure 1-7. A. The resting membrane potential; all cells have a negative intracellular potential. **B.** Generation of a K$^+$ diffusion potential. In this example, K$^+$ is the only permeable ion; a small amount of K$^+$ diffuses to the lower compartment, creating a negative potential in the upper compartment. The Nernst equation predicts the equilibrium potential (voltage), based on the size of the K$^+$ concentration ratio between compartments. **C.** Electrochemical gradients. Membrane potential (V_m) is shown by the dashed line. Downward arrows indicate gradients for cation flux into the cell; the upward arrow indicates a gradient for cation efflux.

2. *Membrane potentials arise because there are stable ion diffusion gradients across the membrane and because cell membranes contain ion channels that provide* **selective ion permeability.**

3. The following steps are involved in the development of a **diffusion potential:**
   a. In the example in Figure 1-7B, two potassium chloride (KCl) solutions are separated by a membrane that is permeable to K$^+$ but not to Cl$^-$.
   b. **K$^+$ diffuses** from the upper to the lower compartment, down its concentration gradient. In this case, Cl$^-$ cannot follow.
   c. A **voltage difference** develops as the K$^+$ ions leave the upper compartment, leaving a net negative charge behind. *A very slight separation of KCl ion pairs is enough to generate physiologic voltages.*
   d. The negative potential in the upper compartment attracts K$^+$ ions and opposes the K$^+$ concentration gradient.
   e. An **equilibrium potential** is established when the voltage difference and the concentration gradient are equal but opposite driving forces. *At the equilibrium potential, there is no net movement of K$^+$.*
   f. This simulated example is analogous to most resting cells, which contain a high [K$^+$] and have numerous open K$^+$ channels at rest (note, however, that the major intracellular anion in cells is protein, not Cl$^-$).

4. The equilibrium potential is a function of the size of the ion concentration gradient (Table 1-3) and is calculated using the **Nernst equation:**

Table 1-3. Ion Concentrations and Equilibrium Potentials

Ion	[Intracellular] mM	[Extracellular] mM	E_{Nernst} mV
Excitable cells (nerve and muscle)			
Na$^+$	12	145	+67
K$^+$	155	4.5	−95
Ca^{2+}	10^{-4}	1.0	+123
Cl$^-$	4	115	−89
HCO$_3^-$	12	24	−19
Nonexcitable cells			
Na$^+$	15	145	+61
K$^+$	120	4.5	−88
Ca^{2+}	10^{-4}	1.0	+123
Cl$^-$	20	115	−47
HCO$_3^-$	16	24	−13

$$E_x = \frac{-61.5}{z}\log\frac{[X]_i}{[X]_o}$$

Equation 1-4

E_x = Equilibrium potential for ion x

z = Ion valence (+1 for K$^+$, −1 for Cl$^-$, +2 for Ca^{2+}, and so on)

$[X]_i$ = Intracellular concentration of X

$[X]_o$ = Extracellular concentration of X

a. **Example.** The only ion channels that open in a resting cell are K$^+$ channels. If the intracellular [K$^+$] = 155 mM/L and the ECF [K$^+$] = 4.5 mM/L, predict the resting membrane potential.

   i. The magnitude of the K$^+$ diffusion potential that develops is calculated using Equation 1-4:

$$E_x = \frac{-61.5}{z}\log\frac{[K]_i}{[K]_o}\,\text{mV}$$

$$E_x = \frac{-61.5}{z}\log\frac{[155]_i}{[4.5]_o}\,\text{mV}$$

$$E_x = -94.5\,\text{mV}$$

5. Resting membrane potential.

  a. *The measured membrane potential (V_m) will usually be a composite of several diffusion potentials because the membrane is usually permeable to more than one ion.*

  b. Ion permeability is best expressed in terms of electrical **conductance** to reflect ion movement through channels.

  c. V_m *can be expressed as the weighted average of ion equilibrium potentials for permeable ions. For example, in the case of a cell with permeability to K$^+$, Na$^+$, and Cl$^-$:*

$$V_m = (g_K/g_m)E_K + (g_{Na}/g_m)E_{Na} + (g_{Cl}/g_m)E_{Cl}$$

Equation 1-5

g_x/g_m = Fractional conductance of ion x

E_x = Equilibrium potential for ion x

i. **Example.** Estimate the membrane potential that will arise, using data in Table 1-3, for a nonexcitable cell and assuming that 80% of the total membrane conductance is due to K^+ channels, 5% is due to Na^+ channels, and 15% is due to Cl^- channels:

$$V_m = (0.80)E_K + (0.05)E_{Na} + (0.15)E_{Cl}$$
$$= (0.80 \times -88) + (0.05 \times 61) + (0.15 \times -47)$$
$$= -74.4 \text{ mV}$$

d. *In most cells, V_m is primarily a function of ECF $[K^+]$ because K^+ conductance predominates in most cells at rest.*

e. Although the **Na^+/K^+-ATPase** is electrogenic (i.e., $3Na^+$ are pumped out for every $2K^+$ pumped into the cell), its direct contribution to the membrane potential is small. *The importance of the Na^+/K^+-ATPase in the development of resting membrane potentials is to maintain resting ion concentration gradients.*

f. According to Equation 1-5, V_m will only change if equilibrium potentials are disturbed (i.e., if ion concentration gradients change), or if the membrane conductance to an ion changes because ion channels open or close.

g. The following terms are used to describe **changes in the membrane potential:**

   i. **Depolarization** is a change to a less negative membrane potential (membrane potential difference is decreased).

   ii. **Hyperpolarization** occurs when the membrane potential becomes more negative (membrane potential difference is increased).

   iii. **Repolarization** is the return of the membrane potential toward V_m following either depolarization or hyperpolarization.

h. ▼ **Hyperkalemia** is a potentially fatal condition in which the serum $[K^+]$ is increased. According to the Nernst equation, an increase in the serum $[K^+]$ will decrease E_K and therefore will depolarize V_m, which can cause fatal cardiac arrhythmias. Using the following example, consider the effects on the heart when a normal serum $[K^+]$ of 4.5 mM is doubled to 9.0 mM.

   i. **Part 1.** Calculate the expected resting membrane potential for cardiac cells using the data in Table 1-3 for excitable cells (note $[K^+]$ = 4.5 mM) and assuming the following fractional membrane conductance values: $g_K/g_m = 0.90$, $g_{Na}/g_m = 0.05$, $g_{Cl}/g_m = 0.05$.

   $$V_m = (0.90)E_K + (0.05)E_{Na} + (0.05)E_{Cl}$$
   $$= (0.90 \times -\mathbf{95} \text{ mV}) + (0.05 \times 67 \text{ mV}) + (0.05 \times -89 \text{ mV})$$
   $$= -\mathbf{87.0} \text{ mV}$$

   ii. **Part 2.** Calculate the expected change in the resting membrane potential when the serum $[K^+]$ is doubled to 9.0 mM. Assume all other variables are unchanged.

   iii. The first step is to calculate the new equilibrium potential based on Equation 1-4 (the Nernst equation):

   $$E_x = \frac{-61.5}{z} \log \frac{[K]_i}{[K]_o} \text{ mV}$$

$$E_x = \frac{-61.5}{z} \log \frac{[155]_i}{[9]_o} \, \text{mV}$$

$$E_x = -76 \, \text{mV}$$

Recalculating the resting membrane potential, using the new value for E_K:

$$\begin{aligned} V_m &= (0.90)E_K + (0.05)E_{Na} + (0.05)E_{Cl} \\ &= (0.90 \times -76) + (0.05 \times 67) + (0.05 \times -89) \\ &= -69.5 \, \text{mV} \end{aligned}$$

iv. Depolarizing excitable cardiac myocytes from a membrane potential of -87 mV to -69.5 mV may be enough to trigger extra cardiac action potentials, which may lead to a fatal arrhythmia. ▼

6. The **electrochemical gradient** for an ion is the *net* driving force for ion flux, which is a combination of the membrane voltage and the ion concentration gradient (Figure 1-7C).
   a. The Nernst equation converts the ion concentration gradient into mV units for combination with the membrane voltage; the electrochemical gradient is defined as $(V_m - E_x)$.
      i. A positive value represents a driving force for outward cation flux or inward anion flux.
      ii. A negative value represents a driving force for inward cation flux or outward anion flux.

Action Potential

1. Excitable tissues (i.e., neurons and muscle) can respond to a stimulus by rapidly generating and propagating electrical signals.
2. An action potential is a constant electrical signal that can be propagated over long distances without decay.
3. Action potentials are an **all-or-none impulse** that occurs when an excitable cell membrane is depolarized beyond a **threshold voltage.**
   a. Once the threshold has been exceeded, there is a phase of rapid depolarization, which ends abruptly at a **peak voltage** greater than 0 mV.
   b. The **overshoot** is the amount that the peak voltage exceeds 0 mV.
   c. A slower **repolarizing phase** returns membrane potential toward V_m.
   d. An **afterhyperpolarization** (undershoot) is observed in nerves (but not in muscle), in which the membrane potential is transiently more negative than the resting membrane potential.
4. *The phases of an action potential are explained by changes in membrane Na⁺ and K⁺ conductance with time* (Figure 1-8A):
   a. **Rapid depolarization** after threshold voltage is exceeded is due to the opening of **voltage-gated Na⁺ channels.**
   b. The **peak voltage** where rapid depolarization abruptly ends and the membrane enters the repolarizing phase has two components:
      i. Closure of **inactivation gates** on Na⁺ channels.
      ii. Opening of **voltage-gated K⁺ channels.**
   c. **Repolarization** of the membrane potential progresses due to the decreasing Na⁺ conductance and the increasing K⁺ conductance.

A.

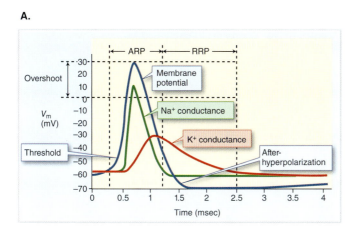

B.

Unmyelinated nerve axon

Continuous conduction

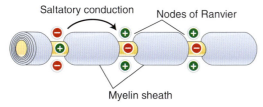

Myelinated nerve axon

Saltatory conduction   Nodes of Ranvier

Myelin sheath

Figure 1-8. A. Nerve action potential. The upstroke of the action potential results from increased Na⁺ conductance. Repolarization results from a declining Na⁺ conductance combined with an increasing K⁺ conductance; afterhyperpolarization is due to sustained high K⁺ conductance. **B.** Action potential propagation. Local current flow causes the threshold potential to be exceeded in adjacent areas of the neuron membrane. Because the upstream region is refractory, an action potential is only propagated downstream. In myelinated axons, action potentials propagate faster by "jumping" from one node of Ranvier to the next node by saltatory conduction. ARP, absolute refractory period; RRP, relative refractory period.

    d. **Afterhyperpolarization** occurs because K^+ conductance is transiently even higher than it is at rest, causing V_m to approach E_K.

5. **Refractory periods.**

    a. *Stimulus intensity (e.g., loudness of a sound) is encoded in the nervous system by action potential frequency since action potentials all have the same amplitude and action potentials never summate.*

    b. The maximum action potential frequency is limited because a finite period of time must elapse after one action potential before a second one can be triggered.

       i. The **absolute refractory period** is the time from the beginning of one action potential when it is *impossible to stimulate another action potential.*

- The absolute refractory period results from closure of **inactivation gates in Na⁺ channels**; inactivated channels must close and the gates must be reset before channels can be reopened.

  ii. The **relative refractory period** is the time after the absolute refractory period when another impulse can occur, but only *if a stronger stimulus is applied*.

  - A stronger stimulus is needed because some of the Na⁺ channels have not yet recovered from inactivation and the membrane is less excitable due to high K⁺ conductance.

6. Action potential propagation (Figure 1-8B).

   a. *Action potentials are only propagated in one direction along a nerve axon or muscle fiber.*

   b. The impulse in one area causes **local current flow,** which depolarizes the adjacent area to threshold, generating a new action potential downstream; conduction is **unidirectional** because the upstream region is in its refractory period.

   c. The speed of *action potential conduction is faster in larger diameter fibers* because they have lower electrical resistance than small diameter fibers.

   d. *Conduction speed is also increased by the* **myelination** *of nerve axons.*

      i. Myelin consists of glial cell plasma membrane, concentrically wrapped around the nerve.

      ii. In the peripheral nerves, the myelin sheath is interrupted at regular intervals by uncovered **nodes of Ranvier.**

      iii. Action potentials are rapidly propagated from node-to-node by "**saltatory conduction**" because *voltage-gated Na⁺ channels are only expressed at the nodes of Ranvier.*

      iv. ▼ Diseases that result in **demyelination** of either the central nervous system (e.g., **multiple sclerosis**) or the peripheral nervous system (e.g., **Guillain-Barré syndrome**) will significantly impede nerve conduction, impairing the function of the nervous system. ▼

Synaptic Transmission

1. Synapses are specialized cell-to-cell contacts that allow the information encoded by action potentials to pass to another cell.

2. There are **two types of synapses:**

   a. **Electrical synapses** occur where two cells are joined by **gap junctions,** which conduct current from cell to cell via nonselective pores. *Cardiac muscle is an example of cells that are electrically coupled via gap junctions.*

   b. **Chemical synapses** involve the release of a chemical transmitter by one cell that acts upon another cell (Figure 1-9).

      i. Action potentials in a presynaptic cell cause the release of the chemical transmitter, which crosses a narrow cleft to interact with specific receptors on a postsynaptic cell.

      ii. Excitatory neurotransmitters depolarize the postsynaptic membrane, producing an **excitatory postsynaptic potential.**

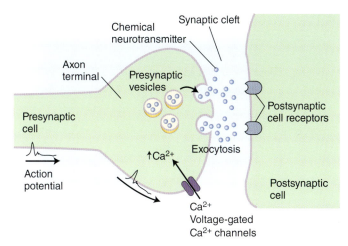

Figure 1-9. Components of a chemical synapse. Action potentials in the presynaptic neuron cause voltage-gated Ca^{2+} channels to open. Ca^{2+} influx triggers exocytosis of neurotransmitter molecules from storage vesicles into the synaptic cleft. Neurotransmitter molecules interact with receptors on the postsynaptic cell membrane to induce either excitatory (depolarizing) or inhibitory (hyperpolarizing) postsynaptic potentials.

     iii. Inhibitory neurotransmitters hyperpolarize the postsynaptic membrane, producing an **inhibitory postsynaptic potential.**

   c. Chemical synapses have the following functional characteristics:

     i. **Presynaptic terminals** contain neurotransmitter chemicals stored in vesicles. Action potentials in a presynaptic terminal cause Ca^{2+} entry through voltage-gated Ca^{2+} channels, triggering the release of neurotransmitter by **exocytosis.**

     ii. There is a **delay** between the arrival of an action potential in the presynaptic terminal and the onset of a response in the postsynaptic cell:

- The delay is short (<1 msec) when the postsynaptic receptor is a ligand-gated ion channel (**ionotropic receptor**).
- The delay is long (>100 msec) if the receptor is linked to an intracellular second messenger system (**metabotropic receptor**).

     iii. Transmitter action is rapidly terminated. One of the following three processes can remove transmitter molecules from the synaptic cleft:

- Diffusion.
- Enzymatic degradation by extracellular enzyme (in the case of **acetylcholine**).
- Uptake of transmitter into the nerve ending or other cell (usually most important).

Skeletal Muscle

1. There are three anatomic types of muscle: **skeletal, cardiac,** and **smooth.**
   a. Both skeletal and cardiac muscles are classified microscopically as **striated muscle.**
   b. Skeletal muscle is also referred to as **voluntary** because it *remains relaxed in the absence of nerve stimulation.*
   c. Cardiac and smooth muscles can function without nerve input and are referred to as **involuntary.**
2. Skeletal muscle structure (Figure 1-10).

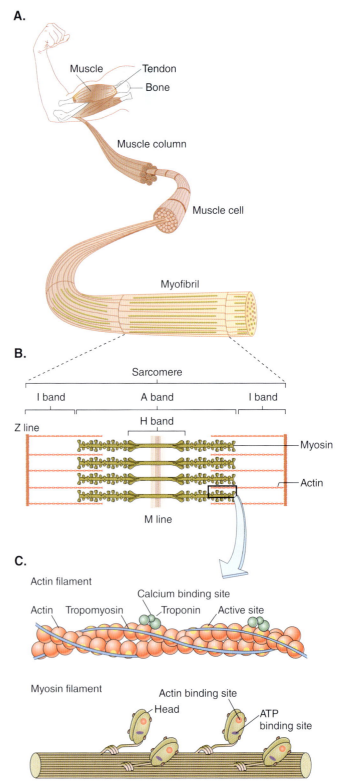

Figure 1-10. A. Structure of skeletal muscle: Muscle cells (fibers) contain a group of myofilaments, each composed of sarcomeres aligned end-to-end. **B.** The sarcomere. A regular array of filament proteins between adjacent Z disks comprises a sarcomere. Thin actin filaments extend from Z disks toward a central M line, partially overlapping thick myosin filaments. Under a microscope, the region of thick filaments (A band) appears darker than adjacent areas with only thin filaments (I band), producing the striated appearance of skeletal muscle. Striations in adjacent myofibrils are also aligned. **C.** Molecular components of thin and thick filaments. Thin filaments are composed of actin, with the associated proteins tropomyosin and troponins; thick filaments are composed of myosin. ATP, adenosine triphosphate.

a. The generation of action potentials in the skeletal muscle cell membrane (**sarcolemma**) triggers a sequence of events that result in force development by the muscle.

b. The ability of muscle to generate force when stimulated results from the presence of **motor proteins** inside muscle cells.

c. Skeletal muscles consist of **muscle columns,** each of which consists of a bundle of muscle cells (also called **fibers** or **myocytes**).

d. Muscle cells are multinucleate and are bounded by the sarcolemma. Each myocyte contains several cylindrical **myofibrils,** which display a distinctive pattern of light and dark bands under the light microscope.

e. Striations are due to the orderly arrangement of structural and contractile proteins. Each repeating motif in the striated pattern is called a **sarcomere,** which is the *fundamental contractile unit of skeletal muscle.* Each sarcomere has the following elements:

   i. A **Z disk** bounds the sarcomere at each end.

   ii. **Thin filaments,** composed of **actin, tropomyosin,** and **troponins,** project from each Z disk toward the center of the sarcomere.

   iii. **Thick filaments,** composed of **myosin,** are present in the center of the sarcomere and are overlapped by thin filaments.

f. Sarcomeres line up end-to-end within a single myofibril.

   i. The darker areas are denoted as **A bands** and correspond to the location of thick filaments.

   ii. Lighter areas at the ends of sarcomeres are denoted as **I bands** and correspond to thin filaments where no overlap with thick filaments occurs.

g. **Thin filaments** have three major components:

   i. The backbone of a thin filament is a double-stranded helix of **actin.**

   ii. The helical groove on the actin filament is occupied by **tropomyosin.** Skeletal muscle contraction is regulated via a protein complex that consists of tropomyosin plus attached troponin subunits.

   iii. **Troponin** is a heterotrimer consisting of troponins T, C, and I:

- **Troponin T** anchors the trimer to tropomyosin.
- **Troponin C** binds Ca^{2+}, which allows muscle contraction to occur.
- **Troponin I** inhibits interaction between actin and myosin if the intracellular Ca^{2+} concentration is low.

h. Thick filaments are composed of **myosin** molecules, which are the molecular motors responsible for the generation of force. Myosin molecules are composed of the following major parts:

   i. The **myosin head** contains the actin-binding site plus elements necessary for ATP binding and hydrolysis. The heads are cross-bridges that bind to actin during muscle contraction.

   ii. Myosin heads are connected to the tail of the molecule via a **hinge.** The hinge allows the movement of cross-bridges, which is the basis of force generation.

i. The protein **titin** is important for maintaining sarcomere structure and runs from the Z disk to the M line at the center of the sarcomere. Titin is extensible and is largely responsible for the passive tension that is measured when a relaxed muscle is stretched (see Muscle Mechanics).

j. ▼ **Dystrophin** is an important scaffolding protein located between the sarcolemma and myofilaments that is mutated in **Duchenne muscular dystrophy** (DMD).
   i. DMD is an X-linked disease causing progressive muscle weakness and, most commonly, death from respiratory failure.
   ii. Milder mutations in the dystrophin gene result in the less severe condition of **Becker's muscular dystrophy.** ▼

3. The sliding filament theory of muscle contraction (Figure 1-11).
   a. *The mechanism of active force generation in all muscle types is based on thin filaments being pulled over thick filaments.*
   b. In a relaxed skeletal muscle, contraction is inhibited by the tropomyosin-troponin complexes, which obscure the active site on actin and prevent cross-bridge binding.
   c. When the muscle is stimulated, the intracellular Ca^{2+} concentration increases and Ca^{2+} **binds to troponin C.** The resulting conformational change exposes active sites on actin.
   d. A cycle of events now occurs in which myosin cross-bridges bind to actin, perform a **powerstroke,** detach, become cocked again, and then reattach. The cycle repeats in the continued presence of Ca^{2+} **and ATP.**
   e. Thin filaments from each end of the sarcomere move toward the center by sliding over thick filaments, causing neighboring Z disks to approach each other. In the example shown in Figure 1-11, muscle shortening has occurred and the sarcomere length is reduced (compare panels 1 and 5).
   f. ▼ When death occurs, ATP production by mitochondria stops and **rigor mortis** (stiffening of the muscles) sets in. *ATP is necessary for the myosin heads to detach from the actin filaments after a powerstroke occurs.* Once ATP production ceases, the cross-bridges are locked in place, which results in stiff muscles. ▼

4. Neuromuscular junction.
   a. *Skeletal muscle does not contract until stimulated by action potentials arriving from a motor neuron.*
   b. Motor neurons branch to activate a group of muscle fibers, known collectively as a **motor unit** (Figure 1-12A).
      i. Muscles that are subjected to fine control (e.g., muscles of the hand) have many small motor units, whereas postural muscles have fewer large motor units. The synapse between a motor neuron and a skeletal muscle cell is called a **neuromuscular junction** or **end plate.**
   c. Every skeletal muscle cell (fiber) has only one neuromuscular junction, near its midpoint.
   d. An individual neuromuscular junction consists of a small, branched patch of bulb-shaped nerve endings, called **terminal boutons** (Figure 1-12B). *Motor neurons release acetylcholine as their neurotransmitter.*
      i. Acetylcholine is synthesized in the cytoplasm of presynaptic terminals from acetyl coenzyme A and choline, via the enzyme **choline acetyltransferase,** and is stored in vesicles within the nerve terminal.
   e. The postsynaptic muscle cell membrane opposite the presynaptic terminals has a high density of **nicotinic acetylcholine receptors.**
      i. Nicotinic receptors are ionotropic receptors that function as **nonselective Na^+ and K^+ channels.**

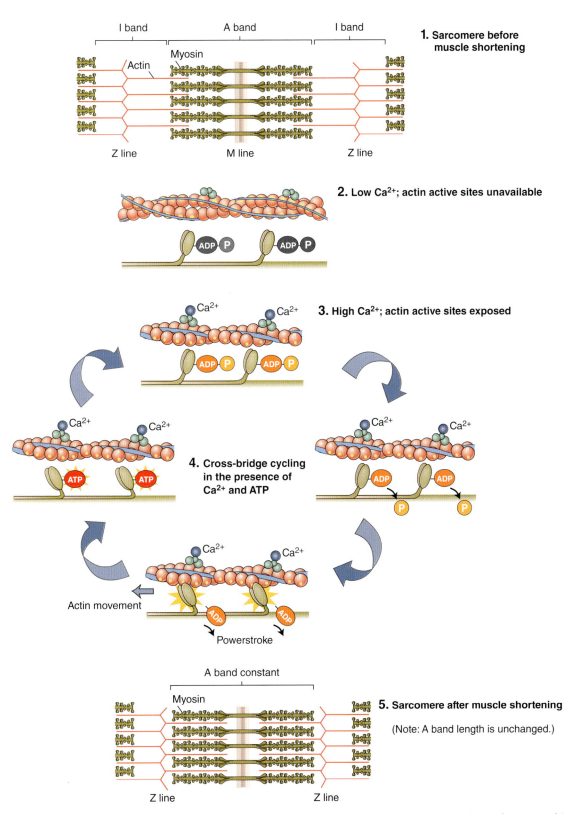

Figure 1-11. Sliding filament theory of muscle contraction. Ca^{2+} binding to troponin C causes actin active sites to be exposed (compare panels 2 and 3). In the presence of adenosine triphosphate (ATP), myosin repeats a cycle of binding to actin, performance of a power stroke, detaching, becoming cocked, and reattaching further along the actin molecule (panel 4). Actin filaments are drawn over myosin. In this example, muscle shortening occurs (compare panels 1 and 5). ADP, adenosine diphosphate.

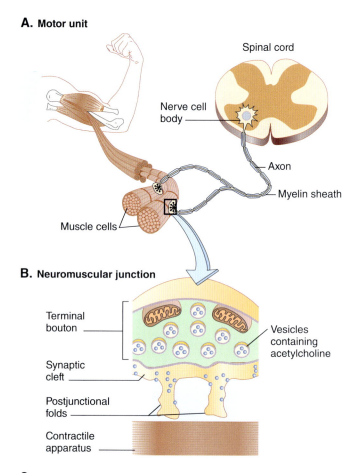

A. Motor unit

Spinal cord

Nerve cell body

Axon

Myelin sheath

Muscle cells

B. Neuromuscular junction

Terminal bouton

Vesicles containing acetylcholine

Synaptic cleft

Postjunctional folds

Contractile apparatus

C. Postsynaptic potentials

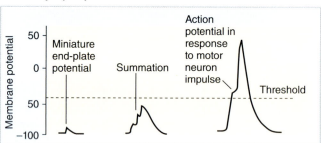

Figure 1-12. Innervation of skeletal muscle. **A.** Motor units include a motor neuron and the group of muscle fibers that are innervated by its branches. **B.** The neuromuscular junction. Acetylcholine release from motor neuron terminals stimulates nicotinic receptors in the muscle membrane, producing an excitatory postsynaptic potential. **C.** End-plate potentials. Acetylcholine in a single presynaptic vesicle (quantum) evokes a miniature end-plate potential. Action potential in a motor neuron triggers the release of many quanta, and miniature end-plate potentials summate to exceed the threshold for action potential in the muscle fiber.

ii. When opened, nicotinic receptors cause skeletal muscle membrane potential to depolarize because the combined equilibrium potential for Na^+ and K^+ (E_{cation}) is approximately 0 mV.

iii. Acetylcholine from a single presynaptic vesicle (a **quantum**) produces a small depolarization of the muscle membrane, called a **miniature end-plate potential.**

   iv. Depolarizations from many quanta summate to produce a full end-plate potential in the muscle membrane, which is an example of an **excitatory postsynaptic potential.**

   v. *A single motor nerve impulse normally produces an end-plate potential that exceeds the threshold for action potential generation in the muscle cell membrane* (Figure 1-12C).

 f. Acetylcholine within the synaptic cleft is rapidly broken down to choline and acetic acid by the enzyme **acetylcholinesterase,** which is anchored to the muscle cell basement membrane.

   i. Choline is taken up by presynaptic nerve terminals and is reused for acetylcholine synthesis.

 g. ▼ **Myasthenia gravis** is an autoimmune disease in which antibodies are directed against nicotinic acetylcholine receptors, reducing the number at the end plate.

   i. Acetylcholine release is normal, but the postsynaptic membrane is less responsive and this results in muscle weakness.

   ii. *Myasthenia gravis is treated with agents that inhibit acetylcholinesterase in the cleft, thereby prolonging the action of acetylcholine at the neuromuscular junction.* ▼

 h. ▼ The neuromuscular junction is the target of several natural venoms and toxins as well as pharmacological agents (see Table 1-4). ▼

Table 1-4. Drugs and Toxins That Affect Neuromuscular Transmission

Agent(s)	Action	Effect
Botulinum toxin	Enters motor nerve terminal, irreversibly inhibits acetylcholine release	Failure of acetylcholine release; flaccid paralysis of muscle
α-**Latrotoxin**	Enters motor nerve terminal, promotes massive release of acetylcholine	Initial surge of acetylcholine release followed by irreversible depletion of acetylcholine; contractions followed by flaccid paralysis
ω-**Conotoxin**	Binds irreversibly to Ca^{2+} channels in motor nerve terminal membrane	Reduced Ca^{2+} entry to nerve terminal, reduced acetylcholine release; flaccid paralysis
d-**Tubocurarine, pancuronium**	Reversible competitive antagonists at nicotinic acetylcholine receptors	Prevents acetylcholine action; flaccid paralysis
α-**Bungarotoxin**	Irreversible antagonist at nicotinic acetylcholine receptors	Prevents acetylcholine action; flaccid paralysis
Neostigmine	Inhibits acetylcholinesterase in synaptic cleft	Prolongs action of acetylcholine at the end plate
Hemicholinium	Choline reuptake blocker in motor neuron terminal	Depletes acetylcholine in nerve terminals; muscle weakness or flaccid paralysis

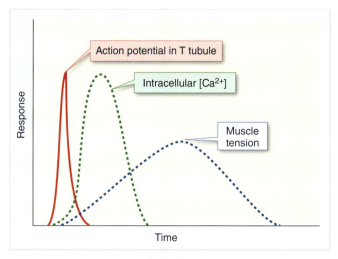

Figure 1-13. E-C coupling sequence in skeletal muscle. Force development depends on increased intracellular Ca²⁺, which is preceded by the muscle action potential.

5. Excitation-contraction coupling.
   a. *In all types of muscle, the key event causing contraction is increased intracellular Ca^{2+} concentration* (Figure 1-13).
   b. In skeletal muscle, the source of Ca^{2+} for contraction is the **sarcoplasmic reticulum (SR).**
   c. The muscle action potential triggers Ca^{2+} release from the SR in skeletal muscle.
   d. *The only physiologic stimulus for skeletal muscle action potentials is the end-plate potential, developed in response to motor nerve impulses.*
   e. The membrane system of the SR is enclosed within the cell and is comprised of **longitudinal tubules,** which surround the contractile apparatus and terminate in **lateral sacs** (terminal cisternae).
   f. Lateral sacs are closely associated with invaginations of the muscle cell plasma membrane called **T tubules.**
   g. The lateral sacs from two neighboring sarcomeres converge on a T tubule to form a structure known as a **triad.** Triads are located at the junction of the A band and the I band of every sarcomere (Figure 1-14A).
   h. Action potentials in T tubules induce Ca^{2+} release from the lateral sacs (Figure 1-14B).
      i. The Ca^{2+} release mechanism involves **voltage sensors** in the T-tubule membrane (L-type Ca^{2+} channels), which are linked to **Ca^{2+} release channels** (ryanodine receptors) in the SR.
      ii. The voltage sensors respond to depolarization in the T tubule with conformational changes that result in the opening of the Ca^{2+} release channels of the SR.
   i. The intracellular $[Ca^{2+}]$ increases from about 10^{-8} M at rest to about 10^{-5} M during a muscle contraction.
   j. To return a muscle to the relaxed state, Ca^{2+} uptake occurs in the longitudinal tubules via **Ca^{2+}-ATPases** of the SR.
   k. Following Ca^{2+} reuptake, most stored Ca^{2+} is found in the lateral sacs, where it is weakly bound to the protein **calsequestrin.**
6. Force of contraction.

A. Sarcotubular system of striated muscle cell

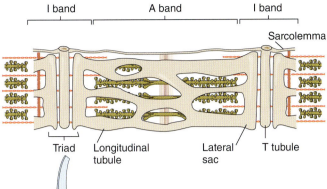

B. Excitation-contraction coupling mechanism

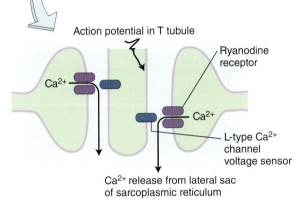

Figure 1-14. A. Muscle triads. Each T tubule is associated with a lateral sac from each of the two neighboring sarcomeres to form a triad. **B.** The excitation-contraction coupling mechanism in skeletal muscle. The close association of membranes in the triad allows muscle action potentials to open the sarcoplasmic reticulum Ca²⁺ release channels through activation of voltage sensors in T tubules.

a. *The force of skeletal muscle contraction is controlled by altering the firing pattern of motor nerves to the muscle.*

b. The effect of increasing action potential frequency to a muscle is known as **temporal summation** (Figure 1-15).

   i. At low stimulation frequency, the muscle briefly generates force and then relaxes.

   ii. At high stimulation frequency, the muscle does not have time to relax between stimuli. Contractions fuse into a plateau of active force called a **tetanic contraction.**

c. If a greater force of muscle contraction is needed, the number of active motor neurons increases. Recruitment of motor units is called **spatial summation.**

   i. Spatial summation is organized according to the "**size principle.**" Small motor neurons, which reach only a few muscle fibers, are more excitable than large motor neurons and are recruited first.

   ii. Large motor neurons are less excitable and require a stronger stimulus from the central nervous system. When large motor neurons are recruited, a large number of muscle fibers are stimulated to produce a strong contraction.

d. ▼ **Tetanus toxin,** which is produced by the bacterium *Clostridium tetani,* can result in tetany throughout all the skeletal muscles of the body.

   i. The bacterium lives in the soil, and once it contaminates a dirty wound, the tetanus toxin is released.

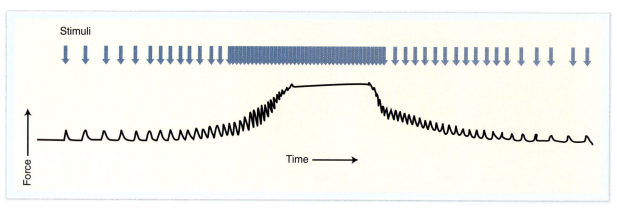

Figure 1-15. Temporal summation. Increased frequency of muscle stimulation (indicated by *downward arrows*) causes increased force of contraction. At low-frequency stimulation, Ca^{2+} reuptake is complete and the muscle relaxes completely between stimuli. With high-frequency stimulation, intracellular Ca^{2+} concentration remains high; the contraction force reaches a plateau (tetanus) when all the troponin C sites are filled with Ca^{2+}.

      ii. The toxin travels to the spinal cord where it blocks inhibitory nerves, allowing the excitatory motor neurons to fire rapidly.

      iii. Rapidly firing motor neurons summate to produce **tetany,** a potentially fatal condition! ▼

7. Skeletal muscle diversity (Table 1-5).
   a. There are two major types of muscle fibers: Slow twitch (type I) and fast twitch (type II).
   b. Expression of different isoforms of myosin and other proteins accounts for different shortening speeds of fast and slow twitch fibers.
   c. Whole muscles are made up of different proportions of slow and fast twitch fibers. For example:
      i. Postural muscles contain a higher proportion of slow twitch fibers because they must maintain tone and resist fatigue.
      ii. Extraocular muscles are required to make fast, brief movements of the eye and therefore contain a high proportion of fast twitch fibers.
   d. There are genetic differences in the general proportions of muscle fiber types that are expressed among individuals, which accounts in part for the tendency for a person to be either a better sprinter (more fast twitch fibers) or to have higher endurance (more slow twitch fibers).
   e. The distribution of fiber types is also affected by the firing patterns of motor neurons and can, therefore, be modified by the type of training a person does (e.g., endurance training increases the proportion of slow twitch fibers).

Table 1-5. Comparison of Slow Twitch and Fast Twitch Muscle Fibers

Characteristic	Slow Twitch (Type I)	Fast Twitch (Type II)
Color	Red (myoglobin)	White (low myoglobin)
Metabolism	Oxidative	Glycolytic
Mitochondria	Abundant	Few
Glycogen content	Low	High
Fatigability	Low	High

8. Muscle mechanics.
   a. There are **two general modes of muscle contraction:**
      i. An **isometric,** or fixed-length contraction, occurs if both ends of a muscle are fixed. The muscle can develop tension but it cannot shorten.
      ii. An **isotonic,** or fixed-load contraction, occurs if a muscle is able to shorten to carry a given load.
   b. *Resting muscle length is an important determinant of the force of contraction.* The **length-tension (length-force) relation** is studied under isometric conditions.
      i. A resting muscle behaves like a rubber band, requiring force to stretch it to different lengths.
      ii. The **preload** is the amount of force applied to a resting muscle before stimulation, creating **passive tension.**
      iii. When the muscle is stimulated, **active tension** is added to the passive tension. The amount of active tension produced is the difference between passive tension and **total tension** (Figure 1-16A).

A.

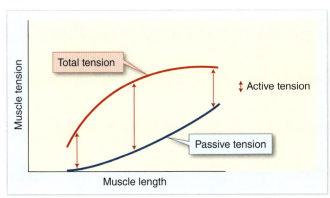

B.

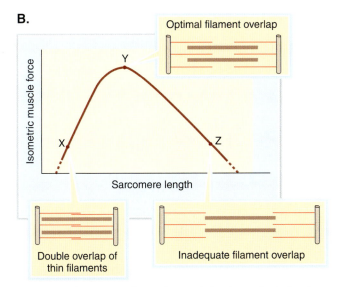

Figure 1-16. The length-tension relationship in skeletal muscle. **A.** Passive tension (preload) is the force required to set the resting length (*blue curve*). Total tension (*red curve*) includes active (developed) tension in addition to passive tension. Maximum active tension is developed from an optimal resting muscle length; short and long resting lengths both reduce developed tension. **B.** Optimal resting muscle length corresponds with optimal overlap of thick and thin filaments in sarcomeres.

      iv. *There is an optimal range of resting muscle length (preload) that produces maximal contraction.*
- At very short or very long muscle lengths, active force development declines, producing the characteristic length-tension relationship of striated muscle.
- *The **plateau** of the length-tension relation* (see Figure 1-16B, point y) *reflects optimal overlap of thin and thick filaments within sarcomeres, providing maximum myosin cross-bridge binding.*
- On the **ascending limb** (see Figure 1-16B, between points x and y), the muscle is too short, resulting in double overlap of thin filaments and attachment of fewer cross-bridges.
- On the **descending limb** of the curve (see Figure 1-16B, points y and z), the muscle is too long, resulting in inadequate overlap of thin and thick filaments.

      v. *Skeletal muscles operate at the plateau of their length-tension relation because preload is set at the optimal level by bony attachments at each end of the muscle.*

c. ▼ *Preload is not fixed in cardiac muscle but varies according to the amount of venous return.*

    i. In a healthy heart, an increased preload will stretch the cardiac myocytes, resulting in a more forceful and speedy contraction.

    ii. However, in a diseased heart (e.g., **left ventricular hypertrophy**), cardiac muscle can become stiff, impairing its ability to stretch. Increasing preload in this setting will mainly increase the pressures in the heart without the benefit of improving contractile force or speed. ▼

d. Muscle performance can be studied under isotonic conditions to produce a **force-velocity relation** (Figure 1-17).

    i. The resting muscle length is set by adding a given preload, and the **initial velocity of shortening** is then measured as the muscle is stimulated to lift a range of additional weights.

    ii. The weight a muscle must lift upon stimulation after resting length has been established is called **afterload.**
- *The speed of shortening decreases as the total load increases.*
- Extrapolating this curve to a theoretical zero load indicates the maximum possible speed of shortening (V_{max}), which reflects the *rate of myosin ATPase activity.*
- If preload is increased, there is an increased speed of shortening for any given total load, but without any change in V_{max}.

    iii. ▼ *In cardiac muscle, increased force and speed of contraction can be produced without changing preload. This is called increased* **contractility** *and can be identified by an increase in* V_{max} *(see Chapter 4).* ▼

Smooth Muscle

1. Smooth muscle lines the walls of most hollow organs, including organs of the vascular, gastrointestinal, respiratory, urinary, and reproductive systems.

A.

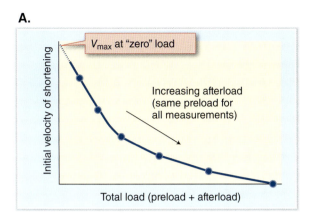

B.

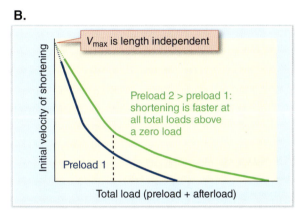

Figure 1-17. The force-velocity relationship in skeletal muscle. **A.** Shortening velocity decreases with increasing total load. The theoretical maximum shortening velocity, V_{max}, indicates intrinsic myosin ATPase activity. **B.** Effect of preload on shortening velocity. Increased preload increases the velocity of muscle shortening in a loaded muscle but does not change V_{max}.

2. Smooth muscle is an important therapeutic target because it regulates variables such as blood flow, ventilation of the lungs, and gastrointestinal motility.
3. Ultrastructure of smooth muscle.
   a. Smooth muscle cells are not striated in appearance (as are skeletal and cardiac muscle) because *thin and thick filaments are not organized as sarcomeres.*
   b. A network of **dense bodies** in the cytoplasm of smooth muscle cells serves as attachment points for actin filaments; thick filaments overlap thin filaments in an irregular array (Figure 1-18A).
   c. *The irregular arrangement of actin and myosin allows smooth muscle cells to generate force over a larger range of preloads than is possible in striated muscle.*
   d. There is no T tubule or muscle triad structure in smooth muscle; SR is present but it has an irregular arrangement.
   e. There are two general **types of smooth muscle:**
      i. **Visceral smooth muscle** is the most common type, in which cells are arranged in large bundles. Cells within a bundle behave as a functional **syncytium** due to the presence of gap junctions between cells.
      ii. **Multiunit smooth muscle** cells function individually since the cells are not connected by gap junctions. There is:
         • A dense nerve supply from autonomic neurons.

A. Morphology of single smooth muscle cells

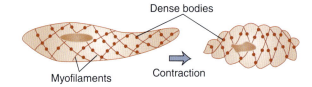

B. Excitation-contraction coupling in smooth muscle

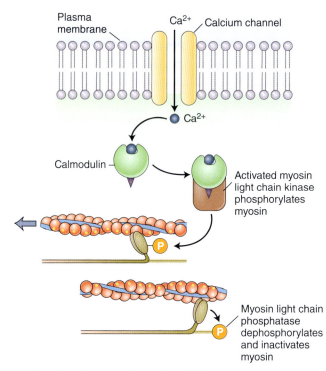

Figure 1-18. A. Structure of a smooth muscle cell. No sarcomeres are present; actin filaments are anchored to dense bodies and overlap myosin in an irregular array; no muscle triads are present. **B.** Excitation contraction coupling in smooth muscle. In most cases, Ca^{2+} enters the cell from the extracellular fluid (ECF) via voltage-gated Ca^{2+} channels. Ca^{2+} binds to calmodulin, resulting in activation of myosin light chain kinase. Phosphorylation of myosin triggers cross-bridge cycling and force development.

- Fine control over force development in a manner similar to spatial summation in skeletal muscle (e.g., control over the diameter of the pupil by the iris).

4. Excitation-contraction coupling in smooth muscle (Figure 1-18B).

   a. The contraction of smooth muscle begins when *the intracellular Ca^{2+} concentration increases.*

   b. *The source of Ca^{2+} is usually from the ECF via* **voltage-gated Ca^{2+} channels** *when the cell membrane becomes depolarized* but can also result from second messenger-stimulated Ca^{2+} release from the SR.

   c. The regulation of smooth muscle contraction involves **myosin phosphorylation** because *smooth muscle myofilaments do not contain troponins.*

   d. The relative activity of the antagonistic enzymes **myosin light chain kinase** and **myosin light chain phosphatase** determines whether myosin is activated.

   e. When smooth muscle is stimulated and the intracellular $[Ca^{2+}]$ increases, the result is the formation of **Ca^{2+}-calmodulin complexes.**

    f. Activated calmodulin stimulates myosin light chain kinase to phosphorylate and thereby activate myosin.

    g. When Ca^{2+} levels decrease, the muscle relaxes because the activity of myosin light chain phosphatase predominates, causing myosin to become dephosphorylated.

    h. An important feature of some smooth muscles (e.g., sphincters) is the *ability to maintain force over long periods* by entering a **latch bridge state,** with slow rates of cross-bridge detachment.

Study Questions

Directions: Each numbered item is followed by lettered options. Some options may be partially correct, but there is only *ONE BEST* answer.

1. The uptake of a novel drug by hepatocytes occurs down an electrochemical gradient. Uptake is independent of other solutes, and the rate of uptake is saturated at high extracellular drug concentrations. Which membrane transport process is most likely to account for all these characteristics of drug uptake?

    A. Antiport with Cl^-
    B. Cotransport with Na^+
    C. Facilitated diffusion
    D. Primary active transport
    E. Simple diffusion through ion channels
    F. Simple diffusion through plasma membrane

Questions 2 and 3

A segment of normal human intestine was perfused in vitro. The lumen was perfused with 150 mM NaCl. The bathing solution contained 300 mM mannitol (an inert sugar). The reflection coefficients of NaCl and mannitol were 0.9 and 1.0, respectively. Assume that NaCl dissociates completely into Na^+ and Cl^-; mannitol does not dissociate in solution.

2. When compared to the osmolarity of the luminal solution, which of the following best describes the osmolarity of the bathing solution?

    A. Isosmotic
    B. Hyperosmotic
    C. Hyposmotic

3. Under the conditions described, what net water movement is expected to occur?

    A. Water moves into the intestine from the bathing solution
    B. Water moves out of the intestine
    C. No net water transport occurs

Questions 4–6

A study of a secretory airway epithelial cell was conducted using methods that allowed the control of ionic composition inside and outside of the cell.

    Intracellular concentrations:

    $[K^+] = 135$ mM
    $[Na^+] = 10$ mM
    $[Cl^-] = 20$ mM

Extracellular concentrations:

$[K^+] = 5$ mM
$[Na^+] = 140$ mM
$[Cl^-] = 110$ mM

Nernst equilibrium potentials were calculated: $E_K = -88$ mV, $E_{Na} = +70$ mV, $E_{Cl} = -46$ mV.

4. Under control conditions, membrane conductance was found to be entirely due to open K^+ channels. Under control conditions, resting membrane potential was closest to

A. -40 mV
B. -50 mV
C. -60 mV
D. -70 mV
E. -80 mV
F. -90 mV
G. -100 mV

5. Treatment of the airway epithelial cells with an agonist caused the opening of many Cl^- selective channels in the plasma membrane. Assuming that K^+ channels were unaffected by the agonist, what change in resting membrane potential will occur in response to the agonist?

A. Depolarization
B. Hyperpolarization
C. Repolarization
D. No change

6. Opening Cl^- channels in the membrane provides a pathway for Cl^- flux across the membrane. In which direction would net Cl^- flux occur?

A. Cl^- moves out of the cell
B. Cl^- moves into the cell
C. There is no net Cl^- flux

7. A 25-year-old man suffered muscle paralysis due to poisoning with ω-conotoxin. This molluscan peptide toxin is known to interfere with voltage-sensitive Ca^{2+} channels at the neuromuscular junction. Which of the following is the most likely explanation for muscle paralysis in this patient?

A. Failure of action potential conduction in the motor nerve terminal
B. Failure of acetylcholine synthesis in the motor nerve terminal
C. Failure of acetylcholine release from the motor nerve terminal
D. Accelerated breakdown of acetylcholine in the synaptic cleft
E. Inhibition of postsynaptic nicotinic acetylcholine receptors

8. A 37-year-old woman with worsening muscle weakness was diagnosed with myasthenia gravis. She was treated with the acetylcholinesterase inhibitor neostigmine, and reported improved muscle strength within 1 day of starting treatment. Which of the following is the most likely reason for improved muscle performance in response to neostigmine treatment?

A. Increased action potential frequency in the motor nerves
B. Increased acetylcholine synthesis in the motor nerve terminals
C. Decreased acetylcholine breakdown at the neuromuscular junctions
D. Decreased reuptake of choline by the presynaptic motor nerves
E. Direct agonism at the nicotinic acetylcholine receptors

9. A skeletal muscle was stimulated to produce an isotonic contraction. Significant muscle shortening was observed. Which part of the sarcomere would retain a constant length during this type of muscle contraction?

A. A band
B. Distance between adjacent Z disks
C. Distance from Z disk to M line
D. Distance between adjacent M lines
E. I band

10. A 49-year-old woman was found to have high blood pressure due to increased vascular smooth muscle tone. Which event occurring inside the vascular smooth muscle cells may contribute to development of high blood pressure in this case?

A. Decreased opening of voltage-sensitive Ca^{2+} channels in the sarcolemma
B. Decreased intracellular concentration of calmodulin
C. Decreased calcium sensitivity of troponin C
D. Decreased myosin light chain kinase activity
E. Decreased myosin light chain phosphatase activity

Neurophysiology

CHAPTER 2

Structural Overview of the Nervous System

1. Anatomical terminology.
   a. Below the level of the midbrain, **rostral** and **caudal** denote toward the "head" and "tail," respectively. Above the midbrain, rostral indicates toward the front of the brain (anterior), and caudal indicates toward the back of the brain (posterior).
   b. Below the level of the midbrain, **dorsal** and **ventral** indicate toward the back and front of the body, respectively. Above the midbrain, dorsal refers to the top (superior) surface of the brain, and ventral refers to the bottom (inferior) surface of the brain.
   c. **Anterior** and **posterior** indicate toward the front or back of the body (or brain), respectively.
   d. **Superior** and **inferior** indicate toward the top of the cerebral cortex or the sacral end of the spinal cord, respectively (Figure 2-1).
   e. The **median sagittal plane** divides the nervous system into two equal halves in the anterior-posterior plane, with the left and right sides being the mirror image of each other.
      i. **Medial** and **lateral** indicate toward or away from the midline, respectively.
      ii. **Ipsilateral** indicates two points on the same side of the midline; **contralateral** indicates two points on opposite sides of the midline.
      iii. **Coronal** "slices" are vertically oriented at ninety degrees to the sagittal plane.
      iv. The **horizontal plane** is perpendicular to both the sagittal and coronal planes.
2. **Neurons** have two general components, the soma and neurites (Figure 2-2):
   a. The **soma** (cell body) contains the cell nucleus and the rough endoplasmic reticulum.
   b. **Neurites** are thin cellular processes extending from the soma:
      i. The **axon** is the cellular process that carries action potentials away from the soma. Axons are often long and may have multiple branches.
      ii. **Dendrites** have a structure similar to axons but receive impulses from other neurons. Many neurons have an extensive set of dendrites, referred to as the **dendritic tree.**
3. Divisions of the nervous system.
   a. The nervous system can be divided into the **central nervous system (CNS)** and the **peripheral nervous system (PNS).**

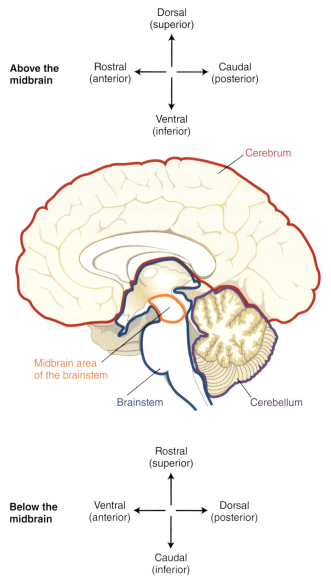

Figure 2-1. Neuroanatomic references. The three major areas of the adult brain are the cerebrum, the cerebellum, and the brainstem. Arrows indicate the different terminology used for anatomic references above and below the midbrain area of the brainstem.

b. *The CNS is enclosed within the meninges* and consists of the **brain** and **spinal cord**.

c. Structures in the PNS are outside the meninges and include spinal nerves, cranial nerves, pre- and post-ganglionic autonomic nerves, and sensory receptors.

d. The **meninges** is the collective term for three membranous layers enclosing the CNS:

   i. The **dura mater** is the outermost layer and consists of tough connective tissue.

   ii. The **arachnoid mater** is the middle layer and lies beneath the dura, which it closely follows. The **subarachnoid space** lies beneath the arachnoid membrane and is filled with **cerebrospinal fluid (CSF).**

   iii. The **pia mater** is the innermost layer. It is a delicate vascular membrane that closely follows the surface of the brain and spinal cord.

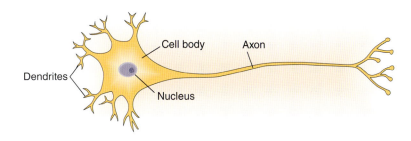

Terms Referring to Collections of Neurons	Description
Gray matter	A general term for neuronal cell bodies in the CNS; the cut surface of the brain appears gray at these sites
Cortex	Thin sheets of neurons, usually at the brain surface and most often used in reference to the cerebral cortex, but there are other examples (e.g., olfactory cortex)
Nucleus (plural: nuclei)	A clearly defined mass of neurons, usually fairly large and deeply placed in the brain (e.g., caudate nucleus of the deep cerebral nuclei)
Locus (plural: loci)	Clearly defined groups of neurons, but smaller than a nucleus (e.g., the locus ceruleus of the brainstem)
Substantia	A less well-defined group of neurons (e.g., the substantia nigra of the midbrain)
Ganglion (plural: ganglia)	Applied to collections of neurons in the PNS (except for the basal ganglia in the CNS)

Terms Referring to Collections of Axons	Description
White matter	A general term for axon groups in the CNS; the cut surface of the brain appears white at these sites
Tract	A collection of axons with a common origin and a common destination (e.g., corticospinal tract)
Capsule	A group of axons connecting the cerebrum and brain stem (e.g., internal capsule)
Commissure	A collection of axons connecting one side of the brain to the other (e.g., anterior commissure connecting the temporal lobes)
Lemniscus	A "ribbon-like" tract (e.g., medial lemniscus that conveys touch sensation through the brain stem)
Nerve	A bundle of axons in the PNS (except the optic nerve)

Figure 2-2. The prototypic neuron and terms used to describe collections of neurons. Many processes (neurites) extend from the neuron cell body. A single process, the axon, carries electrical signals away from the cell body; dendrites are processes receiving information from other neurons. The table summarizes terms that apply to collections of neurons where cell bodies are concentrated and terms used to describe collections of axons.

iv.   ▼ There is normally no space between the cranial dura and the bony skull. The cranial dura has a double layer, with one layer adhered to the inside of the skull bones. Head trauma may force blood between the bone and dura mater, known as an **epidural hematoma.** In contrast, the spinal cord has a single layer of dura mater surrounded by an actual epidural space, which can be used for injection of anesthetic during **epidural anesthesia.** ▼

    v. ▼ Infection (i.e., viral, bacterial, or fungal) of the meninges results in **meningitis,** whereas infection of the brain parenchyma results in **encephalitis.** *The classic clinical triad of meningitis is fever, headache, and nuchal rigidity (stiff neck).* The patient with encephalitis will commonly present with confusion, behavioral abnormalities, an altered level of consciousness, and/or focal neurologic abnormalities. ▼

  e. **Sensory nerves** that convey information from the periphery to the CNS are called **afferent nerves.**

  f. Nerves that carry information from the CNS to the periphery are called **efferent nerves;** the efferent nerves to skeletal muscle are called **motor nerves** and are involved in muscle control.

  g. The **autonomic nervous system (ANS)** is concerned with control of visceral functions such as digestion, blood flow, temperature regulation, and reproduction. The ANS has three divisions:

    i. The **sympathetic nervous system** is generally excitatory and is associated with "fight or flight" responses.

    ii. The **parasympathetic nervous system** usually opposes the sympathetic nervous system and is associated with "rest and digest" functions.

    iii. The **enteric nervous system** (ENS) is a large system of neural networks within the walls of the gastrointestinal tract (see Chapter 7).

  h. The functions of the ANS are contrasted with those of the **somatic nervous system,** in which sensory and motor communication occurs between the CNS and the skin, skeletal muscles, and joints.

  i. The autonomic and somatic nervous systems both consist of afferent and efferent nerves, and both have structures located within the CNS and PNS.

4. Structures of the CNS.

  a. The brain has three major parts:

    i. The **cerebrum** which is divided down the middle into the two large **cerebral hemispheres** by the **longitudinal fissure.** *Each hemisphere receives sensations from, and controls the movements of, the contralateral side of the body.*

    ii. The **cerebellum** lies behind the cerebrum, and is a key part of the motor system that is required for the maintenance of equilibrium and the coordination of muscle actions.

    iii. The **brainstem** is a conduit for the flow of information between the cerebrum and the spinal cord. The brainstem is a site of regulation of vital body functions, including breathing and consciousness. *The loss of brainstem function is fatal.*

  b. The spinal cord (Figure 2-3).

    i. The spinal cord is attached to the brainstem and passes downward within the bony vertebral column.

    ii. The spinal cord is the major conduit of sensory and motor information between the brain and the periphery.

    iii. The spinal cord is connected to the periphery via **spinal nerves.**

A.

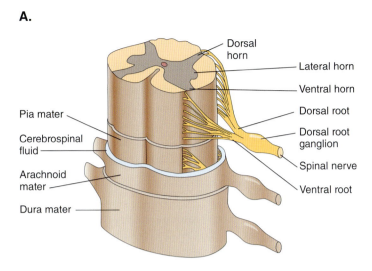

Dorsal horn

Lateral horn

Ventral horn

Dorsal root

Dorsal root ganglion

Spinal nerve

Ventral root

Pia mater

Cerebrospinal fluid

Arachnoid mater

Dura mater

B.

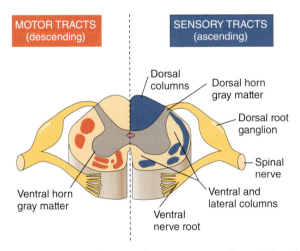

MOTOR TRACTS (descending)

SENSORY TRACTS (ascending)

Dorsal columns

Dorsal horn gray matter

Dorsal root ganglion

Spinal nerve

Ventral and lateral columns

Ventral horn gray matter

Ventral nerve root

Figure 2-3. The spinal cord. **A.** Spinal nerves connect the spinal cord with the periphery. Each spinal nerve has a ventral root containing axons of efferent neurons and a dorsal root containing axons of afferent neurons. The dorsal root ganglion is a swelling containing the cell bodies of sensory neurons. The spinal cord is covered in three membranes that comprise the meninges: the pia, the arachnoid, and the dura mater. **B.** Cross-section through the spinal cord indicating a butterfly-shaped central area of gray matter. Sensory neurons enter the dorsal horn, and motor neurons leave the ventral horn. The surrounding white matter consists of dorsal, lateral, and anterior columns, each containing nerve tracts running to and from the brain. The ascending and descending tracts shown are present on both the left and right sides.

- Each spinal nerve attaches to the spinal cord by two branches: The **dorsal root** brings afferent information into the cord, and the **ventral root** carries efferent information away from the cord.
iv. ▼ *If the spinal cord is transected, there is total loss of sensation and paralysis of muscles below the affected spinal level.* ▼
v. A horizontal view through the **spinal cord** reveals a characteristic pattern of **gray matter** and **white matter:**
  - Gray matter consists of nerve cell bodies; white matter consists of nerve axons covered in **myelin.**

- The gray matter is shaped like a butterfly, with each "wing" having an upper **dorsal horn,** an **intermediate zone,** and a lower **ventral horn.**
- The dorsal horn receives afferent input from the dorsal nerve roots, and the ventral horn sends efferent axons to the ventral nerve roots.
- Cells in the intermediate zone integrate sensory information with descending inputs from higher brain centers to shape the efferent output via the ventral horn.
- The white matter consists of several nerve tracts arranged in **columns** that carry information either to or from the brain.
  - The **dorsal columns** carry only sensory information via ascending tracts.
  - The **ventral** and **lateral columns** convey both sensory and motor information via ascending and descending tracts, respectively.

5. Embryologic development of the brain (Figure 2-4).
   a. The CNS develops from a simple fluid-filled **neural tube.**
   b. The walls of the neural tube become neural tissue, and the tube itself becomes the **ventricular system.**
   c. Early differentiation of the neural tube produces three primary brain vesicles: the **forebrain** (prosencephalon), the **midbrain** (mesencephalon), and the **hindbrain** (rhombencephalon).
      i. The hindbrain connects to the caudal neural tube, which becomes the spinal cord.
   d. ▼ **Neural tube defects** (e.g., anencephaly, spina bifida, meningocele, meningomyelocele, and myelocele) occur as a result of incomplete closure of the neural tube by days 26–28 of embryologic development. *Folic acid supplement prior to conception reduces the incidence of neural tube defects.* ▼

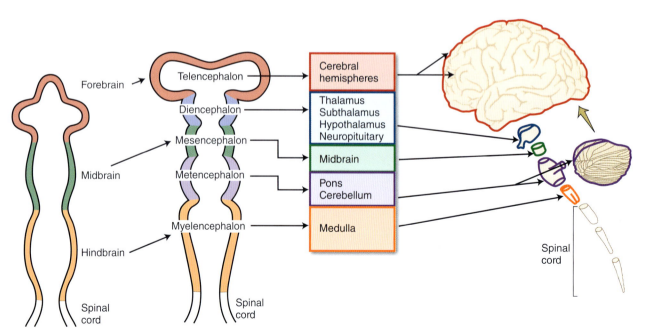

Figure 2-4. Embryologic development of the major anatomic parts of the central nervous system. Early development produces the forebrain, midbrain, and hindbrain vesicles, which subsequently develop into the five vesicles shown in the center of the figure. Differentiation of each of the five vesicles produces the major brain structures indicated in the image on the right side of the figure.

e. Further differentiation of the forebrain and hindbrain produces a tube with five vesicles, which are precursors of the major parts of the adult brain.

6. Forebrain structures.

a. The cerebrum is the largest part of the brain, and is the seat of thoughts, perceptions, and voluntary actions.

b. The term **cortex** refers to the surface layer of gray matter.

c. The surface area of the brain is increased by its many folds (**gyri**), which are separated by fissures (**sulci**).

d. The larger sulci are structures that subdivide the cortex into the **frontal, parietal, occipital,** and **temporal lobes** (Figure 2-5A).

   i. The **insular lobe** is not visible from the surface of the brain, but is seen when the margins of the lateral sulcus are pulled open.

e. Many areas of the cortex can be assigned specific functions (e.g., vision or somatic sensation). **Brodmann's areas** refer to specific brain areas with particular functions (Figure 2-5B).

f. Large areas of cortex *cannot* be assigned specific functions and are called **association cortex;** these areas are involved with interpretation and

A.

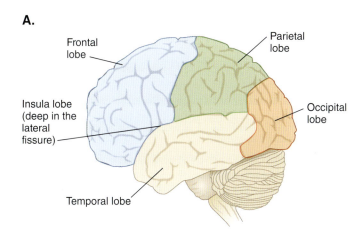

B.

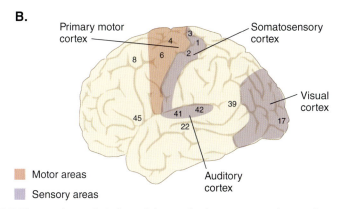

Figure 2-5. The cerebrum. **A.** Lobes of the cerebral cortex, named according to the skull bones under which they are located. **B.** Functional classification of regions of the cerebral cortex showing the location of major functional areas. Selected examples of Brodmann's brain areas are indicated (e.g., areas 1, 2, and 3 are in the primary somatosensory cortex, area 4 is the primary motor cortex, area 6 is the premotor cortex, area 8 is the frontal eye field, area 17 is the primary visual cortex, areas 41 and 42 are the auditory cortex, area 22 and 39 encompass Wernicke's language area, and area 45 is part of Broca's speech area).

meaning of sensory information, formation of intentions, and "higher functions" of the mind.

g. The lower part of the forebrain is the diencephalon, which consists of the thalamus and the hypothalamus:

   i. The **thalamus** is an egg-shaped structure that is a relay station through which each of the sensory pathways for somatic sensation, vision, and hearing synapse as they travel to the cortex.

   ii. Sensory pathways in each side of the thalamus continue to the cerebral hemisphere of the same side of the body but convey information from the opposite side of the body.

   iii. The **hypothalamus** lies ventral to the thalamus. It is a command center for the ANS, and also for much of the endocrine system, through its control of the pituitary gland. In addition, the hypothalamus is a source of several basic motivational drives, including hunger, thirst, and sex.

h. The brain contains extensive white matter formed by myelinated axons (Figure 2-6):

   i. The **internal capsule** is formed from axons running between the thalamus and cortex.

   ii. The internal capsule is continuous with the **cortical white matter,** which mostly consists of **interneurons** that communicate between cortical neurons.

   iii. The **corpus callosum** provides a link between the left and right hemispheres.

i. The **deep cerebral nuclei** or **basal ganglia,** which include the **caudate nucleus, putamen,** and **globus pallidus**, are large collections of gray matter located lateral to the thalamus.

j. Other forebrain structures discussed in later sections include the **amygdala** and **hippocampus** (involved in emotions and memory), the **retina** and **optic nerve** of the eye, and the **olfactory bulb** (involved in the sense of smell).

7. Midbrain structures (Figure 2-7A).

a. The midbrain is a narrow region that is part of the brainstem, and is a conduit for all the nerve tracts passing between the forebrain and hindbrain.

b. The dorsal part of the midbrain is called the **tectum,** which has two pairs of swellings:

   i. The **superior colliculus,** which receives sensory input from the eye, and is involved in the control of eye movements.

   ii. The **inferior colliculus,** which is a relay station for sensory input from the ear before it passes to the thalamus and onward to the cortex.

c. The ventral part of the midbrain is called the **tegmentum** (or **cerebral peduncles**) and contains two areas involved in motor control, the **red nucleus** and the **substantia nigra.**

8. Hindbrain structures.

a. The rostral half of the hindbrain (metencephalon) becomes the pons and the cerebellum.

   i. The **cerebellum** ("little brain") has two hemispheres, which are connected by a midline region called the **vermis.**

   ii. The cerebellum is physically connected to the brainstem via the superior, middle, and inferior **peduncles.**

A.

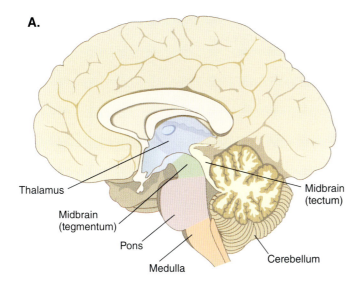

Thalamus

Midbrain
(tegmentum)

Pons

Medulla

Midbrain
(tectum)

Cerebellum

B.

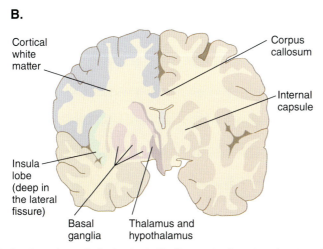

Cortical
white
matter

Insula
lobe
(deep in
the lateral
fissure)

Basal
ganglia

Thalamus and
hypothalamus

Corpus
callosum

Internal
capsule

Figure 2-6. Sections through the brain. **A.** Median sagittal section showing the medial surface of the brain and all the structures of the brainstem from the thalamus superiorly to the medulla inferiorly. **B.** Coronal section at the junction of the thalamus and cerebrum. This view shows the position of the insula lobe; the basal ganglia are visible lateral to the thalamus. Major areas of white matter are visible in this plane, including the internal capsule, the cortical white matter, and the corpus callosum.

iii. The cerebellum receives descending inputs from the forebrain that relay information about the intentions for movements, and ascending inputs from the spinal cord that relay information about the position of the body in space (known as **proprioception**).

iv. The cerebellum determines the correct sequence of muscle contractions needed to coordinate accurate movement. Damage to the cerebellum causes jerky movements that are poorly coordinated and inaccurate, referred to as **ataxia.**

v. The **pons** bulges out from the ventral surface of the brainstem.

vi. The most prominent structural feature of the pons is the massive number of **transverse pontine fibers** that cross from one side to the other (Figure 2-7B). Most of the descending axons from the cortex synapse in the pons and then cross to the opposite side to enter the cerebellum.

A.

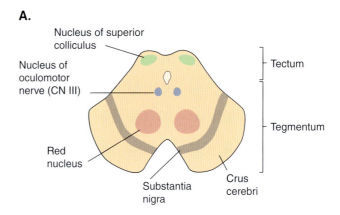

B.

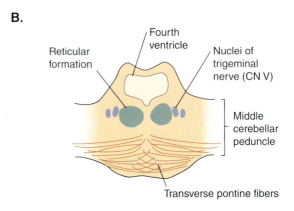

C.

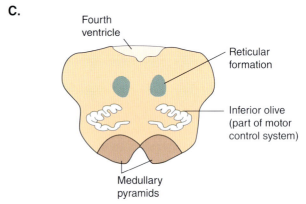

Figure 2-7. Sections through the brainstem at different levels. **A.** The midbrain at the level of the superior colliculus. The midbrain has two major parts, the tectum dorsally and the tegmentum ventrally. The substantia nigra and the red nucleus are part of the motor system. Nuclei of cranial nerves III (oculomotor) and IV (trochlear) are present in the midbrain. **B.** The pons, showing massive crossover of descending fibers in the ventral pons, which are destined for the cerebellum. **C.** The medulla, showing the large medullary pyramids ventrally, which are the site of crossover of the descending corticospinal tracts. Several cranial nerve nuclei, as well as ascending and descending tracts, are present in the medulla but are not shown in the figure.

    b. The **medulla** is the most caudal part of the brainstem and connects the pons superiorly to the spinal cord inferiorly (Figure 2-7C).

        i. The anterior (ventral) surface has prominent swellings on each side called **medullary pyramids.**

ii. Each of the pyramids contains a **corticospinal (pyramidal) tract.** These tracts travel from the motor cortex to the spinal cord and carry axons of motor neurons that command movement.

iii. The medullary pyramids are the site of **decussation** (crossing from one side to the other) of this motor pathway, which explains why *movement of one side of the body is controlled by the opposite cerebral hemisphere.*

c. The midbrain, pons, and medulla also contain the nuclei associated with the **cranial nerves** (Table 2-1).

Table 2-1. The Cranial Nerves

Number of Nerve	Name of Nerve	Type	Major Function(s)
I	**Olfactory**	Sensory	• Smell
II	**Optic**	Sensory	• Vision
III	**Oculomotor**	Motor	• Eye movements and constriction of the pupil
IV	**Trochlear**	Motor	• Eye movements
V	**Trigeminal**		
	• **Ophthalmic division**	Sensory	• Cornea and skin of the forehead, scalp, nose, and eyelid
	• **Maxillary division**	Sensory	• Maxillary facial skin, upper teeth, maxillary sinus, and palate
	• **Mandibular division**	Mixed	• Sensory to skin over mandible, lower teeth, inside of mouth, and anterior part of the tongue • Motor to muscles of mastication
VI	**Abducens**	Motor	• Eye movements
VII	**Facial**	Mixed	• Sensory function includes taste from anterior two-thirds of the tongue • Motor to facial muscles • Parasympathetic secretomotor fibers to salivary and lacrimal glands
VIII	**Vestibulocochlear**		
	• **Vestibular**	Sensory	• Position and movement of the head
	• **Cochlear**	Sensory	• Hearing
IX	**Glossopharyngeal**	Mixed	• Sensory to the pharynx and posterior third of the tongue; carotid sinus baroreceptor and carotid body chemoreceptor • Motor to muscles of swallowing • Parasympathetic secretomotor to salivary gland
X	**Vagus**	Mixed	• Major parasympathetic nerve to heart, lungs, and upper gastrointestinal system
XI	**Accessory**	Motor	• Spinal root: sternomastoid and trapezius muscles • Cranial root: muscles of palate, pharynx, and larynx
XII	**Hypoglossal**	Motor	• Muscles of the tongue

   d. The optic nerve (CN II) can be considered part of the CNS because it is located within the meninges.

   e. The other 11 pairs of cranial nerves exit the brain and pass, via foramina (holes), in the skull. With the exception of the vagus nerve, all of the cranial nerves serve the head and neck region; *the vagus nerve serves visceral structures in the thorax and abdomen.*

9. Structures of the PNS.

   a. *The PNS consists of 31 pairs of spinal nerves and 11 of the 12 pairs of cranial nerves.* The spinal nerves are named according to the segment of the vertebral column they are associated with:

      i. C1–C8 are the **cervical** spinal nerves.

      ii. T1–T12 are the **thoracic** spinal nerves.

      iii. L1–L5 are the **lumber** spinal nerves.

      iv. S1–S5 are the **sacral** spinal nerves.

      v. Coccygeal 1 is the sole **coccygeal** spinal nerve.

Brain Extracellular Fluids

1. ▼ The total volume of the brain, including cells and extracellular fluids, is limited by the bony skull. If the volume of intracellular or extracellular fluid increases, there is a risk that **increased intracranial pressure** will result in reduced brain perfusion. *Increased intracranial pressure can be fatal because it may result in brain herniation into the vertebral canal.* ▼

2. The CNS has **three extracellular fluid compartments** (Figure 2-8):

   a. **Blood plasma** contained inside the vascular system (approximately 70 mL).

   b. **Interstitial fluid** located outside the vascular system in contact with neural cells and glia (approximately 250 mL).

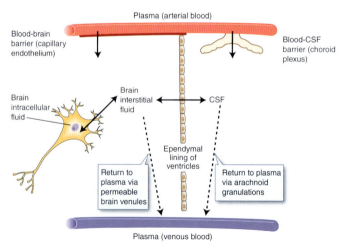

Figure 2-8. Relationships between fluid compartments in the brain. Movement of solutes from arterial plasma into the brain is restricted by the blood-brain barrier and the blood-cerebrospinal fluid (CSF) barrier. There is regulated exchange between the brain interstitial fluid and the brain intracellular fluid compartment across the cell membranes of neurons and glia. There is free exchange between CSF and brain interstitial fluid across ependymal cells lining the ventricles. Brain interstitial fluid can return to the systemic circulation via permeable venules, and CSF returns to systemic venous blood via arachnoid granulations (specialized projections of the arachnoid membrane).

   c. **Cerebrospinal fluid** located within the **ventricular system** and **subarachnoid space** (approximately 150 mL).

3. The composition of brain extracellular fluids is carefully regulated to protect neuronal function:

   a. The brain interstitial fluid is protected from changes in the plasma composition by a **blood-brain barrier.**

   b. The composition of CSF is carefully regulated by actively secreting CSF via the **choroid plexus epithelia.**

   c. *There is free exchange of water and solutes between the brain interstitial fluid (ISF) and the CSF* across the **ependymal cell layer,** which lines the ventricular system.

4. A "**glymphatic system**" has also been described whereby CSF is continuous with a perivascular space (**Virchow-Robin space**) around the penetrating arteries that enter the brain parenchyma. There is rapid CSF-ISF exchange in the brain and drainage into the cervical lymphatics.

   a. ▼ *Glymphatic flow is increased during sleep* facilitating excretion of excess fluid and solutes from the brain, including pathologic proteins such as amyloid and tau tangles that accumulate in **neurodegenerative diseases.** ▼

5. The ventricular system.

   a. The ventricular system is a series of interconnected chambers inside the CNS that are filled with **CSF** (Figure 2-9A). The lumens of the embryonic brain vesicles develop into the ventricular system:

     i. The lumen of the telencephalon becomes the **lateral ventricles** of the **cerebrum.**

       • Each lateral ventricle forms a large C shape as the ventricle curves around from the frontal lobe, through the parietal lobe into the temporal lobe.

     ii. The lumen of the diencephalon becomes the slit-like **third ventricle,** which is located in the midline.

       • The **thalamus** forms the lateral wall of the third ventricle and the hypothalamus forms the floor.

       • The lumen of the third ventricle is continuous with each lateral ventricle through an **interventricular foramen (the foramina of Monro).**

     iii. The lumen of the mesencephalon (midbrain) becomes a narrow channel, called the **cerebral aqueduct,** which connects the third and fourth ventricles.

     iv. The lumen of the hindbrain becomes the **fourth ventricle,** which has the **pons** and **medulla** as its floor and the **cerebellum** as its roof.

       • The fourth ventricle is continuous inferiorly with the **central canal** of the spinal cord.

   b. Each ventricle contains a **choroid plexus** epithelium, which continuously secretes CSF into the ventricles.

     i. CSF exits the ventricular system via holes in the fourth ventricle (the **foramina of Luschka and Magendie**) into the subarachnoid space.

     ii. CSF flows over the surface of the brain and spinal cord and drains back into the venous system at specialized areas of arachnoid membrane called **arachnoid granulations.**

A.

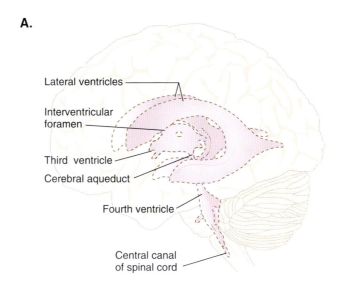

B.

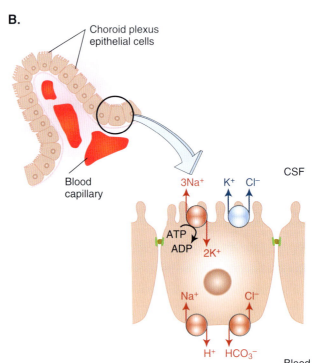

Figure 2-9. The ventricular system. **A.** Location of the ventricles of the brain. **B.** Cerebrospinal fluid secretion by the choroid plexus.

iii. *To maintain a stable CSF volume, the rate of production of CSF by the choroid plexus must be the same as the rate of CSF absorption at arachnoid granulations.*

iv. The circulation of CSF replaces the CSF volume approximately four times a day.

v. ▼ **Hydrocephalus** can be defined in general terms as an increase in CSF volume or pressure as a result of an imbalance in CSF production, flow, or absorption.

- In **communicating hydrocephalus,** there is a free flow of CSF from the ventricles to the subarachnoid space. Communicating hydrocephalus may be caused by oversecretion of CSF (e.g., choroid plexus papilloma) or impaired return of CSF to the venous system (e.g., meningitis can impair the flow of CSF through the arachnoid granulations).

- In **noncommunicating hydrocephalus,** an obstructed path occurs, preventing the free flow of CSF through the ventricular system (e.g., a pineal tumor that occludes the cerebral aqueduct).
- **Normal pressure hydrocephalus** is a special type of communicating hydrocephaly that primarily affects the elderly. The condition is usually painless but results in enlarged lateral ventricles. ▼

c. CSF has three major functions:
  i. To act as a shock absorber to **protect the brain** from contact with the skull during movement.
  ii. To assist in the maintenance of a **constant internal environment** in the CNS.
  iii. To provide a route for **removal of metabolites** from the brain.

d. CSF secretion.
  i. Choroid plexus epithelia have a vascular core surrounded by fronds of epithelial tissue that project into the ventricular lumen.
  ii. The **choroid plexus epithelial cells** actively secrete CSF via a transcellular mechanism (Figure 2-9B).
    - The **Na$^+$/K$^+$-ATPase** drives Na$^+$ secretion across the luminal membrane.
    - Cl$^-$ is secreted into the CSF by **K$^+$-Cl$^-$ cotransport;** K$^+$ is recycled via the Na$^+$/K$^+$-ATPase.
    - Water is secreted by osmosis through **aquaporin water channels** in the cell membranes.

e. The **blood-CSF barrier** is maintained by tight junctions between the choroid plexus epithelial cells.

f. CSF is an isotonic fluid with a composition similar to plasma, *except that there is little protein in CSF.*

g. ▼ CSF can be sampled through a **lumbar puncture.** Changes in CSF composition have diagnostic value:
  i. Yellowing of CSF indicates **subarachnoid hemorrhage** and is caused by red blood cell hemolysis.
  ii. CSF should be sterile and detection of microorganisms is always abnormal.
  iii. Increased white cell count indicates infection and/or inflammation.
  iv. Decreased glucose concentration is detected in acute bacterial infections due to glucose use by neutrophils; glucose is not decreased in viral infections.
  v. Increased protein level is found in many disease states as a sensitive but nonspecific indicator. (For example, in **multiple sclerosis** there is increased IgG and a specific group of proteins called **oligoclonal bands.**)
  vi. *Note: An elevated intracranial pressure is a contraindication to performing lumbar puncture because releasing the pressure from below the opening in the skull can cause the brain to shift downward, inducing herniation.* ▼

A.

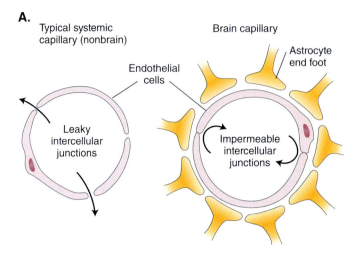

B.

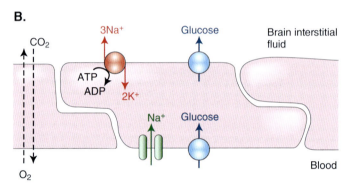

Figure 2-10. The blood-brain barrier. **A.** Comparison between a typical nonbrain systemic capillary, which has spaces between endothelial lining cells that allow free exchange between the plasma and interstitial fluid, and a brain capillary, which has continuous tight junctions that seal the junctions between endothelial cells. Brain capillaries are also surrounded by glia (astrocytes). **B.** Transcellular transport across the blood-brain barrier; oxygen and carbon dioxide can diffuse freely through endothelial cells; glucose enters the brain by facilitated diffusion.

6. The blood-brain barrier (Figure 2-10).
   a. The **capillary endothelial cells** that enclose brain capillaries form the selective blood-brain barrier between the brain interstitium and plasma.
   b. A few highly lipid-soluble substances are able to diffuse through capillary endothelial cell membranes (e.g., O_2, CO_2, urea, nicotine, and ethanol).
   c. Glucose enters the brain by facilitated diffusion via **GLUT1** carriers present in capillary endothelial cell membranes.
   d. A few small areas of the brain, known as **circumventricular organs,** lack a blood-brain barrier: the area postrema, posterior pituitary, subfornical organ, median eminence, pineal gland, and organum vasculosum laminae terminalis (OVLT).
      i. The circumventricular organs allow certain neurons to be directly exposed to solutes in the blood. For example, *in the median eminence of the **hypothalamus,** capillaries must be leaky to take up hypothalamic hormones.*

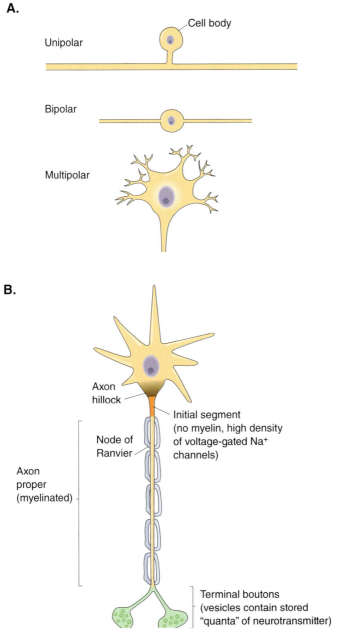

A.

Unipolar

Cell body

Bipolar

Multipolar

B.

Axon hillock

Initial segment (no myelin, high density of voltage-gated Na⁺ channels)

Node of Ranvier

Axon proper (myelinated)

Terminal boutons (vesicles contain stored "quanta" of neurotransmitter)

Figure 2-11. Neuronal structures. **A.** Classification of neurons based on the number of neurites extending from the cell body. Unipolar neurons have a single neurite; bipolar neurons have two neurites; and multipolar neurons are the most common type and have three or more neurites. **B.** Regions of the axon. The axon originates from the soma at a tapering region called the axon hillock. The initial segment lacks myelin and is the site of action potential stimulation. The axon proper may be myelinated or nonmyelinated and may vary greatly in length from one neuron to another; axons may have collateral branches (not shown). The axon terminal is a swollen area called the terminal bouton, which has many vesicles containing neurotransmitter.

Cellular Neuroscience

1. Several overlapping systems of classification are used to describe neurons.
   a. Number of neurites (Figure 2-11A):
      i. **Unipolar neurons** have a single neurite (e.g., primary sensory neurons with the cell body located in the dorsal root ganglia of spinal nerves).

    ii. **Bipolar neurons** have two neurites (e.g., a retinal bipolar cell).

    iii. **Multipolar neurons** have three or more neurites. This is the most common type of neuron (e.g., spinal motor neuron).

    iv. Multipolar neurons usually have a dendritic tree that provides a large number of inputs for that neuron. In contrast, unipolar and bipolar neurons have a highly specific input and are associated with specialized functions (e.g., sensing touch at a specific body location).

  b. Organization of dendrites [e.g., **pyramidal** or **stellate (star-shaped) neurons**]:

    i. *Usually there are tiny dendritic spines at the sites where axons synapse with the dendrite.* The presence or absence of spines is also used to describe neurons as **spiny** or **aspiny.**

  c. Axon length:

    i. **Golgi type I neurons** have long axons and project from one region of the nervous system to another.

    ii. **Golgi type II neurons** have short axons that contribute to local circuits in the region of the cell body.

  d. Neuronal function:

    i. **Primary sensory neurons** have neurites at the body surface, which convey sensory information to the CNS.

    ii. **Motor neurons** end on muscles and initiate muscle contraction.

    iii. **Interneurons** only form connections with other neurons. *Most neurons are interneurons.*

  e. Type of neurotransmitter: For example, neurons that release acetylcholine as the neurotransmitter are "cholinergic" etc.

2. Axons and presynaptic terminals.

  a. *The axon carries the output signal from a neuron after integration of incoming signals by the dendrites and soma.*

  b. There are three major functional axon regions: the axon hillock, the axon proper, and the axon terminal (Figure 2-11B):

    i. The axon hillock is a tapering region of the soma; the initial segment, or *spike initiation zone,* is just beyond the axon hillock. *Action potentials are readily triggered at the initial segment due to a high level of voltage-gated Na^+ channel expression.*

    ii. The **axon proper** has a constant diameter and may extend over a long distance; *the larger the axon diameter, the faster is the conduction velocity.*

    iii. The **axon terminal,** or **terminal bouton**, is the point of synapse formation with the target neuron or effector cell; *axons often branch extensively at their distal end to innervate a group of postsynaptic cells.*

  c. **Axoplasmic transport** between the soma and axon terminals is mediated by the cytoskeleton.

    i. Microtubules function like train tracks and transport material up and down the axon. The movement of materials is driven by **motor proteins** along the microtubule tracks.

      • **Anterograde transport** is movement from the soma toward the axon terminal. An example of anterograde transport is the movement of vesicles containing neurotransmitters from the cell body to the axon terminal.

- **Retrograde transport** is movement from the axon terminal toward the neuron cell body. The uptake of nerve growth factor at the axon terminal by endocytosis and its transport to the soma (where it stimulates protein synthesis) is an example of retrograde transport.
- **Motor proteins** function as "legs" that walk along microtubules carrying a payload such as a vesicle or mitochondrion. The motor protein *kinesin powers anterograde transport and dynein powers retrograde transport.*
- ▼ Some infectious agents (e.g., herpesvirus, polio virus, rabies virus, and tetanus toxin) utilize axonal transport to reach their site of action. For example, the oral **herpesvirus** that causes **cold sores** enters nerve endings at the mouth and is transported back to the cell body, where it is dormant for a period of time. When reactivated, the virus replicates and returns to the axon terminals, causing a cold sore to form.▼

   d. Classification of nerve fibers:

     i. **Type I (Aα)** are myelinated fibers with the largest diameter and fastest conduction speeds (e.g., somatic motor neurons, sensory fibers from muscle spindles, and Golgi tendon organs).

     ii. **Type II (Aβ)** are myelinated fibers with mid-range diameter and fast conduction speeds (e.g., some muscle spindles and fine touch receptors in the skin).

     iii. **Type III (Aδ)** are myelinated fibers with small diameter and moderate conduction speeds (e.g., mediating sharp pain, temperature, and crude touch).

     iv. **Type IV (C)** are unmyelinated fibers with small diameters and have the slowest conduction speeds (e.g., afferent neurons for dull pain, temperature afferents, and postganglionic autonomic neurons).

3. Neuroglia.

   a. There are about ten times more glial support cells than neurons in the brain, and they occupy about half of the brain volume. Three major types of glia are found in the brain: astrocytes, microglia, and oligodendrocytes (Figure 2-12).

   b. **Astrocytes** are highly branched cells that envelope neurons and brain capillaries. Functions include:

     i. To provide a structural **scaffold** for neurons.

     ii. To store glycogen and provide neurons with **lactate** as an energy source.

     iii. To **maintain a stable [K$^+$]** in the brain extracellular fluid by uptake of K$^+$ that is released from active neurons.

     iv. To **remove neurotransmitters** from brain extracellular fluid in the region of synapses (e.g., uptake of glutamate and γ-aminobutyric acid, GABA).

     v. To **synthesize neurotransmitter precursors** for neurons (e.g., glutamine synthesis for glutaminergic neurons).

     vi. To induce and maintain **blood-brain barrier** characteristics of brain capillary endothelial cells.

   c. **Microglia** are highly reactive cells that are activated by injury or infection, which causes them to proliferate and become phagocytic. *Microglia are*

A. Astroycte

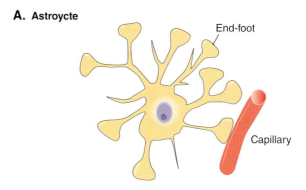

End-foot

Capillary

B. Microglial cell   **Activated microglial cell**

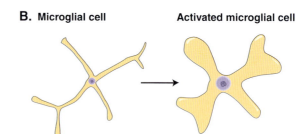

C. Oligodendrocyte

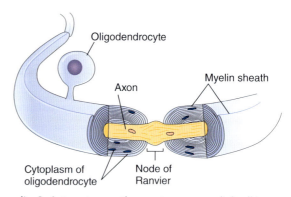

Oligodendrocyte

Axon

Myelin sheath

Cytoplasm of
oligodendrocyte

Node of
Ranvier

Figure 2-12. Neuroglia. **A.** Astrocytes are the most common glial cell type.
B. Microglia are activated by infection and coordinate the brain's immune response.
C. Oligodendrocytes form the myelin sheath around neurons in the central nervous
system.

> *the main antigen-presenting cells in the CNS and function like peripheral*
> ***macrophages.***

   d. **Oligodendrocytes** produce and maintain the **myelin sheaths** around
      neurons in the CNS by wrapping around the axons many times.

      i. A single oligodendrocyte myelinates multiple neurons.

      ii. *Schwann cells are the equivalent of oligodendrocytes in the PNS*; each
          Schwann cell myelinates only a single axon.

4. Neuronal injury.

   a. Injury to the neuron cell body by ischemia, disease, or trauma may result in
      cell death:

      i. **Necrosis** involves cell lysis and inflammation and results from acute
         trauma.

      ii. **Apoptosis** is programmed cell death that does not cause inflammation.

iii. ▼ **Gliosis** is a term used to describe astrocyte proliferation in response to an injury (e.g., stroke) that results in scar formation in the CNS. Gliosis, along with neuronal loss, is a prominent feature in many diseases that affect the CNS, including Alzheimer's disease, multiple sclerosis, and stroke. ▼

b. Axonal injury has several possible outcomes:

   i. **Wallerian degeneration** describes the loss of the axon distal to the site of injury, the axons and myelin degenerate but the endoneurium connective tissue covering remains.

   ii. **Chromatolysis** describes subsequent loss of the cell body.

   iii. **Transneuronal degeneration** is death of either input neurons to the injured neuron (retrograde degeneration) or death of downstream neurons in the circuit (anterograde degeneration).

c. ▼ *Regeneration of neurons is not possible in the CNS.* However, PNS axons may regrow directed along the remaining endoneurial tube and is stimulated by neurotrophic factors from Schwann cells. Axon regrowth occurs at 1–5 mm per day. ▼

5. Synaptic transmission and signal integration.

   a. Complex functions of the nervous system are possible because individual neurons communicate through circuits.

   b. There are several configurations of synaptic inputs that can occur, with the most common being synapses between axon terminals and the dendritic spines of another neuron.

   c. Postsynaptic potentials are **graded potentials** which are not all-or-none like action potentials but vary in size according to the sum of the inputs:

      i. **Excitatory postsynaptic potentials (EPSPs)** result if a neurotransmitter depolarizes the postsynaptic membrane potential.

      ii. **Inhibitory postsynaptic potentials (IPSPs)** result if a neurotransmitter hyperpolarizes the postsynaptic membrane potential.

   d. *The postsynaptic neuron will generate action potentials when the sum of EPSPs and IPSPs in the region of the initial axon segment is depolarized beyond a threshold potential* (Figure 2-13).

   e. Postsynaptic graded potentials decay with time and distance from the point of synaptic contact (Figure 2-14A).

   f. The **time constant (τ)** is the time taken for the membrane potential to decay to 37% of its peak value; if a dendrite has a long time constant, there is more time for individual EPSPs to summate.

      i. *Temporal summation occurs when a series of axon potentials arrive via the same excitatory afferent nerve and the EPSPs summate* (Figure 2-14B).

   g. The **space constant (λ)** is the distance along the dendrite that a postsynaptic potential has traveled when it has decayed to 37% of its maximum value.

      i. *If the space constant is large, then EPSPs from widely spaced synaptic inputs are able to summate, which is known as **spatial summation*** (Figure 2-14C).

   h. Time and space constants vary significantly between dendrites due to differences in their size and shape and ion channel expression.

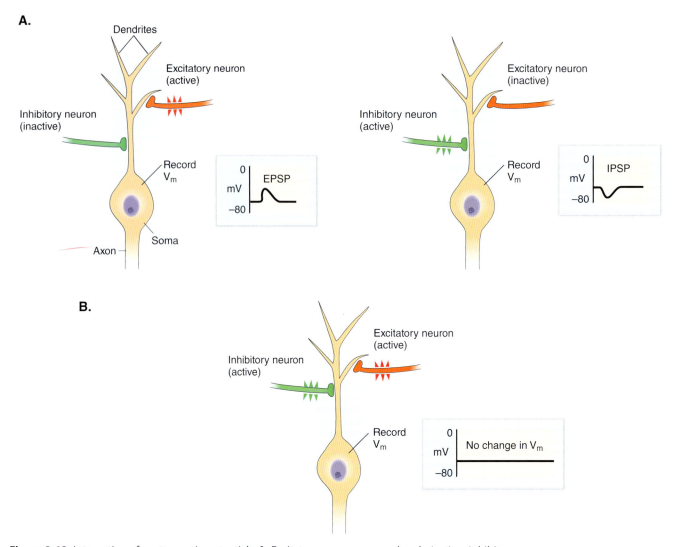

Figure 2-13. Integration of postsynaptic potentials. **A.** Excitatory neurons cause depolarization; inhibitory neurons cause hyperpolarization. **B.** Summation of synaptic inputs occurs to produce a net postsynaptic potential. In this example, a single excitatory input is cancelled out by a single inhibitory input. EPSP, excitatory postsynaptic potential; IPSP, inhibitory postsynaptic potential.

6. Neurochemistry.

   a. *Diversity of nervous system function mainly results from the complexity of neuronal circuits rather than the diversity of neurotransmitters and their postsynaptic receptors.*

   b. Although there are over 100 different neurotransmitters present in the nervous system, many fewer transmitters mediate the majority of synaptic events. There are two major classes of neurotransmitters (Table 2-2):

      i. The **small molecule transmitters,** which include **acetylcholine,** certain **amino acids,** and the **monoamine neurotransmitters.**

      ii. The **large molecule transmitters,** which are **neuropeptides** of various sizes.

   c. ▼ The primary inhibitory neurotransmitters of the CNS are γ-aminobutyric acid (GABA) and glycine, examples of small molecule transmitters. **Sedative-hypnotic drugs** (e.g., benzodiazepines, barbiturates, and alcohols) target the GABA$_A$ receptor, which, through the action of

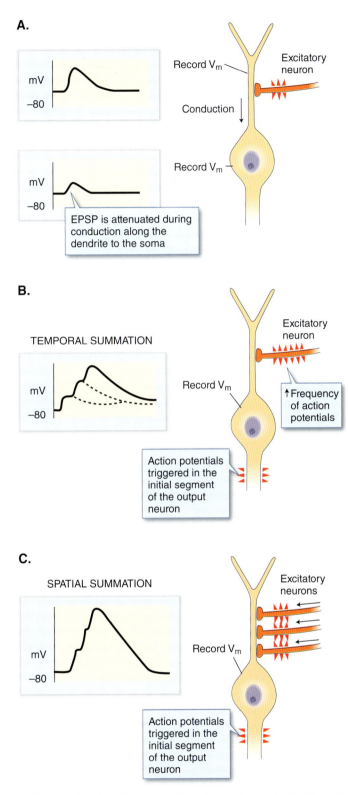

Figure 2-14. Temporal and spatial summation of synaptic inputs. **A.** Attenuation of an excitatory postsynaptic potential (EPSP) during conduction along a dendrite. **B.** Temporal summation of EPSPs produced by a sequence of action potentials in the afferent neuron. **C.** Spatial summation of EPSPs produced by several different afferent neurons.

increased Cl⁻ ion influx, results in membrane hyperpolarization. Caution must be used with these drugs because there is a dose-dependent depression of the CNS: sedation → anxiolysis → hypnosis → anesthesia → medullary depression (respiratory depression) → coma. *Synergism with other CNS depressants occurs, increasing the risk for potentially lethal overdoses.* ▼

Table 2-2. Neurotransmitter Systems

Class	Chemical	Synthesis	Postsynaptic Receptors	Signal Termination	General Function(s) in the Nervous System
Small molecule transmitters					
	Acetylcholine	Choline + acetyl CoA, via the enzyme *choline acetyltransferase*	*Nicotinic* (cation channel) *Muscarinic* (G-protein–coupled)	Extracellular hydrolysis by *acetylcholinesterase*	• Movement control • Cognition
	Glutamate and aspartate	Available from the diet and produced from *glutamine supplied by glia*	*Metabotropic receptors Inotropic receptors* • NMDA (Ca²⁺ permeable channels) • AMPA (Na⁺/K⁺ channel) • Kainate (Na⁺/K⁺ channel)	*Reuptake*	• General excitation (most rapid synaptic events in the brain are mediated by *glutaminergic signaling,* which evokes EPSPs through the opening of cation channels)
	GABA	From the amino acid *glutamate* via the enzyme *glutamic acid decarboxylase*	*GABA_A* (Cl⁻ channel) *GABA_B* (G-protein–coupled)	*Reuptake*	• General inhibition (most rapid inhibitory synapses in the brain use *GABA* to evoke an IPSP)
	Glycine	Available from the diet	Glycine receptor (Cl⁻ channel)	*Reuptake*	• General inhibition
Catecholamines	Dopamine	From the amino acid *tyrosine* via the enzyme *tyrosine hydroxylase* in the *catecholamine pathway*	*D_1* (stimulatory G-protein–coupled) *D_2* (inhibitory G-protein–coupled)	*Reuptake*	• Movement control • General affect
	Norepinephrine	From dopamine in the *catecholamine pathway*	*α- and β-adrenergic receptors*	*Reuptake* or breakdown via the enzymes *monoamine oxidase* and *catechol-O-methyltransferase*	• Alertness • General affect
	Epinephrine*				
	Serotonin (5-HT)	From the amino acid tryptophan via the enzyme *tryptophan hydroxylase*	Several subtypes, both ion channels, and G-protein–coupled	*Reuptake*	• Mood (*5-HT reuptake blockers are commonly prescribed antidepressants*) • General arousal

Table 2-2. Neurotransmitter Systems *(continued)*

Class	Chemical	Synthesis	Postsynaptic Receptors	Signal Termination	General Function(s) in the Nervous System
Large molecule transmitters[**]					
Opioids	β-Endorphin Dynorphin Met-enkephalin Leu-enkephalin	Protein synthesis in the neuron cell body	(β-endorphin) μ-*Receptors* κ-*Receptors* (dynorphin) δ-*Receptors* (enkephalins)	Metabolism by extracellular *neuropeptidase* enzymes	• Control of pain
	Substance P		Neurokinin receptor		• Transmission of pain signals

[*]Epinephrine is produced in the adrenal medulla (see The Autonomic Nervous System).

[**]Only selected neuropeptides are included.

AMPA, α-amino-3-hydroxy-5-methylisoxazole-4-propionic acid; EPSP, excitatory postsynaptic potential; GABA, γ-aminobutyric acid; IPSP, inhibitory postsynaptic potential; NMDA, *N*-methyl-D-aspartate.

Fundamentals of Sensory Neurophysiology

1. Sensory systems provide information about both the external environment (e.g., location of food; sources of danger) and the internal body environment (e.g., arterial blood pressure, body temperature).
2. Sensory systems are each specialized to measure a different type of energy but are organized according to a set of common principles:
   a. The **stimulus** is a distinct type of energy (e.g., light, sound, heat, mechanical, chemical).
   b. ***Receptors** are transducers that convert the stimulus energy into electrical signals in neurons.* Specialized receptors are available to detect each type of stimulus:
      i. **Photoreceptors** for light.
      ii. **Mechanoreceptors** for mechanical stimuli.
      iii. **Thermoreceptors** for heat.
      iv. **Chemoreceptors** for chemical composition.
   c. Specific **neuronal pathways** organize and convey the sensory information to the CNS.
   d. Interpretation of sensory input occurs in specific areas of the CNS; integration of inputs produces the **perception** of a stimulus (Figure 2-15).
      i. The nature of the CNS pathway is important for perception; for example, stimulation of the optic nerve is always perceived as light, even if the stimulation is pressure applied to the eye (a concept referred to as the **labeled line**).
      ii. Subjective factors are important in perception (e.g., physical detection of a stimulus could be disturbing or pleasurable, depending on previously learned information).
3. Any sensory system must be able to encode four attributes of a stimulus:
   a. The **modality** is the type of stimulus. *The five traditional sensory modalities are touch, vision, hearing, taste, and smell.*

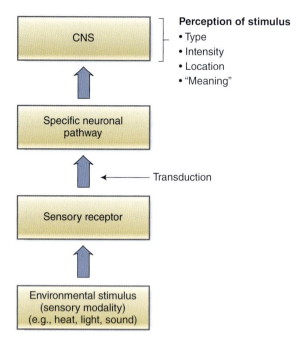

Figure 2-15. General model of sensory perception.

      i. Some sensations require a combination of basic modalities (e.g., detecting that something is wet without seeing the object combines the sensations of touch and temperature).

  b. The **intensity** of stimulus refers to the amount of stimulation (e.g., the loudness of a sound or the pressure applied to the skin).

  c. The **duration** of a stimulus.

  d. The **location** of a stimulus, which might be a position in a three-dimensional space (e.g., source of a sound) or a location could be a site on the body surface.

4. Sensory transduction.

  a. Most sensory receptors preferentially respond to a single type of stimulus.

    i. The **adequate stimulus** is the stimulus for which a receptor has the lowest threshold for detection.

  b. *Receptors transduce the stimulus energy into a graded electrical potential called a **generator potential**,* which will trigger action potentials in the sensory neuron if the threshold potential is exceeded (Figure 2-16).

    i. Receptors encode stimulus duration by producing generator potentials that correspond with the duration of the stimulus.

    ii. *Receptors transduce stimulus intensity by producing larger generator potentials in response to increased stimulus intensity, which is encoded as a higher frequency of action potentials in the sensory neuron.*

  c. Frequency coding about the stimulus intensity is supplemented by **population coding,** which refers to the number of receptors that respond to the same stimulus.

    i. A receptor can only transduce a stimulus that is applied to a restricted area known as the **receptive field.**

    ii. Higher stimulus intensity is perceived if several receptive fields are stimulated at once (e.g., pressing harder on an area of skin stimulates more receptors).

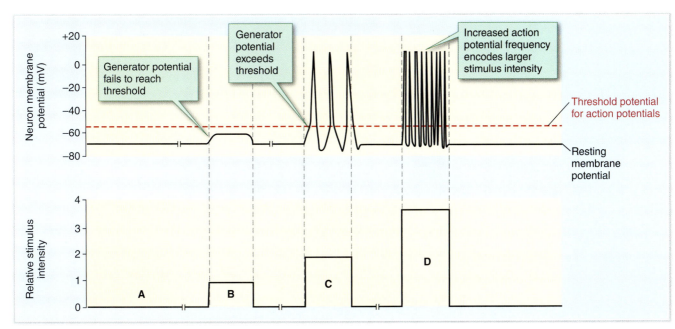

Figure 2-16. Frequency coding of stimulus intensity. The lower part of the figure shows four stimuli (A–D) of increasing intensity (e.g., pressure applied to the skin); the upper part of the figure shows responses in the sensory neuron to this stimulation. **A.** No stimulus; the sensory neuron is at the resting membrane potential. **B.** Weak stimulus; the resulting generator potential does not depolarize the sensory neuron beyond threshold. **C.** Moderate stimulus; action potentials are recorded in the sensory nerve because the generator potential exceeds threshold. **D.** Large (intense) stimulus; the generator potential amplitude and the action potential frequency are increased.

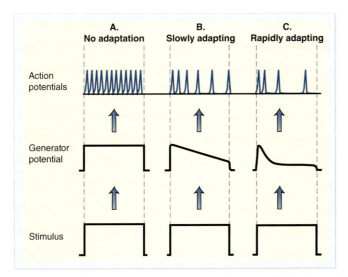

Figure 2-17. Receptor adaptation. An equivalent stimulus is applied to three different sensory receptors. **A.** If there is no receptor adaptation, a constant generator potential and action potential frequency are recorded. **B.** Slowly adapting receptors respond to a constant stimulus with a gradual decline in the generator potential and the action potential frequency. **C.** Rapidly adapting receptors have a generator potential and an action potential frequency that declines rapidly in response to a constant stimulus.

    d. Adaptation of sensory receptors (Figure 2-17).
        i. **Receptor adaptation** refers to a decline in action potential generation when a constant stimulus is applied (producing a **phasic** rather than a tonic response).
        ii. Receptor adaptation is necessary so that constant environmental stimuli can be partially ignored, preventing a flood of sensory information into the CNS.

      iii. The generator potential declines over time with a constant stimulus, causing the frequency of action potentials in the sensory nerve to decrease.

      iv. **Rapidly adapting receptors** are useful in situations where the rate of change of a stimulus is important (e.g., the tension of a working muscle).

      v. **Slowly adapting receptors** are useful where information about a sustained stimulus is important (e.g., application of pressure).

The Somatosensory System

1. The somatosensory system conveys sensations from the skin and muscle; there are four **cutaneous sensory modalities:** touch, vibration, pain, and temperature.

2. The somatosensory system also includes **proprioception,** which relates to sensory information from the musculoskeletal system (see Motor Neurophysiology).

3. The area of skin supplied with afferent nerve fibers by a single dorsal root is referred to as a **dermatome** (Figure 2-18).

4. Touch sensation.

   a. **Discriminative fine touch** is transduced by specialized receptors (Figure 2-19):

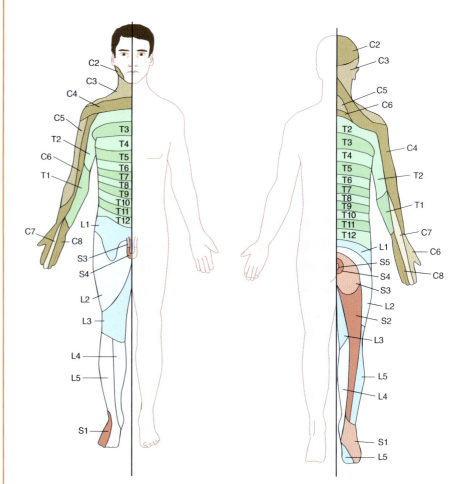

Figure 2-18. Skin dermatomes.

A.

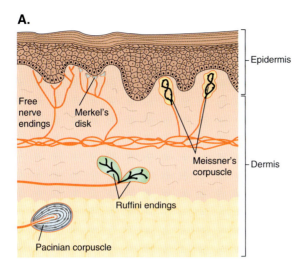

B.

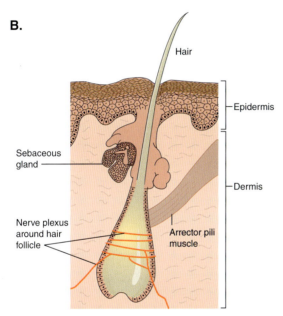

Figure 2-19. Touch receptors in the skin. **A.** Merkel's disks and Meissner's corpuscles just beneath the epidermis mediate discriminative touch. Ruffini's endings sense stretch and Pacinian corpuscles sense vibration. **B.** In hairy skin, the displacement of hairs contributes to touch sensation via a plexus of nerve endings wrapped around the hair root.

    i. **Merkel's disks** and **Meissner's corpuscles** are both located near the skin surface and have small receptive fields allowing fine discrimination. Merkel's disks are slowly adapting and sense steady pressure. Meissner's corpuscles are more rapidly adapting and sense more rapid changes in skin contacts.

    ii. **Ruffini's endings** contribute to the sensation of touch but have large receptive fields and are slowly adapting, making them useful for sensing local stretching of the skin rather than fine discriminative touch.

    iii. **Pacinian corpuscles** are very rapidly adapting receptors that respond to rapidly changing stimuli, and therefore can sense **vibration.**

    iv. **Hair follicles** have a nerve plexus that transduces displacement of the hair.

    b. **A two-point discrimination test** measures the minimum distance between two points of contact that can be perceived as two distinct stimuli.

       i. *The greatest spatial resolution is found on the fingertips and lips, and the lowest spatial resolution is found on the skin of the calf and lower back.*

       ii. The high two-point discrimination of the fingertips is due to a high density of Merkel's disks and Meissner's corpuscles, the large number of neurons in the sensory pathway, and the large representation of these areas in the somatosensory cortex.

    c. The **main pathway for touch, vibration, and proprioception** involves a three-neuron chain (Figure 2-20):

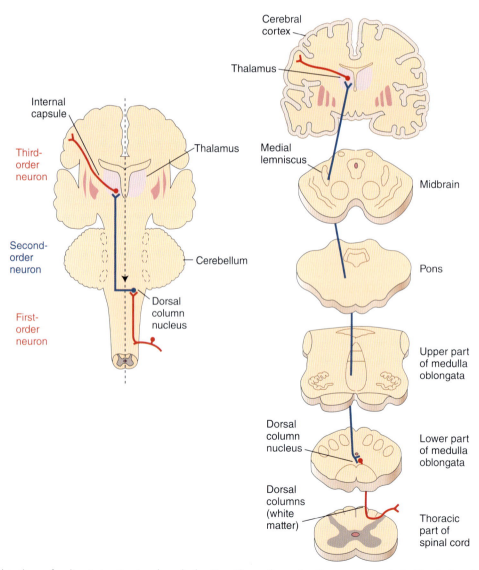

Figure 2-20. Neural pathway for discriminative touch and vibration. The pathway is a three-neuron chain. The first-order neuron ascends in the dorsal column of the spinal cord; the second-order neuron crosses over the midline in the medulla; and the third-order neuron ascends from the thalamus to the somatosensory cortex.

    i. The **first-order neuron** is the somatosensory receptor neuron. The afferent fiber is in the peripheral spinal nerve, the cell body is in the dorsal root ganglion, and the axon ascends the **dorsal column** white matter of the spinal cord to the brainstem.

    ii. The **second-order neuron** is located in the **dorsal column nuclei** of the caudal medulla. *The axon crosses to the opposite side and ascends through the brainstem to the thalamus in a tract called the* **medial lemniscus.**

    iii. The **third-order neuron** is located in the **thalamus** and ascends to the primary somatosensory cortex via the white matter of the internal capsule.

  d. ▼ *The site of decussation for the* **dorsal column-medial lemniscus** (DCML) *tract is at the level of the medulla.* Damage to a DCML tract:

    i. Below the level of the medulla will result in an ipsilateral loss of sensation.

    ii. Above the medulla will result in a contralateral loss of sensation.

    iii. Causes loss of tactile sense; patients lose two-point discrimination and cannot identify objects by touch (**astereognosia**) in the affected areas.

    iv. Causes loss of kinesthetic sense (i.e., position and movement) in the affected areas due to loss of conscious **proprioception.** ▼

  e. The somatosensory cortex.

    i. The **primary somatosensory cortex** is located in the **postcentral gyrus** of the parietal lobe.

    ii. Lesions impair somatic sensations; electrical stimulation evokes sensations in specific parts of the body.

    iii. The body surface is represented as a **somatotopic map** (often called the **homunculus**) in the primary somatosensory cortex (Figure 2-21). The homunculus has two striking features:

- *The somatotopic map is discontinuous,* with the genitals represented below the feet and the hand represented between the head and the face.
- *The amount of cortex representing a given area reflects the importance of the sensory input.* For example, the fingers and mouth occupy a disproportionately large amount of cortex compared to the surface area of skin involved.

    iv. Secondary somatosensory areas include the **posterior parietal cortex,** which integrates the sense of touch with other sensations such as vision.

- ▼ Lesions in the posterior parietal cortex may cause **agnosia,** which is the inability to recognize objects despite the presence of normal sensations. ▼

5. Temperature sensation.

  a. The sensations of "warm" and "cold" reflect two populations of **thermoreceptors** in the skin. Thermoreceptors:

    i. *Are free nerve endings that only respond to temperature.*

    ii. Are rapidly adapting, which explains why a sudden change in temperature (e.g., entering a cold ocean) transmits an initial shock that quickly subsides.

    iii. Protect against exposure to objects or environments that are too hot or too cold.

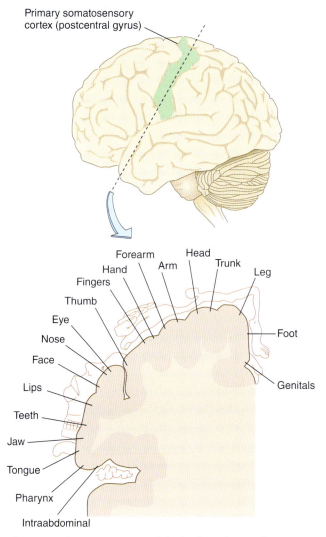

Figure 2-21. Somatotopic representation of the body surface in the primary somatosensory cortex.

    iv. Contribute to the ability to recognize complex modalities like wetness or slipperiness.

  b. *Peripheral thermoreceptors play a minor role in the homeostatic control of core body temperature, which is dominated by hypothalamic thermoreceptors.*

6. Pain sensation.

  a. The term **nociceptor** is used to describe pain receptors, which are free nerve endings. Nociceptors:

    i. Have a high threshold of activation and are silent unless a noxious stimulus is applied.

    ii. Can respond to excessive mechanical, thermal, or chemical stimuli.

    iii. Are slowly adapting so that a constantly applied noxious stimulus continues to be perceived as a painful stimulus.

  b. Somatosensory pain can be described as **superficial pain** (arising from the body surface) or **deep pain** (arising from muscles and joints).

    i. **Superficial pain** has two components:

      • **Initial pain** is a sharp, highly localized pain. *The onset of pain sensation is fast because the nociceptors use myelinated Aδ nerve fibers.*

Table 2-3. Typical Sites of Referred Pain

Pathologic Condition	Site(s) of Referred Pain (Variation in Site Does Occur)
Myocardial infarction	Left chest wall, left neck or jaw, left shoulder, left arm
Diaphragm irritation from cholecystitis or hepatitis	Right shoulder
Diaphragm irritation from ruptured spleen	Left shoulder
Stomach ulcer or cancer	Epigastrium, midback between the scapula
Lower lobe pneumonia	Upper quadrant abdominal pain on the same side as the pneumonia
Appendicitis	Periumbilical area *(note: right lower quadrant pain associated with appendicitis is not referred pain; it indicates somatic pain caused from the inflamed appendix irritating the parietal peritoneum)*
Kidney stone	Flank radiating to groin, including testicle or labia majora

- **Delayed pain** is a diffuse burning sensation that lasts longer than initial pain. *The onset is delayed because the nociceptors involved are unmyelinated C fibers.*

   c. ▼ Inflammation causes **hyperalgesia** around the injured area (e.g., even a minor burn is very sensitive for a prolonged period). Hyperalgesia is caused by inflammatory mediators such as **prostaglandin E$_2$** and leukotrienes. **Nonsteroidal anti-inflammatory drugs (NSAIDs)** are analgesic because they inhibit the production of inflammatory pain sensitizers (e.g., prostaglandins E$_2$). ▼

   d. Pain arising from the internal organs is called **visceral pain,** which is usually a dull, burning sensation that is poorly localized.

      i. Visceral afferent fibers of the ANS are used to convey visceral sensations to the CNS and usually follow the sympathetic distribution.

   e. *Noxious stimuli in the viscera often cause **referred pain**, which is perceived to be on the body surface* (Table 2-3).

      i. The **convergence-projection theory** explains referred pain on the basis that afferent fibers from the viscera converge with somatic pain afferents on the spinal cord; the CNS misinterprets the source of pain by projecting the visceral signal onto the somatic map.

   f. The **main pathway for pain and temperature sensation** via spinal nerves involves a three-neuron chain (Figure 2-22):

      i. The **first-order neuron** is the receptor neuron. *Note: The afferent fiber in the peripheral nerve, which enters the spinal cord via the dorsal root, ascends and descends approximately two spinal segments in the **tract of Lissauer** prior to synapse in the dorsal horn gray matter.*

      ii. The **second-order neuron** is located in the spinal cord in an area of the dorsal horn called the **substantia gelatinosa.** *The second-order neuron crosses immediately to the other side of the midline and ascends in the **anterolateral (spinothalamic) system** of spinal white matter to the thalamus.*

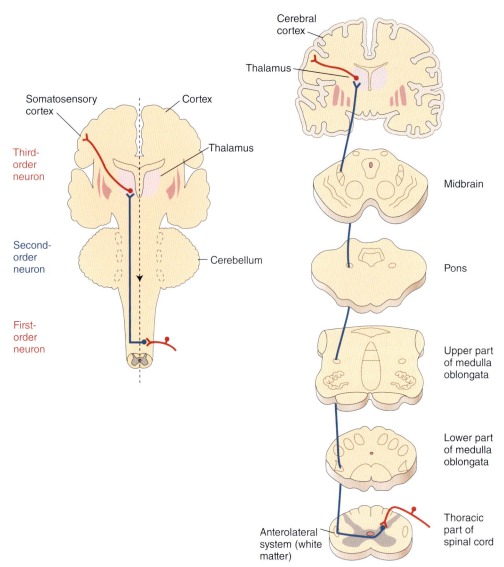

Figure 2-22. Neural pathway for pain and temperature. The pathway is a three-neuron chain. The first-order neuron synapses in the dorsal horn of the spinal cord; the second-order neuron immediately crosses the midline and ascends to the brainstem in the anterolateral white matter of the spinal cord; and the third-order neuron ascends from the thalamus to the somatosensory cortex

    iii. The **third-order neuron** is located in the **thalamus** and ascends to the **primary somatosensory cortex** via the white matter of the internal capsule. This projection is responsible for localizing pain. Other projections to the temporal lobe and brainstem areas contribute to the affective aspects of pain perception as an unpleasant and disturbing sensation.

  g. ▼ *Unilateral damage to the anterolateral system will result in a contralateral loss of sensation beginning 1–2 spinal cord segments below the level of the lesion due to the presence of Lissauer's tract.* ▼

  h. ▼ **Syringomyelia** is characterized by progressive cavitation of the central spinal canal, usually in the cervical region. The decussating second-order neurons associated with the anterolateral system may be damaged as the central canal expands. *Patients present with bilateral loss of pain and temperature in a "cape-like" distribution of the shoulders and upper* *extremities. As the cavitation progresses, motor neurons in the ventral horn of the spinal cord may become compressed, leading to bilateral flaccid paralysis of the upper extremities.* ▼

   i. Neurotransmitters in the pain pathway.

      i. **Glutamate** or **Substance P** is released by the first-order neuron in the afferent pain pathway.

     ii. Pain can sometimes be relieved if nonpainful sensory stimulation is simultaneously applied (e.g., gently rubbing an injured area) by a mechanism known as **pain gating:**

        • Touch fibers entering the same dorsal root as the pain fiber send a collateral branch that synapses on inhibitory interneurons within the spinal gray matter.

        • *The inhibitory interneurons release* **opioids** *(enkephalins) to inhibit transmission in the pain pathway between the first- and second-order neurons.*

        • ▼ **Transcutaneous electrical nerve stimulation (TENS) machines** apply electrical current to the skin and can be effective at relieving pain. The TENS machine is thought to work through the pain gate mechanism. ▼

    iii. Two **descending pathways** can also stimulate the enkephalinergic interneurons to inhibit pain transmission: a serotonergic pathway from the raphe nucleus of the medulla and a norepinephrinergic pathway from the locus ceruleus of the pons.

The Visual System

1. The optics of the eye focus light on specialized retinal **photoreceptor cells,** which transduce light into a neuronal signal.

2. The visual field has a highly ordered representation on the retina and throughout the visual pathway from the retina to the cerebral cortex.

3. Central processing occurs in the primary visual cortex and surrounding visual association cortex and allows interpretation of the complex qualities of vision (e.g., form, color, depth, motion, and distance).

4. The **major structures of the eye** (Figure 2-23A) are organized in three layers:

   a. The outer layer of the eye is made up of the **sclera** and **cornea.**

      i. The sclera is the white of the eye. It is composed of tough connective tissue, which is continuous with the dura mater around the optic nerve.

     ii. The cornea is the curved transparent area where light enters the front of the eye.

   b. The innermost layer of the eye is the **retina.**

      i. The **fovea** is a small depression in the center of the retina, which is surrounded by a region called the **macula.**

     ii. Light is focused on the fovea, which has *the highest level of* **visual acuity** *(i.e., the ability to distinguish between two-point light sources).*

    iii. The **optic nerve** exits the eye posteriorly. The point of exit of the optic nerve causes a discontinuation of the retina and produces a small "**blind spot**" in the visual field.

   c. The middle layer of the eye is the vascular **choroid,** which is continuous with the **iris** and **ciliary body.**

A.

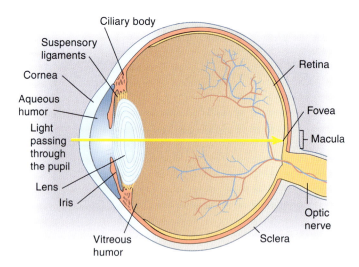

B.

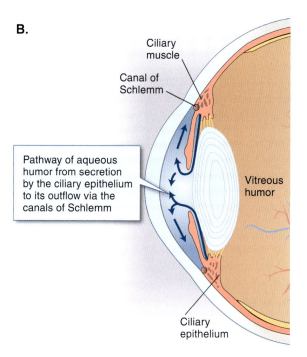

Figure 2-23. A. Anatomy of the eye. **B.** Secretion and reabsorption of aqueous humor. The ciliary epithelium secretes aqueous humor, which enters the anterior compartment of eye via the pupil and drains into the venous system via the canal of Schlemm.

    i. The iris is the colored diaphragm running across the anterior part of the eyeball. The **pupil** is the aperture at the center of the iris, the diameter of which is controlled by muscles of the iris.
- The pupil dilates (**mydriasis**) in the dark to allow more light to enter the eye; *mydriasis is mediated by α_1-adrenergic receptor stimulation.*
- The pupil constricts (**miosis**) in bright light to prevent the excessive entry of light; *miosis is mediated by M_3 cholinergic receptor stimulation.*

Table 2-4. Conditions Involving the Major Structures of the Eye

Major Eye Structure	Disease/Condition
Sclera	**Osteogenesis imperfecta:** The sclera appear blue because the genetic defect in the type I procollagen allows the underlying (blue) choroid layers to be seen.
Retina	**Hypertensive retinopathy:** Severity and duration of hypertension are the key determinants of retinopathy. One classification system is based on funduscopic examination findings: grade 1, arterial narrowing, "copper/silver wiring"; grade 2, arteriovenous (A-V) nicking; grade 3, flame-shaped hemorrhages, cotton-wool spots (infarcted zones), hard exudates (extravasated lipid); grade 4, papilledema.
Macula	**Tay-Sachs disease:** A neurodegenerative disease caused by hexosaminidase A deficiency. Patients have a characteristic macular "cherry-red" spot.
Optic nerve	**Multiple sclerosis:** Optic neuritis is a common initial presenting symptom of multiple sclerosis characterized by decreased visual acuity, ocular pain (especially with movement), and color desaturation.
Cornea	**Herpes:** Dendritic ulcers of the cornea are characteristic of herpetic eye infections.
Iris	**Neurofibromatosis type I:** A genetic condition that results in characteristic neurofibromas (benign Schwann cell tumors), café au lait spots (freckling of non-sun exposed skin), and Lisch nodules (iris hamartomas).
Lens	**Marfan's syndrome:** A genetic defect in fibrillin production that results in the classic clinical triad: ocular lens dislocation, aortic dilation, and long thin extremities.

   ii. The **ciliary body** includes the **ciliary muscle**, which controls the curvature of the lens, and the **ciliary epithelium**, which secretes aqueous humor.

  d. The **lens** lies behind the cornea and consists of a transparent viscous gel encased in a capsule. The lens and cornea together constitute the **optic apparatus** of the eye.

  e. The cavity of the eye contains fluids; the **aqueous humor** is in front of the lens, and the **vitreous humor** is behind the lens.

  f. ▼ Structures of the eye can be adversely affected by a wide range of systemic disease processes (see Table 2-4). ▼

 5. Fluid compartments of the eye.

  a. The intraocular fluids of the eye keep the eyeball distended. Vitreous humor is a stable gelatinous mass, but aqueous humor is continually secreted.

  b. **Intraocular pressure** is maintained within a normal range of approximately 15 mm Hg ($\pm$3 mm Hg) by a balance between the secretion and absorption of aqueous humor.

  c. *The aqueous humor is secreted by the ciliary body and is absorbed via the canal of Schlemm* (Figure 2-23B).

   i. Epithelial cells projecting from the **ciliary body** actively secrete aqueous humor into the space between the iris and the lens (the **posterior compartment**).

      ii. Aqueous humor flows through the pupil into the space between the iris and the cornea (the **anterior compartment**).

      iii. The **canal of Schlemm** leaves the anterior chamber, at the angle between the iris and cornea, and drains into the extraocular veins.

   d. ▼ **Glaucoma** is associated with a pathologic increase in intraocular pressure, which occurs as a result of an imbalance between aqueous humor production and drainage. Glaucoma may result in damage to the optic nerve and progressive loss of vision.

      i. Patients with **acute closed-angle glaucoma,** which results from rapid increases in intraocular pressure, present with a painful, red eye and are at risk of rapid permanent vision loss. *Acute closed-angle glaucoma is considered a medical emergency!*

      ii. **Open-angle glaucoma** is more common and presents as an insidious onset of painless progressive loss of vision; typically, the peripheral vision is affected first, and the central vision is affected later.

      iii. *Glaucoma can be medically treated with* **prostaglandins** *or cholinergic agonists to increase the rate of aqueous humor drainage, or it can be treated with* **beta adrenergic receptor antagonists** *or* **carbonic anhydrase inhibitors** *to decrease the rate of secretion.* ▼

6. Optical principles.

   a. Light rays bend as they enter the eye (known as **refraction**) and become focused at the retina (Figure 2-24).

   b. The cornea and lens are both convex surfaces that cause light to be focused toward a **focal point;** the distance beyond the lens where light focuses is the **focal distance.**

   c. When an image is viewed through a convex lens, *the projected image is turned upside down, with the two sides reversed.* This occurs at the eye, but the brain is able to perceive images in their correct orientation.

   d. The refractive power of a lens is measured using **diopter** ("D") units.

      i. A spherical lens that focuses light 1 m beyond the lens has a power of $+1$ D; a lens with ten times this refractory power ($+10$ D) focuses light 10 cm beyond the lens.

      ii. *Concave lenses disperse light and have refractory powers described in negative dioptric units.*

      iii. The total refractory power of the eye is approximately $+60$ D, with two-thirds of refraction occurring at the cornea and most of the remaining refraction occurring at the lens.

      iv. The lens has a variable curvature contributing between $+13$ D (in its most flattened state) to $+26$ D (in its most curved state).

        • If a lens is isolated from the eye, it becomes almost spherical.

        • Inside the eye, the lens is placed under tension by **suspensory ligaments,** and in the resting condition, the lens remains fairly flat.

        • *Contraction of the ciliary muscles reduces tension in the ligaments and allows the lens to assume a more rounded shape.*

   e. **Accommodation** is the ability to change optical power to maintain focus as the distance to an object varies.

   f. The **accommodation-convergence reflex** occurs when focusing on a near object and has three components:

      i. Convergence of the eyes to maintain a single image.

A.

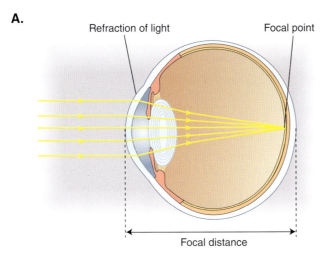

Refraction of light   Focal point

Focal distance

B.

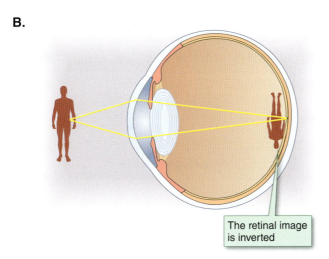

The retinal image is inverted

Figure 2-24. Optical properties of the eye. **A.** The convex cornea and lens cause refraction of light and convergence of light rays to bring objects into focus on the retina. The focal distance is the distance from the front of the eye to the focal point. **B.** Image inversion by the optical apparatus of the eye.

    ii. Constriction of the pupils by contraction of circular muscle in the iris, to prevent excess light scattering that would blur the image.

   iii. Contraction of ciliary muscles to increase refractory power of the lens to focus the object.

   iv. *The reflex is mediated via the parasympathetic nerves to the eye.*

  g. Errors of refraction (Figure 2-25).

    i. People with normal vision (**emmetropia**) focus distant objects clearly, with the ciliary muscle completely relaxed.

    ii. **Myopia** (nearsightedness) occurs when light from distant objects is focused in front of the retina with the ciliary muscle relaxed.

      • There is no way for the maximally flattened lens to refract light any less, resulting in a limiting "far point" for clear vision.

      • Accommodation still occurs to allow clear focus on closer objects.

      • *Myopia is usually caused by an eyeball that is too long; the refraction error can be corrected using eyeglasses with a concave lens.*

A. Normal vision (emmetropia)

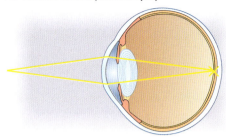

B. Myopia

Myopia correction

Light is focused in front of the retina

Concave lens causes divergence of light before it enters the long eyeball

C. Hyperopia

Hyperopia correction

Light is focused behind the retina

Convex lens causes convergence of light before it enters the short eyeball

Figure 2-25. Myopia (nearsightedness) and hyperopia (farsightedness). **A.** The normal eye focuses light from a distant point on the retina with the ciliary muscles relaxed. **B.** Myopia results when the eyeballs are longer than normal, causing light to be focused on a point in front of the retina. Myopia can be corrected using eyeglasses with a concave lens. **C.** Hyperopia results when the eyeballs are shorter than normal, causing light to be focused behind the retina. Hyperopia can be corrected using eyeglasses with a convex lens.

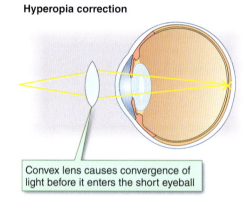

iii. **Hyperopia** (farsightedness) occurs when the resting position of the lens does not refract light from distant objects enough, causing the focal point to lie behind the retina.

- The hyperopic patient is able to voluntarily use the accommodation mechanism to increase the refractive power of the lens and bring distant objects into focus.
- The remaining range of ciliary muscle contraction available to accommodate near objects is reduced, causing the "near point" to recede.
- *Hyperopia is most commonly the result of a short eyeball; the refraction error is corrected using eyeglasses with a convex lens.*

iv. **Presbyopia** is the reduced ability to accommodate near or distant objects due to a decrease in the elasticity of the lens, which occurs with increasing age.

- In most people older than the age of 70, the curvature of the lens becomes fixed, resulting in an inability to focus on near objects (e.g., reading); distance vision is also limited because the lens flattens less than in younger people.
- *Bifocal lenses, which have an upper half of the lens focused for distance vision and a lower part focused for near vision, are often prescribed for presbyopia.*

v. **Astigmatism** is caused by incorrect curvature of the eye in one plane. Two different focal distances are produced, depending on the plane on which light enters the eye.

- *Eyeglasses with a cylindrical lens are needed to correct the refraction error of astigmatism.*

7. The retina is the site of phototransduction and is composed of the several cellular layers (Figure 2-26):

a. The **retinal pigment epithelium** (RPE) is the outermost layer of cells. The functions of the RPE are to:

i. Recycle the visual pigment molecules.

ii. Absorb stray light, preventing reflection of light back into the eye.

b. There are two types of photoreceptor resting on the pigment epithelium: The **rods** and the **cones.**

i. Rods and cones have an outer segment and an inner segment.

ii. The outer segment faces the RPE and is composed of membranous **discs** that contain a high concentration of the visual pigment molecule **rhodopsin.**

iii. The inner segment synapses with bipolar and horizontal cells.

c. **Bipolar cells** form synapses with photoreceptor cells at one pole and with ganglion cells at the other pole.

d. **Ganglion cells** are the innermost layer of cells, and are the output cells of the retina. *The axons of ganglion cells become the optic nerve.*

e. **Horizontal cells** have a radial orientation and form synapses in the outer layer of the retina with the photoreceptors and the bipolar cells.

f. **Amacrine cells** have a similar orientation to horizontal cells but are located in the inner layer of the retina, where they synapse with bipolar cells and ganglion cells.

8. Properties of rods and cones.

a. **Rods** are monochromatic (single color) receptors, which are highly sensitive to light and allow objects to be seen in low-intensity light.

b. **Cones** function best under high light intensity conditions. There are three types, with overlapping sensitivity to light of different wavelength (i.e., blue, green, and red cones).

c. The **fovea** only contains cone cells. High **visual acuity** at the fovea occurs because most cone cells in the fovea synapse with a single bipolar cell, which in turn synapses with a single ganglion cell to produce very small receptive fields.

d. Visual acuity is much lower at the periphery of the eye because there is a high proportion of rod cells, and many rods converge on each ganglion cell.

e. *Therefore, central vision has a high resolution but is poor in dim light, whereas peripheral vision has low resolution but allows vision in low light.*

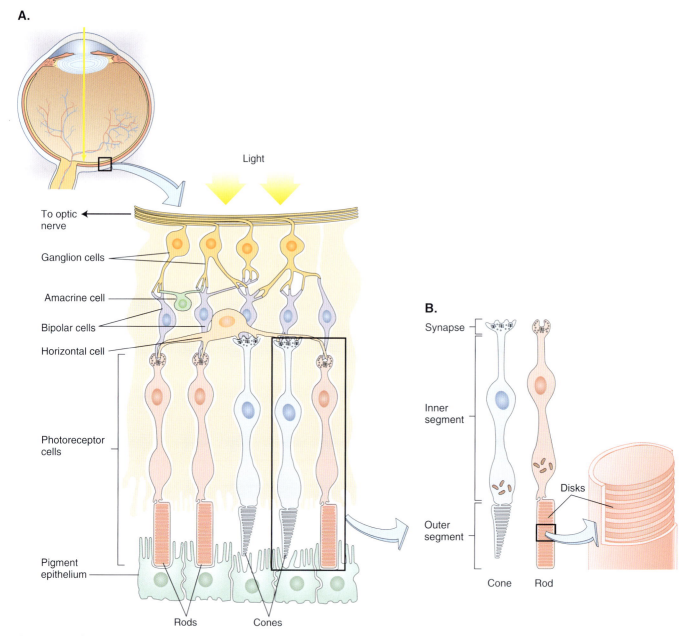

Figure 2-26. The retina. **A.** Incoming light passes through several neuronal layers to reach the photoreceptor cells. The retinal output consists of action potentials in ganglion cells; the axons of ganglion cells are conveyed to the central nervous system via the optic nerve. **B.** Rods and cones. Photoreceptor cells have two major regions: an outer segment resting on the retinal pigment epithelium and an inner segment that synapses with bipolar and horizontal cells. The outer segment contains stacks of membranous discs containing the visual pigment molecule rhodopsin.

9. Mechanism of phototransduction.
   a. Phototransduction is the cascade of chemical and electrical events through which light energy is converted into a receptor potential.
   b. Rods and cones are unusual in that the receptor potential is a **hyperpolarization.**
   c. The **phototransduction mechanism** (Figure 2-27) involves the following steps:
      i. The photoreceptor membrane potential is depolarized in the dark because cGMP-activated cation channels are open. Na^+ influx is measured as the "**dark current**" of photoreceptors.

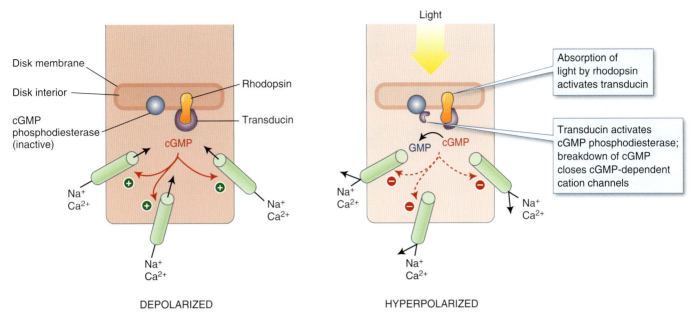

Figure 2-27. Mechanism of phototransduction. The membrane potential of photoreceptors is depolarized in the dark due to sustained opening of cyclic guanosine monophosphate (cGMP)-dependent cation channels. The absorption of light by the visual pigment rhodopsin stimulates the G protein transducin to increase cGMP phosphodiesterase activity. cGMP is broken down to guanosine monophosphate (GMP), which causes cation channels to close and results in a hyperpolarizing receptor potential.

    ii. Light is absorbed by the light receptor molecule **rhodopsin,** which is formed from the transmembrane protein **opsin** and the vitamin A derivative **retinal.**

   iii. A conformational change in opsin activates the rhodopsin pigment resulting in activation of the G-protein **transducin.**

   iv. Transducin stimulates a **cGMP phosphodiesterase.**

    v. The rate of cGMP breakdown increases, closing cGMP-dependent cation channels and inhibiting the dark current.

   vi. The hyperpolarizing receptor potential decreases the rate of **glutamate** release from photoreceptors onto bipolar cells.

  d. Retinal and opsin separate soon after light is absorbed, and must be recycled over a period of several minutes to regenerate rhodopsin for subsequent phototransduction.

10. Dark and light adaptation.

  a. The sensitivity of the retina must be altered in response to changing levels of light or images appear washed out in bright light or invisible in dim light conditions.

  b. In sustained bright light, a large proportion of rhodopsin will dissociate to retinal and opsin. Therefore, *the retina becomes adapted to light by having less visual pigment available for phototransduction.*

  c. Conversely, the retina becomes more sensitive to light with increasing time spent in darkness. Rhodopsin stores are built up as all the available retinal and opsin are combined. *Rods are responsible for the dark adaptation response, which takes 30–40 minutes of continuous darkness to reach a peak.*

  d. ▼ Vitamin A has many important functions in the body, including maintenance of healthy epithelia and vision. **Vitamin A deficiency** results in **night blindness** (rod cell dysfunction), **xerophthalmia** (dry eyes that are prone to ulceration and infection), and **follicular hyperkeratosis** (rough elevations of skin around hair follicles resembling goose bumps). ▼

11. Mechanism of color vision.
    a. *Color is determined by the wavelength of light.*
    b. The phototransduction of light of differing wavelengths is achieved by the three different types of cone receptors.
    c. These receptors are referred to as **blue, green, and red cones,** but they are also called S (short), M (medium), and L (long) to reflect the differences in the wavelengths of light producing the most light absorbance.
    d. *The nervous system decodes color according to the relative stimulation of the three types of cones.*
    e. ▼ **"Color blindness"** is a common condition in which there is a range of possible defects in color vision. Most commonly, a single type of cone receptor is missing. *X-linked recessive mutations are a common cause of defective color vision, resulting in a higher proportion of males than females with this condition.*
        i. **Monochromacy** (true color blindness) is the lack of two out of three of the cone receptor types and is rare.
        ii. **Dichromacy** is the lack of one type of cone receptor. The selective loss of the blue cone (**tritanopia**) is rare. Most commonly, either the red cone (**protanopia**) or the green cone (**deuteranopia**) is missing. The loss of either red or green cones results in difficulty distinguishing between green, yellow, orange, and red colors. *Patients have particular difficulty distinguishing between red and green and are therefore said to have **red-green color blindness.***
        iii. **Anomalous trichromacy** is caused by defective (not missing) L cones with absorbance spectra between the normal L and M ranges. ▼

12. The visual pathway.
    a. The main visual pathway conveys signals from the retina to the primary visual cortex as follows:
        i. Axons from retinal ganglion cells enter the **optic nerve** in each eye.
        ii. The optic nerves meet at the **optic chiasm,** where some axons cross the midline.
        iii. An **optic tract** leads from each side of the optic chiasm to the **lateral geniculate body** of the thalamus, where retinal ganglion cells synapse.
        iv. Second-order sensory neurons follow a course to the primary visual cortex via the **optic radiation.**
    b. The visual fields of each eye overlap extensively to produce binocular vision.
    c. Images from each half of the visual field are processed by the contralateral side of the visual cortex (e.g., the left visual cortex is concerned with information from the right half of the visual field).
    d. *Axons from the nasal half of each retina must cross the midline at the optic chiasm, whereas axons from the temporal half of each retina remain on the ipsilateral side* (Figure 2-28). For example, light from the right half of the visual field projects onto the nasal half of the right retina and will cross at the optic chiasm before continuing on to the left visual cortex, whereas the light that projects on the temporal half of the left retina will not cross at the optic chiasm and will continue on to the left visual cortex.

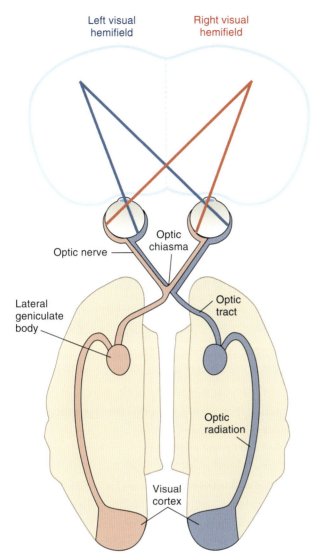

Figure 2-28. The main visual pathway. The binocular visual field is shown, divided into equal left and right halves. Light from the left visual hemifield stimulates the right half of each retina; light from the right visual hemifield stimulates the left half of each retina. Nerve impulses originating from stimuli in the left hemifield are transmitted to the right visual cortex, whereas those from the right hemifield are transmitted to the left visual cortex.

   e.   ▼ Knowledge of the visual pathway allows lesions to be localized based on the patient's visual field defects (see Table 2-5). ▼
   f.   Visual fibers are not restricted to the main visual pathway. Information about light levels and the visual scene project to the following brain areas:
      i.   The **suprachiasmatic nuclei,** for control of circadian rhythms.
      ii. The **superior colliculi** of the midbrain, for the control of eye movements.
      iii. The **pretectal nuclei** of the midbrain, for the reflex control of eye movement associated with changing the focus of vision and for the **pupillary light reflex.**
13. Eye movements.
   a.   The control of eye movement must be able to fix the gaze on objects at different distances, to maintain focus on objects as the head moves, and to follow moving objects in the visual field.

Table 2-5. Visual Field Defects Caused by Lesions in the Visual Pathway

Site of Lesion	Description of Visual Field Defect	Defect	Possible Cause
Optic nerve	Blindness in the affected eye	Monocular blindness	Optic neuritis, retinal artery occlusion
Optic chiasm	Loss of fibers crossing the midline from the nasal half of each retina causes loss of temporal visual field on both sides	Bitemporal heteronymous hemianopia	Pituitary tumor (e.g., craniopharyngioma) pressing on the optic chiasm from below
Optic tract	Loss of fibers for the visual field on the opposite side to the lesion	Homonymous hemianopia	Brain tumor
Optic radiation	Loss of fibers for the visual field on the opposite side to the lesion	Homonymous hemianopia	Brain tumor, occlusion of a branch of the posterior cerebral artery
Visual cortex (one side)	Loss of visual processing for the visual field on the opposite side to the lesion	Homonymous hemianopia with macular sparing	Posterior cerebral artery thrombosis; however, the central (macula) vision is maintained due to collateral circulation between the posterior and middle cerebral arteries

b. The movement of both eyes must be integrated to maintain binocular vision.

c. Movements of the eye are mediated by three pairs of muscles, which receive motor innervation from cranial nerves III (**oculomotor**), IV (**trochlear**), and VI (**abducens**) (see Figure 2-29):

   i. The **medial and lateral rectus** muscles, which move the eyes side to side.

   ii. The **superior and inferior rectus** muscles, which move the eyes upward and downward.

   iii. The **superior and inferior oblique** muscles, which prevent rotation of the eyeball and move the eyes upward and downward.

d. **Fixation movements** of the eye lock the gaze on a specific object, allowing it to be focused on the central part of the retina.

   i. Once a particular object is selected, *the gaze is locked by the **involuntary fixation pathway,*** which begins in the visual association areas surrounding the primary visual cortex.

   ii. Involuntary fixation on the object is maintained by reflexes that are coordinated by the **superior colliculus.**

   iii. *The gaze is unlocked by the **voluntary fixation pathway.*** The voluntary selection of a new object originates from an area in the frontal lobe, close to the premotor cortex.

e. **Saccadic movements** of the eyes are rapid movements in the position of the eyes (saccades). Saccadic movement is necessary when objects in the visual field are moving or when the head is moving.

   i. A succession of fixation points is selected to survey the "highlights" of the moving visual scene.

   ii. Reading is an example of saccadic movement, where the brain becomes trained to use saccades to survey a static visual field for highlights.

   iii. If an object is moving in a regular cycle, saccadic movements quickly become smooth "pursuit" movements as the central visual processing mechanisms adapt and produce programmed eye movements.

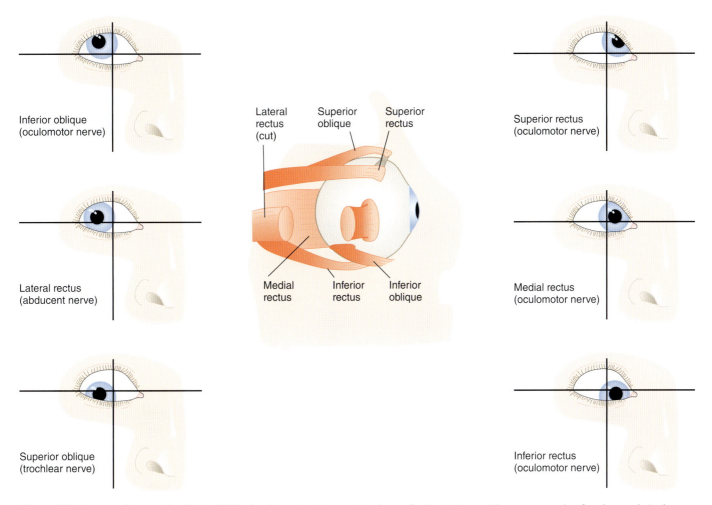

Inferior oblique
(oculomotor nerve)

Lateral rectus (cut)

Superior oblique

Superior rectus

Superior rectus
(oculomotor nerve)

Lateral rectus
(abducent nerve)

Medial rectus

Inferior rectus

Inferior oblique

Medial rectus
(oculomotor nerve)

Superior oblique
(trochlear nerve)

Inferior rectus
(oculomotor nerve)

Figure 2-29. Extraocular muscles. The individual action of each muscle is shown for the right eye. The nerve supply of each muscle is shown in parentheses.

f. ▼ **Nystagmus** is defined as rhythmic oscillations of the eyes characterized by a slow drifting component and a fast saccadic component in the opposite direction.

i. Although nystagmus can be physiologic, it can also indicate underlying serious pathologic conditions, including demyelinating diseases (e.g., **multiple sclerosis**), cerebellar or brainstem lesions, drug intoxication (anticonvulsants or alcohol), or vestibular dysfunction (e.g., **Ménière's disease**).

ii. *A complete neurologic examination should be performed on all patients presenting with nystagmus.* ▼

14. Binocular vision and depth perception.

a. To achieve binocular vision, the visual image of interest must be projected onto the fovea of both eyes simultaneously. The brain fuses the images from each eye into the perception of a single image.

b. Binocular vision improves **depth perception (stereopsis).** Because the eyes are placed about 5 cm apart, the images projected onto the two retinae are not precisely the same. This slight difference is computed by the brain to provide depth perception in the visual scene.

    c. ▼ **Strabismus** refers to misalignment of the eyes, which results in two images being projected to the brain:

        i. In adults strabismus causes **diplopia** (double vision).

        ii. In children uncorrected strabismus can result in **amblyopia** ("lazy eye") resulting in reduced vision of the misaligned eye. The developing brain can suppress the images from the deviated eye, preventing diplopia at the expense of reduced vision in the affected eye. ▼

15. Autonomic innervation of the eye.

    a. The parasympathetic innervation of the eye originates in **oculomotor nucleus,** which has two efferent parts:

        i. A **motor nucleus,** sending motor fibers to the extraocular muscles.

        ii. The **Edinger-Westphal nucleus,** giving origin to parasympathetic preganglionic fibers, which pass via CN III to the **ciliary ganglion.** Postganglionic neurons pass to the eye and innervate the iris and ciliary muscles.

    b. The **pupillary light reflex** is a parasympathetic response that assists the eye in adapting to variable light levels; *reflex constriction of the pupils occurs when light is shone into the eyes:*

        i. **Afferent signals** from some retinal ganglion cells pass (via the **optic nerve**) to the **pretectal nucleus** of the midbrain.

        ii. Interneurons connect the pretectal area to the Edinger-Westphal nucleus on both sides.

        iii. Efferent parasympathetic neurons conveyed via CN III innervate muscles of the iris, resulting in constriction of the pupil.

    c. The pupillary light reflex is **consensual** (i.e., light shone in one eye constricts both pupils). *Brainstem damage can result in an absent pupillary light reflex and/or the presence of different sized pupils.*

    d. ▼ A detailed understanding of the **pupillary light reflex pathway** is essential to diagnosing the location of an associated lesion.

        i. **Afferent (optic nerve, CN II) lesion.** When light is shone in the affected eye, the direct and consensual reflex is absent; when light is shone in the unaffected eye, the direct and consensual reflex is intact.

          • **Explanation.** The afferent nerve must be intact to trigger an efferent (pupillary constriction) response. *Because neurons project from the pretectal area to the Edinger-Westphal nucleus on both sides, any afferent stimulus that reaches the pretectal nucleus will trigger an efferent response in both eyes (assuming an intact efferent pathway).*

        ii. **Efferent (CN III or Edinger-Westphal nucleus) lesion.** Light shone in the eye of the affected side will trigger a consensual reflex but not a direct reflex; light shone in the eye of the unaffected side will trigger a direct reflex not a consensual reflex.

          • **Explanation.** The afferent nerves on both sides are intact and will transmit a stimulus to the pretectal nucleus, which will trigger an efferent response in an intact efferent pathway. *Note: A lesion of CN III will result in weakness of the extraocular muscles, innervated by CN III, in addition to defects in the pupillary light reflex.* ▼

    e. **Sympathetic innervation** to the eye is relayed from the first thoracic segment of the spinal cord and reaches the eye via the **superior cervical ganglion.** Postganglionic fibers travel along the outer surface of blood vessels to the eye. *Sympathetic neurons innervate the iris to cause dilation of the pupil.*

f. ▼ **Horner's syndrome** is caused by the interruption of the sympathetic nerves to the face and head and therefore has the following consequences:

    i. **Persistent constriction of the pupil** on the affected side, due to loss of the sympathetic dilator response.

    ii. **Persistent vasodilation** of blood vessels on the affected side, due to loss of sympathetic vasoconstriction.

    iii. **Loss of sweating** in the affected area, due to sweat glands being stimulated by sympathetic innervation.

    iv. **Droop of the upper eyelid,** due to loss of contraction of smooth muscle fibers in the eyelid, which receive sympathetic innervation. ▼

The Auditory System

1. The auditory and vestibular systems are concerned with the sense of hearing (**audition**) and the sense of **balance,** respectively.
2. The auditory and vestibular systems both use **hair cells** to transduce mechanical forces into action potentials.
3. Hair cells are located in a fluid-filled sensory organ called the **membranous labyrinth** (Figure 2-30). There is a labyrinth inside a hollowed out part of the temporal skull bone on each side of the head. Each labyrinth has two parts:
   a. The **cochlea** is the auditory part of the labyrinth. Afferent neurons exiting the cochlea form the **auditory (cochlear) nerve.**

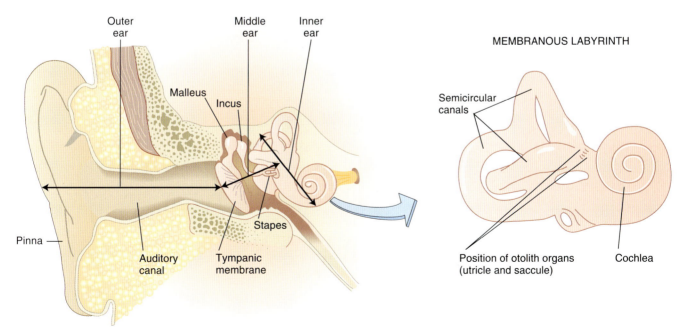

Figure 2-30. Anatomy of the auditory and vestibular apparatus. The outer ear is comprised of the pinna and auditory canal; the middle ear consists of the tympanic membrane and the three ossicles, the malleus, incus, and stapes. The inner ear is comprised of the membranous labyrinth; the cochlea is the auditory part of the labyrinth; and the semicircular canals and the otolith organs form the vestibular part of the inner ear.

b. The **otolith organs** and the **semicircular canals** form the vestibular part of the labyrinth. Afferent neurons from these organs form the **vestibular nerve.**

c. The auditory and vestibular nerves combine to form **the vestibulocochlear nerve (CN VIII).**

4. The physical nature of sound.

a. Sounds are caused by variations in air pressure that travel as a **sound wave.**

b. All sound waves travel at the same speed through air (343 m/s, or 768 m/h), but they have the variable properties of **frequency** and **amplitude** (Figure 2-31).

c. The frequency is the number of cycles of peaks and troughs in air pressure per second, measured in **hertz (Hz).** *The sound frequency determines the pitch (high or low tone) that we perceive.*

    i. ▼ Age-related hearing loss (**presbycusis**) commonly affects older adults. Whereas children can hear sound frequencies ranging from 20 Hz to 20 kHz, older adults often lose high-frequency hearing above 15–16 kHz, making speech hard to hear against ambient noise. ▼

d. *The amplitude of pressure cycles in a sound wave reflects the **intensity** of the sound and is perceived as its loudness.* A **decibel (dB)** scale is used to describe sound intensity.

5. The outer and middle ear.

a. The visible outer ear (**pinna**) funnels sound down the **auditory canal** to the **tympanic membrane** (eardrum).

b. The middle ear is an air-filled space beyond the tympanic membrane, containing a chain of three small bones (**ossicles**) called the **malleus,** the **incus,** and the **stapes.**

c. Sound waves cause movements of the tympanic membrane, which are transferred across the middle ear by the ossicles to a second membrane, the **oval window.**

d. *The structures of the middle ear transfer sound waves into vibrations of fluid in the inner ear.*

e. The middle ear amplifies the force of sound waves because the **oval window** has a smaller surface area than that of the tympanic membrane and because the ossicles act as mechanically efficient **levers.**

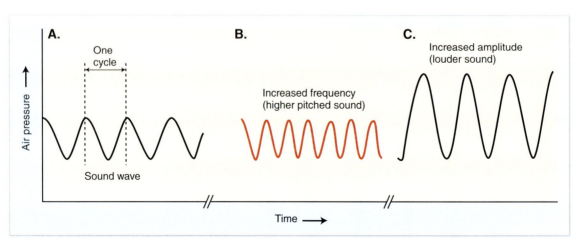

Figure 2-31. The physical nature of sound. **A.** Sound waves produced by cyclic variation in air pressure. **B.** Increased frequency of sound waves is perceived as a higher pitch sound. **C.** Increased amplitude of sound waves is perceived as a louder sound.

f. The **eustachian tube** links the cavity of the middle ear to the nasal cavity and provides a route to drain fluid and to equalize air pressure between the middle ear and the atmosphere (e.g., during ascent and descent of an airplane).

g. The **tensor tympani** and **stapedius** are muscles of the middle ear that mediate the **attenuation reflex** in response to excessively loud sounds. Contraction of the muscles stiffens the ossicles and reduces transmission of vibrations to the inner ear. The attenuation reflex has several functions:

    i. **Protection of hair cells** from damage due to excessive vibrations. However, the reflex has a long latency, approximately 0.1 s, so that sudden loud sounds are still damaging.

    ii. **Prevention of saturation** of the hair cell transduction mechanism by a prolonged loud noise.

    iii. **Discernment of speech** against ambient noise. Compared to higher frequency speech sounds, the attenuation reflex dampens ambient noise by suppressing lower frequency sounds.

    iv. ▼ Vibration of the stapes is regulated by the stapedius muscle, which is innervated by the facial nerve (CN VII). *A lesion of CN VII can result in paralysis of the stapedius,* resulting in **hyperacusia** (excessive sensitivity to sounds). ▼

6. The inner ear.

a. The inner ear includes all of the structures of the membranous labyrinth, although only the cochlea is concerned with the transduction of sound.

b. The cochlea consists of three coiled tubes, located side by side: the **scala vestibuli,** the **scala media,** and the **scala tympani** (Figure 2-32).

c. The spiral coils of the cochlea are encased in a bony shell and are wrapped around a central bony pillar (the **modiolus**).

d. The scala vestibuli is separated from the scala media by **Reissner's membrane,** and the scala media is separated from the scala tympani by the **basilar membrane.**

e. At the base of the cochlea, the **oval window** meets the scala vestibuli, and the **round window** meets the scala tympani.

    i. When the oval window bulges inward and compresses fluid in the cochlea, the round window can bulge outward to prevent excessive pressure changes within the cochlea.

    ii. Movement of the oval window sets up a "**traveling wave**" that flexes the basilar membrane. *Movement of the basilar membrane is the key mechanical event that excites hair cells and results in action potentials in auditory neurons.*

f. The auditory receptors are located in the **organ of Corti,** which sits on top of the basilar membrane.

    i. The sensory hair cells rest on the basilar membrane and extend upward to a supporting membrane, the **reticular lamina,** which is anchored to the basilar membrane by **the rods of Corti.**

    ii. The roof of the organ of Corti is formed by the gelatinous **tectorial membrane.**

g. When a traveling wave passes along the basilar membrane, the hair cells, reticular lamina, and rods of Corti move as one unit toward the tectorial membrane.

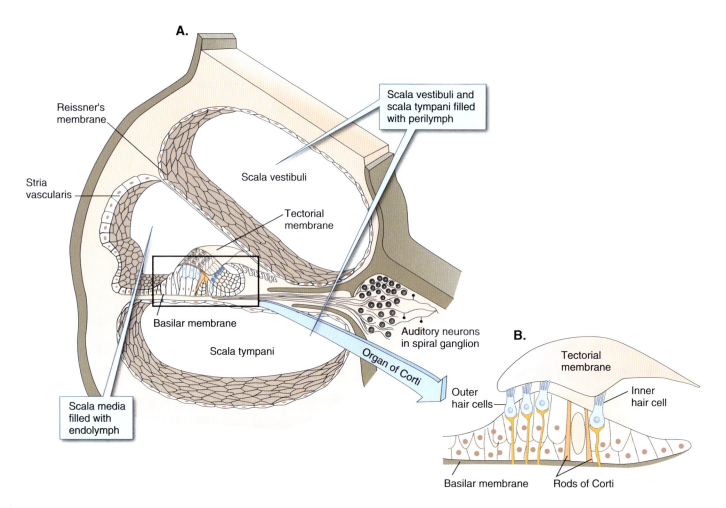

Figure 2-32. The cochlea and organ of Corti. **A.** Cross-section through the cochlea. **B.** The organ of Corti.

h. Traveling waves in the basilar membrane bend the stereocilia that project from the surface of hair cells; *the bending of stereocilia is the crucial event in the transduction of sound waves into a receptor potential.*

7. Fluids of the inner ear.

   a. The inner ear is filled with fluid that facilitates the generation of traveling waves in the basilar membrane in response to movements of the oval window.

   b. Differences in the composition of the cochlea fluids are important for generation of receptor potentials in response to the traveling wave.

      i. The scala vestibuli and scala tympani are both filled with **perilymph,** which has a similar composition to other extracellular fluids; that is, low $[K^+]$ and high $[Na^+]$.

      ii. The scala media is a blind-ended structure that contains **endolymph,** *an unusual extracellular fluid because it has a high $[K^+]$ of 150 mM and a low $[Na^+]$ of 1 mM.*

         • Endolymph is actively secreted by a layer of endothelial lining cells called the **stria vascularis.**

      iii. *The difference in $[K^+]$ between perilymph and endolymph creates an* **endocochlear potential** *difference across Reissner's membrane of about +80 mV in the endolymph.*

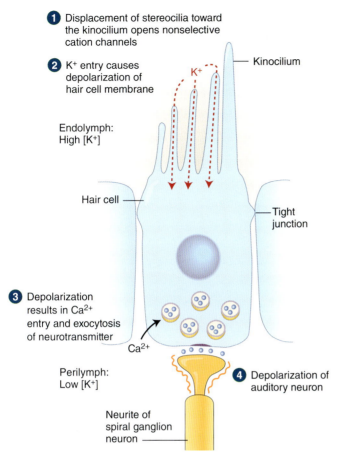

1 Displacement of stereocilia toward the kinocilium opens nonselective cation channels

2 K⁺ entry causes depolarization of hair cell membrane

K⁺

Kinocilium

Endolymph: High [K⁺]

Hair cell

Tight junction

3 Depolarization results in Ca²⁺ entry and exocytosis of neurotransmitter

Ca²⁺

Perilymph: Low [K⁺]

4 Depolarization of auditory neuron

Neurite of spiral ganglion neuron

Figure 2-33. Mechanotransduction of sound by a hair cell. Deformation of the stereocilia toward the large kinocilium results in the opening of mechanically gated cation channels. The resulting entry of K⁺ from the K⁺-rich endolymph causes depolarization of the hair cell and Ca²⁺ entry. Release of neurotransmitter by exocytosis from the base of the cell excites the neurites of auditory neurons.

iv.   ▼ **Jervell and Lange-Nielsen syndrome** is a rare condition caused by a K⁺ channel mutation that results both in congenital deafness and the risk of sudden cardiac death! In the inner ear there is decreased [K⁺] in the endolymph that disrupts the endocochlear potential difference. Patients also have a prolonged cardiac action potential, which results in a long Q-T segment on the electrocardiogram. ▼

8. Transduction of sound.
   a. When vibration of the oval window causes a traveling wave in the basilar membrane, hair cells are pushed against the tectorial membrane.
   b. Hair cells have a tall **kinocilium** at one edge of the cell, which is surrounded by approximately 100 stereocilia.
   c. *Displacement of the stereocilia laterally toward the kinocilium opens mechanically gated, nonselective cation channels in the tips of stereocilia, resulting in membrane depolarization* (Figure 2-33).
   d. The hair cell body is bathed in perilymph, whereas the tips of stereocilia pierce the reticular lamina and are bathed in endolymph. *Influx of K⁺ from the K⁺-rich endolymph causes depolarization.*

e. A depolarizing receptor potential causes influx of Ca^{2+} and exocytosis of neurotransmitter (probably glutamate) from storage granules at the base of the cell.

f. Conversely, displacement of stereocilia away from the kinocilium closes cation channels, thereby hyperpolarizing the hair cell membrane potential and decreasing neurotransmitter release.

9. Functions of inner and outer hair cells.

a. The hair cells located between the rods of Corti and the modiolus are referred to as inner hair cells, and those lateral to the rods of Corti are referred to as outer hair cells.

b. *Inner hair cells are responsible for the transduction of sound.*
   i. The neurites that contact inner hair cells extend from neurons located in a swelling on the auditory nerve, called the **spiral ganglion.**
   ii. *Axons from spiral ganglion neurons form the auditory nerve and enter the auditory pathway.*

c. Outer hair cells are collectively referred to as the **cochlear amplifier** because they amplify the traveling wave that passes along the basilar membrane.
   i. Outer hair cells respond to sound by producing a receptor potential and by changing length, known as **electromotility.**
   ii. The mechanism involves the membrane protein **prestin.** *Selective damage to outer hair cells or mutations in the prestin gene can lead to deafness, demonstrating the importance of the cochlear amplifier.*

d. ▼ **Ototoxicity** is a potential adverse effect of the **aminoglycoside antibiotics.** These antibiotics are directly toxic to the hair cells of the inner ear and can lead to permanent hearing loss. ▼

10. Central auditory pathways.

a. *There are several alternative neuronal pathways from the cochlea to the cortex that synapse at intermediate brainstem nuclei.*

b. Axons of the auditory nerve synapse first in the **cochlear nuclei** of the medulla.

c. Many second-order neurons pass via the **lateral lemniscus** directly to the **inferior colliculi,** whereas others synapse in the **superior olivary nucleus** of the pons first.

d. Third- (or fourth-) order neurons pass from the inferior colliculus to the **medial geniculate nucleus** of the thalamus, where the signal is relayed via the white matter of the **acoustic radiation** to the **auditory cortex** in the temporal lobe.

e. *Note: There are multiple crossover points from the left and right auditory pathways as well as binaural neurons, which receive inputs from both ears, such that no single focused brainstem lesion can cause unilateral deafness.*

f. The auditory cortex is located in the region of the superior temporal gyrus.
   i. The **primary auditory cortex** is referred to as **Brodmann area 41.**
   ii. *The secondary auditory association areas include **Wernicke's area** (**Brodmann area 42**), which is critical to the interpretation of speech* (see Language and Speech).

11. Encoding the properties of sound.

a. The basic properties of sounds that must be encoded to allow higher level processing are **intensity, frequency,** and **location.**

b. **Loudness** correlates with the number of active auditory neurons and their rate of firing.
   i. More intense sounds cause larger vibrations of the basilar membrane, thereby involving more hair cells and activation of more auditory neurons.
   ii. Larger distortions of hair cells produce larger receptor potentials, which increase action potential frequency in auditory neurons.
c. **Pitch** is related to the frequency of sound waves.
   i. Frequency encoding depends on the mechanical properties of the basilar membrane. At the base of the cochlea, the basilar membrane is narrow and stiff, whereas at the apex it is wider and more compliant.
   ii. High-frequency sounds produce traveling waves that peak near the base, and low-frequency sounds produce traveling waves that propagate all the way to the apex.
   iii. Each section of the basilar membrane has a **characteristic frequency** that produces a maximal deflection and a large hair cell response (known as the "**place code,**" see Figure 2-34).
   iv. Auditory nerves have a systematic organization known as the **tonotopic map** in which the location of an active neuron reflects the frequency of the sound that excited it.
d. The ability to localize the origin of a sound is important for survival (e.g., locating a moving vehicle).

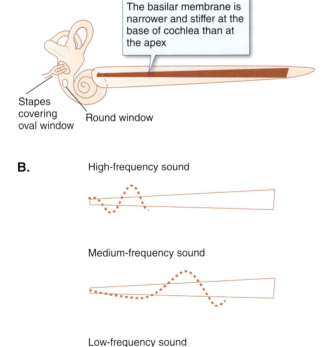

Figure 2-34. Place code for sound frequency. A. An uncoiled cochlea showing the nonuniform geometry of the basilar membrane. **B.** Representations of traveling waves produced in the basilar membrane by sounds of different frequencies. High-frequency sounds produce a traveling wave toward the base of the cochlea, whereas low-frequency sounds are represented by traveling waves reaching the apex of the cochlea.

    i. Unless a sound occurs directly ahead or behind a person it takes slightly longer for the sound to reach one ear compared to the other, known as the **interaural time delay,** which is a major location cue.

    ii. The second cue to location is the **interaural intensity difference,** which occurs because the head obstructs the passage of sound waves and casts a "sound shadow."

    iii. *The outer ear is important in locating sounds moving in the vertical plane for which there are no differences in interaural timing or intensity.* Sounds are reflected off the folds of the pinna, creating delays between sound waves that enter the auditory canal directly and those that are reflected off the pinna.

12. **Deafness** can be characterized as either conductive or sensorineural hearing loss.

    a. **Conductive hearing loss** can be caused by a defect in any of the sound-conducting structures (e.g., auricle, external auditory canal, tympanic membrane, or the middle ear).

    b. **Sensorineural hearing loss** can be a result of a lesion of the inner ear or CN VIII (vestibulocochlear nerve).

    c. ▼ The **Weber and Rinne tuning fork tests** are used to differentiate conductive hearing loss from sensorineural hearing loss.

        i. The **Weber test** is performed by placing the stem of a vibrating tuning fork on top of the patient's skull, an equal distance from each ear. *The normal response is to hear the sound equally with both ears.*

        ii. The **Rinne test** is performed by initially placing the vibrating tuning fork against the mastoid process behind the ear until the sound is no longer heard; the fork is then immediately placed in the air just outside the ear. *The normal response is to detect sound by air conduction better than bone conduction.*

        iii. *In **unilateral conductive hearing loss,** the Weber test will result in lateralization of the vibrations toward the affected side because the ambient room noise is absent on this side; the Rinne test will indicate bone conduction greater than air conduction.*

        iv. *In **unilateral sensorineural hearing loss,** the Weber test will result in lateralization of the vibrations to the unaffected side; the Rinne test will indicate air conduction greater than bone conduction.* ▼

The Vestibular System

1. The functions of the vestibular system are to provide a sense of balance and equilibrium and to aid in control of eye movement and body posture.

2. *Vestibular dysfunction is manifested by uncontrolled eye movements and feelings of **nausea** and **vertigo.***

3. There are two types of structures in the inner ear that provide vestibular sensation:

    a. The **otolith organs** detect tilting of the head and linear acceleration.

    b. The **semicircular canals** detect angular acceleration produced by rotation of the head.

4. The otolith organs.

    a. The otolith organs include two endolymph-filled chambers within the labyrinth, the **utricle** and the **saccule** (Figure 2-35).

    b. Hair cells are located in a sensory epithelium called the **macula.**

A.

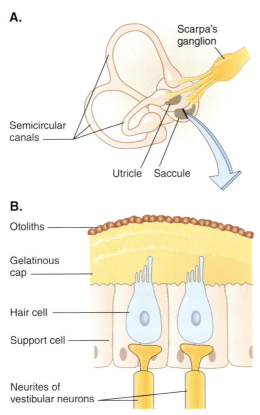

Scarpa's ganglion

Semicircular canals

Utricle   Saccule

B.

Otoliths

Gelatinous cap

Hair cell

Support cell

Neurites of vestibular neurons

Figure 2-35. The otolith organs. **A.** Location of the utricle and saccule (cochlea removed). **B.** Cross-section through an otolith organ showing the sensory epithelium (macula). Stereocilia of vestibular hair cells are embedded in a gelatinous cap, which is covered in otolith crystals. Tilting of the head, or linear acceleration forces, displaces the stereocilia resulting in the generation of a hair cell receptor potential.

   c. The tips of hair cell stereocilia project into a gelatinous cap, which is covered in small calcium carbonate crystals called **otoliths.**

   d. Movement of the head displaces otoliths and bends the stereocilia, resulting in development of a receptor potential in the same way as that described for auditory hair cells.

   e. *The otolith organs transduce two types of information, the static angle (tilting) of the head and the presence of linear acceleration.*

     i. **Tilting of the head** changes the angle between the otolith organs and the direction of the force of gravity. Different degrees of tension are placed on hair cell stereocilia, depending on their orientation. *All possible angles are represented because the macula of each utricle is oriented horizontally and the macula of each saccule is oriented vertically.*

     ii. **Linear acceleration** (e.g., starting and stopping when riding in a vehicle) also displaces the otoliths and excites hair cells in the maculae. *(Note: When traveling at a **constant velocity,** there is no acceleration, resulting in the sensation of being perfectly still.)*

5. The semicircular canals.

   a. *There are three semicircular canals, arranged at right angles to each other.*

   b. The hair cells of each canal are located in a swelling called the **ampulla;** the cilia of the hair cells project into a gelatinous mass called the **cupula.**

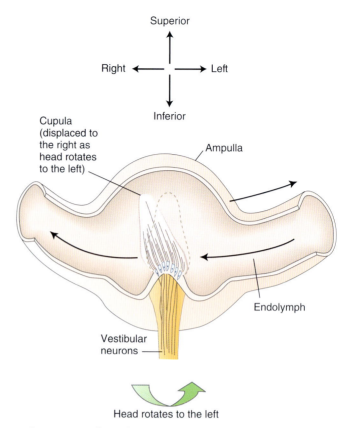

Figure 2-36. Cross-section through the ampulla of a semicircular canal. The movement of the cupula in the horizontal canal is shown as the head rotates to the left.

    c. Movements of the cupula cause generation of receptor potentials in the hair cells. The presence of three semicircular canals provides information about all possible orientations.

    d. Rotation of the head produces **angular acceleration forces.** When the head begins to rotate, there is a lag in the movement of the endolymph, causing the cupula to be deflected like a sail being hit by the wind (Figure 2-36). The semicircular canals respond to rotation in different planes as follows:

        i. The **superior canal** senses rotation front to back (e.g., nodding the head for "yes").

        ii. The **horizontal canal** senses rotation left to right (e.g., shaking the head for "no").

        iii. The **posterior canal** senses rotation in the plane from the left to the right shoulder.

    e. The position of the semicircular canals on one side of the head is the mirror image of those on the other side. In this arrangement, any rotation will cause stimulation on one side and inhibition on the other side, thereby augmenting the vestibular stimulus to the brain.

    f. If constant rotation occurs for approximately 30 seconds, the movement of endolymph "catches up" so that the canal and endolymph move together at the same speed. The angular acceleration is now zero, and the cupula is no longer deflected.

    g. If a constant rotation is suddenly stopped, inertia causes the endolymph to bend the cupula in the opposite direction, which is accompanied by the sensation of spinning in the opposite direction.

6. The central vestibular pathways.
    a. The primary afferent vestibular neurons are located in a swelling on the vestibular nerve called **Scarpa's ganglion.**
    b. Neurites extend to the vestibular hair cells, and action potential firing is modulated by the depolarizing or hyperpolarizing receptor potentials produced by hair cells.
    c. Axons of primary afferent neurons travel in the vestibular part of CN VIII to the **vestibular nuclei** of the brainstem.
    d. The vestibular nuclei send **neuronal projections** to the following targets above and below the brainstem:
        i. **Projections to the cortex** occur via the thalamus, as with other sensory pathways, although there is no equivalent "vestibular cortex" to the auditory and visual areas.
        ii. There is a rich supply of second-order vestibular neurons to the **cerebellum** to coordinate movements.
        iii. Vestibular input to motor neurons of the **lower limb** occurs via the **vestibulospinal tract,** which assists in the automatic maintenance of balance.
        iv. Vestibular input to motor neurons of the **neck** facilitates independent maintenance of head position.
        v. Projections to the motor neurons for **extraocular muscles** keep the eyes focused on an object as the body moves.
            • The **vestibuloocular reflex** causes the eyes to turn in the direction opposite that of the rotation of the head.
            • For example, if the gaze is fixed on a particular object, turning to the right causes both eyes to move toward the left, thereby keeping the object in view.
            • The vestibuloocular reflex relies on projections from the vestibular nucleus to nuclei of CN III, IV, and VI, which control eye movements.
    e. ▼ **Vertigo,** often imprecisely referred to as dizziness, is the sensation that either the body or the environment is moving when actually both are stationary, and is classically described as a spinning sensation.
        i. Spatial orientation and posture are controlled by three sensory systems: Vestibular, visual, and somatosensory. A mismatch between any of these three systems can result in vertigo.
        ii. *Vestibular dysfunction is the most common cause of pathologic vertigo.*
        iii. Vertigo is commonly accompanied by nausea, nystagmus, postural unsteadiness, and gait ataxia. Several clues obtained during the physical examination can help to differentiate peripheral causes of vertigo (e.g., **Ménière's disease, benign positional vertigo,** or **labyrinthitis**) from central causes of vertigo (e.g., **cerebellar infarct or mass**):
            • A finding in **peripheral vertigo** is nystagmus that is unidirectional and has fast saccadic eye movements in the opposite direction to the lesion; nystagmus may be suppressed with visual fixation. Tinnitus and/or deafness are often present, but other neurologic signs are typically absent.
            • In **central vertigo,** nystagmus may be bidirectional or unidirectional, vertical or purely horizontal, and does not suppress with visual fixation. Tinnitus and/or deafness are absent, but other neurologic findings are often present. ▼

Gustation and Olfaction

1. *Taste (gustation) and smell (olfaction) are examples of chemoreception.*
2. Numerous chemical odors can be detected because there are hundreds of different **olfactory receptor proteins** in the olfactory neurons. In contrast, there are only five basic qualities of taste: **salty, sour, sweet, bitter,** and **umami.**
3. *The ability to perceive the subtleties of flavor depends on the normal functioning of both taste and smell.*
4. Taste sensation.
   a. Taste receptors are located on projections from the surface of the tongue called **papillae,** which each have numerous **taste buds.**
   b. Taste buds open onto the surface of the tongue at a small depression called the **taste pore.** Each taste bud contains approximately 100 **taste receptor cells** bearing microvilli that project into the taste pore.
   c. The microvilli are the chemically sensitive region of the taste receptor cell. Sensory neurons form synapses at the base of taste receptor cells.
5. There are different transduction mechanisms underlying the **five primary qualities of taste** (Figure 2-37).
   a. **Salt** receptors use a Na^+ channel to sense the $[Na^+]$ in the mouth. Na^+ enters the receptor cell, causing a graded receptor potential; an increase in $[Na^+]$ in the mouth drives more Na^+ entry, resulting in a larger depolarization.
   b. **Sourness** receptors respond to *acidity.* H^+ binds to and inhibits K^+ channels in the cell membrane, resulting in reduced K^+ conductance and membrane depolarization.
   c. **Sweetness** receptors use intracellular second messengers. For example, binding of a sugar may stimulate formation of cyclic adenosine monophosphate (cAMP), which inhibits a K^+ channel and depolarizes the receptor cell membrane.
   d. **Bitterness** receptors use more than one transduction mechanism, depending on the tastant. Mechanisms include direct binding to K^+ channels and changes in second messengers.
   e. **Umami** (Japanese word for "delicious") receptors respond to amino acids, particularly glutamate. An ionotropic glutamate receptor mediates depolarization. The umami receptor accounts for the desirable flavor of amino acids, such as the culinary additive **monosodium glutamate (MSG).**
   f. *Every taste transduction mechanism causes depolarization of the receptor cell,* which causes Ca^{2+} entry into the cell and exocytosis of neurotransmitters.
   g. Taste receptors release one of several neurotransmitters to stimulate gustatory afferent neurons (e.g., serotonin, glutamate, acetylcholine, norepinephrine and others).
6. The central taste pathway.
   a. *Taste sensation from the anterior two-thirds of the tongue is carried in the* **facial nerve (CN VII);** *taste sensation from the posterior one-third of the tongue is carried in the* **glossopharyngeal nerve (CN IX).**
   b. Primary sensory neurons synapse in the **gustatory nucleus** of the medulla.

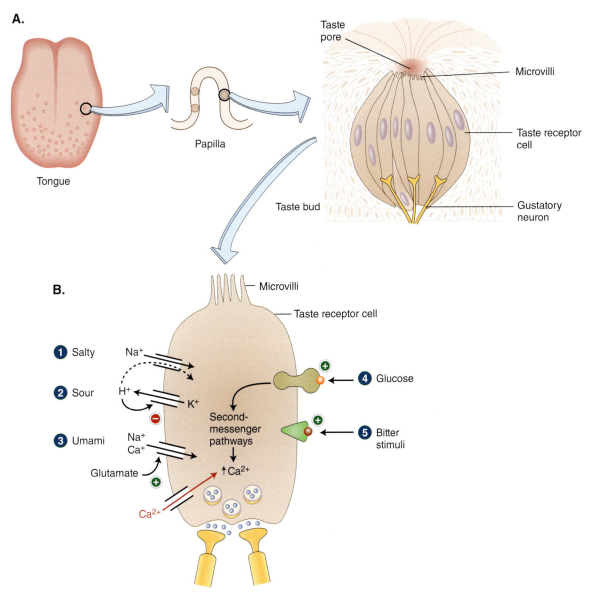

Figure 2-37. Taste receptors. **A.** Location of taste receptors within taste buds on the tongue, which are located on various types of papillae. Taste buds consist of a collection of taste receptor cells, each of which communicates with a sensory neuron. **B.** Sensory transduction mechanisms for the primary qualities of taste (*note: some taste receptors do not express every transduction mechanism*).

    c. Second-order neurons cross the midline and ascend to the thalamus; third-order neurons are relayed to the primary **gustatory cortex** in the postcentral gyrus of the **parietal lobe** and then to the **insular lobe.**

7. Olfaction.

    a. The **olfactory receptor cells** are bipolar neurons.

       i. A peripheral neurite extends into a patch of nasal membrane in the upper part of the nasal cavity called the **olfactory epithelium.**

      ii. A central axon joins an olfactory nerve and enters the brain through one of many small holes in the **cribriform plate** of the skull.

    iii. The peripheral neurite bears cilia, called **olfactory hairs,** which project into the mucus covering the nasal membrane.

    iv. Nasal mucus contains soluble **odorant-binding proteins,** which help odorants to diffuse to the surface of the olfactory hairs.

   b. The **sensory transduction mechanism** that detects the odorant functions as follows:

      i. The odorant binds to an **olfactory receptor protein** (a transmembrane receptor) in an olfactory hair; each olfactory neuron expresses only one type of olfactory receptor protein.

      ii. All olfactory receptor proteins stimulate the G protein G_{olf} when occupied by an odorant.

      iii. Adenylyl cyclase is stimulated, which increases the intracellular concentration of **cAMP.**

      iv. cAMP causes depolarization due to opening of **nonselective cation channels, voltage-gated Ca^{2+} channels,** and **Ca^{2+}-activated Cl^- channels.**

      v. When the receptor potential reaches threshold, action potentials are generated in the cell body and axon of the olfactory neuron.

      vi. The olfactory response is terminated when odorants diffuse away and when enzymes within the mucus break down the odorants.

   c. The central olfactory pathway.

      i. *The main olfactory pathway includes only two neurons and does not synapse in the thalamus.*

      ii. Axons of the olfactory receptor neurons enter the **olfactory bulb,** an ovoid structure on the inferior surface of the frontal lobe, where they synapse with second-order neurons (Figure 2-38).

      iii. The second neuron in the chain sends axons via the **olfactory tract** to the **olfactory cortex** in the temporal lobe.

      iv. There are projections to the limbic system underlying the affective and emotional components of smell.

      v. Some second-order neurons cross the midline via a band of white matter, called the anterior commissure, to synapse in the opposite olfactory bulb.

   d. ▼ **Kallmann syndrome** is an X-linked disorder characterized by congenital anosmia (lack of smell) and gonadotropin-releasing hormone (GnRH) deficiency. During embryologic development, anosmin, the mutated protein associated with this syndrome, is needed to mediate migration of the olfactory bulb and GnRH-producing neural progenitor cells. The lack of neural migration results in this syndrome. ▼

Motor Neurophysiology

1. The motor system is comprised of skeletal muscles and the neurons that control them.

2. *Muscle contraction only occurs in response to action potentials in **alpha motor neurons**, which originate in the ventral gray matter of the spinal cord (and brainstem nuclei of certain cranial nerves) and constitute the **final common pathway** for motor control.*

3. The **hierarchy of motor control** within the CNS is as follows:

   a. The **association cortex** and the **basal ganglia** determine the goal of movements.

   b. The **primary motor cortex** and **cerebellum** determine the correct sequence of commands that will allow the goal to be achieved.

   c. Neuronal circuits in the **spinal cord** implement descending commands.

A.

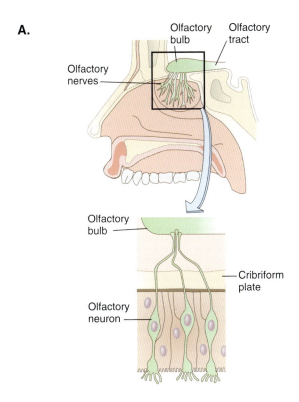

B.

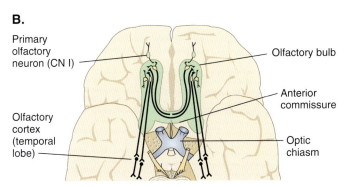

Figure 2-38. The olfactory system. **A.** The olfactory epithelium is located in a patch of nasal membrane. Primary sensory neurons pass via small holes in the cribriform plate of the skull to enter the olfactory bulb. **B.** The main central olfactory pathway conveys second-order neurons from the olfactory bulb directly to the olfactory cortex in the temporal lobe. Some fibers pass between olfactory bulbs by crossing the midline via the anterior commissure.

4. Spinal control of movement.
   a. *There are three inputs to alpha motor neurons that determine which muscle fibers will contract: upper motor neurons, spinal interneurons, and sensory neurons.*
      i. **Upper motor neurons** from the cortex or brainstem regulate voluntary movements and are *mainly inhibitory in nature.*
      ii. **Spinal interneurons** may be excitatory or inhibitory and form an extensive circuitry within the spinal cord.
         • Basic motor programs (e.g., walking) are encoded in spinal circuits known as **central pattern generators.**
      iii. **Sensory neurons from muscle proprioceptors** provide feedback about muscle length and tension.

5. Sensory feedback in motor control.
   a. Sensory information and feedback is needed at every stage of motor control to ensure smooth, coordinated, and accurate movements.
   b. Sensory information about body position and its relationship to the environment is relayed from the **vestibular, visual, and auditory systems.**
   c. Feedback about body position (**proprioception**) includes conscious sensation derived from receptors in the skin and joint capsules (e.g., Pacinian corpuscles).
   d. *Unconscious sensation about muscle length and tension is relayed from muscle spindles and Golgi tendon organs (GTOs):*
   e. **Muscle spindles** consist of specialized muscle fibers called **intrafusal fibers** contained in a fibrous capsule (Figure 2-39A).
      i. Intrafusal fibers are connected at both ends to the force-generating extrafusal muscle fibers.
      ii. The muscle spindle is expanded in the middle where sensory axons are wrapped around the intrafusal fibers.
      iii. The sensory fibers are large myelinated axons, known as **type Ia,** and have very fast conduction speeds.
      iv. *Muscle spindles provide information to the CNS about muscle stretch (length) and the speed with which muscle length is changing.*
   f. Gamma motor neurons.
      i. The motor supply to contractile filaments within muscle spindles is from gamma motor neurons and is referred to as the **fusimotor system.**
      ii. The cell bodies of gamma motor neurons are located in the ventral gray matter of the spinal cord.
      iii. *Contraction of intrafusal fibers alters the sensitivity of muscle spindles.* For example, intrafusal fibers and extrafusal fibers must shorten at the same time to prevent the muscle spindles from becoming slack.
   g. **GTOs** are sensory nerve terminals that are encapsulated within tendons.
      i. GTOs are arranged *in series* with extrafusal muscle fibers, with one end attached to the extrafusal muscle fibers and the other end attached to the collagen fibers of the tendon (Figure 2-39B).
      ii. Sensory axons from GTOs are smaller than type Ia fibers and are designated **type Ib.**
      iii. *GTOs provide information about muscle force.*
6. The **muscle stretch (myotactic) reflex.**
   a. The muscle stretch reflex is demonstrated by tapping a tendon with a reflex hammer (Figure 2-40). For example, when testing the **knee jerk reflex:**
      i. Tapping the patellar tendon causes a small degree of **stretch in the quadriceps muscle,** which results in the generation of action potentials in Ia afferents from muscle spindles.
      ii. A **monosynaptic reflex arc** is formed when sensory afferents enter the spinal cord, via the dorsal root, and synapse directly on the alpha motor neurons; reflex contraction of the quadriceps causes the knee jerk response.
      iii. *The physiologic function of the monosynaptic myotactic reflex is to resist gravity.* When a load is placed on a muscle, it is stretched, which results in reflex contraction of the muscle to take up the load.

A.

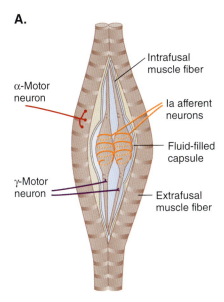

α-Motor neuron

Intrafusal muscle fiber

Ia afferent neurons

Fluid-filled capsule

γ-Motor neuron

Extrafusal muscle fiber

B.

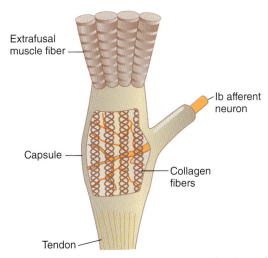

Extrafusal muscle fiber

Ib afferent neuron

Capsule

Collagen fibers

Tendon

Figure 2-39. Muscle proprioceptors. **A.** Muscle spindle. Intrafusal muscle fibers are arranged in parallel with the extrafusal muscle fibers. Muscle length is monitored by myelinated Ia afferent neurons coiled around the midsection of intrafusal fibers. Gamma motor neurons contract intrafusal fibers to maintain spindle tension when surrounding extrafusal fibers contract. **B.** A Golgi tendon organ arranged in series with muscle fibers at the junction between the muscle and tendon. Sensory endings of Ib afferent neurons are intertwined with collagen filaments and detect the force of muscle contraction.

b. ▼ A lesion in any part of the myotactic reflex circuit will result in **areflexia.** The following deep tendon reflexes (and their associated spinal segments) are important to know when performing a neurologic examination: brachioradialis (C5–C6), biceps (C5–C6), triceps (C6–C7), knee (L2–L4), ankle (S1). ▼

c. Reciprocal inhibition.

    i. Many muscles work in antagonistic pairs (e.g., the biceps and triceps muscles of the arm, or the quadriceps and hamstring muscles of the thigh).

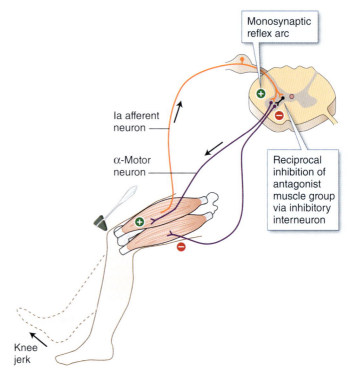

Figure 2-40. The knee-jerk reflex, an example of the myotactic (stretch) reflex. Muscle contraction is stimulated by a monosynaptic pathway following activation of muscle spindle afferents. Reciprocal inhibition of antagonist muscles occurs simultaneously, via inhibitory spinal interneurons.

      ii. When a muscle produces movement by shortening, it is referred to as an **agonist;** muscles that oppose the action of the agonist are **antagonists.**

     iii. In a simple movement (e.g., flexion of the elbow), the contraction of biceps is accompanied by relaxation of its antagonist, the triceps muscle; this phenomenon is known as **reciprocal inhibition** and is mediated by spinal interneurons.

     iv. Reciprocal inhibition also occurs in the myotactic reflex because collateral branches of the Ia afferents synapse on inhibitory interneurons that supply alpha motor neurons of the antagonist muscle.

7. The **flexor withdrawal reflex.**

  a. The flexor withdrawal response rapidly removes a limb from an injurious stimulus (Figure 2-41). For example, when a painful stimulus is applied to one leg the following steps occur:

     i. **Pain receptors** are activated at the site of stimulation.

     ii. **Afferent pain fibers** enter the dorsal root and send collaterals to several spinal segments.

     iii. **Excitatory interneurons** that synapse with alpha motor neurons serving flexors are stimulated. *Contraction of flexors removes the limb from the aversive stimulus.*

     iv. **Reciprocal inhibition** suppresses contraction of the extensors of the affected limb.

  b. The **crossed extensor reflex** is an additional component of the flexor withdrawal response to support the body using the opposite limb.

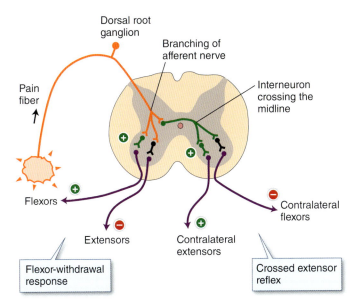

Figure 2-41. The flexor-withdrawal reflex pathway. If a painful stimulus is applied to one side of the body, flexors contract and extensors relax on that side to rapidly remove the body part from the stimulus. The opposite response occurs on the contralateral side of the body to maintain posture; this crossed-extensor reflex is mediated by spinal interneurons.

    i. In the example, where one leg would suddenly be lifted, the person would rarely fall down because extensors on the opposite side of the body contract to provide postural support.

    ii. Spinal interneurons cross the midline to stimulate extensors and relax flexors on the opposite side.

8. Descending motor tracts (Figure 2-42A).

  a. The brain communicates with the spinal motor circuitry through **two major groups of descending pathways,** named according to their location in the spinal white matter:

    i. The **lateral pathways** are concerned with voluntary movement of the distal muscles (e.g., muscles of the arm and hand). The two major lateral pathways are the **corticospinal (pyramidal) tract** and the **rubrospinal tract.**

    ii. The **ventromedial pathways** originate in the brainstem and innervate the proximal and axial muscles to help maintain head position and posture. The major ventromedial pathways are the **vestibulospinal, tectospinal,** and **reticulospinal tracts.**

  b. The **corticospinal tract** contains fibers that mostly originate from the motor cortex; the fibers descend through the internal capsule and upper brainstem to the medullary pyramids, where the tract crosses the midline.

    i. ▼ Similar to the sensory pathways, the site of decussation of the **lateral corticospinal tract** has significant clinical implications. *Lesions above the medullary pyramids will result in contralateral muscle weakness; lesions below the pyramidal decussation will produce an ipsilateral muscle weakness.* ▼

  c. The **rubrospinal tract** originates in the red nucleus of the midbrain, which in turn receives input from the motor cortical areas.

A.

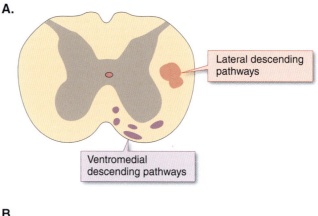

Lateral descending pathways

Ventromedial descending pathways

B.

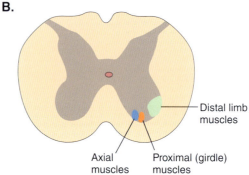

Distal limb muscles

Axial muscles

Proximal (girdle) muscles

Figure 2-42. A. Descending motor pathways in the spinal white matter. **B.** Organization of alpha motor neurons in the ventral gray matter of the spinal cord. Note that a major function of the lateral pathways is to mediate voluntary control of the (laterally placed) alpha motor neurons to the distal limb muscles.

    i. ▼ Many rubrospinal tract neurons are redundant in humans but they are active in mediating flexion, which can help to diagnose the site of neurologic injury in comatose patients where "posturing" can clue the physician to the site of neurologic damage:
- **Decorticate posturing,** characterized by flexion of the elbows and wrists and supination of the arms, indicates damage immediately rostral to the red nucleus of the midbrain. *An intact red nucleus allows the upper extremities to undergo flexion via the rubrospinal neurons.*
- In contrast, **decerebrate posturing,** characterized by extension of the elbows and wrists with pronation, indicates a midbrain lesion that involves the level of the red nucleus. ▼

  d. The **ventromedial pathways** provide sensory information from the visual and vestibular systems about the body position and balance:

    i. The **vestibulospinal tract** originates in the vestibular nuclei and provides one of the links between the sensors for balance and the extensor muscles, which are important for maintaining posture.

    ii. The **tectospinal tract** originates in the superior colliculus of the midbrain, which receives input from the retina and visual cortex and has reciprocal connections with the vestibular nuclei. *The main function of the tectospinal tract is to direct the head and eyes to move toward a selected object in the visual field.*

    iii. The **reticulospinal tract** originates in the reticular formation and consists of two antagonistic pathways: one from the pontine reticular area and the other from the medullary reticular area. A balance between the activities of these pathways facilitates fine control of posture through actions on the extensor muscles of the lower limb.

9. Organization of spinal motor neurons (Figure 2-42B).
   a. The group of lower (alpha) motor neurons that serves a single muscle is known as the **motor neuron pool.**
   b. Motor neuron pools that control a particular action (e.g., flexion of the wrist) are located close to each other in the **ventral horn** of the spinal cord.
   c. Organization of the lower motor neurons is consistent with the function and location of the descending motor tracts, with a **medial to lateral organization:**
      i. Distal muscles of the limbs are represented most laterally.
      ii. Axial muscles of the trunk are represented medially.
      iii. Motor neurons for the proximal limb (girdle) muscles are located in an intermediate position.
   d. ▼ *Interpreting the cause of motor weakness necessitates distinguishing an upper motor neuron lesion from a lower motor neuron lesion:*
      i. **Upper motor neuron lesions** are characterized by spastic paresis (an incomplete paralysis), hyperreflexia, hypertonia, and a positive Babinski sign (up-going toes when the lateral edge of the sole is stroked with a blunt object; the normal response is down-going toes and is referred to as the plantar response).
      ii. *Note: Upper motor neurons typically work through inhibitory spinal interneurons. Thus, a lesion that disrupts upper motor neurons will remove the inhibition, resulting in* **spasticity.**
      iii. **Lower motor neuron lesions** are characterized by flaccid paralysis, areflexia, hypotonia, absent Babinski sign, fasciculations (visible muscle twitches), and atrophy. ▼
   e. ▼ **Poliomyelitis** is an example of a pure lower motor neuron lesion. The poliovirus infects and selectively destroys the motor neuron cell bodies located in the ventral horn of the spinal cord, typically in the lumbar region. ▼
   f. ▼ **Amyotrophic lateral sclerosis** (also known as ALS or Lou Gehrig's disease) is a progressive motor neuron disease that affects both upper and lower motor neurons. Although cranial nerve involvement does occur, this disease typically begins in the cervical spine. Patients with both an upper and a lower motor neuron lesion at the level of the cervical spine can present with *flaccid paresis of the upper extremities* and *spastic paresis of the lower extremities.* ▼

10. The motor cortex.
    a. The creation of instructions for movement engages many areas of the cerebral cortex, allowing perceptions about the spatial relations of the body to be combined with abstract thought and decision making.
    b. The **primary motor cortex:**
       i. Is located in the precentral gyrus.
       ii. Is organized in a detailed **somatotopic map** (similar to that of the primary sensory cortex); destruction of cortex in this area produces specific movement deficits.
       iii. Provides a large fraction of neurons in the corticospinal tract.
       iv. *Produces movements in the contralateral side of the body.*

c. ▼ The **middle cerebral artery** supplies the majority of the lateral surface of the cortex, including the section of primary motor cortex (and primary sensory cortex) responsible for movement (and sensation) of the face and upper extremities. The area responsible for the lower extremities is supplied by the **anterior cerebral artery.** *An occlusion of the middle cerebral artery will cause contralateral spastic paresis (and impaired sensation) of the face and upper extremities, whereas occlusion of the anterior cerebral artery will have similar effects of the lower extremities.* ▼

d. Additional motor cortical areas involved in the programming and sequencing of movements include:

   i. The **supplementary motor cortex,** which is located medially and directs many axons to distal limb muscles via the corticospinal tract.

   ii. The **premotor cortex,** which is located laterally and communicates with the reticulospinal neurons controlling the proximal muscles.

   iii. The **posterior parietal cortex,** which integrates somatosensory and visual information about objects in the visual field.

e. ▼ Lesions in the posterior parietal cortex in particular can cause **apraxia** and **sensory neglect:**

   i. In apraxia the person has difficulty performing a motor task (e.g., brushing hair) when asked, despite understanding the request, being willing to perform the task, having intact sensory and muscle functions and previously knowing how to do the task.

   ii. Injury to the posterior parietal cortex (especially the nondominant cortex) may cause sensory neglect of objects or activities on the contralateral side; neglect may include **anosognosia** where the person lacks awareness of disability in the affected limb. ▼

11. The basal ganglia.

a. The basal ganglia are forebrain structures that consist of several interconnected deep cerebral nuclei: the **striatum** (divided into the **caudate nucleus** and **putamen**), the **globus pallidus,** and **subthalamic nucleus** (Figure 2-43A).

b. The **substantia nigra** of the midbrain (although not part of the forebrain) is a functional part of the basal ganglia.

c. The basal ganglia are a key part of a **motor loop,** which begins and ends in the cortex and is important in the initiation of voluntary movements (Figure 2-43B).

   i. Excitatory input from large areas of cortex involved in developing the strategy for a voluntary movement are funneled into the basal ganglia via the **striatum.**

   ii. The final excitatory output from the basal ganglia back to the cortex arrives at the supplemental motor area, via the **ventral lateral nucleus (VLN)** of the thalamus.

   iii. The output from the basal ganglia to the VLN is a tonic inhibitory stimulus, which is mainly conveyed via the **internal segment of the globus pallidus.** *Stimulation of the VLN occurs when the tonic inhibitory signal from the output nuclei is suppressed.*

A.

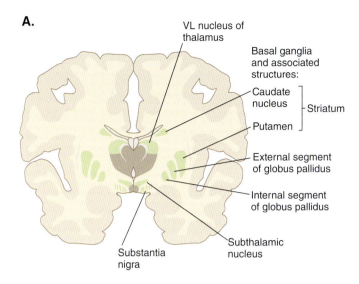

B.

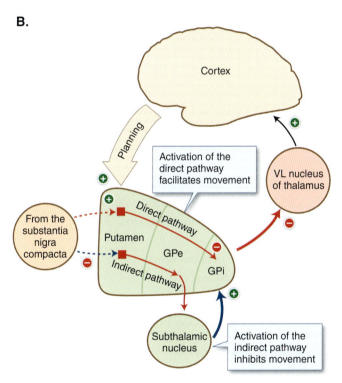

Figure 2-43. The basal ganglia. **A.** Coronal section through the forebrain at the midthalamic level, showing the position of the basal ganglia. **B.** The major motor loop mediates a cycle of positive feedback from the cortex, through the basal ganglia, and back to the cortex via the ventrolateral (VL) nucleus of the thalamus. Excitatory cortical input to the basal ganglia is via the putamen; output from the basal ganglia is inhibitory via the internal segment of the globus pallidus and the pars reticulata of the substantia nigra (not shown). The direct pathway through the basal ganglia inhibits the output nuclei, leading to disinhibition of the VL nucleus and facilitation of movement. The indirect pathway through the basal ganglia passes, via the external segment of the globus pallidus and subthalamic nucleus, and augments the inhibitory output nuclei. Dopaminergic inputs from the pars compacta of the substantia nigra promote motor behaviors by stimulating the direct pathway and inhibiting the indirect pathway.

iv. There are two pathways connecting the input and output nuclei of the basal ganglia:

- The **direct pathway** from the putamen to the internal segment of the globus pallidus is an inhibitory connection via GABAergic neurons that suppresses the tonic inhibitory output nuclei. *Activation of the direct pathway therefore facilitates movement by allowing positive feedback through the thalamocortical pathways.*
- The **indirect pathway** is conveyed to the output nuclei of the basal ganglia via the external segment of the globus pallidus and the subthalamic nucleus. Excitatory neurons from the subthalamic nucleus boost the activity of the output nuclei. *Stimulation of the indirect pathway therefore inhibits movement by suppressing the VLN.*

12. Disorders of the basal ganglia.

a. A fine balance between the activity of the direct and indirect pathways is necessary to ensure normal motor function.

b. Overactivity of the indirect pathway will result in paucity of movement (**hypokinesia**); underactivity will lead to uncontrollable movements that lack purpose (**hyperkinesia**).

c. ▼ *In **Parkinson's disease,** there is degeneration of the dopaminergic neurons that project from the substantia nigra to the striatum.*

   i. Dopaminergic input to the striatum *stimulates the direct pathway* via activation of D_1-**receptors,** which facilitates movement; dopamine *inhibits the indirect pathway* via activation of D_2-**receptors,** which facilitates movement circuitously by inhibiting an inhibitory pathway.

   ii. *Thus, when dopaminergic input to the striatum decreases (as occurs in Parkinson's disease), the resulting imbalance favors paucity of movement (bradykinesia).*

   iii. The cardinal signs of **parkinsonism** are bradykinesia, rigidity, and a resting "pill-rolling" tremor.

   iv. *The goal of therapy in Parkinson's disease is to rebalance the direct and indirect basal ganglia pathways to favor movement, achieved by stimulating the direct pathway and/or inhibiting the indirect pathway:*

- Administering **levodopa,** the metabolic precursor to dopamine, accomplishes this goal.
- Utilization of direct dopamine-receptor agonists (e.g., bromocriptine) also improves symptoms.
- Another approach in therapy is to alter the cholinergic influence on the striatum. *Acetylcholine drives the indirect pathway, decreasing movement.* Use of anticholinergics (e.g., benztropine) will reduce indirect pathway stimulation, shifting the balance toward direct pathway output and improved motor function. ▼

d. ▼ **Huntington's disease** is a fatal autosomal dominant disorder affecting the **huntingtin gene;** multiple additional **CAG repeats** are added to the gene resulting in an abnormal protein with a long N-terminal **polyglutamine chain.**

   i. Patients present with an insidious onset of **chorea** (quick random involuntary movements, often of the extremities), progressive **dementia,** and **behavioral disorders.**

ii. The key pathologic lesion that characterizes this condition is severe idiopathic degeneration of **GABAergic neurons,** particularly affecting the indirect pathway of the basal ganglia. ▼

e. ▼ **Hemiballismus** is clinically characterized by wild violent flinging movements, typically of the upper extremities.

i. Hemiballismus is caused by injury to a subthalamic nucleus (e.g., hypertensive lacunar infarct).

ii. *Note: The subthalamic nuclei normally stimulate the inhibitory output nuclei of the globus pallidus; this is another example of loss to the indirect pathway that results in excessive motor system function.* ▼

13. The cerebellum ("little brain").

a. The cerebellum is located caudal to the occipital lobe and is attached to the posterior aspect of the brainstem by the paired inferior, middle, and superior **cerebellar peduncles.**

b. The cerebellum receives a large input from the motor cortical areas as well as from the somatosensory, vestibular, visual, and auditory systems.

i. There are two types of input (afferent) fibers within the cerebellum: **mossy fibers** and **climbing fibers,** both of which are excitatory.

c. The cerebellum has **three major functions:**

i. To coordinate movements by adjusting motor cortical output based on sensory feedback.

ii. To maintain muscle tone.

iii. To achieve motor learning tasks.

d. The cerebellum has two **lateral hemispheres** that are separated by a midline ridge called the **vermis** (Figure 2-44). These structures correlate with **functional divisions** as follows:

i. Output from the **vermis** is directed mainly to the ventromedial descending pathways controlling the axial musculature.

ii. Output from the **lateral hemispheres** is directed to the cerebral cortical areas, which control limb movements via the lateral descending pathways.

e. Anatomic descriptions of the cerebellum utilize surface fissures to further define cerebellar lobes and lobules. The major lobes are the **anterior, posterior,** and **flocculonodular lobes.**

f. Output from the cerebellum is relayed via three pairs of **deep cerebellar nuclei:** the **fastigial, interposed,** and **dentate** nuclei.

i. All efferent cerebellar output to the deep nuclei are from **Purkinje cells,** which have massive dendritic trees to achieve integration.

g. An alternative description of the cerebellum is based on the evolution of cerebellar functions:

i. The **vestibulocerebellum** correlates with the flocculonodular lobe. *It is the most primitive system and contributes to the control of balance and eye movements.* Input arrives from the vestibular and visual systems and output is relayed to the vestibular nuclei of the brainstem.

ii. The **spinocerebellum** correlates with the vermis and medial areas of the lateral hemispheres (referred to as the **intermediate zone**).

- Output from the vermis projects to the fastigial nucleus, and output from the intermediate zones projects via the interposed nucleus.

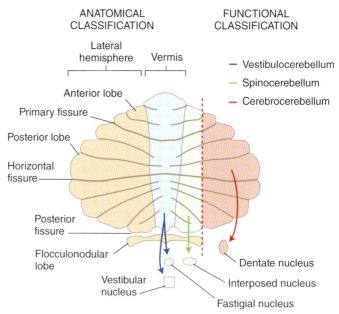

Figure 2-44. The cerebellum. The cerebellum is divided into anterior, posterior, and flocculonodular lobes by surface fissures (shown on the left). The functional regions of the cerebellum are the vestibulocerebellum, spinocerebellum, and cerebrocerebellum (shown on the right); the output pathways of the functional cerebellar areas via the cerebellar nuclei are shown (*note: the nuclei are bilateral but are only shown on the right*).

- *The spinocerebellum contributes to the control of posture and walking, and modulates spinal reflex activity.*

iii. The **cerebrocerebellum** represents the highest level of evolution and occupies most of the lateral hemispheres.
- The motor cortical areas provide a massive neuronal projection via the pons to the lateral cerebellum.
- A **motor loop** is completed by output from the lateral cerebellum back to the motor cortex and premotor cortex via the dentate nucleus and VLN of the thalamus.
- *The cerebrocerebellum is crucial for the detailed sequence and timing of muscle contractions needed to effect a coordinated movement.*

h. ▼ *Cerebellar lesions produce a characteristic movement disorder called **ataxia**, in which movements become inaccurate and are poorly coordinated; there is also decreased muscle tone (**hypotonia**).*
  i. **Friedreich's ataxia** is the most common inherited form of ataxia and usually includes degeneration of the spinocerebellar tracts, lateral corticospinal tracts, and dorsal columns.
  ii. **Chronic alcohol abuse** can cause cerebellar degeneration, most profoundly seen in the vermis and presenting with ataxia. ▼

i. ▼ *In addition to ataxia, **cerebellar dysfunction** commonly presents with an intention tremor, dysmetria, and dysdiadochokinesia.*
  i. An **intention tremor** is absent at rest and most prominent during voluntary movement toward a target.
  ii. **Dysmetria** (past pointing) is the inability to estimate distance as it relates to a voluntary movement and is assessed during the finger to

nose test. Patients with dysmetria will often overshoot or undershoot their intended target.

   iii. **Dysdiadochokinesia** is the impaired ability to perform rhythmic, rapid alternating movements, such as rapidly alternating supination and pronation of the hands; the movements become slow, poorly timed, and uncoordinated.

   iv. *Note: Physical findings are ipsilateral to the cerebellar lesion (i.e., a patient will fall toward the side of the cerebellar lesion).* ▼

The Autonomic Nervous System

1. The CNS has only two output systems: The somatic motor system, which controls skeletal muscles, and the ANS, which controls **involuntary functions.**

2. The **functions of the ANS** can be categorized in three areas:
   a. **Maintenance of homeostasis** in response to the normal fluctuations of controlled variables (e.g., the negative feedback regulation of blood pressure).
   b. **Integration of the stress response,** including the response to exercise and the classic "fight or flight" response.
   c. **Integration of visceral function** (e.g., coordination of organs in the digestive system after the ingestion of food).

3. The functions of the ANS are integrated with the endocrine system because *the hypothalamus controls both efferent ANS activity and the secretion of hormones by the pituitary gland* (see Chapter 8).

4. The divisions of the ANS are the **sympathetic, parasympathetic,** and **enteric nervous systems** (see Chapter 7).

5. The actions of the sympathetic and parasympathetic divisions usually oppose each other (Table 2-6).
   a. *The activation of the sympathetic division occurs in a widespread pattern in* **response to stress.**
   b. *The functions of the parasympathetic division generally conserve and restore energy reserves.*

6. In some cases, the sympathetic and parasympathetic divisions act cooperatively; for example, during the male sexual response, penile erection is mediated by parasympathetic neurons, whereas ejaculation is coordinated by the sympathetic division (see Chapter 9).

7. The hierarchy of ANS control includes all levels of the nervous system:
   a. Motivational behaviors and responses to emotions are driven by the hypothalamus and the **limbic system** (see Overview of Integrative and Behavioral Functions).
   b. Brainstem nuclei coordinate basic homeostatic functions; for example, the **nucleus of the solitary tract** in the medulla is a site of cardiovascular, respiratory, and gastrointestinal control.
   c. Reflexes at the level of the **spinal cord** contribute to autonomic control (e.g., micturition, defecation, and ejaculation).
   d. The cell bodies of lower motor neurons in the ANS are located outside the CNS, in **autonomic ganglia.** These neurons are referred to as **postganglionic neurons,** and are controlled by **preganglionic** neurons located either in the spinal cord or the brainstem.

Table 2-6. Effects of the Autonomic Nervous System on Effector Organs

Organ	Sympathetic Response	Adrenergic Receptor Type	Parasympathetic Response	Muscarinic Receptor Type
Heart				M2
Sinoatrial node	Increased heart rate	β_1	Decreased heart rate	
Atrioventricular node	Increased conduction speed	β_1	Decreased conduction speed	
Myocardium	Increased contractility	β_1	–	
Vascular smooth muscle	Constriction in skin, abdominal viscera, and kidney	α_1	–	
	Dilation in skeletal muscle	β_2	–	
Bronchiolar smooth muscle	Relaxation	β_2	Constriction	
Gastrointestinal tract				M2, M3
Circular smooth muscle	Reduced motility	α_2, β_2	Increased motility	
Sphincters	Constriction	α_1	Relaxation	
Secretion	Inhibition	α_2	Stimulation	
Liver	Glycogenolysis and gluconeogenesis	β_2	–	
Adipose tissue	Lipolysis	β_1, β_3	–	
Kidney	Renin secretion	β_1	–	
Urinary bladder				M2, M3
Detrusor	Relaxation of bladder wall	β_2	Contraction of bladder wall	
Sphincter	Constriction	α_1	Relaxation	
Genitalia	Ejaculation; vaginal contraction	α_1	Erection	M3
Eye				M3
Pupil	Dilation	α_1	Constriction	
Ciliary muscle	–		Contraction (accommodation)	

    e. The neurotransmitter released by preganglionic neurons is **acetylcholine:**

       i. Acetylcholine binds to **nicotinic (ionotropic) receptors** on the postganglionic neuron (*note: this is a different receptor than that expressed at the neuromuscular junction*).

       ii. The binding of acetylcholine results in depolarization of the postganglionic neuron.

    f. Postganglionic fibers in the parasympathetic nervous system are also cholinergic but act via **muscarinic receptors** at the target organs.

    g. Postganglionic fibers in the sympathetic nervous system release different transmitters, most commonly norepinephrine, acting via **adrenergic receptors.**

8. The sympathetic nervous system.

    a. Preganglionic sympathetic neurons originate in the **lateral horn** of the spinal cord.

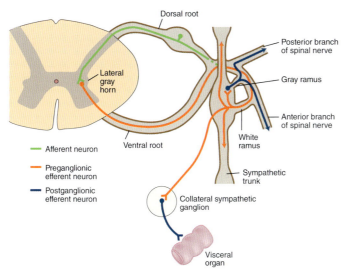

Figure 2-45. Organization of neurons in the sympathetic nervous system. Preganglionic neurons arise from the lateral horn of the spinal cord; myelinated fibers enter the sympathetic trunk via the white ramus. Preganglionic fibers may synapse in the sympathetic trunk at the same spinal level; they may ascend or descend within the sympathetic trunk or pass to collateral ganglia. Postganglionic fibers are unmyelinated and leave the sympathetic trunk via the gray ramus.

b. Preganglionic neurons may synapse either in the **paravertebral ganglia,** which are arranged in a chain called the **sympathetic trunk,** or in the **collateral ganglia.**

c. A preganglionic fiber can follow one of three pathways to its synapse with a postganglionic neuron (Figure 2-45):

  i. Most sympathetic preganglionic axons are short; *the myelinated axons exit the spinal cord via ventral nerve roots to join a spinal nerve and pass, via **white rami communicantes,** to synapse in a paravertebral ganglion.*

  ii. Some fibers ascend or descend within the sympathetic trunk because ***preganglionic sympathetic neurons** only arise from spinal segments T1 to L2.* Therefore, some preganglionic axons from the upper thoracic spinal segments must ascend to the **cervical ganglia.** Some fibers from the lower lumbar spine descend to serve pelvic organs (e.g., bladder and reproductive organs) via the **sacral ganglia.**

  iii. Some fibers in the thoracic region pass through the sympathetic trunk without synapsing. These neurons form the **splanchnic nerves,** which pass to the collateral ganglia associated with major abdominal blood vessels (i.e., the **celiac, superior mesenteric, inferior mesenteric,** and **renal arteries**).

d. There are three possible routes taken by postganglionic sympathetic neurons:

  i. Postganglionic fibers destined for somatic structures in the body wall (e.g., skin, blood vessels, and sweat glands) are distributed in **spinal nerves.** *Postganglionic fibers are unmyelinated and exit the paravertebral ganglia via **gray rami communicantes** to rejoin the spinal nerve.*

  ii. Fibers from paravertebral ganglia, which are destined for internal organs, may form anatomically distinct nerves (e.g., **cardiac nerves**).

Table 2-7. Signaling Mechanisms and Basic Pharmacology of Autonomic Receptor Subtypes

Adrenergic Receptor Type	Physiologic Agonist	Signaling Mechanism	Pharmacologic Agonist	Pharmacologic Antagonist
α_1	Norepi $\geq$ Epi	IP_3/DAG/Ca^{2+}	Phenylephrine	Prazosin
α_2	Norepi $\geq$ Epi	$\downarrow$ [cAMP]	Clonidine, methyldopa	Yohimbine
β_1	Epi > Norepi	$\uparrow$ [cAMP]	Dobutamine, isoproterenol ($\beta_1 = \beta_2$)	Metoprolol
β_2	Epi > Norepi	$\uparrow$ [cAMP]	Albuterol, isoproterenol ($\beta_1 = \beta_2$)	Propranolol (nonselective β_1 and β_2)
β_3	Epi > Norepi	$\uparrow$ [cAMP]	Isoproterenol	
Cholinergic Receptor Type				
nAChR$_{muscle}$	Acetylcholine	Ionotropic receptor	Nicotine	D-Tubocurarine
nAChR$_{neuron}$	Acetylcholine	Ionotropic receptor	Nicotine	Hexamethonium, mecamylamine
M$_{1-5}$	Acetylcholine	Various	Bethanechol, methacholine, pilocarpine	Atropine, benztropine, ipratropium

cAMP, cyclic adenosine monophosphate; DAG, diacylglycerol; Epi, epinephrine; IP_3, inositol 1,4,5-triphosphate; M_{1-5}, muscarinic receptors (five subtypes); nAChR$_{muscle}$, nicotinic receptor at the neuromuscular junction; nAChR$_{neuron}$, nicotinic receptor at autonomic ganglia and CNS; Norepi, norepinephrine.

    iii. Postganglionic fibers may also be distributed in nerves that pass along the outside of the **arteries.** For example, fibers passing to the head via cervical ganglia and fibers originating in the collateral ganglia utilize this pathway.

  e. *Norepinephrine is the primary neurotransmitter released by postganglionic sympathetic neurons, with the exception of the cholinergic postganglionic sympathetic neurons serving the sweat glands.*

  f. The responses of target cells to norepinephrine depend on the specific **adrenergic receptor type** that is expressed (i.e., α_1, α_2, β_1, β_2, or β_3) (Table 2-7).

  g. The adrenal medulla.

    i. The adrenal medulla is an **endocrine gland** located at the core of the adrenal (suprarenal) gland.

    ii. The endocrine (chromaffin) cells are modified postganglionic sympathetic neurons.

    iii. *Sympathetic preganglionic neurons pass to the adrenal gland via the splanchnic nerves and release acetylcholine as their neurotransmitter.*

    iv. Medullary endocrine cells respond to acetylcholine by secreting **epinephrine** and norepinephrine into the circulation, in a 4:1 ratio.

    v. The hormonal actions of epinephrine are complementary to those elicited by norepinephrine acting as a neurotransmitter at synapses between postganglionic neurons and target cells (see Chapter 8).

    vi. *The increased plasma concentration of epinephrine stimulates target cells that receive little sympathetic innervation (e.g., hepatocytes and adipose tissue).*

9. The parasympathetic nervous system.
   a. In general, the *parasympathetic preganglionic fibers are long and synapse with postganglionic neurons that are either in ganglia close to the target organ or are within the target organ itself.*
   b. Most preganglionic fibers originate in brainstem nuclei. Axons are contained in **four cranial nerves** (Figure 2-46):
      i. The **oculomotor nerve** (CN III) conveys axons from the **Edinger-Westphal nucleus** in the midbrain to the ciliary ganglion; most postganglionic neurons supply the **ciliary muscles of the eye.**
      ii. The **facial nerve** (CN VII) relays preganglionic fibers from the **superior salivary nucleus** of the medulla; postganglionic neurons are relayed to the submandibular and sublingual salivary glands via the submandibular ganglion. Other preganglionic fibers pass via the pterygopalatine ganglion, which gives origin to postganglionic neurons serving the **lacrimal and nasal glands.**
      iii. The **glossopharyngeal nerve** (CN IX) contains preganglionic fibers from the **inferior salivary nucleus** of the medulla. A complex pathway relays fibers via the otic ganglion to the **parotid salivary gland.** The *glossopharyngeal nerve also carries visceral afferent neurons from the sensory organs that monitor blood pressure (the **carotid sinus**) and blood gas composition (the **carotid body**).*
      iv. *The **vagus nerve** (CN X) carries the largest collection of preganglionic parasympathetic fibers.* The neurons originate in the **nucleus ambiguous** and **dorsal motor nucleus** of the medulla. Vagal fibers terminate in the heart and lungs and the gastrointestinal system.
   c. *Parasympathetic innervation of the pelvic organs originates in the gray matter of the sacral spinal cord, from segments **S2 to S4** (Figure 2-46).*
      i. Preganglionic axons exit the spinal cord via the ventral nerve roots and exit the spinal nerves to form the **pelvic splanchnic nerves.**
      ii. Preganglionic fibers terminate in the **hypogastric nerve plexuses** of the pelvis.
      iii. Unmyelinated postganglionic fibers pass to the **distal large intestine,** the **bladder,** and the **reproductive organs.**

Overview of Integrative and Behavioral Functions

1. The nervous system is capable of highly complex phenomena such as emotions, motivated behavior, consciousness, language, memory, and cognition.
2. Three areas of the brain are particularly important for the implementation of integrative functions:
   a. The **hypothalamus** is the major controller of the endocrine and autonomic nervous systems. It is a key site for the control of homeostatic functions and motivated behaviors, including eating, circadian rhythms, and the sex drive.
   b. The **reticular formation** consists of several well-defined nuclei that give origin to monoaminergic neurons; the widespread connections of these neurons form the **diffuse modulatory systems** of the brain. The functional concept is one of an **ascending reticular activating system** for the forebrain, which is essential for determining the level of consciousness and general arousal.

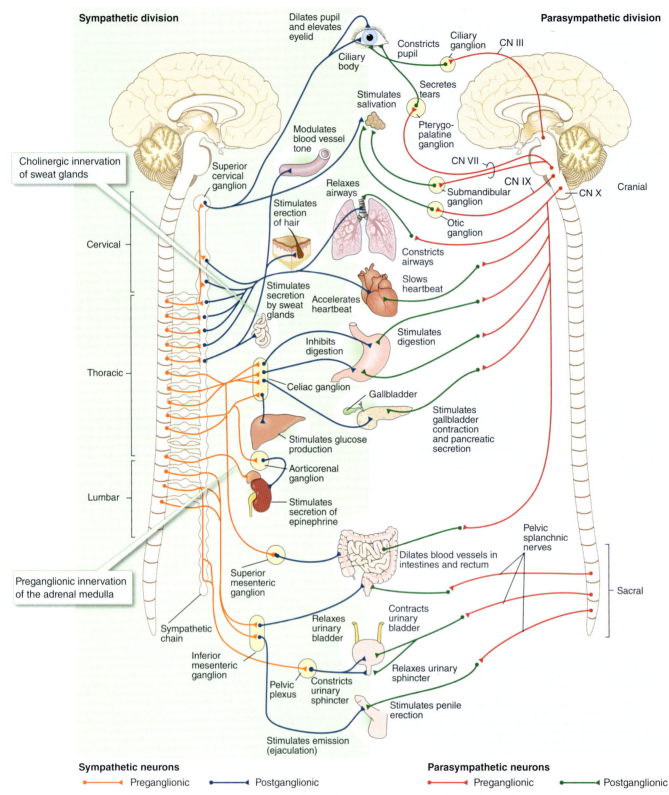

Sympathetic division

Parasympathetic division

Dilates pupil and elevates eyelid

Constricts pupil

Ciliary ganglion

CN III

Ciliary body

Secretes tears

Stimulates salivation

Pterygo-palatine ganglion

Modulates blood vessel tone

CN VII

Superior cervical ganglion

CN IX

Submandibular ganglion

CN X

Cranial

Cholinergic innervation of sweat glands

Relaxes airways

Stimulates erection of hair

Otic ganglion

Cervical

Constricts airways

Stimulates secretion by sweat glands

Slows heartbeat

Accelerates heartbeat

Stimulates digestion

Inhibits digestion

Thoracic

Celiac ganglion

Gallbladder

Stimulates gallbladder contraction and pancreatic secretion

Stimulates glucose production

Aorticorenal ganglion

Stimulates secretion of epinephrine

Lumbar

Preganglionic innervation of the adrenal medulla

Pelvic splanchnic nerves

Dilates blood vessels in intestines and rectum

Superior mesenteric ganglion

Sacral

Sympathetic chain

Relaxes urinary bladder

Contracts urinary bladder

Inferior mesenteric ganglion

Relaxes urinary sphincter

Pelvic plexus

Constricts urinary sphincter

Stimulates penile erection

Stimulates emission (ejaculation)

Sympathetic neurons

◀ Preganglionic   ●━━◀ Postganglionic

Parasympathetic neurons

━━◀ Preganglionic   ●━━◀ Postganglionic

Figure 2-46. Organ-specific autonomic innervation. Acetylcholine is the neurotransmitter released from all preganglionic neurons and from parasympathetic postganglionic fibers. Sympathetic postganglionic fibers release norepinephrine (with the exception of cholinergic neurons to sweat glands). (*Note: The names of the parasympathetic ganglia serving the head and those of the collateral sympathetic ganglia are shown in the figure.*)

c. The **limbic system** is the seat of emotions, and is formed from a series of cortical and subcortical structures that have reciprocal connections with the reticular formation and hypothalamus.

d. *Dysfunction of the limbic system and diffuse modulatory systems underlie psychiatric diseases such as major depression, bipolar disorder, and schizophrenia.*

The Hypothalamus

1. The hypothalamus is the small area below the thalamus, from the optic chiasm anteriorly to the mammillary bodies posteriorly; the lower part of the third ventricle lies at its center.

2. The hypothalamus consists of groups of nuclei that orchestrate homeostatic functions via the autonomic and endocrine systems and are a key output pathway for the limbic system, playing a role in the expression of emotions (Figure 2-47).

3. The major afferent inputs to the hypothalamus include:

a. Collaterals from the **visceral** and **somatic sensory pathways** (e.g., via the medial lemniscus and the reticular formation) to integrate homeostatic and visceral functions.

b. Afferent fibers from the **frontal lobe** and parts of the **limbic system** to link the hypothalamus with the higher centers for mood and emotion.

4. The hypothalamus has several **major efferent connections:**

a. Output to the **endocrine system** is via connections with the pituitary gland, via the **hypothalamohypophyseal tract** to the posterior pituitary, and via the **hypophyseal portal blood supply** to the anterior pituitary (see Chapter 8).

b. *Efferent neurons pass to the brainstem nuclei to influence parasympathetic outflow and to the lateral horn of the spinal cord for sympathetic outflow.*

c. Output to the reticular formation and **limbic system** also occurs through several pathways (e.g., the **mammillothalamic tract**).

5. Body temperature regulation.

a. Body temperature is an example of a key physiologically controlled variable that is regulated by the hypothalamus.

b. The normal set-point value for core body temperature is approximately $37.0\pm0.6°C$ ($98.6\pm1.0°F$) and is determined by the hypothalamus.

c. *A negative feedback response occurs if body temperature deviates from the set point; active regulation of heat transfer is controlled by the hypothalamus.*

d. Afferent input regarding body temperature is derived from two sources:

   i. **Peripheral thermoreceptors** in the skin provide information about body surface temperature.

   ii. **Central thermoreceptors** are temperature-sensitive neurons in the hypothalamus that monitor the core body temperature. Warm receptors are most abundant and are localized in the **preoptic area** of the hypothalamus.

   iii. *Physiologic responses are mostly driven by changes in core temperature rather than by changes in skin temperature.*

e. There are several **effectors for body temperature regulation:**

   i. **Skin circulation.**

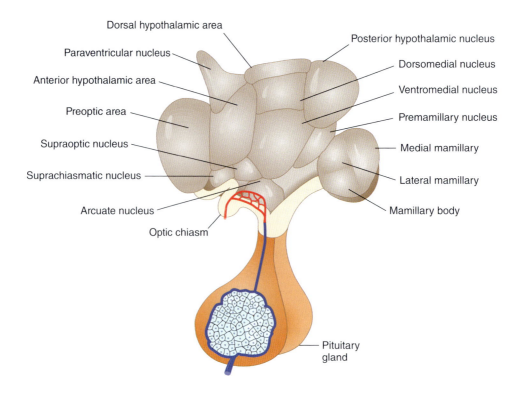

Function of the Hypothalamus	Area of the Hypothalamus
Secretion of hormonal release factors controlling the pituitary gland	Arcuate and paraventricular nuclei; periventricular area
Activation of sympathetic nervous system	Dorsal and posterior areas
Eating behavior	Ventromedial and arcuate nuclei; lateral area
Drinking behavior and thirst	Lateral area
Water and electrolyte balance	Supraoptic and paraventricular nuclei
Body temperature regulation	Preoptic area
Sexual behavior	Preoptic and anterior area
Circadian rhythms	Suprachiasmatic nucleus

Figure 2-47. Anatomy of the hypothalamic nuclei and the homeostatic functions of the hypothalamus.

- Vasoconstriction mediated by adrenergic tone minimizes heat loss in response to cold.
- Decreased sympathetic tone when the body is hot vasodilates blood vessels in the skin and results in increased heat loss.

ii. **Metabolic rate.**
- A low body temperature increases cellular metabolism via activation of the sympathetic nervous system and through increased thyroid hormone secretion.
- **Shivering** occurs when the core body temperature falls below approximately 35°C (95°F); it is coordinated by the hypothalamus and occurs first in the proximal muscles. *Shivering generates a large amount of heat from muscle but is a short-term response.*

iii. **Sweating.**
   - Sweating effectively decreases body temperature due to the large amount of heat needed to evaporate water.
   - *Sweat is a **hypotonic saline solution** secreted by the eccrine sweat glands in the skin in response to **cholinergic** postganglionic sympathetic innervation.*
   - The corelease of other peptide transmitters along with acetylcholine, or possibly the local generation of **bradykinin** by the sweat glands, also causes vasodilation.
   - ▼ **Sweating** can be viewed as a symptom of many underlying pathologic conditions. *Cholinergic sweating occurs in response to increased core temperature but the action of circulating epinephrine on **beta-adrenergic receptors** in sweat glands means that sweating can occur in any condition that drives sympathetic output.* For example, excessive sweating (**diaphoresis**) is a prominent feature during a myocardial infarction, amphetamine intoxication, or hypoperfusion states, such as hypovolemic shock. ▼

iv. **Behavioral changes** that minimize both heat and cold stress occur in response to thermal discomfort; for example, changing the amount of physical activity, clothing, or food ingestion.

f. *Fever is a regulated increase in body temperature in response to infection or inflammation* (Figure 2-48). The mechanism of fever is as follows:

   i. **Cytokine** secretion by immune cells in response to an infection or inflammatory process; cytokines function as **circulating pyrogens** (e.g., interleukin 6).

   ii. Capillary endothelial cells in the blood-brain barrier generate **prostaglandin E$_2$** (PGE$_2$) in response to cytokines.

   iii. *PGE$_2$ stimulates the hypothalamus to raise the set point for body temperature.*
      - ▼ Cyclooxygenase inhibitors (e.g., NSAIDs) are effective at reducing fever because PGE$_2$ formation is reduced. Glucocorticoids can also reduce fever by inhibiting inflammatory processes. ▼

   iv. Fever begins with sensations of cold discomfort ("**the chills**") because the body temperature is temporarily below the new set point temperature; there may be vasoconstriction and even shivering.

   v. When a fever "breaks," and the set point returns to normal, there is heat discomfort associated with sweating and vasodilation as the body temperature is temporarily above the set point temperature.

   vi. ▼ **Non-febrile hyperthermia** is an unregulated increase in body temperature due to a heat gain in excess of heat loss (e.g., exercise, heat stroke, seizure). *Timely diagnosis of hyperthermia relies on the medical history; unlike true fever, non-febrile hyperthermia is also unresponsive to NSAIDs since it is not caused by pyrogens.* ▼

g. Cold stress may cause **hypothermia,** which is defined as core body temperature below 35°C (95°F) (i.e., the point at which compensatory heat conserving mechanisms begin to fail). To prevent significant morbidity and mortality, patients should be removed from the cold environment and rewarmed.

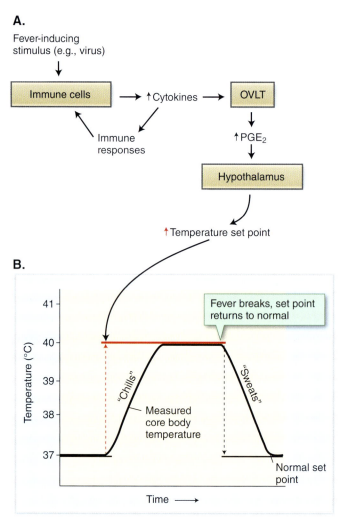

Figure 2-48. A. The mechanism of fever generation. Infections cause cells of the immune system to secrete cytokines, which cross the blood-brain barrier at the organum vasculosum laminae terminalis (OVLT). Endothelial cells of the OVLT produce prostaglandin E_2 (PGE_2) in response to cytokines, resulting in an increase in the hypothalamic set point for body temperature. **B.** The phases of fever. Changes in the hypothalamic set point during episodes of fever induce effector responses that cause the measured body temperature to change. At the beginning of a fever, the body temperature is initially below the set point; the patient feels cold and experiences "chills" (vasoconstriction and possible shivering) until the fever is established. When a fever "breaks," the body temperature is suddenly above the set point temperature; the patient feels hot and experiences vasodilation and sweating until the body cools.

6. Circadian rhythms.
   a. The hypothalamus generates the cyclical variation seen in most variables throughout a 24-hour period (e.g., body temperature varies by about 1°C, and is lowest in the early morning and highest in the evening).
   b. Circadian rhythms are generated by an **endogenous body clock** because they persist in people who are isolated from all time and light and dark cues.
   c. The body clock is created by neurons of the **suprachiasmatic nucleus** of the hypothalamus, the activity of which oscillates spontaneously in a daily cycle.
   d. Several **clock genes** interact to cause oscillating cycles of transcription and translation that underlie circadian rhythms.

e. The endogenous clock has a free running period of about 25 hours, and is entrained to a 24-hour period by the normal light and dark cycle and other social cues called "**zeitgebers.**"

   i. The suprachiasmatic nucleus receives afferent fibers directly from the retina via the **retinohypothalamic tract,** which provides information about daylight to entrain the circadian rhythm.

   ii. The pineal gland secretes the hormone **melatonin** in the hours of darkness, which helps to synchronize the day/night and sleep cycles.

   iii. ▼ Air travel across time zones produces the unpleasant sensations of "**jet lag**" (e.g., fatigue and being unable to eat and sleep properly when in the new time zone). Jet lag is caused by the mismatch between the endogenous circadian rhythms and the new time zone, and several days are required to entrain the body clock to the new time. A similar problem is faced by shift workers who are expected to suddenly switch their routines from nights to days or vice versa. ▼

The Reticular Formation and Diffuse Modulatory Systems

1. The reticular formation is an anatomic concept that describes columns of neurons that extend throughout the core of the brainstem. *Neurons in the reticular formation have very widespread connectivity throughout the CNS.*

2. The reticular formation has a strong influence on wakefulness, referred to as the concept of a **reticular activating system.**

3. ▼ Consciousness requires proper functioning of the reticular activating system and both cerebral hemispheres. Therefore, the **principal causes of unconsciousness or coma** are lesions that damage the reticular activating system or when there is diffuse damage to both cerebral hemispheres. *Note: Global suppression of the cerebrum and/or reticular activating system by drugs (e.g., sedative-hypnotics or alcohol) or metabolic derangements (e.g., anoxia, hypercapnia, hypoglycemia, or hepatic encephalopathy) is a common cause of unconsciousness or coma.* ▼

4. The reticular formation utilizes **diffuse modulatory systems,** which are categorized according to the principal neurotransmitter that is used. There are four major diffuse modulatory systems:

a. The **serotonergic system** originates in the **raphe nuclei,** which form a seam on either side of the midline throughout much of the brainstem and release the neurotransmitter serotonin (5-hydroxytryptamine, known as 5-HT). *Serotonergic neurons of the raphe nucleus are central to the control of wakefulness and sleep-wake cycles and to the control of mood and emotions.*

b. The **noradrenergic system** originates in the **locus coeruleus** of the pons, which functions as an "alarm center" that becomes most active when new environmental stimuli appear. Noradrenergic neurons are widely distributed throughout the CNS and increase the general state of arousal. *The noradrenergic system, taken together with the serotonergic system, correlates with the concept of a reticular activating system.*

c. **Cholinergic neurons** are widespread in the CNS and include diffuse modulatory systems originating in the basal forebrain and brainstem. *Cholinergic neurons are involved in the ability to direct selective attention to a particular task and are important for learning and memory.*

    d. **Dopaminergic neurons** are widespread in the CNS; several dopaminergic systems have been identified, including:

        i. The **nigrostriatal system,** which is a functional part of the basal ganglia and connects the substantia nigra of the midbrain to the striatum. Dopaminergic neurons are important in the initiation of **voluntary movement** (see Disorders of the Basal Ganglia).

        ii. The **mesocorticolimbic system,** which originates in the **ventral tegmental area (VTa)** of the midbrain and ramifies throughout the limbic system. Dopaminergic neurons play an important role in the brain's **reward system.**

5. The primary reward circuit has the following elements:

    a. The **VTa** is the primary receiving area for pleasurable stimuli.

    b. Dopaminergic neurons project to the **nucleus accumbens,** which mediates pleasure and initiates motor functions related to the reward.

    c. Projections to the **amygdala and hippocampus** promote learning and memory about the pleasurable experiences.

    d. The **prefrontal cortex** initiates executive control and motivation to seek the reward.

    e. ▼ Drugs of **addiction** such as cocaine and amphetamines both increase dopaminergic transmission in the mesocorticolimbic system by inhibiting dopamine reuptake. *The reward system is short circuited by **addictive drugs,** including cocaine, amphetamines, alcohol, nicotine, and opiates, which all increase dopaminergic transmission in the nucleus accumbens.* ▼

6. ▼ The two major **affective (mood) disorders** are **major depression** and **bipolar disorder.**

    a. Bipolar disorder is expressed by periods of depression alternating with bouts of mania (sustained emotional highs). *Drugs that enhance the diffuse serotonergic and noradrenergic modulatory systems are among the most effective treatments available for mood disorders.*

    b. The **monoamine oxidase inhibitors (MAOIs)** reduce the rate of norepinephrine and serotonin breakdown, which elevates the levels of these transmitters in the brain; **serotonin-selective reuptake inhibitors (SSRIs)** such as fluoxetine (e.g., Prozac) are effective in mood disorders. ▼

7. ▼ **Schizophrenia** is a group of **psychotic disorders** characterized by a loss of the normal perceptions of reality, evidenced by delusions, hallucinations, and disordered speech and behavior.

    a. **Dopamine antagonists** are effective when used as **antipsychotic (neuroleptic) drugs** due to the inhibition of dopamine signaling in the mesocorticolimbic system.

    b. *The antipsychotic actions of dopamine antagonists are mediated by blocking D_2-receptors. The use of nonselective dopamine antagonists inhibits the nigrostriatal dopaminergic system, resulting in adverse effects that resemble Parkinson's disease.* ▼

The Electroencephalogram (EEG) and Sleep

1. The **electroencephalogram (EEG)** is a method that measures cortical activity and is an extracellular voltage recording produced by placing electrodes at several locations on the patient's scalp.

A.

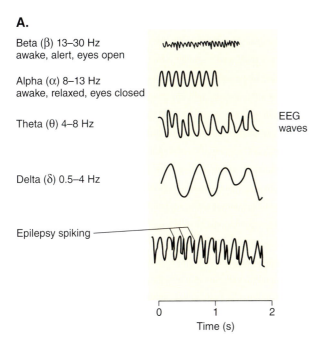

Beta (β) 13–30 Hz
awake, alert, eyes open

Alpha (α) 8–13 Hz
awake, relaxed, eyes closed

Theta (θ) 4–8 Hz

EEG
waves

Delta (δ) 0.5–4 Hz

Epilepsy spiking

Time (s)

B.

Increasing depth of sleep

Sleep stages
reverse through
4-3-2-1 before
REM sleep begins

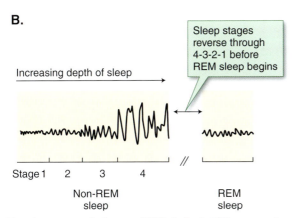

Stage 1   2   3   4

Non-REM
sleep

REM
sleep

Figure 2-49. The electroencephalogram (EEG). **A.** Basic EEG wave patterns and a spiking pattern associated with epileptic brain activity. **B.** EEG patterns observed during the five stages of sleep. REM, random eye movement.

a. The voltage differences measured between selected pairs of electrodes reflect the summation of electrical activity in the cortical neurons.

b. The size of EEG waves reflects synchronized activity of large groups of neurons. The diffuse modulatory systems play an important role in the overall level of cortical activation.

c. **EEG rhythms** are highly variable but can be categorized based on their frequency, and they can be correlated to general states of alertness (Figure 2-49A).

d. The EEG is particularly useful in diagnosing **seizures,** in which neurons in a given area fire synchronously to produce large spikes or waves. *Patients who regularly suffer seizures are described as having **epilepsy.***

e. ▼ Many treatment modalities exist for the **management of epilepsy.** The goals of therapy follow three main mechanisms:

    i. **Reduce seizure initiation** by inducing hyperpolarization via stimulating GABA-mediated inhibitory tone (e.g., using **barbiturates** or **benzodiazepines**).

    ii. **Decrease axonal conduction** via blockade of Na^+ channels, thereby inhibiting seizure propagation (e.g., using **phenytoin** or **carbamazepine**).

    iii. **Inhibit depolarization** by blocking presynaptic T-type Ca^{2+} channels in the thalamus (e.g., using **valproic acid** or **ethosuximide**). ▼

2. Sleep.

    a. *Sleep is largely controlled by the diffuse modulatory systems.*

    b. The serotonergic and noradrenergic systems are most active during an awake cycle; activity in these neurons decreases at the onset of sleep.

    c. Waking involves a general increase in activity of the serotonergic and noradrenergic systems as well as in cholinergic pathways in the basal forebrain.

    d. The **sleep cycle** has several defined phases, each of which has its own distinct EEG rhythm (Figure 2-49B).

        i. **Non-rapid eye movement (non-REM) sleep** is characterized by a decreasing level of consciousness and an increasing level of rest. The parasympathetic nervous system is active and the heart rate and respiration are reduced; muscles are relaxed and movement is minimal. Non-REM sleep progresses through **four stages;** stages 3 and 4 are the most restful and correlate with **slow-wave sleep,** which can be recorded on an EEG.

        ii. **REM sleep** is dreaming sleep, which occurs after non-REM sleep has progressed in a cycle through stages 1–4, then back in reverse to stage 1.

        iii. ▼ *REM sleep features an awake brain and a paralyzed body.* In addition to these classic features, vivid visual imagery and sexual arousal also occur during this time of the sleep cycle. Evaluation of nocturnal penile tumescence can help to determine whether the cause of **erectile dysfunction** is psychogenic (nocturnal penile tumescence does occur) or organic (nocturnal penile tumescence is limited or does not occur). ▼

    e. ▼ The normal adult generally sleeps 7–8 hours per night; each sleep cycle typically is about 90–120 minutes, with approximately 25% of the time spent in REM sleep.

        i. **Young children** sleep for longer periods and have a higher proportion of REM sleep.

        ii. **Elderly persons** have reduced sleep time and an absent stage 4, often leaving them with the complaint that they do not feel as rested as they used to feel. ▼

The Limbic System

1. The **limbic *lobe*** is an anatomic concept that describes the cortical areas surrounding the brainstem, including the **cingulate and parahippocampal gyri.**

2. The **limbic *system*** is a functional concept, which includes a series of structures that are intimately associated with the experience and control of emotions and with learning and memory.

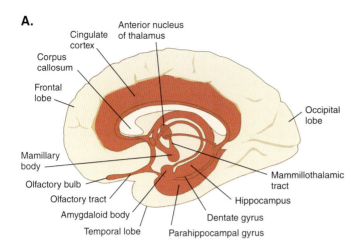

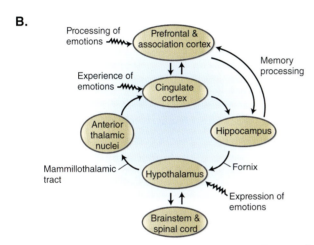

Figure 2-50. The limbic system. **A.** Major anatomic structures forming the limbic system. **B.** The main circuit of the limbic system.

3. The limbic system consists of **several cortical structures** with extensive connections to the hypothalamus and reticular formation (Figure 2-50A):

   a. The **cingulate cortex** is connected to the highest centers of cognition in the prefrontal and association areas of cortex, and is a site where the "sensations" of emotions are perceived.

   b. The **hippocampus** is a curved elevation of gray matter on the medial surface of the temporal lobe and interacts with the cingulate cortex and the higher association cortex. *The hippocampus is important in the conversion of short-term memory to long-term memory.*

   c. The **amygdaloid nucleus (amygdala)** is located lateral to the hippocampus and just below the basal ganglia. *The amygdala is involved in strong emotions, including fear and aggression, and linking emotions with memories.*

4. The circuits of the limbic system include fiber tracts passing between cortical and subcortical areas (Figure 2-50B):

   a. The **hypothalamus** is an important output route of the limbic system for the expression of emotions because its efferent connections coordinate autonomic and visceral functions. *The hypothalamus is connected to higher parts of the limbic system, via the hippocampus, by tracts passing in the* **fornix.**

   b. The activity of the hypothalamus is relayed back to the cortex, via the **mammillothalamic tract,** from the mammillary bodies to the **anterior thalamic nuclei,** thereby providing a pathway linking the expression with the sensation of emotions.

5. Fear and anxiety.

   a. The *amygdala is a central structure in mediating the fear response and in learning and memory about fears or emotional events;* lesions in this area can prevent fear.

   b. There are both cognitive and reactive fear circuits:

      i. In the **cognitive fear** pathway, higher areas in the prefrontal and cingulate cortices integrate sensory information with learned experience and produce descending input to the amygdala, which results in the sensation of fear.

      ii. In the **reactive fear** circuit, lower centers from the periaqueductal gray of the midbrain contribute to rapid fear activation to address an immediate threat.

   c. *Output from the amygdala to the hypothalamus results in activation of the "fight or flight" response by the sympathetic nervous system.*

   d. The hippocampus has a calming effect on activation of the stress response and provides a negative feedback pathway to limit the stress response:

      i. Increased plasma concentration of **cortisol** is part of the stress response.

      ii. Cortisol stimulates areas of the **hippocampus.**

      iii. The hippocampus inhibits activation of the stress response by the **hypothalamus.**

      iv. *Note: This mechanism becomes less effective in states of **chronic stress.***

   e. **Aggression** is an emotion related to fear and is also mediated by the amygdala and hypothalamus.

      i. Lesions in the amygdala can result in a flattening of emotions, loss of fear, and also produce a placid state.

      ii. Aggression is normally suppressed by higher parts of the limbic system in the frontal cortex, which, if severed, may result in uncontrolled rage.

   f. ▼ **Klüver-Bucy syndrome** is a rare neurologic disorder that occurs as a result of bilateral lesions of the amygdala (e.g., herpes encephalitis). Patients exhibit **hypersexuality** (lack of social sexual restraint), **hyperorality** (strong compulsion to place objects in the mouth), **visual agnosia** (able to see objects, but unable to identify them), **flat affect,** and **placidity** (able to approach danger without anger or fear). ▼

Learning and Memory

1. The learning process requires that information is stored and can be retrieved (remembered).

2. **Declarative memory** relates to facts and events that can be consciously recalled.

3. **Nondeclarative memory** uses different mechanisms to store information that is generally not consciously recalled. There are **three types of nondeclarative memory:**

   a. The ability to learn a skill or procedure (e.g., riding a bicycle) is called **procedural memory.**

   b. The ability to form emotional associations in the memory is called **learned emotion.**

   c. **Conditioned reflexes** are a simple form of memory; for example, the habit of hearing a lunchtime alarm may be sufficient to induce reflex gastrointestinal activity.

4. The working model for memory includes sensory, working, and long-term memory:

   a. **Sensory memory** holds only 3–7 units and is very brief unless we pay attention to the stimulus and promote it to the working memory.

   b. **Working memory** holds around 7–9 chunks of information but these will also be forgotten quickly (e.g., remembering a telephone number) unless there is *rehearsal to maintain the memory.*

   c. The conversion of short-term memory into a **long-term memory** is called **memory consolidation,** and is strongly enhanced by memory **retrieval** (do quizzes rather than re-reading these notes!) or by adding emotional context.

   d. *Memory consolidation requires the hippocampus; damage in this area causes* **anterograde amnesia** *(the inability to form new declarative memories).*

   e. *The ability to recall long-term memories that are already stored does not require the hippocampus. The inability to recall previous memories is called* **retrograde amnesia.**

5. ▼ **Alzheimer's disease** is the most common cause of dementia in the United States.

   a. Alzheimer's disease manifests as an insidious onset of progressive memory loss followed by a slowly progressive course of dementia, aphasia (loss of language skills), and apraxia (loss of learned motor skills).

   b. Late in the disease, there is a loss of judgement, reason, and cognitive ability. This disease typically is fatal within 10 years of onset, with death occurring due to secondary causes (e.g., pneumonia).

   c. Alzheimer's disease is associated with decreased levels of **acetylcholine,** thought to be the result of *degeneration of cholinergic neurons in the* **nucleus basalis of Meynert.**

   d. Key pathologic findings include diffuse cerebral cortical atrophy resulting in enlarged ventricles and *hippocampal atrophy associated with memory loss.*

   e. Microscopic findings include senile plaques (Aβ **amyloid**) and **neurofibrillary tangles.** ▼

6. The cellular basis of learning.

   a. **Memory engrams** are located in the large areas of the association cortex, where it is thought *there is no limit to memory storage.*

   b. Learning and memory is associated with changes in the structure and function of synapses and is known as **synaptic plasticity.**

   c. Repeated synaptic stimulation can result in a persistent increase in the sensitivity of a neuron, called **long-term potentiation (LTP).**

   d. LTP is associated with remodeling of synaptic contacts as well as functional changes including ion channel phosphorylation, altered intracellular second-messenger activity, and gene expression.

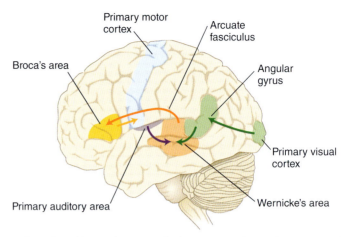

Figure 2-51. Broca's and Wernicke's areas for language and speech. Arrows indicate the Wernicke-Geschwind model for speech production; information about spoken or written words is conveyed from the auditory and visual cortices respectively to Wernicke's area where language comprehension occurs. Output from Wernicke's area, via the arcuate fasciculus, directs Broca's area to develop a motor program for the generation of speech, which is conveyed to the neighboring motor cortex.

Language and Speech

1. *Language is a **lateralized brain function** and is dominated by centers in the left hemisphere.* There are **two cortical areas specialized for language** (Figure 2-51):
    a. **Broca's area** is in the frontal lobe, just anterior to the motor cortical areas that control the mouth.
    b. **Wernicke's area** is in the upper part of the temporal lobe, near the auditory cortex.
2. The **Wernicke-Geschwind model** for language has the following elements:
    a. Inputs of spoken or written words arrive from the **auditory and visual cortex,** respectively, and are relayed to Wernicke's area.
    b. *Understanding the meaning of words is achieved by processing in **Wernicke's area.***
    c. Output from Wernicke's area to Broca's area occurs via a tract called the **arcuate fasciculus.**
    d. ***Broca's area** generates the commands needed to instruct the neighboring motor cortex to produce the movements of the mouth and tongue needed to speak.*
    e. ▼ The Wernicke-Geschwind model is based on clinical findings in patients with defects in understanding or producing words (i.e., **aphasia**).
        i. **Broca's aphasia** is characterized by an *inability to produce speech or "find a word,"* whereas comprehension is generally preserved.
        ii. **Wernicke's aphasia** is characterized by fluent production of speech, but the sentences lack meaning and *comprehension of language is poor.* ▼

Study Questions

Directions: Each numbered item is followed by lettered options. Some options may be partially correct, but there is only *ONE BEST* answer.

1. A novel drug produced by screening snake venoms was found to kill glial cell tumors in culture. However, initial in vivo studies showed that the drug did not enter the brain of experimental animals and therefore could not access glial cells in the intact brain. Which structure is most responsible for preventing the entry of this drug into the brain?

   A. Arachnoid mater
   B. Brain capillary endothelium
   C. Choroid plexus epithelium
   D. Dura mater
   E. Pia mater

2. A 28-year-old woman was prevented from traveling by air to a family wedding due to an acute episode of vertigo. Over the next few months, she experienced several transient, neurologic problems, including blurred vision, sudden muscle weakness in her legs, loss of perineal sensations, and urinary incontinence. What cellular defect is most likely to account for these clinical findings?

   A. Atrophy of skeletal muscles
   B. Demyelination of central nervous system (CNS) neurons
   C. Destruction of preganglionic sympathetic neurons
   D. Loss of CNS dopaminergic neurons
   E. Proliferation of Schwann cells

3. In a laboratory experiment, a cortical neuron was electrically stimulated to produce action potentials. The stimulated neuron made synaptic contact with another neuron in which a recording electrode was located. The recording electrode detected a small depolarization following the electrical stimulation of the first neuron. Which neurotransmitter was most likely to be released at the synapse between these neurons?

   A. GABA
   B. Glutamate
   C. Glycine
   D. Met-enkephalin
   E. Somatostatin

4. A 53-year-old man suffered a vascular lesion to a small area of the lower lumbar spinal cord, which resulted in the loss of touch sensation from his left leg. Sensations of pain and temperature were not affected. Damage to which part of the spinal cord accounts for this pattern of sensory loss?

   A. Right anterolateral tract
   B. Right dorsal column
   C. Right dorsal horn
   D. Right ventral horn
   E. Left anterolateral tract
   F. Left dorsal column
   G. Left dorsal horn
   H. Left ventral horn

5. A 13-year-old boy was referred to a pediatrician due to his unusual height of 196 cm (6 ft 5 in). The boy recently reported visual disturbances. A pituitary tumor was discovered using MRI scans, and was found to be pressing on the center of the optic chiasm from below. What visual field defects are expected in this patient?

A. Binasal hemianopia
B. Bitemporal hemianopia
C. Left homonymous hemianopia
D. Right homonymous hemianopia

6. A 41-year-old woman was taken to the emergency department after being involved in a motor vehicle accident. Neurologic examination showed that the pupillary light reflex was absent in both eyes when light was shone in the left eye, but was normal in both eyes when light was shone in the right eye. At which location could a lesion account for this pattern of deficit in the pupillary light response?

A. Left oculomotor nerve (CN III)
B. Left optic nerve
C. Right Edinger-Westphal nucleus
D. Right visual cortex
E. Superior colliculi

7. A 19-year-old girl visited her family doctor, concerned about poor hearing in her right ear. She had no family history of deafness and could not remember having any ear infections as a child. She admitted listening to loud music through a personal music player, and while at her work in a launderette, she usually listened in her right ear only so that she could still hear the customers. What are the most likely results of the Weber and Rinne tuning fork tests performed by her doctor?

A. Weber test lateralizes to the left; Rinne test shows air conduction > bone conduction
B. Weber test lateralizes to the left; Rinne test shows bone conduction > air conduction
C. Weber test lateralizes to the right; Rinne test shows air conduction > bone conduction
D. Weber test lateralizes to the right; Rinne test shows bone conduction > air conduction

8. A functional magnetic resonance imaging (fMRI) study of the thalamus showed changes in neuronal activity in the thalamus in response to various sensory stimuli. Which of the following sensory modalities would be associated with the lowest level of thalamic neuronal activity?

A. Audition
B. Conscious proprioception
C. Gustation
D. Olfaction
E. Vision

9. A 68-year-old man visits his doctor complaining about a tremor in his hands, which is particularly bad when he tries to perform a task. He demonstrates past-pointing when asked to perform a finger to nose test, and has difficulty producing rapidly alternating supination and pro-nation movements of the hands. The doctor also notes a wide, awkward gait. Based on these clinical findings alone, in which part of the motor system is a dysfunction expected?

   A. Basal ganglia
   B. Cerebellum
   C. Lateral spinal pathways
   D. Primary motor cortex
   E. Ventromedial spinal pathways

10. A 17-year-old girl was taken to the emergency department because of a drug overdose. She was unconscious and remained comatose for 2 weeks. Her friend reported that she had started taking an unknown recreational drug 1 month earlier. In the days after regaining consciousness, the girl was profoundly depressed and developed unrelenting insomnia. Which of the following nuclei is most likely to have been damaged by her drug abuse?

   A. Amygdaloid
   B. Arcuate
   C. Caudate
   D. Dentate
   E. Edinger-Westphal
   F. Fastigial
   G. Paraventricular
   H. Raphe
   I. Suprachiasmatic
   J. Supraoptic

Blood

CHAPTER 3

The Composition of Blood

1. Blood is composed of **cellular elements** (i.e., red blood cells, white blood cells, and platelets) suspended in blood **plasma.**
   a. A person who weighs 70 kg has approximately 5 L of blood with about 2 L of cellular elements and 3 L of plasma.
2. Plasma composition.
   a. Plasma is the part of the ECF contained within the cardiovascular system.
   b. It is approximately 92% water, 7% protein, and 1% small dissolved solutes (e.g., ions, urea, glucose, amino acids, and lipids).
   c. Plasma concentrations of ions and small molecules are similar to those in the interstitial fluid, due to the free exchange of water and small solutes across most blood capillaries (Table 3-1).
   d. Protein concentration is higher in plasma than interstitial fluid because *most capillaries are impermeable to plasma proteins.*
      i. The protein concentration gradient creates the colloid osmotic (oncotic) pressure gradient that opposes the filtration of plasma out of the capillaries (see Chapter 4).
      ii. **Albumin** is the most abundant type of plasma protein and is the greatest contributor to the plasma oncotic pressure (Table 3-2).
      iii. ▼ **Hypoalbuminemia** has many causes, including nephrotic syndrome, liver failure, and severe malnutrition. Regardless of the cause, hypoalbuminemia can result in **anasarca** (generalized massive edema). ▼
3. There are three main cell types in circulating blood (Table 3-3):
   a. **Red blood cells (erythrocytes)** are essential for the transport of O_2 and CO_2 in blood. *There are approximately 5×10^{12} red blood cells per liter of blood.*
   b. **Platelets (thrombocytes)** are small cellular fragments that play a key role in **hemostasis**. *There are approximately 300×10^9 platelets per liter of blood.*
   c. **White blood cells (leukocytes)** are the only fully functional nucleated cells in circulating blood. White cells play a defensive role in destroying infecting organisms and in the removal of damaged tissue. *The total white cell count is approximately 5×10^9 cells per liter of blood.*

Hematopoiesis

1. The formation of blood cells (hematopoiesis) occurs in the **bone marrow.**
   a. In neonates, most of the skeleton contains active bone marrow, but in adults it is found in the vertebrae, ribs, skull, pelvis, and the proximal femurs.

Table 3-1. Normal Plasma Composition

Substance	Normal Value	Normal Range
Sodium	140 mM	136–146 mM
Potassium	4.5 mM	3.5–5.5 mM
Chloride	100 mM	96–106 mM
Bicarbonate	24 mM	22–28 mM
Calcium*	2.5 mM	2.2–2.8 mM
pH (arterial)	7.40	7.35–7.45
PCO_2 (arterial)	40 mm Hg	38–42 mm Hg
PO_2 (arterial)	90 mm Hg	80–100 mm Hg
Glucose (fasting)	80 mg/dL	70–99 mg/dL
Urea (BUN)	12 mg/dL	9–18 mg/dL
Protein	7 g/dL	6–8 g/dL

*Approximately 50% is protein bound.

BUN, blood urea nitrogen.

Table 3-2. The Major Types of Plasma Proteins

Plasma Protein	Major Source	Examples and Functions
Albumin	Liver	Main component of plasma oncotic pressure; binding of various substances
α-Globulins and β-globulins	Liver	Examples (there are many) include hormone-binding proteins and the iron carrier protein transferrin
Coagulation proteins	Liver	Examples include plasminogen, prothrombin, antithrombin III, and fibrinogen
Immunoglobulins	Lymphoid tissue	Host defense reactions
Complement proteins	Liver	Host defense reactions

2. Blood cells are derived from **stem cells** in the bone marrow after several stages of cell division and differentiation.
   a. **Erythropoiesis** is the process of red blood cell formation.
   b. **Thrombopoiesis** is the process of platelet production.
   c. **Leukopoiesis** describes white blood cell production.
3. Blood-forming cells may be divided into four groups, depending on their capacity for self-renewal, cell division, and the ability to form different cell types (Figure 3-1):
   a. **Pluripotent hematopoietic stem cells** can form any type of blood cell but are few in number.
   b. **Multipotential progenitor cells** can form a specific but wide range of blood cells. There are two types of multiprogenitor cells.
      i. Lymphoid progenitor cells.
      ii. The granulocyte-erythroid-monocyte-megakaryocyte (GEMM) progenitor cell that differentiates into all the other types of blood cells.

Table 3-3. Types of White Blood Cells

Cell Type	Relative Abundance (%)	Characteristic Feature(s)	Major Function(s)
Neutrophils	50–70	• Multilobed nucleus • Cytoplasmic granules containing antibacterial, digestive, and proinflammatory agents	• Ingest and destroy invading microorganisms • Coordination of the early phase of acute inflammation
Eosinophils	5	• Acidophilic granules in cytoplasm	• Phagocytic, especially against parasitic infestation
Basophils	0.5	• Basophilic granules in cytoplasm; contents include histamine	• Migrate to tissues to become mast cells; release of histamine contributes to inflammation • Degranulation is a key feature in allergic reactions mediated by immunoglobulin E
Monocytes	1–5	• Large cell with numerous small lysosomes in the cytoplasm	• Respond chemotactically to invading microorganisms and sites of inflammation • Part of a cell network, called the monocyte-macrophage system; called macrophages when outside the vascular system • Key part of cell-mediated immune response, in concert with lymphocytes
Lymphocytes	20–40	• Small cells with variable morphology	• Generate specific immune responses • B lymphocytes become plasma cells and secrete antibodies, mediating humoral immunity • T cells provide cell-mediated immunity (e.g., destruction of virally infected cells)

   c. **Committed progenitor cells** are capable of self-renewal but are only able to form one or two cell types.

      i. Neutrophils and monocytes are both derived from a single type of committed progenitor cell.

      ii. All other mature cell types have their own committed progenitor cell.

   d. **Maturing cells** do not divide again and are undergoing structural differentiation to form a specific type of blood cell.

   e. ▼ **Bone marrow (hematopoietic cell) transplant** may be used in the treatment of many different hematologic and immunologic diseases, including acquired conditions such as leukemia, lymphoma, and aplastic anemia, and inherited conditions such as sickle cell anemia and severe combined immunodeficiency.

      i. **Hematopoietic stem cell** transplant is possible because these cells can survive cryopreservation, have an innate ability to "home" to the bone marrow of the recipient, and have a remarkable regenerative capacity.

      ii. *Only a small percentage of the donor's bone marrow is needed for complete replacement of the recipient's entire lymphohematopoietic system.* ▼

4. Erythropoiesis.

   a. The **erythron** is a dispersed organ that consists of the whole mass of mature red blood cells and their progenitors in the bone marrow.

   b. The production of red blood cells is regulated to provide an adequate O_2-carrying capacity in blood.

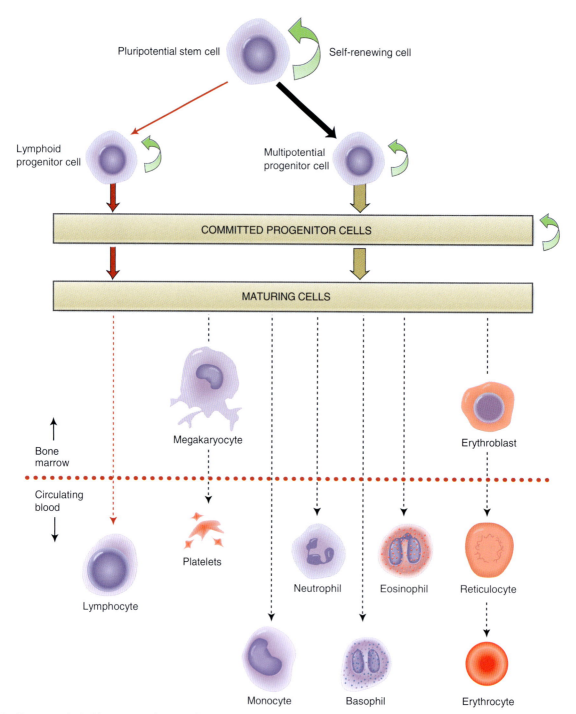

Figure 3-1. Hematopoiesis. Pluripotential stem cells in the bone marrow are self-renewing cells that have the potential to differentiate into any type of blood cell. Cell division and differentiation produces stem cells that are committed to produce particular types of blood cell. Most bone marrow cells are in a phase of maturation, on the way to becoming one of the cell types in circulating blood.

    i. *The hormone **erythropoietin (EPO)** is the primary regulator of erythropoiesis, and is released from the kidney when O_2 tension in the renal parenchyma is reduced* (see Chapter 6).

    ii. Committed erythroid stem cells in the bone marrow respond to EPO with increased rates of cell division and differentiation into mature red cells.

  c. The maturation of red cells in the bone marrow requires several factors; most notably **iron,** for the synthesis of the O_2-carrying pigment **hemoglobin,** and the essential nutrients **folic acid** and **vitamin B_{12}**.

   d. Stem cell differentiation into mature red cells involves a decrease in cell size, production of **hemoglobin,** and the eventual disappearance of cell **organelles.**

   e. In the final stage of differentiation, immature red cells are called **reticulocytes,** which are characterized by the presence of organelle remnants.

      i. *There is normally less than 1% of circulating red blood cells in the immature reticulocyte stage.*

      ii. Larger numbers of reticulocytes reflect a rapid increase in the demand for red blood cells (e.g., after acute hemorrhage). *The reticulocyte count is an index of the rate of red blood cell production.*

5. Thrombopoiesis.

   a. **Platelets** have the following properties:

      i. Are small disk-shaped cell fragments without a nucleus.

      ii. Have an extensive cytoskeleton, which allows the shape of a platelet to change upon activation.

      iii. Have many secretory granules containing factors that regulate hemostasis.

   b. Platelet production occurs in the bone marrow by the cytoplasmic fragmentation of **megakaryocytes.**

      i. Megakaryocytes are the largest cells in the bone marrow and are formed when committed progenitor cells undergo repeated nuclear division without cell division.

   c. The rate of platelet formation is regulated by the cytokine **thrombopoietin (TPO)** (*note: the term "cytokine" is used to describe peptide hormones that regulate cell differentiation or immune functions*).

      i. TPO is constitutively secreted by the liver and kidneys.

      ii. Platelets regulate TPO levels by removing it from the circulation; for example, high levels of TPO will result when there is a low platelet count (**thrombocytopenia**).

      iii. TPO stimulates platelet production to restore a normal platelet count.

6. Leukopoiesis.

   a. The development of **lymphoid progenitor cells** in bone marrow only yields primitive precursor cells. *The final differentiation of lymphocytes occurs in peripheral lymphoid tissues as part of a specific immune response:*

      i. **T lymphocytes** differentiate in the thymus gland.

      ii. **B lymphocytes** mainly differentiate in the lymph nodes.

   b. **Myelopoiesis** is the formation of the nonlymphoid white blood cells through immature **myeloid cell** stages in the bone marrow into fully differentiated cells.

      i. The **granular white blood cells** (i.e., neutrophils, eosinophils, and basophils) all have morphologically similar stages of cell differentiation in the bone marrow.

        • Granulocytes are released from the bone marrow as mature cells.

        • *A large pool of neutrophils is maintained in the bone marrow and can be rapidly mobilized in response to an infection.*

      ii. **Monocytes** leave the bone marrow soon after their formation.

        • There is no pool of mature monocytes in the bone marrow.

        • *Monocytes spend 2–3 days in the circulation before entering the tissues to become macrophages.*

      iii. ▼ Leukopoiesis is regulated by cytokines known as **colony-stimulating factors.** Patients undergoing cancer chemotherapy are at risk of severe infection due to **neutropenia** (neutrophil count <500 per μL) and can be treated with colony-stimulating factors to stimulate neutrophil production, allowing chemotherapy to continue. ▼

      iv. ▼ Active white blood cells can direct white cell production causing changes in the **differential white cell count:** For example, *bacterial infections are usually associated with an increased proportion of neutrophils and monocytes, whereas viral infections increase the proportion of lymphocytes.* ▼

  c. ▼ If a malignant transformation occurs in a white blood cell lineage, a person can develop **leukemia** or **lymphoma.**

      i. *Leukemia is a general term used to describe a malignancy that is primarily based in the bone marrow and blood; lymphomas are solid tumors that are primarily based in the lymph nodes.*

      ii. In **acute leukemia,** the bone marrow becomes infiltrated with malignant blast cells (immature white blood cells).

        • Blast cells of myeloid lineage cause **acute myeloid leukemia;** blast cells of lymphoid lineage cause **acute lymphoblastic leukemia.**

        • *The symptoms associated with acute leukemias are typically due to bone marrow failure, which includes suppressed red blood cells (presenting as anemia), suppressed white blood cells (presenting as infection), and suppressed platelet formation (presenting as bleeding tendency).*

      iii. **Chronic leukemia** has a more gradual onset and results in very high leukocyte counts with cells that have a mature appearance (e.g., **chronic myeloid leukemia** and **chronic lymphocytic leukemia**). ▼

Red Blood Cells

1. Mature **erythrocytes** are:
  a. Disk-shaped anucleate cells, approximately 7–8 μm in diameter.
  b. Flexible due to an extensive cytoskeleton so that they can pass through the microcirculation.
  c. Able to withstand large osmotic pressure differences, which are encountered when they pass through the renal circulation.

2. Key cytoplasmic proteins in erythrocytes include:
  a. The O_2-carrying pigment **hemoglobin,** which is the major protein present and is responsible for the red cell color.
  b. **Glycolytic enzymes,** needed because *red cells have no mitochondria and must synthesize adenosine triphosphate (ATP) via glycolysis.*
  c. **Carbonic anhydrase,** used to catalyze the following equilibrium reaction, which is essential for CO_2 carriage in blood (see Chapter 5):

$$H_2O + CO_2 \leftrightarrow H_2CO_3 \leftrightarrow HCO_3^- + H^+$$

3. The normal lifespan of a red blood cell in the circulation is approximately 100–120 days (i.e., *erythropoiesis must replace approximately 0.8–1.0% of the circulating red cells daily*).

a. Aging red cells become progressively more fragile and are ultimately removed from the circulation by macrophages, particularly in the spleen.

b. The end product of hemoglobin breakdown in macrophages is **bilirubin,** which is conjugated in the liver and excreted in the bile (see Chapter 7).

4. *Balance must be maintained between the rate of red cell production and the rate of red cell loss from the circulation;* imbalance results in either decreased red cell mass (**anemia**) or increased red cell mass (**polycythemia**).

5. Several **red blood cell indices** are routinely reported in a **complete blood count (CBC)** to characterize the red cell mass (Table 3-4).

a. The **size of the total red cell mass** is described by three variables:

   i. **Hemoglobin concentration (Hb)** is the amount of hemoglobin in a volume of blood.

   ii. **Hematocrit (Hct) or packed cell volume (PCV)** is the ratio of the volume of red cells to the volume of whole blood. It may be determined by centrifuging a sample of blood and comparing the height of the column of packed red cells at the bottom of the tube to the total height of the column.

   iii. **Red cell count (RBC)** is the number of red cells per liter of blood.

b. The average size of a red blood cell is described using the **mean cell volume (MCV),** which is the average volume of a single red cell expressed in femtoliters (fL = 10^{-15} L).

   i. MCV is calculated by dividing the hematocrit by RBC.

   ii. *MCV <80 fL indicates that red cells are small (**microcytosis**).*

   iii. *MCV >100 fL indicates that red cells are large (**macrocytosis**).*

c. Two derived variables describe the **adequacy of hemoglobin synthesis:**

   i. **Mean cell hemoglobin (MCH)** is the average amount of hemoglobin in the average red cell, expressed in picograms (pg = 10^{-12} g). MCH is calculated by dividing the hemoglobin concentration by RBC.

   ii. **Mean cell hemoglobin concentration (MCHC)** is the average concentration of hemoglobin in red cells, calculated by dividing MCH by MCV.

   iii. ▼ Patients with abnormal MCH and MCHC will have altered red cell color (i.e., **chromicity**) when viewed under the microscope.

Table 3-4. Red Blood Cell Indices

Index	Units/Calculation	Normal Range
Hemoglobin concentration (Hb)	g/dL	• Adult man, 14–18 g/dL • Adult woman, 11–15 g/dL
Hematocrit (Hct)	%	• Adult man, 40–54% • Adult woman, 34–46%
Red cell count (RBC)	10^{12}/L	• Adult man, 4.5–6.5 • Adult woman, 3.9–5.6
Mean cell volume (MCV)	(%*Hct* ÷ 100)/*RBC* (fL)	82–98 fL
Mean cell hemoglobin (MCH)	(*Hb* × 10)/*RBC* (pg)	27–33 pg
Mean cell hemoglobin concentration (MCHC)	(100 × MCH)/MCV (g/dL)	30–35 g/dL (g %)

- Low MHC and MCHC cause pale **hypochromic** cells.
- High MHC and MCHC result in more intensely colored **hyperchromic** cells. ▼

d. **Example:** A 42-year-old woman visits her family doctor complaining of recent heavy menses and a constant feeling of fatigue. A CBC reveals Hb of 8 g/dL, Hct of 24%, and RBC of 2.6×10^{12}/L. Calculate the MCV, MCH, and MCHC.

$$MCV = (\%Hct \div 100)/RBC \text{ L}$$
$$= 24 \div 100/2.6 \times 10^{12} \text{ L}$$
$$= 92 \times 10^{-15} \text{ L} = 92 \text{ fL (normal range} = 82 - 98)$$

$$MCH = (Hb \times 10)/RBC \text{ g}$$
$$= (8 \times 10)/2.6 \times 10^{12} \text{ g}$$
$$= 30.8 \times 10^{-12} \text{ g} = 30.8 \text{ pg (normal range} = 27 - 33)$$

$$MCHC = (100 \times MCH)/MCV \text{ g/dL}$$
$$= (100 \times 30.8)/92 \text{ g/dL}$$
$$= 33.5 \text{ g/dL} = (g\%) \text{ (normal range} = 30 - 35)$$

    i. This patient has anemia, as defined by her low hemoglobin concentration and low hematocrit; her RBC is decreased in proportion to the decreased hematocrit. Therefore, the reduced red cell mass consists of normally sized cells (rather than abnormally sized cells), which contain a normal concentration of hemoglobin. If viewed under the microscope cells would have normal size and chromicity.

    ii. ▼ A **blood smear** viewed under the microscope may be used with the CBC to investigate variations in cell size and in cell shape. When defects in red cell production are indicated, or abnormal cells are identified, an aspirate of the bone marrow may also be studied. ▼

6. Anemia and polycythemia.
   a. *Anemia is defined as a reduced red cell mass* (Figure 3-2).
   b. The symptoms of advanced anemia include fatigue, dizziness, and shortness of breath.
   c. A physical examination may indicate signs of compensatory increases in cardiac output, such as strong peripheral pulses and tachycardia. Upon auscultation, flow murmurs may be heard over the branch points of large arteries due to the low viscosity of the blood.
   d. *A high reticulocyte count suggests an increased rate of erythropoiesis, which reflects physiologic compensation for an increased rate of red cell loss.* There are two general causes of red cell loss:
      i. **Hemorrhage** causes immediate loss of red cells. *When plasma volume is restored, the reduced red cell mass is revealed by a low hematocrit.*
      ii. **Hemolytic anemia** (increased rate of red cell breakdown) is caused by a wide range of conditions, for example:
         - **Hereditary spherocytosis,** where a defective cytoskeleton causes increased red cell fragility.

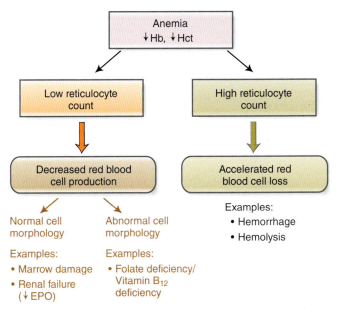

Figure 3-2. General causes of anemia. Accelerated loss of red blood cells stimulates red blood cell production, increasing the proportion of reticulocytes in circulating blood. Anemia caused by inadequate red blood cell production is characterized by a reduced reticulocyte count. EPO, erythropoietin; Hb, hemoglobin concentration; Hct, hematocrit.

- **Hemoglobinopathies** (e.g., **sickle cell disease**), which are inherited defects in hemoglobin structure that can result in the deformation and increased destruction of red cells.
  e. *In cases of anemia where the reticulocyte count is normal or reduced, a defect in red cell production or maturation is indicated.* There are three requirements for normal red cell production:
    i. Functional bone marrow. Hypoproliferation of red cells may result if the bone marrow is damaged (e.g., **aplastic anemia**).
    ii. **Erythropoietin.** Secretion of EPO is needed to stimulate the bone marrow. *Low EPO levels are found in patients with renal insufficiency.*
    iii. Adequate nutrient supply:
      - **Iron** is needed to make hemoglobin. *The most common cause of anemia worldwide is iron deficiency, which causes a **microcytic anemia.***
      - **Vitamin B$_{12}$** and **folic acid** are needed for DNA synthesis and red cell maturation; deficiencies cause **macrocytic (megaloblastic) anemia.**
  f. *Polycythemia is an abnormally high level of circulating red blood cells and is less commonly encountered than anemia.*
    i. A high red cell mass increases the viscosity of blood and increases the risk of thrombosis (formation of an intravascular blood clot).
    ii. The most common causes of polycythemia are associated with increased levels of EPO. For example, conditions that result in reduced arterial O_2 content, such as **lung disease, carbon monoxide poisoning,** or living at a **high altitude,** all stimulate EPO secretion.

Hemostasis

1. *A fine balance must be achieved between the activation of hemostatic mechanisms to prevent **bleeding,** and excessive activation, which can cause intravascular **thrombosis** and **embolism** (blood vessel occlusion).*

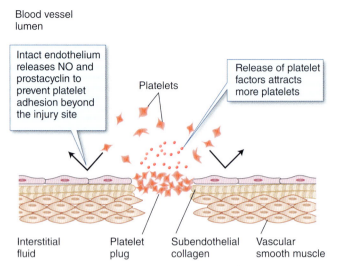

Figure 3-3. Primary hemostasis. A platelet plug is rapidly formed to stop blood loss from an injured vessel. Adhesion of platelets to subendothelial collagen is accompanied by the release of platelet factors, resulting in recruitment and aggregation of more platelets. Intact endothelial cells release factors such as nitric oxide (NO) and prostacyclin, which prevent platelet adhesion beyond the site of injury.

2. Three physiologic mechanisms interact to **prevent hemorrhage:**
   a. **Vasoconstriction** of small vessels reduces blood flow and increases the likelihood of vessel closure.
      i. At a site of injury, platelets release the vasoconstrictors **serotonin and thromboxane A$_2$.**
      ii. The clotting protein thrombin stimulates endothelial cells to secrete the potent vasoconstrictor **endothelin-1.**
   b. **Platelet plug formation** occurs at the site of damage in capillaries, arterioles, and venules. Plug formation is called **primary hemostasis** and involves three overlapping phases: **platelet adhesion, activation,** and **aggregation** (Figure 3-3).
   c. **Clot formation (coagulation)** occurs in which a fibrin mesh forms together with platelets and other trapped blood cells. Clot formation is called **secondary hemostasis** and is closely coordinated with primary hemostasis.
3. **Platelet adhesion** to the exposed subendothelial extracellular matrix occurs at a site of injury. Adhesion is mediated by a variety of different platelet receptors, including:
   a. The **von Willebrand factor** (vWF), which:
      i. Is a glycoprotein present in plasma and is released by endothelial cells and by activated platelets.
      ii. Binds to glycoprotein receptors on platelets and to collagens in the subendothelium to act as a key bridging molecule between platelets and sites of endothelial injury.
   b. Receptors of the **integrin family,** which bind platelets directly to extracellular matrix proteins (e.g., collagen).
   c. Other platelet receptors that promote platelet adhesion and activation include ligands associated with platelet activation (e.g., **thromboxane A$_2$**) as well as blood coagulation (e.g., **thrombin**).
   d. ▼ **von Willebrand's disease (vWD)** is the most common inherited bleeding disorder and is characterized by a deficiency or a defect in vWF. ▼

i. In addition to its role in platelet adhesion, vWF is carrier molecule for the procoagulant factor VIII in plasma and is needed to maintain normal factor VIII concentrations.

ii. *Therefore, a defect in vWF will result in both platelet dysfunction and coagulopathy, a characteristic feature of this disease that is shared with very few other conditions* (e.g., **disseminated intravascular coagulopathy**).

4. **Platelet activation** involves exocytosis of the contents of platelet granules and morphologic changes from a smooth membrane surface to one with finger-like cytoplasmic projections that increase adhesion and aggregation with other platelets. Activated platelets release many factors that promote hemostasis, including:

   a. **Adenosine diphosphate (ADP)**—A potent activator of other platelets to amplify the platelet activation response.

   b. **Serotonin** and **thromboxane A$_2$** to assist in hemostasis as vasoconstrictors.

   c. **vWF** to augment platelet adhesion and aggregation.

   d. **Ca^{2+}** and the clotting factors **fibrinogen** and **factor V** to facilitate coagulation.

   e. **Platelet-derived growth factor** to promote wound healing.

5. **Platelet aggregation** completes the formation of a platelet plug.

   a. The signaling molecules released during platelet activation amplify the platelet adhesion and activation responses and recruit more platelets to the site of injury.

   b. The platelet plug is prevented from extending beyond the site of injury by **prostacyclin** and **nitric oxide,** which are secreted from intact endothelial cells and inhibit platelet activation.

   c. ▼ **Antiplatelet drugs** are used to prevent thrombosis and target many of the steps of platelet activation and adhesion. A few examples include:

      i. **NSAIDs** (e.g., **aspirin**), which inhibit the production of thromboxane A$_2$ by blocking the key enzyme cyclooxygenase (COX), inhibiting platelet activation and secretion.

      ii. **Purinergic receptor inhibitors** (e.g., **clopidogrel** and **ticlopidine**), which antagonize the actions of ADP, and therefore inhibit platelet activation.

      iii. **Glycoprotein IIb/IIIa inhibitors** (e.g., **eptifibatide**). Glycoprotein IIb/IIIa is a platelet-specific adhesion molecule in the integrin family. *Blockade of this important adhesion receptor prevents the binding of fibrinogen, vWF, and other adhesion molecules to activated platelets.* ▼

6. ▼ **Thrombocytopenia** (low platelet count) has many causes, which can be broadly classified into three categories:

   a. Decreased platelet production by the bone marrow (e.g., **leukemia** or tumor infiltration of the marrow).

   b. Splenic sequestration of platelets (e.g., **splenomegaly** secondary to portal hypertension).

   c. Increased destruction of platelets (e.g., antibody-mediated platelet destruction in **idiopathic thrombocytopenic purpura**).

   d. *Regardless of the cause, thrombocytopenia results in an increased bleeding tendency.* ▼

7. ▼ Bleeding that results from defective platelet function typically occurs superficially in sites such as the skin (e.g., **petechiae and ecchymosis**)

and mucous membranes. In contrast, patients who bleed secondary to clotting factor dysfunction will suffer "deep" bleeds, such as in the deep subcutaneous tissues or muscles causing a **hematoma,** or in the joints causing **hemarthrosis.** ▼

8. **Blood coagulation** and blood clot formation occur when the plasma protein **fibrinogen** is proteolytically cleaved to produce **fibrin,** which subsequently becomes cross-linked into a stable mesh.

   a. Clotting can occur in the absence of platelet activation, but there is usually parallel activation of primary and secondary hemostasis and crosstalk between the pathways to ensure coordinated activation.

   b. In the classic description of coagulation, clotting may be initiated by one of two pathways: the **intrinsic pathway** or the **extrinsic pathway** (Figure 3-4).

   c. Each pathway consists of a cascade of reactions, in which inactive circulating precursor proteins ("**clotting factors**") become activated, in most cases by proteolytic cleavage.

   d. These chain reactions normally are not activated in the circulation because clotting factors are present at low concentration in plasma.

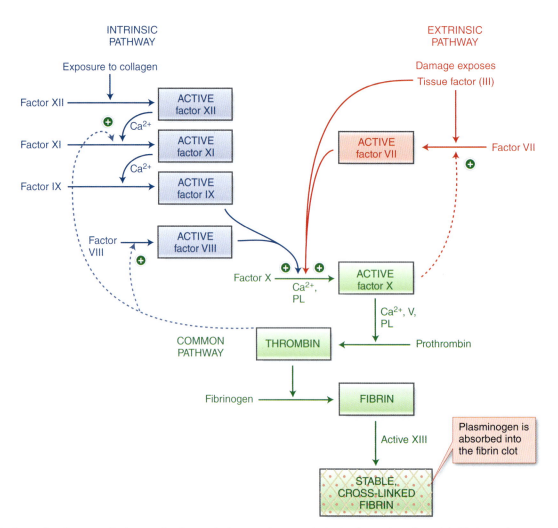

Figure 3-4. Secondary hemostasis. A cascade of coagulation reactions results in the formation of a stable fibrin mesh to prevent bleeding from a site of injury. The intrinsic pathway for coagulation is triggered by the exposure of subendothelial collagen; the extrinsic pathway is activated when tissue factor (a cell membrane lipoprotein) is exposed in injured tissue. The intrinsic and extrinsic pathways converge at the activation of factor X resulting in the generation of thrombin, which converts fibrinogen to fibrin.

e. *The intrinsic pathway is triggered when blood contacts a negatively charged surface (e.g., exposed subendothelial collagen; aggregations of platelets).*

f. *The extrinsic pathway is activated when blood contacts cells outside the vascular endothelium:*
   i. Nonvascular cells express a membrane protein called **tissue factor.**
   ii. *Exposure to tissue factor activates **factor VII,** triggering the final common pathway.*

g. The intrinsic and extrinsic pathways converge at the **common pathway** for coagulation, which begins with the activation of factor X.
   i. *Factor V is a key cofactor needed for activation of factor X.*
   ii. The plasma protein **prothrombin** (factor II) is cleaved by activated factor X to produce the protease **thrombin.**
   iii. Thrombin cleaves **fibrinogen** (factor I) and activates factor XIII, which cross-links **fibrin** into a stable mesh.

h. *The extrinsic pathway is the most important pathway for initiating thrombin activation; the intrinsic pathway is more important for maintaining thrombin generation.*

i. The classic descriptions of an intrinsic, extrinsic, and common pathway being independent is outdated since they form a network with reciprocal connections. For example:
   i. Activated factor IX of the intrinsic pathway activates factor VII of the extrinsic pathway.
   ii. In the reverse direction, a complex formed from tissue factor, activated factor VII, and Ca^{2+} in the extrinsic pathway activates factors IX and XI of the intrinsic pathway.
   iii. *Thrombin plays a central role in the coordination of the clotting cascades* because it stimulates formation of a fibrin clot, and it mediates positive feedback stimulation upstream in the intrinsic and extrinsic pathways.

9. Several **clotting indices** are used to assess the function of primary and secondary hemostatic mechanisms, including:

a. The **bleeding time,** which is a sensitive test of platelet function. A small standardized incision is made in the underside of the forearm, and the amount of time it takes for bleeding to stop is recorded. *Drugs such as aspirin, which inhibits platelet function, increase the bleeding time.*

b. The **prothrombin time (PT)** evaluates the extrinsic coagulation pathway. A sample of blood plasma is incubated with tissue factor in the presence of an excess of Ca^{2+}. Because there are variations between assays, corrections may be applied that normalize the prothrombin time of a sample to that of a normal sample (e.g., the **prothrombin ratio** and **international normalized ratio [INR]**). *The anticoagulant drug warfarin increases the PT.*

c. The **partial thromboplastin time (PTT)** indicates the performance of the intrinsic pathway. The intrinsic pathway is triggered by adding an activator surface (e.g., silica) plus phospholipid and Ca^{2+} to a plasma sample. *The anticoagulant drug heparin increases the PTT.*
   i. ▼ The bleeding disorders **hemophilia A** (classic hemophilia) and **hemophilia B** (Christmas disease) are X-linked recessive disorders that result in the deficiency of clotting factors VIII and IX, respectively. *An increase in PTT is expected in both conditions because both factors VIII and IX are part of the intrinsic pathway.* ▼

10. ▼ **Clotting factors II, VII, IX, and X** (and the anticoagulant proteins C and S) are produced in the liver and rely upon a **vitamin K-dependent** enzymatic reaction, γ-carboxylation of a glutamyl residue.

    a. In select patients (e.g., those at risk of developing a blood clot secondary to atrial fibrillation), it can be advantageous to block the function of γ-glutamyl carboxylase to induce a coagulopathy.

    b. The anticoagulant medication **warfarin** (Coumadin) inhibits the enzyme vitamin K epoxide reductase, making vitamin K unavailable for the γ-carboxylation reaction, which will halt the production of the vitamin K-dependent coagulation factors.

    c. *Careful monitoring of the PT/INR is required to ensure that excessive anticoagulation does not occur.* ▼

11. **Anticoagulation factors** are needed in the circulation to prevent random blood clotting. *The capillary endothelium is the main source of anticoagulant factors.*

    a. **Tissue factor pathway inhibitor (TFPI)** is anchored to the endothelial cell membrane and blocks the action of activated factor VII in the extrinsic pathway.

    b. **Antithrombin III** inhibits coagulation by binding to activated factor X and thrombin.

       i. ▼ **Heparin** is another important anticoagulant that is released endogenously from **mast cells** and **basophils** and is widely used as an anticoagulant drug. *Heparin functions by augmenting the anticoagulant effects of antithrombin III.* ▼

    c. **Thrombomodulin** inhibits coagulation by binding to thrombin.

    d. **Proteins C and S** act together to inactivate activated factors V and VIII.

       i. ▼ **Hypercoagulable states** occur when there is a defect in the anticoagulant pathway. The most common inherited cause of hypercoagulability is the **factor V Leiden** mutation. In this condition, factor V undergoes a mutation that renders it *resistant to the anticoagulant actions of protein C*, which allows factor V to remain activated, prolonging its thrombogenic effect. ▼

12. Fibrinolysis (Figure 3-5).

    a. *Fibrinolysis begins soon after a clot is formed* because the plasma protein **plasminogen** is among the serum proteins that are adsorbed into the clot at the time of its formation.

    b. The cleavage of plasminogen produces the protease **plasmin,** which breaks down fibrin and fibrinogen; the breakdown products of the fibrin mesh are scavenged by macrophages.

    c. The activation of plasminogen is mainly regulated by two factors, which are released from capillary endothelial cells: **tissue plasminogen activator (tPA)** and **urokinase.**

    d. ▼ **D-dimer** is a fibrin breakdown product not normally present in blood. *Levels are increased in thromboembolic diseases such as deep vein thrombosis, pulmonary embolism, and disseminated intravascular coagulation; absence of D-dimer helps to rule out thrombosis.* ▼

    e. *Plasmin must not become active in the circulation because it can also break down fibrinogen.* If plasmin escapes from the clot, it is rapidly bound and inactivated by the circulating plasma protein α_2-**antiplasmin.**

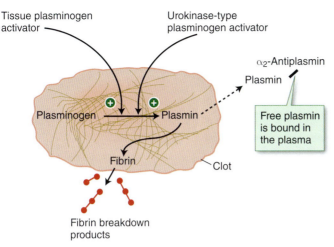

Figure 3-5. Fibrinolysis. The plasma protein plasminogen is incorporated into the fibrin mesh when a clot forms. The cleavage of plasminogen produces the protease plasmin, which breaks down fibrin. Tissue plasminogen activator and the urokinase-type plasminogen activator are factors secreted from endothelial cells, which catalyze the conversion of plasminogen to plasmin.

f.   ▼ In addition to the pharmacologic approaches to decreasing bleeding of antiplatelet drugs or anticoagulants, the **fibrinolytic agents** (**thrombolytics** or "**clot busters**") are used in some patients suffering from acute clotting emergencies such as **stroke, coronary thrombosis, pulmonary embolism,** or **deep vein thrombosis.** Agents include tPA, urokinase, streptokinase, and other synthetic agents. *The mechanism of action is activation of plasmin to break the clot down.* ▼

Study Questions

Directions: Each numbered item is followed by lettered options. Some options may be partially correct, but there is only *ONE BEST* answer.

1. A 61-year-old woman visits her family doctor complaining of severe fatigue, which has become progressively worse over the past 6 months. She is referred to a hematologist following the results of a complete blood cell count, which shows decreased hematocrit (24%), decreased hemoglobin concentration (8 g/dL), and decreased red blood cell count (2.6×10^{12}/L). The mean cell volume and reticulocyte counts are normal. Which type of anemia does the patient have?

   A. Macrocytic anemia (large red cells)
   B. Microcytic anemia (small red cells)
   C. Normocytic, hypoproliferative anemia
   D. Normocytic, hyperproliferative anemia
   E. No anemia is present

2. A 21-year-old woman returns to the United States from a student exchange visit to Australia. The morning after her flight, she is awakened because she is experiencing a pain throughout her right leg, which is of pale blue color. She is taken to the emergency department, where a clinical diagnosis determines that she has deep vein thrombosis. Which of the following laboratory findings would be consistent with this history?

A. Antithrombin III defect

B. Decreased hematocrit

C. Decreased fibrinogen

D. Decreased platelet count

E. Factor VIII defect

3. The addition of sodium citrate to banked blood inhibits coagulation. By what mechanism do citrate ions inhibit coagulation?

A. Antagonist to adenosine diphosphate

B. Antagonist to thromboxane A_2

C. Binds to factor VII

D. Binds to factor X

E. Chelates Ca^{2+} ions

4. A 42-year-old man with a family history of stroke and heart attack decides to take a daily aspirin tablet, having seen a television commercial. What is the main mechanism by which aspirin reduces the likelihood of intravascular blood clot formation?

A. Inhibition of the extrinsic clotting pathway

B. Inhibition of the intrinsic clotting pathway

C. Inhibition of platelet function

D. Stimulation of anticoagulant synthesis

E. Stimulation of fibrinolysis

F. Vasodilation

5. A 29-year-old woman with Crohn's disease develops mild vitamin K deficiency despite trying to eat a healthy diet. How will this vitamin deficiency manifest when blood clotting indices are measured?

A. Decreased platelet count

B. Decreased international normalized ratio (INR)

C. Prolonged bleeding time

D. Prolonged prothrombin time (PT)

E. Prolonged partial thromboplastin time (PTT)

The Cardiovascular System

CHAPTER 4

Fundamentals

1. The cardiovascular system consists of the heart, blood vessels, and the blood, which transports materials to and from all parts of the body.
2. *The heart pressurizes blood and provides the driving force for its circulation through the blood vessels.* Blood moves away from the heart in the arteries and returns to the heart in the veins.
3. Substances transported throughout the cardiovascular system can be categorized as:
   a. Materials entering the body from the external environment (e.g., O_2 and nutrients).
   b. Materials moving between cells within the body (e.g., hormones and antibodies).
   c. Waste products from cells requiring elimination (e.g., heat and CO_2).
4. *The exchange of materials between blood and interstitial fluid occurs across capillaries in the microcirculation.*

Organization of the Cardiovascular System

1. The heart has four chambers. The two **atria** are reservoirs for blood returning to the heart. The two **ventricles** are pumps that propel blood through the circulation (Figure 4-1).
2. A **septum** divides the heart into right and left sides.
   a. The right atrium is the reservoir serving the right ventricle, which pumps blood to the **pulmonary circulation** via the pulmonary artery.
   b. Blood returns from the lungs to the left atrium via the pulmonary veins.
   c. The left ventricle propels blood, via the aorta, to all other organs in the body through the **systemic circulation.**
   d. Circulation of blood is completed as the blood from the systemic circulation drains into the right atrium via the superior and inferior venae cavae.
3. The pulmonary and systemic circulations are referred to as the right and left sides:
   a. The "**right side**" is the pulmonary circulation, which is served by the right ventricle.
   b. The "**left side**" is the systemic circulation, which is served by the left ventricle.
   c. *The right side of the heart propels deoxygenated blood to the lungs, and the left side of the heart propels oxygenated blood to the tissues.*
4. ▼ **Heart failure** results from conditions that impair the ability of the heart to fill with, or to pump out, sufficient blood. Either side of the heart may be affected, or both sides may be affected in some patients.

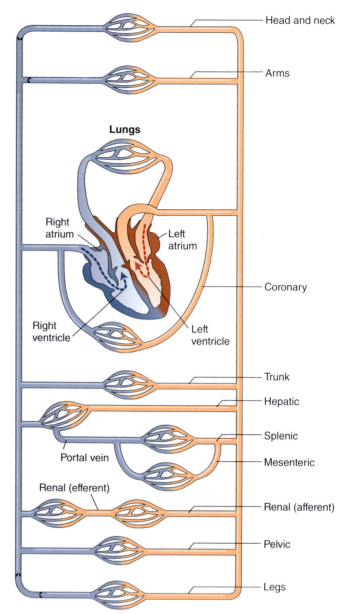

Figure 4-1. Overview of the cardiovascular system. Systemic and pulmonary circulations are arranged in series. Organ blood supply in the systemic circulation is arranged in parallel. Blue indicates deoxygenated blood; red indicates oxygenated blood.

a. In **right-sided heart failure,** there is a buildup of pressure that begins with the failing right ventricle and then moves to the right atrium and back to the systemic veins. Clinical signs include **jugular venous distention** and peripheral edema.

    i. *The most common cause of right-sided heart failure is preexisting left-sided heart failure.*

    ii. In **pulmonary hypertension** the increased pulmonary artery pressure strains the right ventricle, which can cause right-sided heart failure.

b. In **left-sided heart failure,** pressure begins to build in the left ventricle, then back to the left atrium and into the lungs. Clinical signs include **pulmonary edema** and shortness of breath. *The most common cause of left-sided heart failure is myocardial infarction.* ▼

5. *The pulmonary and systemic circulations are in series with each other, and all blood passing through one system must flow through the other system.*
   a. In the pulmonary circulation, blood flows at low pressure and receives the entire output of the right ventricle.
   b. Output from the left ventricle is distributed at higher pressure through organ systems arranged in parallel.
   c. One-way **valves** between the atria and the ventricles, between the ventricles and their receiving arteries, and within the systemic veins ensure that *blood flows in one direction around the circulation.*

Hemodynamics

1. Blood flow depends on the pressure difference between arteries and veins and on how much resistance to flow is offered by the vascular system.
2. **Pressure** is defined as a force exerted per unit area. Units of mm Hg are used clinically—1 mm Hg is equivalent to a pressure exerted by a 1 mm Hg column of mercury acting on an area of 1 cm^2.
3. In a closed system of fluid-filled tubes, such as the cardiovascular system, *the difference in pressure between the aorta and the large central veins drives blood flow through the systemic circulation.*
4. Blood is an incompressible fluid, and its volume cannot decrease when the ventricles contract. Instead, blood is pressurized, creating the potential energy for blood flow.
5. Blood pressure decreases over distance as potential energy is lost through **friction** between blood and blood vessel walls and between blood cells. For a given pressure difference between two points, the amount of flow that occurs depends on **resistance.**
6. According to **Ohm's law,** flow is proportional to the driving pressure gradient (ΔP) and is inversely proportional to resistance (R):

$$Q = \Delta P / R \qquad \text{Equation 4-1}$$

Q = Flow
ΔP = Difference in pressure, $P_1 - P_2$
R = Resistance

   a. ▼ Ohm's law may be applied in many situations. For example, **stenosis (severe narrowing) of the aortic valve** increases resistance to ejection of blood from the left ventricle. According to Ohm's law, left ventricular pressure must increase to maintain sufficient cardiac output. Chronically high left ventricular pressures can result in left ventricular hypertrophy and heart failure. ▼

7. Resistance.
   a. A tube will offer greater resistance (R) to fluid flow if its length (L) increases or if the radius (r) is decreased. Resistance is also greater if the fluid moved has a higher viscosity (η). **Poiseuille's law** describes the determinants of resistance:

$$R = 8L\eta/\pi r^4 \qquad \text{Equation 4-2}$$

R = Resistance

L = Length of tube
η = Viscosity of fluid
r = Radius of tube

b. *Radius is the dominant variable that determines resistance because radius is raised to the fourth power;* for example, doubling the vessel radius increases flow by a factor of 16 (Figure 4-2).

c. Physiologic control of vascular resistance is achieved by altering the blood vessel diameter through **vasoconstriction** and **vasodilation.**

d. ▼ Poiseuille's law is also applied when selecting an appropriate sized intravenous catheter to achieve **rapid fluid infusion.** For example, when attempting resuscitation of a hemodynamically unstable patient, a catheter is selected that maximizes radius and minimizes length to reduce its resistance. In this situation, a large-bore intravenous catheter placed in a peripheral vein is preferable to placing a long central venous line. ▼

e. *Resistance in the circulation can occur in series or in parallel.*

   i. When resistances are arranged in series, the total resistance (R_T) is the sum of individual resistances: $R_T = R_1 + R_2 + R_3 \ldots + R_n$.

   ii. When resistances are arranged in parallel, such as in organ systems in the systemic circulation, individual resistances contribute as reciprocals: $1/R_T = 1/R_1 + 1/R_2 + 1/R_3 \ldots + 1/R_n$, and the total resistance is much less than for serial resistances.

8. Compliance.

a. **Compliance** describes the distensibility of a structure and is defined as the volume change produced by a given pressure change:

$$C = \Delta V / \Delta P \qquad \text{Equation 4-3}$$

C = Compliance
ΔV = Volume change
ΔP = Pressure change

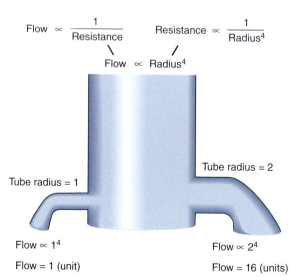

Flow $\propto \dfrac{1}{\text{Resistance}}$ Resistance $\propto \dfrac{1}{\text{Radius}^4}$

Flow $\propto$ Radius^4

Tube radius = 1

Tube radius = 2

Flow $\propto 1^4$

Flow = 1 (unit)

Flow $\propto 2^4$

Flow = 16 (units)

Figure 4-2. Effect of changing vessel radius on flow. If radius is doubled, resistance decreases by a factor of $2^4 = 16$. Flow increases 16-fold, assuming the driving pressure stays the same.

b. If a structure has low compliance (i.e., it is stiff), applying a normal pressure change (ΔP) will produce a small volume change (ΔV). Alternatively, delivering a normal volume will be associated with a large pressure change.

c. ▼ Low compliance is the central pathology in **diastolic heart failure.** Chronic hypertension makes the left ventricular wall thicker and noncompliant, impairing relaxation and diastolic filling. Ventricular compliance may be improved by treatment with calcium channel blockers to aid relaxation of the cardiac myocytes during diastole. ▼

Structure and Function of Cardiac Muscle

1. Atria and ventricles are composed of cardiac muscle cells, together with supporting connective tissue.
2. The atria are electrically isolated from the ventricles by a fibrous ring that is perforated by **four valve openings** (Figure 4-3):
   a. The **tricuspid valve** permits blood flow from the right atrium to the right ventricle.
   b. The **pulmonic valve** conveys blood from the right ventricle to the pulmonary artery.
   c. The **mitral valve** allows blood to flow from the left atrium into the left ventricle.
   d. The **aortic valve** conducts blood from the left ventricle into the aorta.
   e. The mitral and tricuspid valves are termed **atrioventricular** (AV) valves; the pulmonic and aortic valves are referred to as **semilunar** valves.
3. Cellular anatomy of ventricular muscle.

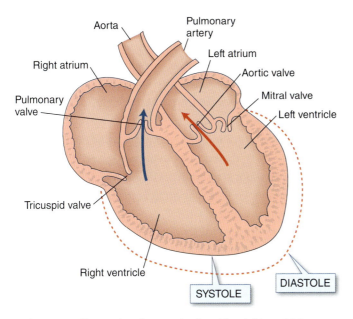

Figure 4-3. Anatomy of heart chambers and valves. The right ventricle pumps deoxygenated blood (*blue arrow*) to the lungs via the pulmonary arteries. The left ventricle pumps oxygenated blood (*red arrow*) to the systemic circulation via the aorta. Systole, in which the semilunar valves are open and the atrioventricular valves are closed, is shown.

Table 4-1. Comparison of Muscle Types

Characteristic	Cardiac Muscle	Skeletal Muscle	Smooth Muscle
Histologic appearance	Striated	Striated	Not striated
Stimulus for excitation	Pacemaker potentials and electrical coupling via gap junctions	Transmission at the neuromuscular junction	Variable: • Synaptic • Hormonal • Pacemakers • Coupling via gap junctions
Electrical activity	Long action potential plateau	No action potential plateau	Variable
Excitation-contraction coupling	Ca^{2+}-induced Ca^{2+} release from sarcoplasmic reticulum	Voltage sensor triggers Ca^{2+} release from sarcoplasmic reticulum	Variable: • Ca^{2+} entry via L-type channels • IP_3-mediated Ca^{2+} release from stores
Molecular basis of contraction	Ca^{2+}-troponin C	Ca^{2+}-troponin C	Ca^{2+}-calmodulin
Ending contraction	Repolarization of action potential	Breakdown of acetylcholine in neuromuscular junction	Myosin light-chain phosphatase activity
Control of force developed	Regulation of Ca^{2+} entry	Spatial and temporal summation	Latch bridge state
Metabolism	Oxidative	Oxidative and glycolytic fiber types	Oxidative

a. Cardiac muscle is striated and has an intracellular sarcomere structure that is similar to that of skeletal muscle. *Unlike skeletal muscle, cardiac muscle cells (myocytes) form a highly branched network* (Table 4-1 and Figure 4-4).

b. Myocytes are surrounded by a sarcolemma (plasma membrane), with transverse tubules (T tubules) that extend into the cell interior.

c. Sarcoplasmic reticulum is associated with every T tubule.

d. Myocyte-to-myocyte connections occur at structures called **intercalated disks.** *Gap junctions in intercalated disks provide low electrical resistance.*

e. A single adequate stimulus for action potential in one myocyte results in the rapid spread of excitation to all myocytes via gap junctions. This is known as the **all-or-none** electrical response of the heart.

f. ▼ In the patient with **coronary ischemia,** areas of heart muscle can begin to randomly depolarize. These myocytes are referred to as "irritable." Depolarization of one irritable myocyte rapidly propagates via the all-or-none principle, which can lead to a fatal **arrhythmia** (ventricular fibrillation or ventricular tachycardia). *Fatal arrhythmias are the most common cause of sudden death during a myocardial infarction.* ▼

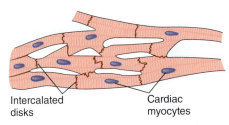

Intercalated   Cardiac
disks   myocytes

Figure 4-4. Electrical coupling of cardiac myocytes. Gap junctions in the intercalated disks provide a low-resistance pathway for the spread of electrical excitation.

4. Excitation-contraction coupling.
   a. *Cardiac muscle cells contract without nervous stimulation.*
   b. Pacemaker cells spontaneously generate action potentials, which spread through gap junctions.
   c. Action potentials conducted along T tubules open voltage-gated Ca^{2+} channels causing entry of extracellular Ca^{2+} into the cells.
   d. **Ca^{2+}-induced Ca^{2+} release** is triggered from internal sarcoplasmic reticulum stores.
   e. Almost all Ca^{2+} that interacts with **troponin C** to initiate contraction is derived from internal stores.
   f. Contraction occurs via the same **sliding filament** mechanism as was described in Chapter 1.
   g. *Relaxation depends on the removal of free cytosolic Ca^{2+}:*
      i. Ca^{2+} is moved back into the extracellular fluid via the **Na^+/Ca^{2+} exchangers** in the sarcolemma, which couple the inward transport of three Na^+ ions from the extracellular fluid to the outward transport of one intracellular Ca^{2+} ion.
      ii. **Ca^{2+}-ATPase** is used by all types of muscle and pumps Ca^{2+} back into the sarcoplasmic reticulum.
      iii. More rapid sequestration of Ca^{2+} causes faster muscle relaxation referred to as **positive lusitropy,** which occurs with sympathetic nerve stimulation when the heart rate (HR) is increased and ventricular ejection time is shorter.
   h. ▼ Drugs that increase the availability of intracellular free Ca^{2+} cause an increase in myocardial contractility referred to as **positive inotropy. Digitalis** (active agent digoxin) is the classic prototype **cardiac glycoside** with multiple cardiac effects, one of which is to increase myocardial contraction via greater loading of intracellular Ca^{2+} stores. This is accomplished via the following steps:
      i. Digitalis blocks the Na^+/K^+-ATPase on the myocyte of the cardiac cell membrane, yielding an increase in intracellular $[Na^+]$.
      ii. Increased intracellular $[Na^+]$ alters the electrochemical driving force for Na^+/Ca^{2+} exchange and results in the reversal of the normal transport direction, bringing Ca^{2+} into the cell.
      iii. Increased intracellular $[Ca^{2+}]$ causes more Ca^{2+} to be stored in the sarcoplasmic reticulum.
      iv. Subsequent excitation releases more Ca^{2+}, resulting in increased contractility.
      v. *Note: Although cardiac glycosides can reverse symptoms of heart failure they are now used with caution due to increased risk of sudden death.* ▼

Cardiac Electrophysiology

1. The **sinoatrial (SA) node** is the normal **pacemaker** of the heart and the origin of each normal heartbeat.
   a. The SA node is a collection of specialized myocytes near the site where the superior vena cava enters in the wall of the right atrium (Figure 4-5).
   b. Spontaneous depolarization of the SA node occurs, resulting in the generation of action potentials.
   c. Action potentials from the SA node spread rapidly throughout the atria via gap junctions between adjacent myocytes.
2. The **atrioventricular (AV) node** is the only electrical communication between the atria and the ventricles.
   a. *The AV node has very slow electrical conduction, ensuring that atrial contraction is completed before the ventricles are activated.*
   b. The AV node is continuous with the ventricular conducting system, which consists of the **atrioventricular bundle** (bundle of His), the left and right **bundle branches**, and the **Purkinje fiber** system.
3. The **ventricular conducting system** is composed of columns of specialized myocytes containing a small amount of contractile protein.
   a. The cells have large diameter and low electrical resistance for rapid conduction.
   b. A thick connective tissue sheath insulates the ventricular conducting system, ensuring that the *first electrical connection with working ventricular muscle occurs through* **Purkinje fibers.**
   c. Action potentials spread rapidly through the ventricular muscle via gap junctions between the adjacent myocytes.

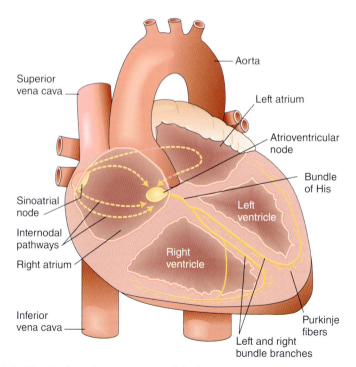

Figure 4-5. Electrical conducting system of the heart. Sinoatrial node → atrial muscle → atrioventricular node → bundle of His → bundle branches → Purkinje fibers → ventricular muscle.

Table 4-2. Ionic Currents Responsible for Ventricular Muscle and Nodal Action Potentials

Location	Phase 4	Phase 0	Phase 1	Phase 2	Phase 3
Ventricular muscle	Stable resting potential: I_K only	$I_{Na} \uparrow$ (fast)	$I_{Na} \downarrow$ I_{Cl} and $I_K \uparrow$	Plateau phase: $I_{Ca} \uparrow$ $I_K \downarrow$	Repolarization: $I_{Ca} \downarrow$ $I_K \uparrow$
Sinoatrial and atrioventricular nodes	Unstable pacemaker potential: I_f and $I_{Ca} \uparrow$ $I_K \downarrow$	$I_{Ca} \uparrow$ (slow)			Repolarization: $I_{Ca} \downarrow$ $I_K \uparrow$

d. The typical sequence of ventricular activation is:

   i. From the left side of the ventricular septum near the apex of the heart, and then to the inner surface of the myocardium in both ventricles in the region of the apex.

   ii. *Excitation spreads from the inner (endo-)myocardium to the outer (epi-) myocardium and from the apex toward the base.*

e. ▼ In **Wolff-Parkinson-White syndrome,** there is an accessory conduction pathway that creates a bidirectional link between the atria and the ventricles.

   i. A normal impulse that conducts from the atria down the AV node to the ventricles can travel up the accessory pathway to reexcite the atria.

   ii. Alternatively, an atrial impulse can first conduct down the accessory pathway, depolarizing the ventricles, and then travel up the AV node (retrograde) and reactivate the atria.

   iii. Either can lead to **paroxysmal supraventricular tachycardia,** which manifests as palpitations, syncope, hypotension, and sometimes heart failure. ▼

4. Ventricular muscle action potential.

   a. Action potentials arriving at the ventricular muscle from the ventricular conducting system trigger the rapid spread of action potentials in all ventricular myocytes.

   b. The ventricular muscle action potential has a very long duration (250 ms) with the following **five phases** 0 through 4 (Table 4-2 and Figure 4-6):

      i. **Phase 4** is the interval between action potentials when the ventricular muscles are at their stable **resting membrane potential.**

      ii. **Phase 0** is the **initial rapid upstroke** that occurs immediately after stimulation. Membrane potential moves from its resting value of about -90 mV to a peak of about $+30$ mV during phase 0.

      iii. **Phase 1** is a **partial repolarization** of the membrane potential from its peak value of $+30$ mV to about 0 mV.

      iv. **Phase 2,** also known as the **plateau phase,** is a dramatic slowing of repolarization.

      v. **Phase 3** is the **repolarization** of membrane potential back to the resting value.

5. SA node action potential.

   a. SA nodal cells are pacemakers because their membrane potential depolarizes spontaneously during phase 4, which is called the **pacemaker potential** or **diastolic depolarization** (Table 4-2 and Figure 4-7).

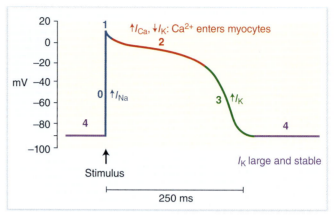

Figure 4-6. Ventricular action potential. Phase 4 = stable resting membrane potential; phase 0 = rapid depolarization upon stimulation; phase 1 = partial repolarization; phase 2 = plateau phase; and phase 3 = repolarization. I_{Na}, Na$^+$ current; I_{Ca}, Ca^{2+} current; I_K, K$^+$ current.

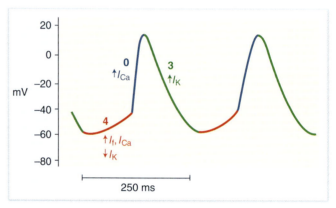

Figure 4-7. Nodal action potential. Phase 4 = unstable pacemaker potential; phase 0 = slow depolarization upon stimulation; and phase 3 = repolarization. I_f, nonselective cation current; I_{Ca}, Ca^{2+} current; I_K, K$^+$ current.

      i. The maximum membrane potential difference in pacemaker cells is about -60 mV, but *there is no stable period of resting membrane potential.*

     ii. When the pacemaker potential reaches a threshold voltage of about -40 mV, the action potential is triggered in the cells of the SA node.

   iii. When compared with ventricular muscle, phase 0 in the SA node is slow and the action potential duration is shorter.

  b. Action potential generation in the AV node is similar to the SA node but has a slower phase 4 depolarization.

6. ▼ A knowledge of the cardiac action potential helps in the understanding of the mechanism of antiarrhythmic agents.

  a. There are **four classes of antiarrhythmics,** based on their site of action, class I, sodium channel blockers; class II, beta blockers; class III, potassium channel blockers; and class IV, calcium channel blockers.

  b. The SA node and AV node action potential upstroke (phase 4) is Ca^{2+} dependent, whereas the ventricular upstroke (phase 0) is Na$^+$ dependent. As such, class I antiarrhythmics are effective in the treatment of ventricular ectopy (additional heart beats of ventricular origin), and class II and class

IV antiarrhythmics are effective in slowing conduction in the SA and AV nodes. ▼

7. Hierarchy of pacemakers.

   a. *The SA node is the normal pacemaker of the heart because it has the most rapid rate of phase 4 (diastolic) depolarization.*

   b. A person is in **normal sinus rhythm** when cardiac excitation progresses from the SA node through the entire conduction pathway.

   c. The intrinsic rate of SA node firing is about 100 beats/min. Normal **parasympathetic tone** reduces the SA node firing rate to about 70 beats/min at rest.

      i. Endurance athletes have enhanced parasympathetic tone, which results in the classic finding of a slow resting HR in trained individuals.

   d. The AV node becomes the pacemaker if the SA node fails or transmission to the AV node fails. These patients are in **nodal rhythm** and typically have resting heart rates of 45–55 beats/min.

   e. ▼ In patients with **complete heart block** (see normal and abnormal heart rhythm), there is no transmission through the AV node; the His-Purkinje fibers pace the heart between 20 and 40 beats/min.

      i. Slower pacemaker activity in distal parts of the conducting system allows the heart to continue beating if the SA node fails. However, these patients have **bradycardia** (slow HR) and reduced cardiac output.

      ii. For example, **sick sinus syndrome** occurs when the SA node becomes fibrotic and loses its ability to spontaneously depolarize. Patients have bradycardia and symptoms of hypoperfusion such as dizziness, syncope, weakness, and fatigue. ▼

8. Refractory periods (Figure 4-8).

   a. The normal mechanical pumping cycle of the heart requires a single excitation event.

   b. Any additional action potentials spread rapidly through coupled myocardial cells and produce **arrhythmias** (inappropriate heart beats).

   c. If the ventricular rate is excessive, there is insufficient time between beats for the ventricles to fill.

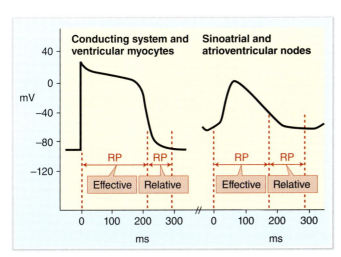

Figure 4-8. Cardiac action potentials. Cardiac action potentials have long refractory periods (RP). No stimulus can produce another action potential during the effective refractory period.

d. ▼ **Circular (reentry) conduction** occurs when control by the pacemaker fails and each spread of excitation through the ventricles triggers the next.

   i. Reentry is normally prevented because ventricular muscle cells have a long **effective (absolute) refractory period** from the onset of phase 0 to midway through phase 3.

   ii. Treatment with drugs such as beta blockers and calcium channel blockers, which extend the refractory period, can be effective at preventing reentry arrhythmias. ▼

e. ▼ The long refractory period of the AV nodal cells also protects against conduction of rapid atrial arrhythmias to the ventricles. For example, in **atrial fibrillation,** the atrial rate is between 350 and 500 impulses per minute. Without the refractory properties of the AV node, the ventricular rate would correspond with the atrial rate, which would be incompatible with life. ▼

9. Autonomic regulation of HR (Figure 4-9).

a. If the autonomic nerves to the heart are cut (such as may occur during a heart transplant), the spontaneous HR at rest is approximately 100 beats/min.

b. Parasympathetic tone reduces the typical resting HR to approximately 70 beats/min, and parasympathetic stimulation reduces the HR further, referred to as a **negative chronotropic effect.**

   i. Parasympathetic nerves release acetylcholine, which acts via **M2-muscarinic receptors** on the nodal cells.

   ii. ▼ The muscarinic receptor antagonist **atropine** can be used to treat symptomatic bradycardia. Atropine blocks parasympathetic tone, allowing sympathetic tone to continue unchecked. ▼

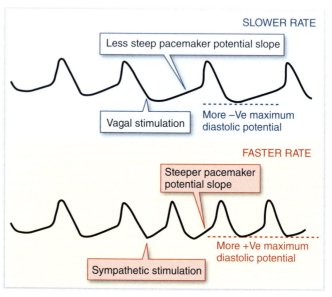

Figure 4-9. Effects of autonomic nerve stimulation on nodal action potentials. Parasympathetic (vagal) stimulation reduces the heart rate by hyperpolarizing the nodal cells and reducing the slope of pacemaker potentials. Sympathetic stimulation increases the heart rate by depolarizing the nodal cells and increasing the slope of pacemaker potentials.

c. Sympathetic nerve stimulation or circulating catecholamines increase the HR and produce a **positive chronotropic effect.**

   i. Sympathetic nerves release norepinephrine, acting on the β_1-adrenergic receptors.

   ii. Conduction speed through the AV node is also increased, known as **positive dromotropy.**

d. ▼ Activation of the sympathetic nervous system occurs in response to **stress.** Signs include tachycardia as well as pale cool skin, sweating, and dilation of the pupils. It is important to identify the cause of sympathetic drive, which may be intrinsic or extrinsic. Examples of intrinsic activation include pain, fear, anxiety, or hypotension; examples of extrinsic activation include use of drugs such as caffeine, cocaine, methamphetamines, or ephedrine. ▼

10. The electrocardiogram (ECG).

a. The spread of action potentials through the myocytes produces small voltages that can be measured on the surface of the body with an ECG.

b. A standard ECG is obtained by placing an electrode on each limb and at six specific locations on the anterior chest wall.

c. In a **lead,** one electrode is regarded as the positive side of a voltmeter and another is the negative side. A lead reports changes in voltage difference between the positive and negative electrodes.

d. By varying which electrode is regarded as positive or which is negative, a standard set of **12 leads** provides a range of views of electrical events in the heart.

e. Figure 4-10 illustrates the major waves on an ECG, together with standard intervals and segments and standard calibrations of time and voltage.

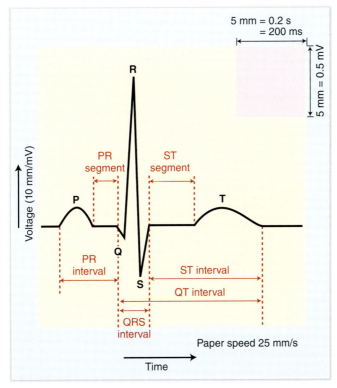

Figure 4-10. Electrocardiogram (ECG). Typical recording from lead II showing ECG waves, segments, and intervals, and standard calibrations for time and voltage.

f. **ECG waveforms** are produced by momentary changes in voltage differences during the spread of cardiac excitation.

　　i.   The **P wave** represents atrial depolarization.

　　ii. The **QRS complex** is produced by ventricular depolarization.

　　iii. The **T wave** results from ventricular repolarization.

　　iv. Atrial repolarization is obscured by the QRS complex.

g. ▼ *Heart muscle mass is depicted as amplitude on the ECG.* For example:

　　i.   Electrical activity in nodal and conducting tissue is not seen on an ECG because the amount of tissue is too small to produce measurable voltage differences at the body surface.

　　ii. The P wave is smaller than the QRS complex because atria have less mass than ventricles.

　　iii. **Left ventricular hypertrophy** is identified if the sum of voltage deflections for the S wave in lead V_1 and the R wave in leads V_5 or V_6 $\geq$35 mm.

　　iv. **Right ventricular hypertrophy** is characterized by an R wave that is larger than the S wave in V_1. ▼

h. ▼ *The QT interval corresponds to the duration of phase 2 of the ventricular action potential.* A longer phase 2 is represented on the ECG as a **prolonged QT interval,** which may set up a dangerous form of ventricular tachycardia called **torsade de pointes.**

　　i.   Class III antiarrhythmic drugs cause a prolonged phase 2 of the action potential because *repolarization is delayed when the K^+ channels are blocked.* Careful monitoring of the QT interval is a must when initiating therapy with a class III drug (e.g., amiodarone). ▼

i. There are two **ECG lead systems** (Table 4-3):

　　i.   The frontal (vertical) plane is defined by **six limb leads.**

　　ii. The transverse plane is perpendicular to the frontal plane and is defined by six **precordial chest leads.**

j. Every lead has a unique axis within its plane. Frontal plane leads are composed of three **bipolar limb leads** (I, II, and III), and three **augmented unipolar limb leads** (aV_R, aV_L, and aV_F) (Figure 4-11A).

　　i.   In bipolar leads the positive electrode placed on one limb is compared to a negative electrode placed on another limb.

　　ii. Augmented unipolar limb leads are defined by using each limb electrode as a positive electrode referenced to a null point obtained by adding the potential from the other two limb leads.

　　iii. The bipolar limb leads alone, with electrode connections to the left arm, the right arm, and the left leg form an equilateral triangle with the heart at its center, called **Einthoven's triangle.**

k. All six frontal plane leads together can be represented as a circle in which each lead occupies one axis to produce the **hexaxial reference system,** which is used to report the direction of electrical vectors (Figure 4-11B).

l. Each precordial chest electrode is a positive electrode terminal, and can be compared to the virtual center of the heart, estimated electronically from the average of the limb leads.

m. Figure 4-12 illustrates the concept of an **electrical vector** and how one may appear on different ECG leads.

Table 4-3. Placement and Polarity of Electrocardiogram (ECG) Electrodes

Lead System	Lead Name	+Ve Electrode	−Ve (or Reference) Electrode
Frontal plane leads	I	LA	RA
	II	LL	RA
	III	LL	LA
	aV$_R$	RA	LA and LL combined
	aV$_L$	LA	RA and LL combined
	aV$_F$	LL	RA and LA combined
Transverse plane precordial leads	V$_1$	Fourth intercostal space to the right of the sternum	
	V$_2$	Fourth intercostal space to the left of the sternum	Virtual reference to center of heart
	V$_4$	Fifth intercostal space in the midclavicular line	
	V$_3$	Midway between V$_2$ and V$_4$	
	V$_6$	Fifth intercostal space in the midaxillary line	
	V$_5$	Midway between V$_4$ and V$_6$	

LA, left arm; LL, left leg; RA, right arm.

i. The ECG is an extracellular recording that views cells from the outside. Resting myocytes have a negative voltage on the inside or, stated differently, they have a positive voltage on the outside of the cell membrane.

ii. A region of myocytes that has depolarized is negative on the outside when compared to neighboring cells at rest, creating a voltage difference between adjacent regions, which is a vector quantity (i.e., has size and direction).

iii. Vectors are represented using an arrow to illustrate their size and direction. By convention, the head of the vector (arrow) points toward the positive voltage (i.e., toward tissue not yet depolarized).

iv. The average vector changes in size and direction from moment to moment to produce the waves seen on an ECG.

v. Each of the 12 leads view cardiac excitation from different angles so that the waveform looks different in each lead.

n. When estimating the direction of vectors by assessing the ECG, *the largest net deflection occurs in the lead that is roughly parallel to the electrical event; if a lead shows no net deflection (i.e., the event is **isoelectric**), then*

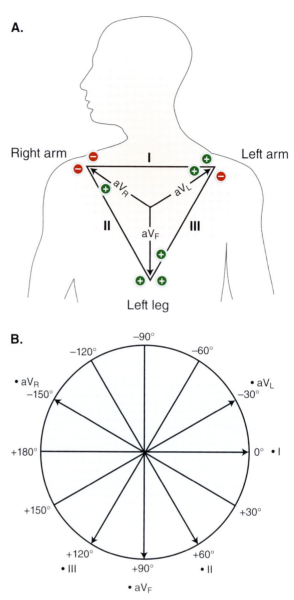

Figure 4-11. Frontal plane electrocardiogram leads. **A.** Einthoven's triangle, formed by bipolar limb leads I, II, and III. Directions of the unipolar limb leads aV_R, aV_L, and aV_F are also shown. **B.** Hexaxial reference circle, showing the axis of each frontal plane lead.

the electrical vector is perpendicular to the axis of that lead. Knowledge of the orientation of leads in the frontal plane is necessary to estimate vector direction in this way.

o. The mean axis of ventricular depolarization (i.e., the QRS complex) is the vector most commonly evaluated. The following ranges are described on the hexaxial system:

   i. **Normal axis** = QRS axis between −30° and +90°.

   ii. **Left axis deviation** = QRS axis less than −30°.

   iii. **Right axis deviation** = QRS axis greater than +90°.

   iv. **Extreme axis deviation** = QRS axis between −90° and 180°.

   v. Occasionally all leads show biphasic waves causing an **indeterminate axis.**

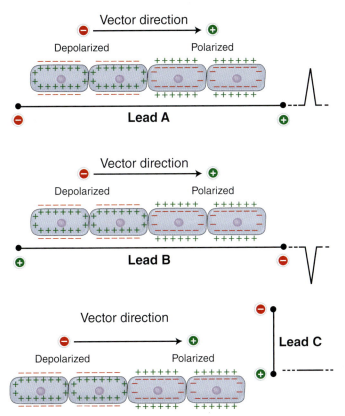

Figure 4-12. An electrical vector recorded by different leads. Adjacent areas of cells at different potentials produce a vector. A large positive recording in lead A is seen because the vector is parallel to lead A and is directed at its positive terminal. A large negative recording is seen in lead B because the vector is parallel to lead B but directed at its negative terminal. No net signal is recorded in lead C because it is perpendicular to the vector.

p. ▼ **Ventricular hypertrophy** is the thickening (or enlargement) of the myocardium and is a common cause of axis deviation.

   i. An increased left ventricular mass biases the direction of the net QRS vector toward the left. **Left axis deviation** can also occur when the abdominal contents physically push the heart up and to the left, such as that which occurs in patients who are **obese or pregnant.**

   ii. Patients with **right ventricular hypertrophy** usually have a **right axis deviation.** ▼

q. Figure 4-13 shows an example of left axis deviation.

   i. The sum of all deflections (net deflection) in the QRS complex of lead aV_R is near zero. The mean axis is, therefore, approximately perpendicular to this lead, corresponding to the axis of lead III.

   ii. There is a large net QRS deflection recorded in lead III, confirming that the electrical vector in this case is roughly parallel to lead III.

   iii. Because the net deflection is negative in lead III, the QRS vector is directed at the negative end of lead III at an angle of approximately $-60°$ on the hexaxial reference system.

11. Normal and abnormal heart rhythm.

   a. In **normal sinus rhythm,** a P wave is followed at normal intervals by a QRS complex and a T wave (see Figure 4-14A).

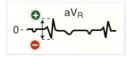

When there is no net recording in a lead (the isoelectric lead), this indicates that the direction of the QRS vector is perpendicular to the lead (aV$_R$ in this case).

LEFT AXIS DEVIATION

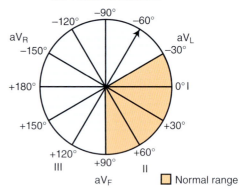

When the direction of the QRS vector is roughly parallel to a lead, this produces a large net QRS recording (lead III in this case).

A net negative (downward) recording indicates that this vector is directed toward the negative terminal of the lead III (−60°).

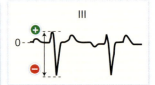

Figure 4-13. Inspection method to assess the mean QRS axis (mean electrical axis of the heart).

    i. HR, in beats/min, is calculated by dividing the R-R interval (expressed in seconds) into 60.

    ii. *HR above 100 beats/min is described as* **tachycardia;** *a HR below 60 beats/min is described as* **bradycardia.**

  b. A **premature atrial beat** is revealed when a P wave occurs earlier than expected and is followed by the usual QRS complex and T wave (see Figure 4-14B).

  c. **Paroxysmal atrial tachycardia** is a rapid run of heart beats that begins suddenly and ends abruptly; P waves precede each QRS complex, showing that beats originate in the atria (see Figure 4-14C).

  d. In **atrial fibrillation** (see Figure 4-14D), there is chaotic electrical activity; no P waves can be defined, and QRS complexes occur at irregular intervals, reflecting random depolarization of the AV node.

    i. The pulse is classically described as "irregularly irregular."

    ii. ▼ *In atrial fibrillation, stasis of blood often occurs in the atrial appendages due to the loss of atrial contraction.* Anticoagulation therapy may be needed to counter the risk of **thromboembolism.** ▼

  e. **Heart block** is due to varying degrees of impaired conduction through the AV node.

    i. In **first-degree heart block,** the PR interval is abnormally long at a normal HR, indicating delayed conduction through the AV node (see Figure 4-14E).

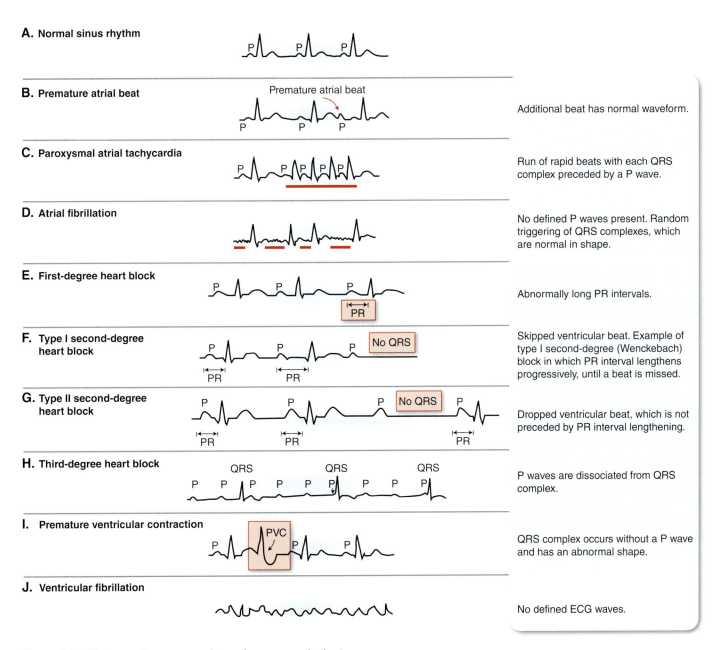

A. Normal sinus rhythm

B. Premature atrial beat
Premature atrial beat

Additional beat has normal waveform.

C. Paroxysmal atrial tachycardia

Run of rapid beats with each QRS complex preceded by a P wave.

D. Atrial fibrillation

No defined P waves present. Random triggering of QRS complexes, which are normal in shape.

E. First-degree heart block

Abnormally long PR intervals.

F. Type I second-degree heart block

Skipped ventricular beat. Example of type I second-degree (Wenckebach) block in which PR interval lengthens progressively, until a beat is missed.

G. Type II second-degree heart block

Dropped ventricular beat, which is not preceded by PR interval lengthening.

H. Third-degree heart block

P waves are dissociated from QRS complex.

I. Premature ventricular contraction

QRS complex occurs without a P wave and has an abnormal shape.

J. Ventricular fibrillation

No defined ECG waves.

Figure 4-14. Electrocardiogram recordings of common arrhythmias.

ii. In **second-degree heart block** there is intermittent failure of the AV node so that not every P wave is followed by a QRS complex. There are two types of second-degree heart block:
- **Mobitz type I,** or **Wenckebach,** block is a benign rhythm whose origin is the AV node (see Figure 4-14F). It is characterized by progressive lengthening of the PR interval on consecutive beats, followed by a dropped QRS complex.
- **Mobitz type II** second-degree heart block is a more ominous rhythm and has its origin in the distal His-Purkinje system. *Dropped ventricular beats are not preceded by PR interval lengthening* (see Figure 4-14G). The block may persist for two or more beats, yielding an atrial to ventricular ratio of 2:1, 3:1, and so on. *Type II heart block may progress quickly to complete heart block.*

iii. **Third-degree (complete) heart block** occurs when the atrial rhythm is completely dissociated from the ventricular rhythm (see Figure 4-14H).

- When a period of block begins, there is often an interval of 5–30 seconds before the ventricular conducting system takes over as the pacemaker, which may cause fainting due to lack of cerebral blood flow. This pattern of periodic fainting is called **Stokes-Adams syndrome.**
- *Treatment of third-degree heart block includes implanting a pacemaker to maintain an adequate HR and blood pressure.*

iv. **Premature ventricular contractions (PVCs)** occur with no preceding P wave (see Figure 4-14I). The origin of the ventricular excitation is within the ventricular conducting system or from a ventricular muscle focus. The QRS complex from a PVC has an irregular shape, due to the abnormal direction of electrical excitation.

v. Abnormal ventricular pacemakers, which are often damaged or unstable areas of ventricular myocardium, can drive **ventricular tachycardia.** This is a dangerous type of arrhythmia because the beating frequency may be too high to allow adequate ventricular filling.

vi. Ventricular tachycardia may degenerate into **ventricular fibrillation** associated with random chaotic electrical activity (see Figure 4-14J). *Ventricular fibrillation is fatal within a short period of time due to lack of coordinated ventricular contraction.*

- ▼ *The most common cause of death during a **myocardial infarction** is fatal arrhythmia (ventricular fibrillation or ventricular tachycardia).* ▼

vii. ▼ *Arrhythmias are often caused by electrolyte abnormalities.* For example, as plasma K^+ concentration increases, **hyperkalemia** produces the following sequence of cardiotoxic effects: peaked T waves → prolonged PR interval → widening of QRS complex → AV node conduction block → loss of P waves → merging of the QRS complex with the T wave to produce a "**sine wave**" **pattern** that can degenerate into ventricular fibrillation or asystole. ▼

The Cardiac Cycle

1. The cardiac cycle is the repetitive electrical and mechanical events that occur with each beat of the heart. Electrical events precede mechanical events, which result from the entry of Ca^{2+} into the myocytes during cardiac action potentials. ECG waves can be correlated with mechanical events:
   a. The P wave precedes atrial contraction.
   b. During the PR segment, there is no apparent electrical activity in the ECG. During this time, there is conduction through the AV node and the ventricular conducting system.
   c. The QRS complex precedes contraction of the ventricle.
   d. The T wave of ventricular repolarization precedes ventricular relaxation.

2. Blood is pressurized by ventricular contraction and then ejected into the circulation during systole. Muscle relaxation is followed by ventricular filling during diastole. Mechanical events of the cardiac cycle occur in five phases (Figure 4-15):

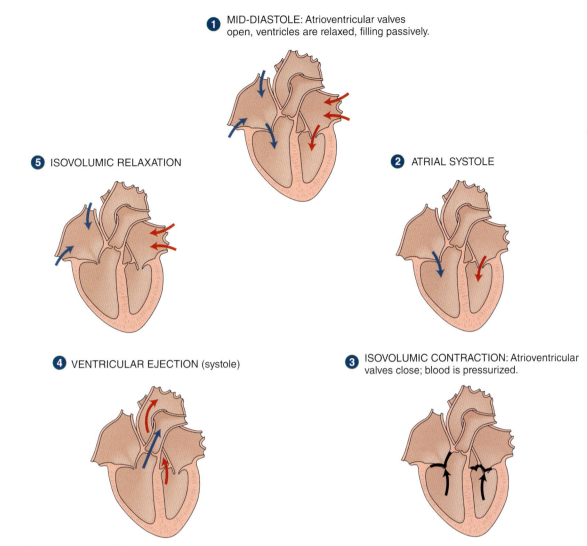

Figure 4-15. Major phases of the cardiac cycle.

a. **Ventricular diastole.** Throughout most of ventricular diastole, the atria and ventricles are relaxed. The AV valves are open, and the ventricles passively fill.

b. **Atrial systole.** During atrial systole, a small amount of additional blood is pumped into the ventricles.

c. **Isovolumic ventricular contraction.** Initial contraction increases ventricular pressure, closing the AV valves. Blood is pressurized during isovolumic ventricular contraction.

d. **Ventricular ejection (systole).** The semilunar valves open when ventricular pressures exceed pressures in the aorta and pulmonary artery. Ventricular ejection of blood follows.

e. **Isovolumic relaxation.** The semilunar valves close when the ventricles relax and pressure in the ventricles decreases. The AV valves open when pressure in the ventricles decreases below atrial pressure.

f. Atria fill with blood throughout ventricular systole, allowing rapid ventricular filling at the start of the next diastolic period.

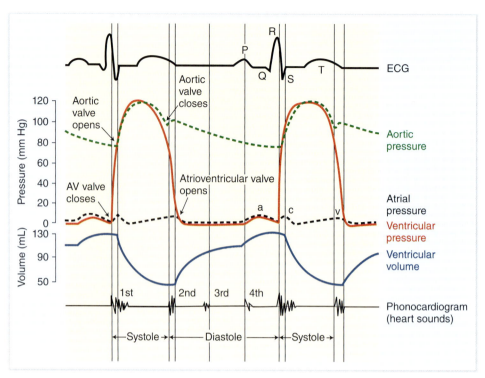

Figure 4-16. Wiggers diagram, a correlation of electrical and mechanical events during the cardiac cycle. A phonocardiogram records heart sounds.

3. The **Wiggers diagram** allows correlation of the following electrical and mechanical events during the cardiac cycle (Figure 4-16):

a. **Left ventricular pressure:**

   i. Is normally 0–10 mm Hg at the end of diastole but increases rapidly as the ventricles contract.

   ii. The **mitral valve** closes when the left ventricular pressure exceeds left atrial pressure.

   iii. AV valves are not forced back into the atria during ventricular contraction because they are anchored to the papillary muscles via the fibrous **chordae tendineae.**

   iv. The **aortic valve** opens when the left ventricular pressure increases above the aortic diastolic pressure, typically about 80 mm Hg.

   v. Forceful contraction during early ventricular ejection increases the left ventricular pressure to a peak value of about 120 mm Hg, corresponding to the **aortic systolic blood pressure.**

   vi. As the ventricular contraction weakens, the left ventricular pressure decreases. When the left ventricular pressure decreases just below the aortic blood pressure, the aortic valve closes.

   vii. Left ventricular pressure decreases rapidly as the muscle relaxes; when the pressure decreases just below the left atrial pressure, the mitral valve opens. Ventricular filling occurs at low pressures, reflecting the left atrial pressure.

b. **Aortic pressure:**

   i. *Aortic pressure increases in concert with the left ventricular pressure during ventricular ejection.*

   ii. Vibration caused by closure of the aortic valve causes a deviation in the aortic pressure, called the **dicrotic notch.**

iii. The aortic pressure decreases between ventricular beats as blood continues to flow from the aorta into the circulation.

iv. *Diastolic blood pressure is the aortic pressure minimum recorded just before the next ventricular ejection.*

c. **Left atrial pressure:**

i. Is normally no greater than 10 mm Hg at any time during the cardiac cycle.

ii. Three small peaks, or waves, are identified and denoted as a, c, and v:

- The **a wave** is produced by atrial systole.
- The **c wave** occurs when the mitral valve bulges into the left atrium during ventricular contraction.
- The **v wave** reflects passive atrial filling during ventricular systole.

d. ▼ Atrial pressure waves also occur on the right side of the heart. Inspection of the **external jugular vein** during physical examination provides information about right atrial pressure.

i. A "**cannon**" **a wave** is seen in jugular venous pulsations if the atria contract when the AV valves are closed. This occurs in **complete heart block** when the atria and the ventricles contract independently.

ii. A large v wave can be seen in the jugular vein during **tricuspid regurgitation** as additional blood enters the right atrium from the right ventricle. ▼

e. ▼ *Right-sided heart failure results in increased right-sided heart pressures and* **jugular venous distention (JVD).** *In the* **abdominojugular reflux test** *the examiner presses on the liver to increase venous return to the right side of the heart. JVD is observed if the patient has right ventricular failure.* ▼

f. **Left ventricular end-diastolic volume (LVEDV):**

i. LVEDV is about 140 mL in a normal heart at rest.

ii. *Ventricular systole normally ejects a little over one-half of the end-diastolic volume at rest,* producing a typical **end-systolic volume** of about 60–70 mL.

iii. *The* **stroke volume** *(SV) is the difference between end-diastolic volume and end-systolic volume.*

iv. Ventricular filling is rapid in early diastole. Ventricular volume reaches a plateau during passive filling, called **diastasis,** because ventricular compliance decreases as the chamber fills.

v. **Atrial systole** normally contributes about 10% of ventricular filling at rest.

- As the HR increases, the amount of time available for passive ventricular filling decreases, and the contribution of atrial systole can increase to over 30% of end-diastolic volume.
- ▼ Patients with atrial fibrillation lack this "**atrial kick**" and may have inadequate ventricular filling, particularly during physical activity.
- *Patients with cardiovascular disease may rely on the atrial kick to maintain adequate cardiac output; without it, they may develop heart failure.* ▼

4. Normal heart sounds.

a. **AV valves** prevent backflow of blood into the atria during ventricular contraction.

b. **Semilunar valves** prevent backflow of blood from the aorta and pulmonary artery to the ventricles during diastole.

c. Heart valves open and close passively in response to pressure differences across the valves. *Valve opening is silent in the normal heart.*

d. Closure of the valves produces vibrations that are heard as heart sounds (Figure 4-17A). A **phonocardiogram** is a recording of sounds that occur during the cardiac cycle.

e. The **first heart sound (S_1)**, a "**lub,**" is generated by the closing of the mitral (M_1) and tricuspid (T_1) valves.

   i. Closure of the tricuspid valve follows so closely after mitral valve closure that these sounds are perceived as a single sound.

   ii. The larger diameter of the AV valves produces a low-pitched sound that is best heard with the bell of a stethoscope.

   iii. The anatomic complexity of the AV valve apparatus contributes to the longer duration of the first heart sound compared to the second.

f. The **second heart sound (S_2)**, a "**dup,**" occurs when the semilunar valves snap close at the onset of diastole.

   i. The second heart sound has a crisper, higher pitch and shorter duration, and is best heard with the diaphragm of a stethoscope because the pressure gradients producing valve closure are larger.

   ii. The second sound is composed of aortic (A_2) and pulmonic (P_2) valve closures.

g. During inspiration, A_2 and P_2 are often heard as separate sounds. The **splitting of S_2** is caused by delayed closure of the pulmonic valve and earlier closure of the aortic valve (Figure 4-17B).

   i. Decreased intrathoracic pressure on inspiration allows the distensible pulmonary circulation to receive a greater SV from the right ventricle, prolonging right ventricular systole and delaying the P_2 sound.

   ii. Increased pulmonary vascular capacitance during inspiration also reduces venous return to the left atrium, which shortens left ventricular systole and produces an earlier A_2 sound.

   iii. ▼ **Paradoxical splitting of S_2** occurs when closure of the aortic valve is delayed, causing P_2 to occur first, followed by A_2. The most notable causes are **aortic stenosis** (which prolongs left ventricular systole) and **left bundle branch block** (which delays the onset of left ventricular contraction). ▼

h. A **third heart sound (S_3)** is sometimes heard in normal persons. It is a low-pitched, early diastolic sound heard best at the apex of the heart and is caused by vibrations due to rapid ventricular filling. S_3 may be normal in children and in adults after exercise.

i. A **fourth heart sound (S_4)** can be caused by atrial systole. It is a low pitched, late diastolic or presystolic sound.

   i. S_4 may be heard normally in young children but is usually associated with cardiovascular pathology in adults.

   ii. In atrial fibrillation, there is no atrial kick; these patients, therefore, cannot have an S_4.

   iii. In patients with tachycardia, S_4 may be fused with an S_3 sound, producing a **summation gallop.**

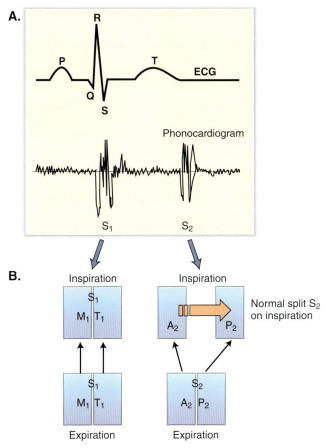

Figure 4-17. **A.** First (S_1) and second (S_2) heart sounds. **B.** Physiologic splitting of S_2. S_1 is caused by the closure of the atrioventricular valves; S_2 is caused by the closure of the semilunar valves. Physiologic splitting mainly results from the delayed closure of the pulmonic valve on inspiration. M_1, mitral valve closure; T_1, tricuspid valve closure; A_2, aortic valve closure; P_2, pulmonic valve closure.

5. Common valvular abnormalities and murmurs.
   a. Blood flow through blood vessels is normally silent because flow is laminar (i.e., blood flow is smoothly distributed throughout the vessel, with the fastest flow in the center of the lumen).
   b. *Sounds in the vascular system are produced by turbulent blood flow which is more likely with high blood flow velocity.*
      i. Velocity of flow is accelerated across narrow areas of blood vessels or heart valves creating turbulent flow
   c. Noises are known as **bruits** in blood vessels and as **murmurs** in the heart.
      i. *Murmurs are best heard "downstream" from their origin along the course of the turbulent blood flow.*
   d. There are two types of valve abnormalities that produce heart murmurs.
      i. **Stenosis** is a narrowing of the valve that creates higher velocity blood flow through the partially constricted opening and *produces a murmur when the valve is normally open.*
      ii. **Insufficiency** (also called incompetence or regurgitation) is failure of a valve to close completely. When valves do not close properly, there is some backflow of blood when the valve should be closed.
   e. **Aortic stenosis** is a systolic murmur that occurs when the velocity of blood flow accelerates through the narrowed valve (Figure 4-18).

Aortic Stenosis

A. Phonocardiogram: paradoxical split S₂

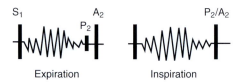

Expiration   Inspiration

B. Elevated left ventricular pressure

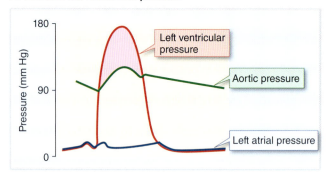

Note high left ventricular pressure to maintain cardiac output through narrow aortic valve.

Figure 4-18. Systolic murmur of aortic stenosis. **A.** Paradoxical splitting of the second (S₂) heart sound occurs because the aortic valve (A₂) closes later than the pulmonic valve (P₂) due to prolonged left ventricular systole. **B.** Pressure gradient across the narrowed aortic valve.

    i. The murmur is loudest in the middle of systole when the pressure gradient across the valve is greatest.

    ii. Pressure in the left ventricle is increased above normal to eject the SV.

    iii. Aortic stenosis leads to reduced SV and a decrease in systolic pressure in the aorta.

    iv. ▼ Aortic stenosis is most common in elderly patients and is caused by calcification of the valve. *Three cardinal symptoms of aortic stenosis are angina, syncope, and congestive heart failure.* ▼

f. **Mitral insufficiency** is a systolic murmur produced by blood flowing backward through the valve when it is normally closed. This produces a soft, **holosystolic (throughout systole) murmur** (Figure 4-19).

    i. There is an increased volume load to the left atrium and ventricle.

    ii. Forward flow into the aorta usually does not change significantly unless congestive heart failure occurs late in the course of the disease.

    iii. Increased left atrial pressure and large atrial v waves are expected due to the backflow of blood from the left ventricle during systole, but they often are absent due to increasing compliance of the left atrium during the course of the disease.

g. **Mitral valve prolapse** is billowing of floppy, redundant mitral leaflets back into the left atrium during ventricular systole.

    i. Sudden tensing of floppy leaflets produces the classic auscultatory finding of **midsystolic click.**

    ii. Mitral valve prolapse can be accompanied by mitral insufficiency if the prolapsing leaflets do not come together properly; a late systolic murmur is then heard, due to backflow of blood into the atrium.

h. **Aortic insufficiency** allows regurgitation of blood through the valve during diastole, when it should normally be closed (Figure 4-20).

Mitral Insufficiency

A. Holosystolic murmur, early aortic valve closure

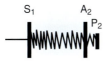

B. Possible elevated left atrial pressure

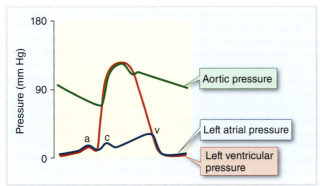

Note large v wave due to regurgitation of blood from left ventricle to left atrium.

Figure 4-19. Systolic murmur of mitral insufficiency. **A.** The early aortic valve (A_2) sound indicates the shortened systole due to retrograde blood flow into the left atrium. **B.** The large atrial v wave due to regurgitation of blood from the left ventricle into the left atrium during systole.

Aortic Insufficiency

A. Decrescendo murmur

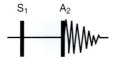

B. "Water-hammer" pulse: increased systolic blood pressure and decreased diastolic blood pressure

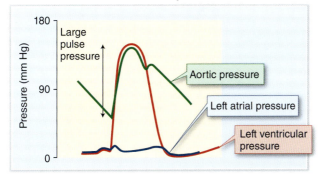

Figure 4-20. Diastolic murmur of aortic insufficiency. **A.** Sound intensity of the murmur decreases during diastole as a function of aortic blood pressure. S_1 is the first heart sound; A_2 indicates timing of the closure of the aortic valve. **B.** Pathologic runoff of blood from the aorta into the left ventricle decreases aortic diastolic blood pressure and increases left ventricular filling, increasing stroke volume and systolic blood pressure.

i. The murmur decreases in intensity as the pressure gradient across the valve decreases in late diastole.

ii. Retrograde flow from the aorta into the left ventricle during diastole increases the ventricular end-diastolic volume.

iii. This subsequently increases the SV and the aortic systolic blood pressure.

iv. The abnormal blood flow runoff from the aorta into the ventricle during diastole causes the aortic diastolic pressure to decrease.

v. ▼ *Increased systolic pressure and decreased diastolic pressure produce a large arterial pulse* that is the basis of several physical findings:

- **Corrigan's pulse,** the "water-hammer pulse" that collapses rapidly.
- **Quincke's pulse,** when pulsations are noted in the root of the fingernail bed while lightly pinching the tip of the fingernail.
- **de Musset's sign,** when the head bobs with each pulsation. ▼

vi. *Aortic insufficiency may result from valve disease (e.g., rheumatic heart disease) or aortic root dilation (e.g., syphilis or Marfan's syndrome).*

i. **Mitral stenosis** causes high resistance across the mitral valve and produces turbulent blood flow into the left ventricle during diastole (Figure 4-21).

i. The murmur is a **soft crescendo murmur.**

ii. There may also be an "**opening snap,**" created by rapid movement of the contracted mitral valve apparatus and heard as a sharp sound immediately after S_2.

Mitral Stenosis

A. Presystolic murmur (PSM) and opening snap (OS)

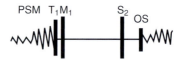

B. Continually elevated left atrial pressure

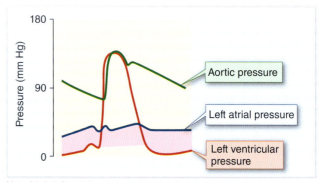

Note high left atrial pressure due to obstructed flow through mitral valve.

Figure 4-21. Diastolic murmur of mitral stenosis. **A.** An opening snap (OS) is a unique sound that is characteristic of mitral stenosis. The sound produced by obstructed flow through the mitral valve is described as a presystolic murmur (PSM). Obstructed ventricular filling may delay closure of the mitral valve (M_1) relative to closure of the tricuspid valve (T_1). **B.** Obstruction of the mitral valve causes a sustained increase in left atrial pressure.

    iii. Systemic blood pressure may be reduced in mitral stenosis because of decreased filling of the left ventricle, leading to a decrease in SV.

    iv. *Left atrial pressure is often elevated, causing pulmonary congestion.*

    v. ▼ *Mitral stenosis is the most common valvular lesion caused by* **rheumatic heart disease.** However, proper treatment of streptococcal pharyngitis with penicillin can prevent the valvular complications of rheumatic fever. ▼

  j. **Patent ductus arteriosus** produces a characteristic continuous murmur in neonates.

    i. The ductus arteriosus is a normal fetal connection between the aorta and the pulmonary artery, which normally closes near the time of birth. *The incidence of patent ductus arteriosus is high in premature infants.*

    ii. **Prostaglandin E** and low arterial partial pressure of O_2 (Pao_2) maintain patency of the ductus, so that *administering O_2 and prostaglandin inhibitors (e.g., indomethacin) promotes closure of the patent ductus arteriosus.*

    iii. A patent ductus allows blood flow from the high pressure in the aorta to the lower pressure in the pulmonary artery causing increased pulmonary blood flow and greater filling of the left atrium and ventricle.

    iv. There is a large arterial pulse wave similar to that seen in aortic insufficiency because a large SV increases systolic aortic blood pressure; in addition, runoff of blood from the aorta through a patent ductus during diastole decreases aortic diastolic blood pressure.

    v. The murmur of patent ductus is continuous because there is a pressure gradient from the aorta to the pulmonary artery throughout the entire cardiac cycle.

  k. ▼ **Anemia** can cause flow murmurs because cardiac output is increased to maintain delivery of O_2 to the tissues. The increased velocity of blood flow plus decreased blood viscosity can cause turbulent flow that is heard mostly at the cardiac valves and at bifurcations of the larger arteries. ▼

6. Pressure-volume (PV) loops.

  a. Plotting left ventricular pressure against volume produces a loop (see Figure 4-22).

    i. At point A, the ventricle contains the end-systolic blood volume, and the mitral valve opens.

    ii. The ventricle fills until end-diastolic volume is achieved at point B, where the mitral valve is closed by the onset of ventricular contraction.

    iii. Isovolumic contraction increases pressure to point C, which corresponds to diastolic blood pressure and opening of the aortic valve.

    iv. Ventricular ejection propels pressure through its peak value at point D, corresponding to aortic systolic pressure, until the aortic valve closes at point E.

    v. Pressure decreases back to point A during isovolumic relaxation, completing one cardiac cycle.

    vi. The width of the PV loop is the **stroke volume** (the difference between end-diastolic volume and end-systolic volume).

    vii. The area within a PV loop is an index of **stroke work.**

A. Left ventricular pressure and volume

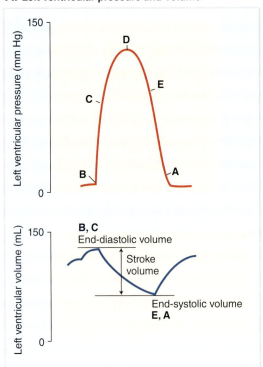

B. Pressure-volume loop

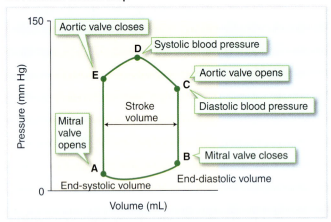

Figure 4-22. Left ventricular pressure-volume loop. **A.** Correlation between changes in left ventricular pressure (upper panel) and left ventricular volume (lower panel) during a single cardiac cycle. **B.** Left ventricular pressure is plotted as a function of left ventricular volume. Landmark events of valve opening and closure and the point where peak systolic blood pressure occurs are noted in both figures at points A–E.

Cardiac Output

1. *Cardiac output is the volume of blood pumped by each ventricle per minute* and is the product of HR and SV. In adults, cardiac output is usually expressed in liters per minute:

$$Q_T = (SV \times HR) / 1000 \qquad \textbf{Equation 4-4}$$

Q_T = Cardiac output (L/min)

SV = Stroke volume (mL/min)

HR = Heart rate (beats/min)

Example. If resting SV is 70 mL and HR is 70 beats/min, then

$$Q_T = (70 \text{ mL} \times 70 \text{ beats/min}) / 1000 = 4.9 \text{ L/min}$$

2. The Fick principle is a traditional physiologic method for calculating cardiac output, which derives blood flow from variables related to O_2 consumption.

   a. The O_2 consumption (Vo_2) of a specific organ is the product of blood flow and the drop in arterial O_2 content (Cao_2) between the artery and the vein ($Cao_2 - Cvo_2$). In the Fick equation (Equation 4-5), these terms are rearranged to determine blood flow.

   b. Cardiac output can be calculated by applying the Fick concept to the entire body, relating total body O_2 consumption to the difference in O_2 content between blood in the systemic arteries and the mixed venous blood sampled from the pulmonary artery or the right ventricle:

$$Q_T = Vo_2 / (Cao_2 - Cvo_2) \qquad \text{Equation 4-5}$$

Q_T = Cardiac output

Vo_2 = O_2 consumption

Cao_2 = Arterial O_2 content

Cvo_2 = Mixed venous O_2 content

Example. A person consumes 250 mL of O_2 per minute. Arterial O_2 content is 20 mL of O_2 per dL of blood, and the O_2 content of mixed venous blood is 15 mL of O_2 per dL of blood:

$$Q_T = 250 (\text{mL/min}) \div (20 \text{ mL/dL} - 15 \text{ mL/dL})$$
$$= 50 \text{ dL/min} = 5 \text{ L/min}$$

   c. Cardiac output can also be measured clinically in the cardiac catheterization laboratory, using a **thermodilution method** whereby a cold saline solution of known temperature and volume is injected into the right atrium. The reduction in blood temperature measured downstream in the pulmonary artery is a function of cardiac output. Newer noninvasive methods including Doppler ultrasound are also being developed to measure cardiac output.

3. **Ejection fraction** is a simple measurement of ventricular performance and describes the fraction of end-diastolic volume ejected from the ventricle during systole:

$$EF = SV \div EDV \qquad \text{Equation 4-6}$$

EF = Ejection fraction

SV = Stroke volume

EDV = End-diastolic volume

Example. A healthy man of average size is found to have a resting end-diastolic volume of 140 mL and a resting SV of 80 mL:

$$EF = 80 / 140 = 0.57 \ (57\%)$$

a. ▼ **Congestive heart failure** is classified as either systolic dysfunction (loss of contractility) or diastolic dysfunction (impaired compliance). *The ejection fraction is decreased in patients with systolic dysfunction due to the loss of contractility, but it is maintained in patients with diastolic dysfunction.* ▼

4. **Cardiac index.**

   a. Cardiac index expresses the cardiac output relative to the body surface area (BSA), providing approximate indexing to tissue metabolic demand.

$$CI = Q_T / BSA \qquad \textbf{Equation 4-7}$$

CI = Cardiac index (L/min/m²)
Q_T = Cardiac output (L/min)
BSA = Body surface area (m²)

Example. A 24-year-old woman is found to have a resting cardiac output of 4.0 L/min. Her BSA is 1.40 m²:

$$CI = 4.0/1.40 = 2.86 \ \text{L/min/m}^2$$

5. The **Frank-Starling principle** describes the relationship between SV and end-diastolic volume (Figure 4-23).

   a. Increased diastolic filling produces greater stretch of heart muscle, resulting in a larger SV by two mechanisms:

      i. Optimizing overlap between the thin and thick muscle filaments.

      ii. Increased sensitivity of troponin C to Ca^{2+}.

   b. *As a result, end-diastolic volume is the most important determinant of SV in the healthy heart.*

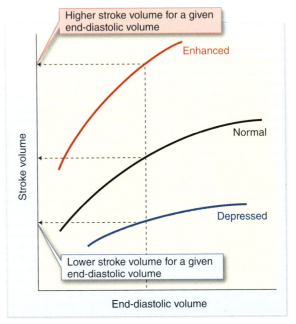

Figure 4-23. Frank-Starling relationship. End-diastolic volume is the most important determinant of stroke volume. Increased contractility of ventricular muscle produces a left shift in the Frank-Starling relationship; decreased contractility produces a right shift.

    c. Another result of the Frank-Starling principle is that left and right heart outputs are equalized since output of one side becomes the venous return of the other side.

6. Assessment of ventricular function.

    a. **Stroke volume** is determined by three factors:

        i. Ventricular **preload** is the end-diastolic volume created by venous return.

        ii. Ventricular **afterload** is the sum of factors that oppose ejection of blood during systole.

        iii. **Contractility** is the intrinsic vigor of muscle contraction related to the biochemical state of the cell.

    b. In a healthy heart, increasing preload results in increased SV (Figure 4-24). **Preload** is enhanced by several factors:

        i. Increased blood volume.

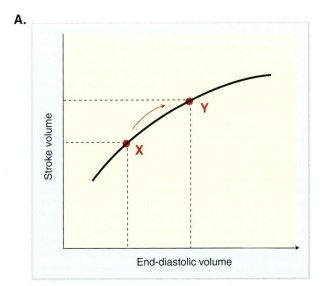

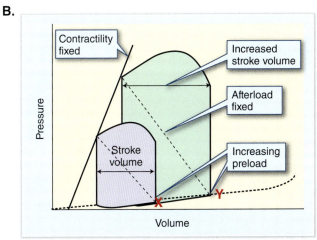

Figure 4-24. Effect of increased preload on ventricular performance. **A.** Increase in the end-diastolic volume from point X to point Y increases stroke volume due to greater force of ventricular contraction via the Frank-Starling mechanism. **B.** Higher preload moves the end-diastolic pressure-volume point to the right from point X to point Y. The increased left ventricular systolic pressure and stroke volume result from greater force of ventricular contraction.

    ii. Rhythmic skeletal muscle contraction, which propels blood toward the heart due to the presence of one-way valves in veins.

   iii. Deep inspiration, which decreases intrathoracic pressure and increases abdominal pressure, promoting venous return to the thorax.

   iv. Atrial systole.

    v. Venoconstriction, which reduces venous pooling and promotes the return of blood to the central circulation.

   vi. ▼ Preload can be quickly increased at the bedside by placing the patient in the **Trendelenburg position** (supine with the head lower than the feet), as well as by using intravenous fluids. ▼

   vii. ▼ *Acute myocardial infarction is an example where increasing preload may not be indicated.* The O_2 supply to the myocardium is disrupted, and treatments that reduce myocardial O_2 consumption are desirable. **Nitrates** are dilators that reduce preload, decreasing the ventricular wall tension and, as a result, decrease the myocardial O_2 consumption. ▼

  c. Afterload.

    i. The major component of afterload is normally the resistance to blood flow created by small muscular arteries and arterioles.

      • *Aortic diastolic blood pressure is often used as an index of afterload because it is created by blood flow through vascular resistance.*

    ii. Other sources of afterload could be low compliance (stiffness) of the ventricle or great vessels, or stenosis of the semilunar valves.

   iii. Afterload is represented using a PV loop, as shown in Figure 4-25, by a line drawn from the end-diastolic pressure volume point (B) to the end-systolic PV point (E).

      • *The slope of this line represents all factors opposing the volume change that occurs in systole.*

      • If the slope of the line is increased, there is higher systolic pressure or reduced SV, or both.

   iv. ▼ **Afterload reduction** is an important therapeutic approach in the treatment of heart failure to allow higher SV without increasing

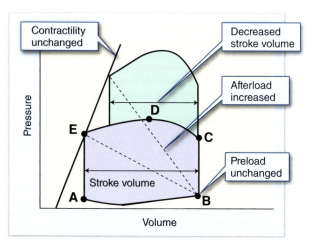

Figure 4-25. Effect of increased afterload on ventricular performance. Dashed lines indicate the afterload slope, which becomes steeper when the ventricle develops more pressure but delivers a smaller stroke volume, reflecting higher impedance opposing blood flow (increased afterload).

myocardial O_2 consumption. **Angiotensin-converting enzyme (ACE) inhibitors** or **angiotensin-receptor antagonists** not only reduce afterload but also inhibit the maladaptive effects of angiotensin II on cardiac remodeling in congestive heart failure. ▼

d. Contractility.

   i. In isolated muscle, altered contractility is indicated as a change in the maximal velocity of shortening (V_{max}) (see Figure 4-26A).

   • V_{max} is obtained by extrapolating the load-velocity relation to a theoretic zero load. *An increase in* V$_{max}$ *implies faster myosin crossbridge cycling.*

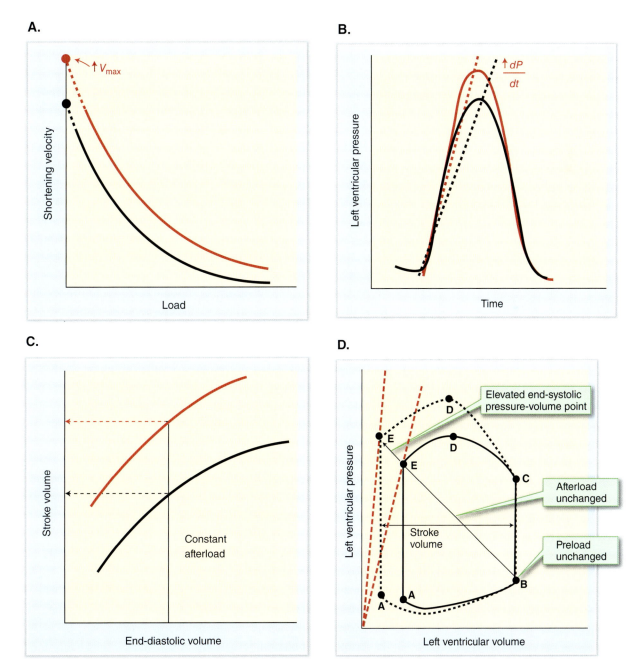

Figure 4-26. Representations of increased ventricular contractility. **A.** Increased velocity of muscle shortening at zero muscle load (V_{max}) in isolated muscle. **B.** Increased rate of pressure development in the left ventricle (*dP/dt*). **C.** Left shift of Frank-Starling relation. **D.** Elevation of the end-systolic pressure-volume point.

Table 4-4. Mechanisms of Increased Myocardial Contractility Following β-Adrenergic Stimulation

Cellular Mechanism	Effect
L-type Ca^{2+} channel activation	↑ Ca^{2+} entry in phase 2 of action potential → ↑ Ca^{2+}-induced Ca^{2+}-release → ↑contractility
Phosphorylation of phospholamban (Ca^{2+}-ATPase suppressor protein)	↓ Phospholamban → ↑ Ca^{2+}-ATPase → ↑ Ca^{2+} reuptake into sarcoplasmic reticulum → ↑ Rate of muscle relaxation
Phosphorylation of troponin I	↑ Rate of Ca^{2+} dissociation from troponin C → ↑ Rate of muscle relaxation

    ii. Another indicator of contractility in the intact heart is the rate of pressure change in the left ventricle at the onset of isovolumic contraction (see Figure 4-26B).

    iii. *A left shift in the Frank-Starling relation also indicates greater contractility,* whereas a right shift indicates depression of function (see Figure 4-26C).

    iv. Contractility can be also assessed using a PV loop by examining the rate at which the end of systole is reached.

       • *The slope of a line drawn from a zero pressure point to the end-systolic pressure volume point (E) is an index of contractility* (see Figure 4-26D).

       • For a given preload and afterload, an increase in the slope of this line yields greater SV and higher systolic pressure, indicating increased contractility.

  e. ▼ Agents that increase contractility are called **positive inotropes,** and those that decrease contractility are called **negative inotropes.** ▼

  f. **Catecholamines** are the most important physiologic examples of positive inotropes.

    i. Catecholamines occupy myocardial β_1-**adrenoceptors**, causing the generation of intracellular cyclic adenosine monophosphate (cAMP) and activation of protein kinase A.

    ii. Cellular mechanisms that underlie increased contractility are summarized in Table 4-4.

    iii. ▼ "Sympathomimetic" drugs that are positive inotropes include **dobutamine**, dopamine, and isoproterenol. *Using positive inotropes to treat heart failure may increase mortality; therefore, these drugs must be used with caution.* ▼

7. Left ventricular failure (Figure 4-27).

  a. **Systolic dysfunction** occurs when myocardial contraction is weak, most commonly following a **myocardial infarction.**

    i. Patients have reduced SV despite normal preload; contractility is reduced and tachycardia is present to maintain cardiac output.

    ii. *Afterload reduction treatments are used to increase SV.*

  b. In **diastolic dysfunction,** there is low cardiac muscle compliance and poor filling.

    i. Patients have a right shift of the end-diastolic PV point. Increased ventricular diastolic pressure at any given volume indicates low compliance.

A. Systolic dysfunction

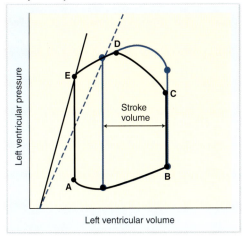

B. Diastolic dysfunction

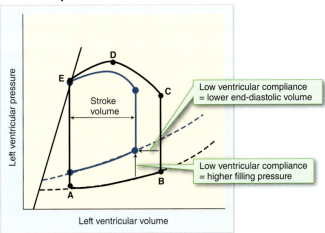

Figure 4-27. Reduced ventricular performance. **A.** Low stroke volume at a given preload and afterload shows lower ventricular contractility and defines systolic dysfunction. **B.** Low ventricular compliance in diastolic dysfunction reduces end-diastolic volume and increases end-diastolic pressure.

   ii. Common causes include **ischemic heart disease** and **ventricular hypertrophy** from longstanding hypertension.
   iii. *Treatment is aimed at reducing blood volume and preload and promoting ventricular relaxation.*

Vascular Function

1. Blood flows through a circuit of vessels:
    a. **Large arteries** (e.g., the aorta) are high-pressure reservoirs that store energy in their elastic walls during ventricular ejection and release it during diastole to maintain blood flow.
    b. **Small muscular arteries and arterioles** are the *site of greatest vascular resistance in the circulation,* accounting for the large drop in blood pressure that occurs across this segment of the circulation (see Figure 4-28).
        i. *Neurohumoral regulation of arteriolar tone controls vascular resistance and has a major effect on arterial blood pressure.*

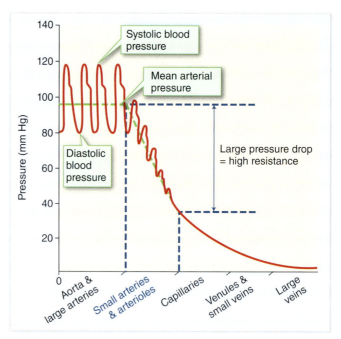

Figure 4-28. Blood pressures throughout the systemic vasculature. Pressure is highest in the central arteries and lowest in the central veins. The largest pressure decrease occurs across the arterioles, indicating that they are the site of highest vascular resistance.

    c. **Capillaries** are thin-walled vessels that provide a *large surface area for the exchange of gases, nutrients, and wastes.*

       i. Imbalances of hydrostatic and osmotic pressure gradients across the capillary walls are the most common causes of **edema** (swelling due to excess interstitial fluid volume).

    d. **Venules and veins** present little resistance to flow. *The venous system is a high capacitance, low-pressure reservoir.*

       i. The largest blood volume in the cardiovascular system (about two-thirds) is in the systemic veins (the second largest blood volume is in the pulmonary vasculature).

       ii. Small muscular veins assist in the regulation of venous return. *Increased venous tone reduces the capacitance of veins, causing increased venous return.* Larger cardiac preload results in increased cardiac output via the Frank-Starling mechanism.

2. Systemic arterial blood pressure (Figure 4-29).

    a. *The pressure difference across the circulation from the arteries to the veins drives blood flow.*

    b. **Systolic blood pressure** (SBP) is the peak pressure recorded in the central arterial system and occurs during ventricular ejection.

    c. **Diastolic blood pressure** (DBP) is the minimum pressure recorded in the central arterial system and occurs just before the start of ventricular systole.

    d. **Pulse pressure** (PP) is the difference between SBP and DBP. *PP is reflected by the strength of the arterial pulse wave palpated in the peripheral arteries.*

    e. **Mean arterial pressure (MAP)** is a time-weighted average of SBP and DBP. Systole occupies about one-third of the cardiac cycle under resting conditions and diastole occupies about two-thirds, giving rise to the following estimate of MAP:

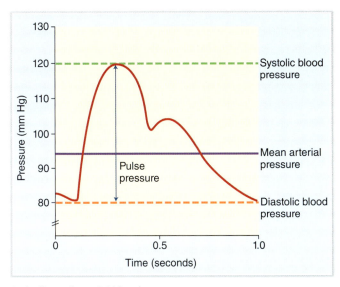

Figure 4-29. Indices of arterial blood pressure.

$$MAP = DBP + \frac{1}{3}PP \qquad\qquad \textbf{Equation 4-8}$$

MAP = Mean arterial blood pressure

DBP = Diastolic blood pressure

PP = Pulse pressure

Example. Blood pressure measured by cuff inflation in the upper arm of a healthy person is 120/80 mm Hg; SBP = 120 mm Hg; DBP = 80 mm Hg; and PP = 120 – 80 = 40 mm Hg.

$$MAP = 80 + 1/3(40)$$
$$= 93.3 \, mm \, Hg$$

f. ▼ **Hypertension,** or high blood pressure, is a risk factor associated with several diseases, including heart attack, stroke, and renal failure.

   i. **Normal blood pressure** is defined as SBP <120 mm Hg but >90 mm Hg, and DBP <80 mm Hg but >60 mm Hg.

   ii. SBP between 120 and 129 mm Hg with DBP <80 mm Hg is considered "**elevated**" **blood pressure.**

   iii. SBP between 130 and 139 mm Hg or DBP between 80 and 89 mm Hg is **Stage 1 hypertension.**

   iv. SBP >140 mm Hg or DBP >90 is **Stage 2 hypertension.**

   v. SBP >180 mm Hg or DBP >120 mm Hg is **hypertensive crisis.**

   vi. *Hypertension causes end-organ damage,* and may be an asymptomatic disease for many years before being diagnosed. To assess the severity and duration of hypertension, the physician can examine the interior of the eye using an ophthalmoscope to assess the extent of retinal artery damage. ▼

g. SBP has three determinants:

   i. **Stroke volume.** Increased SV increases SBP and PP.

      ii. **Diastolic blood pressure.** The absolute value of SBP must be interpreted with respect to DBP, since this is the baseline pressure before systole. *For this reason, PP is a useful guide to SV.*

      iii. **Aortic compliance.** If compliance is low (i.e., stiff aorta), the SV produces a large SBP.

- Aortic compliance is not physiologically regulated but often declines with age due to loss of elastic tissue, atherosclerosis, and calcification; *SBP typically increases 1 mm Hg for each year after age 60.*

h. DBP has three determinants:

      i. *Vascular resistance is the main determinant of DBP.*

- Blood flow through the circulation continues throughout diastole because the arterial pressure exceeds the venous pressure and due to recoil of the elastic aorta.
- DBP is determined by the size of arteriolar resistance encountered by blood flow. *Higher arteriolar resistance (vasoconstriction) increases DBP.*

      ii. **Runoff of blood from the aorta.** DBP decreases if blood flow into the circulation during diastole is reduced.

- **Aortic valve insufficiency** is an example where aortic pressure rapidly decreases during diastole because backflow of blood into the left ventricle reduces forward flow into the circulation.

      iii. **Diastolic time interval.** Aortic pressure decreases with time between heart beats because blood continues to flow into the circulation from the aorta throughout diastole.

- DBP is lower when the HR is slow because more time elapses between beats. DBP is higher at faster heart rates because there is less time for a decline in aortic pressure between beats (Figure 4-30).

i. ▼ **Isolated systolic hypertension** is mainly a disease of elderly patients. It occurs because of a gradual decline in arterial compliance (a component of SBP, not DBP), so that SBP increases and DBP decreases. Treatment adds an additional challenge because reducing DBP further may increase cardiovascular events, which occur because *most coronary perfusion occurs during diastole, not systole.* ▼

3. Regulation of systemic vascular resistance.

a. The collective resistance to blood flow presented by the systemic vasculature is called systemic vascular resistance, or **total peripheral resistance.**

b. *Systemic vascular resistance is mainly determined by changes in the diameter of the arterioles.*

      i. Arterioles are partially constricted under normal physiologic conditions, called **vascular tone,** and are the sites of active regulation of blood flow in the circulation.

      ii. Arteriolar tone is affected by many factors, including sympathetic tone and hormones and endothelial and metabolic factors.

      iii. *Systemic vascular resistance is increased by vasoconstriction and reduced by vasodilation.*

4. Venous return.

a. **Venous return** is the volume of blood returning to the central venous compartment (i.e., thoracic venae cavae and right atrium) per minute.

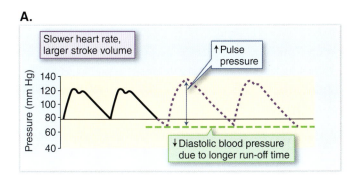

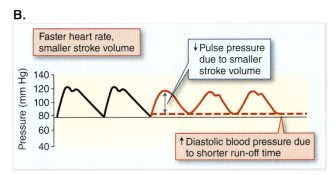

Figure 4-30. Effect of heart rate on diastolic blood pressure. **A.** Decrease in diastolic blood pressure at a reduced heart rate due to increased run-off time. **B.** Increase in diastolic blood pressure at a faster heart rate due to reduced run-off time. Cardiac output is the same in A and B, but there is a faster heart rate and a smaller stroke volume in B compared to A.

    b. **Central venous pressure** (CVP) is the pressure of venous blood in the thoracic vena cava and the right atrium.

       i. Low CVP promotes venous return into the central venous compartment, whereas *high CVP reduces venous return.*

      ii. CVP has a strong influence on cardiac preload and, through the Frank-Starling mechanism, determines ventricular SV.

    c. ▼ Measuring or estimating CVP in the hemodynamically unstable patient can guide management.

       i. In **hypovolemia,** a low CVP indicates the need for aggressive intravenous fluid resuscitation. Intravenous fluid replacement will increase preload, thereby increasing cardiac output, blood pressure, and tissue perfusion.

      ii. By contrast, giving intravenous fluid loading to patient in **heart failure** with high CVP is likely to worsen edema and is contraindicated. ▼

    d. During **dynamic exercise,** mechanisms to support venous return are needed because ventricular diastolic filling time is reduced by rapid heart rates:

       i. The "**muscle pump**" describes rhythmic contraction of skeletal muscles, which promotes venous return by compressing veins in the limbs, forcing venous return back toward the thorax. *Retrograde flow is prevented by one-way valves in the veins.*

      ii. The "**inspiratory pump**" describes the effect of increasing the rate and depth of ventilation, which causes the intrathoracic pressure to become more negative and increases blood flow from the abdomen to the thorax.

e. **Transmural pressure** is a general concept sometimes used to explain phenomena such as the inspiratory pump.

   i. Transmural pressure is the pressure exerted across the wall of a structure and is calculated by subtracting the external pressure from the internal pressure. *Transmural pressure can be thought of as the pressure acting to distend or dilate a structure* (Figure 4-31A).

   ii. In the example of deep inspiration increasing venous return, transmural pressure across the wall of the vena cava and right atrium increases because the external pressure becomes more negative during inspiration (Figure 4-31B).

f. ▼ In the healthy heart, a deep inspiration (i.e., more negative intrathoracic pressure) will collapse the jugular veins as the blood is pulled into the right side of the heart. In **right-sided heart failure,** the pressures on the right side of the heart are high and unable to accommodate the increased volume

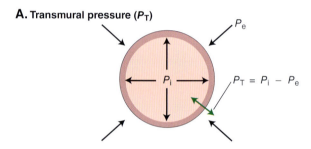

A. Transmural pressure (P_T)

$$P_T = P_i - P_e$$

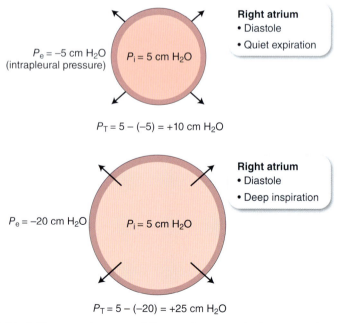

B. Example of the change in transmural pressure across the wall of the right atrium during deep inspiration

$P_e = -5$ cm H_2O (intrapleural pressure) $P_i = 5$ cm H_2O

Right atrium
- Diastole
- Quiet expiration

$$P_T = 5 - (-5) = +10 \text{ cm } H_2O$$

$P_e = -20$ cm H_2O $P_i = 5$ cm H_2O

Right atrium
- Diastole
- Deep inspiration

$$P_T = 5 - (-20) = +25 \text{ cm } H_2O$$

Figure 4-31. A. Transmural pressure difference (P_T). **B.** Worked example of altered transmural pressure difference across the right atrium during deep inspiration.

coming from the venae cavae. This is detected clinically as increased JVD, known as **Kussmaul's sign.** ▼

5. Vascular and cardiac function curves.

   a. Vascular and cardiac function curves describe factors affecting venous return and cardiac output, respectively.

   b. The curves must intersect at a single operational point because venous return equals cardiac output.

   c. A systemic vascular function curve plots venous return as a function of right atrial pressure (Figure 4-32).

      i. Venous return decreases if the right atrial pressure increases because there is a smaller pressure gradient allowing venous return into the atrium.

      ii. At the point where venous return (flow) becomes zero, the right atrial pressure is typically between 6 and 12 mm Hg.

      iii. If blood flow in the circulation stops, the arterial pressure decreases and the venous pressure increases until the pressure equalizes at all points in the cardiovascular system. This pressure is called **systemic function pressure (P_{SF}), or mean circulatory filling pressure.**

   d. *P_{SF} is not measured clinically but can be thought of as the amount of pressure in the vascular system that drives venous return.*

      i. P_{SF} is determined by the relationship between blood volume and vascular compliance.

      ii. P_{SF} increases if blood volume is high or if vascular compliance is low. *The overall compliance of the vascular system is determined by venous tone because the venous system is 10–20 times more compliant than the arterial system.*

      iii. Increasing blood volume or reducing venous compliance shifts the venous return curve upward to the right, thereby increasing P_{SF} and venous return.

   e. *Arteriolar vasoconstriction reduces venous return because blood flow into the microcirculation, and into the venous system beyond it, is reduced.* Vasodilation has the opposite effect.

   f. There is no change in P_{SF} when the arteriolar tone changes because the arterioles contribute little to overall vascular compliance.

   g. Cardiac function curves represent the **Frank-Starling relationship** because an increase in the right atrial pressure drives more ventricular filling (preload), which increases SV and cardiac output (Figure 4-33).

   h. When described using cardiac and venous function curves, **dynamic exercise** increases venous return and cardiac output for three reasons (Figure 4-34A):

      i. Activation of the sympathetic nervous system increases **cardiac contractility** (shifting the cardiac function curve left).

      ii. Sympathetic activation increases venous return due to **venoconstriction** (shifting the vascular function curve right).

      iii. Release of local metabolites in working muscle causes **vasodilation** (increasing the slope of the vascular function curve).

A.

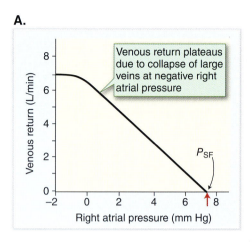

B.

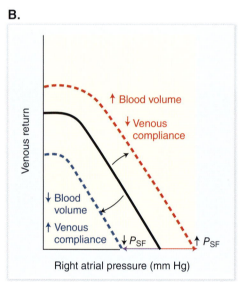

C.

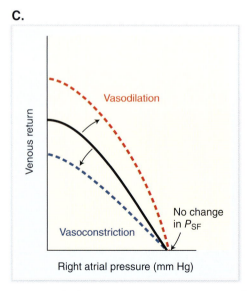

Figure 4-32. Systemic vascular function curves. **A.** Systemic vascular function curve, indicating the determination of mean circulatory filling pressure (P_{SF}) at zero blood flow. **B.** Changes in the mean circulatory filling pressure (P_{SF}) and venous return caused by altered blood volume or venous tone. **C.** Effects of changes in the arteriolar tone on venous return.

A.

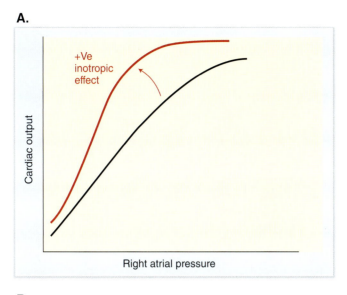

B.

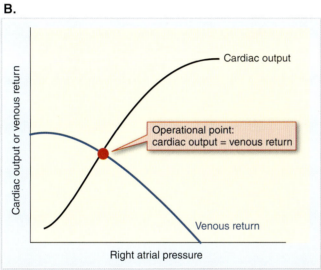

Figure 4-33. Cardiac function curves. **A.** Frank-Starling curve representing cardiac function. A left shift indicates increased ventricular contractility. **B.** The cardiac function curve and the systemic vascular function curve plotted together, showing a single operational point where cardiac output equals venous return.

i. Cardiac and venous function curves can also illustrate how **compensation** occurs in patients with **heart failure** (Figure 4-34B).

   i. The primary problem of heart failure shifts the cardiac function curve downwards and to the right.

   ii. Chronic salt and water retention by the renal system increase blood volume (shifting the vascular function curve right).

   iii. Therefore, in compensated heart failure venous return is restored at the expense of higher right atrial pressure, which in turn increases the venous blood pressure.

   iv. *Note: The risk of edema formation is increased when venous blood pressure increases (see The Capillary Microcirculation).*

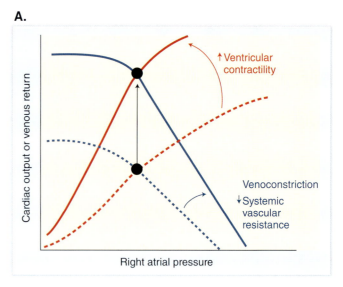

A.

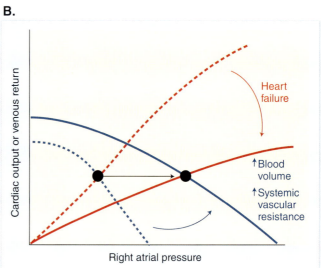

B.

Figure 4-34. A. Increased cardiac output and venous return in dynamic exercise. The sympathetic nervous system activation increases ventricular contractility, producing a left shift in the cardiac function curve. Venoconstriction causes a right shift in the vascular function curve, with increased mean circulatory filling pressure and venous return. Vasodilation in working muscle causes systemic vascular resistance to decrease, increasing the slope of the venous return curve. A new operating point at higher venous return and cardiac output is achieved. **B.** Cardiac output and venous return in compensated heart failure. Decreased ventricular performance causes a right shift in the cardiac function curve. Mean circulatory filling pressure is increased by fluid retention but venous return is restricted by increased systemic vascular resistance. Cardiac output and venous return are almost maintained in this patient, but at the cost of high right atrial pressure.

Neurohumoral Regulation of the Cardiovascular System

1. *The main homeostatic goal of cardiovascular regulation is to maintain adequate cardiac output.*
2. Wall stretch provides information about blood pressures, which is used as an index of blood flow:
   a. **Carotid sinus baroreceptors** monitor arterial blood pressure.
   b. **Low-pressure baroreceptors** in the venous system and cardiac atria monitor blood volume.

c. The **renal juxtaglomerular apparatus** senses *effective* circulating blood volume.

3. Input from sensors is coupled to changes in autonomic nervous tone and endocrine axes such as **renin-angiotensin-aldosterone, atrial natriuretic peptide,** and **vasopressin** (see Chapters 6 and 8).

4. Changes in vascular resistance and compliance, cardiac performance, and renal handling of sodium and water are integrated to maintain normal blood pressure and flow.

5. The autonomic nervous system.

   a. *The primary site of cardiovascular control within the central nervous system is the medulla oblongata.*

      i. Sensory inputs enter the **nucleus tractus solitarius.**

      ii. Inhibitory interneurons project to sympathetic nerve cell bodies, and excitatory interneurons project to parasympathetic nerve cell bodies so that *basal baroreceptor input results in tonic activation of parasympathetic outflow and suppression of sympathetic outflow.*

   b. Parasympathetic (vagal) fibers innervate the SA and AV nodes, the conduction pathways, and the cardiac myocytes.

      i. Acetylcholine acts via muscarinic (M_2) receptors *to slow HR and conduction velocity and to reduce the force of atrial contraction.*

      ii. Parasympathetic activation also causes vasodilation in erectile tissue but has no significant overall effect on systemic vascular resistance.

   c. Sympathetic innervation in the heart and vasculature is extensive.

      i. **Norepinephrine** is the primary neurotransmitter.

      ii. Increased HR, conduction velocity, and contractility are mediated via β_1 **receptors.**

      iii. Generalized vasoconstriction and venoconstriction are mediated via α_1 **receptors.**

      iv. Vascular beds such as skeletal muscle also express β_2 **receptors,** which mediate local vasodilation.

      v. *The net effect of sympathetic nerve stimulation is vasoconstriction and an increase in systemic vascular resistance* because:

         • α_1 receptors are more widely expressed in vascular smooth muscle than β_2 receptors.

         • Norepinephrine has a higher affinity for α than β receptors.

   d. When the sympathetic system is activated, **epinephrine** is also secreted into the circulation from the adrenal medulla.

      i. Effects are similar to norepinephrine.

      ii. Epinephrine infusion alone produces a smaller change in systemic vascular resistance because it has a higher affinity for β_2 receptors and, at low doses, produces a mixture of vasoconstriction and vasodilation in different parts of the circulation.

6. The **baroreceptor reflex** protects against acute changes in the systemic arterial blood pressure. *MAP must be maintained because it is the driving pressure for cardiac output.*

   a. The primary stretch sensors are located in the **carotid sinus,** with secondary sensors in the **aortic arch.**

   b. Afferent nerve impulses are carried from the **carotid sinus nerve** to the brainstem via the glossopharyngeal nerves.

c. Increased stretch of the carotid sinus, caused by a rise in MAP or PP, increases the action potential frequency in the carotid sinus nerve.

d. In the medulla oblongata, this *input inhibits sympathetic outflow and stimulates parasympathetic outflow* (the opposite occurs when MAP or PP decreases).

  i. ▼ Activation of the baroreceptor reflex can be used to terminate **supraventricular tachycardia.** Carotid massage or an intravenous fluid bolus both increase wall stretch in the carotid sinus, activating parasympathetic outflow, which can terminate supraventricular tachycardia. ▼

e. The adequacy of the baroreceptor reflex can be assessed by the **tilt-table test:**

  i. If a patient is moved from a supine to a standing position, the normal response is an initial decrease in MAP due to venous pooling in the lower limbs, which reduces venous return and cardiac output.

  ii. Decreased action potential frequency in the carotid sinus nerve results in reduced parasympathetic tone and increased sympathetic tone.

  iii. Several effector mechanisms restore MAP to prevent reduced brain perfusion and fainting (Figure 4-35):

    • **Heart rate** is increased by withdrawal of vagal tone and by increased sympathetic stimulation of the SA node.

    • **Ventricular contractility** and SV are increased by sympathetic stimulation of cardiac myocytes.

    • **Vasoconstriction,** mediated by the sympathetic nerves, increases the systemic vascular resistance and thereby increases the DBP and MAP.

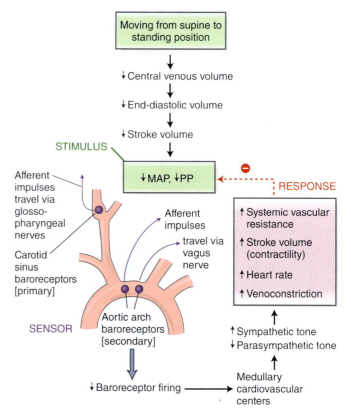

Figure 4-35. Baroreceptor reflex response to a decrease in mean arterial blood pressure. MAP, mean arterial pressure; PP, pulse pressure.

- **Venoconstriction,** due to sympathetic stimulation, reduces vascular compliance, increasing venous return and restoring cardiac preload.

  f. ▼ Patients with poor vascular or neural tone or low blood volume may sustain a decrease in MAP of more than 20 mm Hg when moving to a standing position; this is defined as **postural (orthostatic) hypotension.**

    i. Patients with **diabetes mellitus** may develop neuropathy, causing autonomic nervous system dysfunction. When moving from a supine to a standing position, these patients do not combat postural hypotension with reflex tachycardia—they will have a decrease in blood pressure and a slow to normal HR. ▼

Regional Blood Flow

1. *Blood flow is not distributed equally to all organs and tissues and depends on the control of relative vascular resistance between organs* (Table 4-5).
   a. Some organs have wide variation in blood flow, for example, in the gastrointestinal tract during digestion of a meal or in muscle during exercise.
   b. In other organs, such as the brain and the kidney, blood flow is relatively constant.

Table 4-5. Regional Control of Systemic Blood Flow

Organ	% Cardiac Output at Rest	Blood Flow (per min/100 g)	Major Vascular Resistance Control Mechanism
Heart	15	55 mL	• Local metabolic control • Nitric oxide • Autoregulation
Brain	4	70 mL	• Autoregulation • Arterial blood gases • Local metabolic control
Splanchnic organs	26	100 mL	• Sympathetic control (α_1-mediated vaso- and venoconstriction)
Kidneys	20	400 mL	• Autoregulation • Sympathetic control (α_1-mediated vasoconstriction)
Skeletal muscle	20	6 mL	• Local metabolic control (active muscle) • Sympathetic control (synaptic norepinephrine release mediates α_1-mediated vasoconstriction)
Skin	5	10 mL	• Sympathetic control • Medullary cardiovascular centers: α_1-mediated vasoconstriction • Hypothalamic thermoregulation: sweating and vasodilation via cholinergic sympathetic nerves
Others	10	—	—

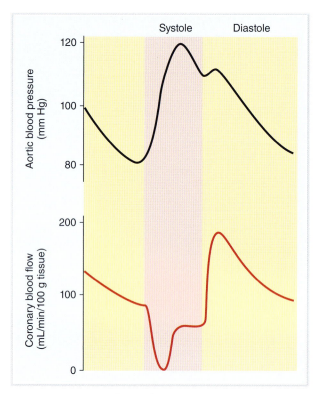

Figure 4-36. Variation in coronary blood flow throughout the cardiac cycle.

2. Coronary blood flow (Figure 4-36).
    a. Unlike blood flow to other organs, *blood flow to the myocardium is higher during diastole than during systole.*
        i. Contraction of the myocardium during systole compresses coronary blood vessels, limiting coronary blood flow.
        ii. *Tachycardia may present a problem for coronary perfusion in patients with heart disease because most blood flow occurs during diastole, which becomes shorter as HR increases.*
    b. **Coronary perfusion pressure** is estimated clinically as the difference between DBP and left ventricular end-diastolic pressure.
        i. *Patients with low DBP or high filling pressures in the heart therefore have a reduced driving force for coronary perfusion.*
    c. O_2 extraction from arterial blood in the myocardium is maximal at rest and the only means of increasing O_2 supply to the heart is to increase coronary blood flow.
        i. *Coronary arteriolar resistance is mostly regulated by metabolic demand of myocytes.*
        ii. An increase in myocardial metabolism causes a local release of vasodilator metabolites such as **adenosine** and CO_2, K^+, and H^+ into the interstitial fluid.
    d. *Autonomic nerves have little direct effect on coronary vascular resistance.* However, sympathetic stimulation indirectly results in coronary vasodilation by increasing cardiac work, causing greater production of local vasodilator metabolites.
    e. When cardiac activity increases, **nitric oxide** is also produced by the vascular endothelial cells.

       i. The stimulus for nitric oxide release is mechanical distortion (shearing forces) acting on the **vascular endothelial cells.**

      ii. Nitric oxide diffuses into nearby vascular smooth muscle cells, where it acts through cyclic guanosine monophosphate (**cGMP**) to produce vasodilation.

     iii. Nitric oxide donors (e.g., nitroglycerin) are used to provide relief from **angina pectoris.**

  f. ▼ Cardiac O_2 consumption is closely related to the amount of ventricular wall tension developed during contraction. Patients with **dilated cardiomyopathy** have an increased myocardial O_2 demand because a dilated heart must develop more wall tension to pressurize the blood. This is a consequence of **Laplace's law ($P = 2T/r$),** which states that the amount of wall tension (T) in a sphere is proportional to both the amount of luminal pressure developed (P) and the radius (r). ▼

  g. ▼ Patients with **atherosclerotic coronary artery disease** have maximal arteriolar dilation at rest and are unable to further increase coronary blood flow.

    • These patients are at risk of developing cardiac ischemia when local O_2 demand increases. Myocardial O_2 consumption is increased by increased HR, increased contractility, and increased afterload (aortic blood pressure).

    • The severity of coronary artery disease can be assessed using a **treadmill stress test,** which may produce angina pectoris and changes that can be seen on an ECG that indicate coronary ischemia. ▼

3. Cerebral blood flow (Figure 4-37).

  a. The brain requires a constant supply of O_2 and its blood flow is relatively independent of MAP and autonomic nervous system activity.

  b. *Cerebral blood flow is mainly determined by **myogenic autoregulation,** in which blood flow is relatively constant over a wide range of MAP, from approximately 60 mm Hg to 130 mm Hg.*

    i. Cerebral arterioles respond directly to the degree of distention by varying smooth muscle tone.

    ii. When MAP decreases, there is less wall distention on arterioles; thus, smooth muscle relaxes and increases vessel diameter, which reduces resistance and restores blood flow.

  c. ▼ *In patients with **chronic hypertension,** the autoregulation curve shifts to the right.*

    i. When these patients are treated with antihypertensive drugs, the corrected blood pressure may be below their range of autoregulation, in which case cerebral blood flow decreases, causing dizziness or altered cognitive function. ▼

  d. *Cerebral blood flow also responds to changes in local metabolic demand and arterial CO_2 partial pressure (Pa_{CO_2}).*

    i. Increased neuronal activity and O_2 consumption cause local vasodilation. [*Note: This is the basis of functional magnetic resonance imaging (fMRI) studies of the brain.*]

    ii. Blood gases, particularly Pa_{CO_2}, strongly influence cerebral blood flow.

      • For example, dizziness associated with hyperventilation is caused by cerebral vasoconstriction resulting from increased CO_2 excretion and reduced Pa_{CO_2}.

A.

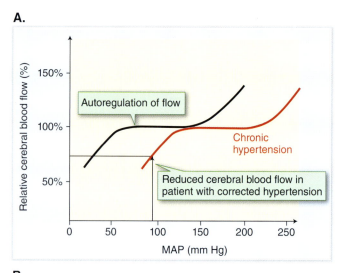

B.

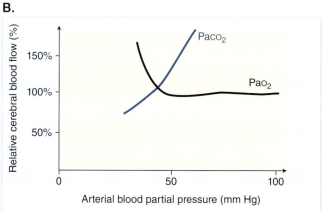

Figure 4-37. Control of cerebral blood flow. **A.** The red curve shows adaptation in the autoregulatory range in a patient with chronic hypertension. If the normal mean arterial pressure (MAP) is below the patient's autoregulatory range, a correction of hypertension may reduce the cerebral blood flow. **B.** The effect of arterial blood gases on cerebral blood flow. MAP, mean arterial pressure.

- Conversely, increased $Paco_2$ causes cerebral vasodilation.
- Variations in Pao_2 have little effect unless severe hypoxemia (low Pao_2) occurs, resulting in pronounced cerebral vasodilation.

e. The brain is the only circulation encased in bone, which limits the total volume of brain tissue, cerebrospinal fluid, and blood.

   i. **Intracranial pressure** increases if there is a tumor, bleeding, or cerebral edema, in which case compression of the blood vessels increases vascular resistance and reduces blood flow.

   ii. **Cerebral perfusion pressure** is estimated as the difference between MAP and intracranial pressure.

f. ▼ Reducing intracranial pressure in the patient with a **head injury** is critical:

   i. In the mechanically ventilated patient, **hyperventilation** can be used to decrease $Paco_2$, causing cerebral vasoconstriction and reducing cerebral blood volume and intracranial pressure.

ii. Intravenous infusion with **hypertonic saline** or mannitol is also used to draw water from the brain by osmosis, decreasing cerebral volume and intracranial pressure. ▼

4. Renal blood flow.

   a. *To supply enough plasma for glomerular filtration, the kidneys have one of the highest rates of organ blood flow.*

   b. Renal perfusion pressure is the difference between MAP and venous pressure and is therefore similar to most other organs.

   c. High rates of blood flow are achieved with normal perfusion pressure because renal vascular resistance is low; vascular resistance is shared equally by afferent and efferent glomerular arterioles (see Chapter 6).

   d. *Renal blood flow is most strongly influenced by **autoregulation** and **sympathetic tone.***

      i. Under most circumstances, renal blood flow is relatively constant because myogenic autoregulation operates over a MAP range of 60–160 mm Hg.

      ii. However, increased sympathetic tone occurs during exercise or if the baroreceptor reflex is stimulated by reduced MAP, resulting in renal vasoconstriction.

      iii. Unlike cerebral blood flow, renal blood flow is not controlled by metabolic factors.

   e. ▼ Despite high tissue O_2 consumption rates, the kidney normally has the lowest O_2 extraction (i.e., AV O_2 concentration difference) of the major organs because normal renal blood flow rates are very high and easily exceed tissue O_2 demand. *However, the kidney is at a high risk of ischemia (e.g., **acute tubular necrosis**) in states of shock due to strong sympathetic vasoconstriction.* ▼

5. Splanchnic blood flow.

   a. The splanchnic circulation receives the highest proportion of cardiac output at rest and is shared among the liver, the spleen, and the digestive organs (see Chapter 7).

   b. *The sympathetic nervous system exerts dominant control over splanchnic blood flow,* causing vasoconstriction and venoconstriction.

   c. Splanchnic blood flow increases significantly after eating due to:

      i. Release of enteric nervous system transmitters (e.g., vasoactive intestinal polypeptide).

      ii. Production of vasodilator local metabolites (*note: parasympathetic stimulation of multiple digestive organs indirectly causes vasodilation through increased local metabolism*).

6. Cutaneous blood flow.

   a. Blood flow to skin is regulated in response to both thermoregulatory signals and general cardiovascular control of MAP.

   b. Activation of **norepinephrinergic sympathetic neurons** by such means as pain, cold, fear, or low MAP leads to cutaneous vasoconstriction, directing blood to more vital organs.

   c. Increased core body temperature causes hypothalamic activation of **cholinergic sympathetic neurons,** resulting in sweating and cutaneous vasodilation to increase heat loss.

7. Skeletal muscle blood flow.

   a. Skeletal muscle has a large flow reserve; at rest, there is relatively high vascular tone and a high proportion of the capillaries are not perfused.

b. Blood flow to **resting muscle** is strongly influenced by norepinephrinergic sympathetic vasoconstriction.

c. During **dynamic exercise,** more than 75% of cardiac output may be directed to working skeletal muscle. *Local metabolism now exerts dominant control over vascular resistance in working skeletal muscle,* and there is recruitment of capillaries that were not perfused at rest.

The Capillary Microcirculation

1. Capillaries are the site for exchange of nutrients and wastes between the blood and tissues.
   a. Capillaries have the largest collective **surface area** in the vascular system.
   b. The **velocity of flow** is least in the capillaries because blood flow is shared among many parallel vessels, with a large collective cross-sectional area.

2. **Diffusion** is the most important mechanism for exchange:
   a. Lipid-soluble substances and gases diffuse readily.
   b. Lipid-insoluble substances such as peptides have low permeability and are restricted to openings between adjacent endothelial cells or transport through cells using vesicular pathways.

3. Transcapillary fluid flux.
   a. Bulk fluid movement occurs between plasma and interstitium across capillary walls; a circuit is formed as interstitial fluid drains via the lymphatic system back into the venous system in the neck.
   b. Understanding factors that determine transcapillary fluid movement is clinically important as the basis for understanding **edema formation** (tissue swelling caused by excessive accumulation of interstitial fluid).
      i. Cerebral edema is dangerous because it increases intracranial pressure, leading to brain compression.
      ii. Pulmonary edema is dangerous because it presents a diffusion barrier for O_2 uptake into the blood.
      iii. However, in other organs a large amount of edema fluid can usually accumulate before organ function is compromised.
   c. Net fluid movement is a function of the driving pressure for filtration and the capillary permeability.
      i. The net driving force for filtration consists of a gradient of hydrostatic pressure that pushes fluid out of plasma and is opposed by a gradient of oncotic pressure:

$$J_v = K_f[(P_c - P_i) - \sigma(\pi_c - \pi_i)] \qquad \textbf{Equation 4-9}$$

J_v = Net fluid flux
K_f = Filtration coefficient
P_c = Capillary hydrostatic pressure
P_i = Interstitial fluid hydrostatic pressure
π_c = Capillary oncotic pressure
π_i = Interstitial fluid oncotic pressure
σ = Protein reflection coefficient

   d. Equation 4-9 is called the Starling equation, and the individual components of the net driving pressure are referred to as **Starling's forces:**

i. **Capillary hydrostatic pressure** (P_c) is a force pushing fluid out of the capillaries. Hydrostatic pressure is usually about 35 mm Hg at the arteriolar end of a capillary, decreasing to about 15 mm Hg at the venous end of a capillary.

ii. **Interstitial fluid hydrostatic pressure** (P_i) is usually near zero or is slightly subatmospheric, favoring fluid movement into the interstitial space.

iii. **Capillary oncotic pressure** (π_c) is an osmotic force exerted by plasma proteins, and pulls fluid into the plasma from the interstitium and is approximately 25 mm Hg.

iv. **Interstitial fluid oncotic pressure** (π_i) is normally low because proteins have reflection coefficients of 0.8–1.0 and interstitial protein concentration is low (see Chapter 1 for a discussion of reflection coefficient).

Example. The following Starling forces were measured in a systemic capillary: capillary hydrostatic pressure = 30 mm Hg, interstitial hydrostatic pressure = 1 mm Hg, capillary oncotic pressure = 25 mm Hg, interstitial oncotic pressure = 2 mm Hg

$$\text{Net pressure} = (P_c - P_i) - (\pi_c - \pi_i)\,\text{mm Hg}$$
$$= (30 - 1) - (25 - 2)\,\text{mm Hg}$$
$$= +6\,\text{mm Hg (favors net filtration)}$$

e. Capillary hydrostatic pressure decreases as blood flows from the arterial to the venous end of a systemic capillary. *Net fluid filtration out of plasma typically occurs at the arterial end of capillary beds, and net fluid reabsorption into plasma occurs toward the venous end* (Figure 4-38).

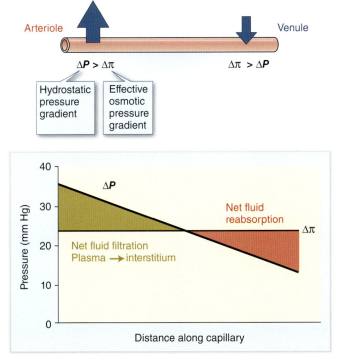

Figure 4-38. Balance of Starling's forces along a normal systemic blood capillary.

Table 4-6. Common Causes of Edema

Mechanism of Edema	$\uparrow P_c$	$\downarrow \pi_c$	$\downarrow \sigma$	Lymphatic Blockage
Some conditions that cause edema	Heart failure	Malnutrition	Sepsis	Tumor
	Hypervolemia	Liver disease	Inflammation	Surgery
	Venous thrombosis or other obstruction	Nephrotic syndrome (renal protein loss)	Burns	Inflammation
	Gravity			Parasite (e.g., filariasis)
	Sustained vasodilation			

4. Lymphatics.
   a. Lymphatic capillaries are permeable to fluid and to protein.
   b. There is net formation of 3–4 L/day of interstitial fluid, which enters the lymphatic capillaries and is delivered back to the venous system through larger lymph vessels, lymph nodes, and lymphatic ducts.
   c. Uptake of lymphatic fluid resists edema formation and can increase as interstitial fluid hydrostatic pressure (P_i) increases.
   d. *Proteins that enter the interstitium from plasma are removed by the lymphatic system.*
   e. Most causes of **edema** (see Table 4-6) can be explained in terms of changes in one or more of the variables noted in Equation 4-9:
      i. The most common causes of edema result from **increased venous pressure** due to heart failure or venous obstruction.
      ii. **Generalized edema** may also result from low serum protein concentration due to reduced capillary oncotic pressure (π_c). For example, this can occur in liver failure when insufficient albumin is synthesized and in nephrotic syndrome when plasma protein is excreted in the urine.
      iii. In **inflammation or sepsis,** generalized edema may occur because inflammatory mediators reduce protein reflection coefficient (σ) and proteins leak into the interstitium, thereby increasing interstitial fluid oncotic pressure.
      iv. **Lymphatic blockage** causes edema because the tissue fluid that has formed is trapped in the interstitium when the outflow pathway is blocked.
   f. ▼ Pulmonary capillaries are normally surrounded by negative intrathoracic pressures, which promote net fluid filtration. Patients with **acute respiratory distress syndrome** may develop pulmonary edema. The edema occurs because the patient must inspire forcefully to breathe, causing intrathoracic pressure and interstitial fluid oncotic pressure to become more negative. ▼
   g. ▼ Assessing whether edema is unilateral or bilateral is important in determining the cause. For example, **congestive heart failure** typically results in bilateral edema (e.g., bilateral pulmonary edema, pleural effusions, and ankle swelling). In contrast, edema caused by blockage of lymphatic drainage that occurs from parasitic infection (e.g., **Wuchereria bancrofti**) is often unilateral. ▼

Study Questions

Directions: Each numbered item is followed by lettered options. Some options may be partially correct, but there is only *ONE BEST* answer.

1. A 14-year-old boy with sickle cell disease received a blood transfusion that caused his blood volume to increase significantly above normal. What changes in cardiac contractility and total peripheral resistance (TPR) would occur within a few minutes of receiving this transfusion?

   A. Increased contractility and increased TPR
   B. Increased contractility and decreased TPR
   C. Decreased contractility and increased TPR
   D. Decreased contractility and decreased TPR

2. A 29-year-old elite endurance athlete completes a medical examination as part of her registration for a triathlon event. Her resting HR is measured at 36 beats/min. Compared with untrained individuals, what change in the cardiac conduction system or autonomic nervous tone is most responsible for this woman's low resting HR?

   A. Decreased automatic rate of (SA) node discharge
   B. Decreased sympathetic neural tone
   C. Decreased vagal tone
   D. Increased automatic rate of SA node discharge
   E. Increased sympathetic neural tone
   F. Increased vagal tone

3. Paramedics were called to attend to a 74-year-old man who fainted while watching a baseball game. When they arrived, the man was conscious but confused. He was noticeably short of breath, had profound bradycardia (HR 25 beats/min), and appeared to be complaining of chest pain. An ECG showed normal P waves that were regularly spaced. QRS complexes were wide and regularly spaced but were dissociated from P waves. What is the most likely origin for electrical stimulation of this patient's ventricles?

   A. SA node
   B. Atrial internodal conduction pathways
   C. AV node
   D. Bundle of His
   E. Purkinje fibers

4. A 40-year-old woman from a remote rural area is transferred to a city hospital for treatment of a longstanding heart valve abnormality. Her chief current complaint is the inability to perform any physical work, although she also reports waking several times each night with severe shortness of breath. Auscultation reveals a long rumbling diastolic murmur and an opening snap. Which valve abnormality does this patient most likely have?

   A. Aortic stenosis
   B. Aortic insufficiency
   C. Mitral stenosis
   D. Mitral insufficiency

5. An 80-year-old man visits a new family physician. He has not visited a physician for 15 years, but is presently having trouble sleeping and is seeking a prescription for sleeping pills. Upon physical examination, the man seems in good physical health but his blood pressure is 160/80 mm Hg, and his HR is 66 beats/min. The patient has never been treated for hypertension and recalls no previous blood pressure problems. What is the most likely cause of elevated blood pressure in this patient?

   A. Decreased aortic compliance
   B. Decreased parasympathetic nerve activity
   C. Increased sympathetic nerve activity
   D. Increased vascular smooth muscle tone

6. A 64-year-old woman with hypertension (blood pressure of 160/110 mm Hg) and coronary artery disease was treated with angiotensin-converting enzyme (ACE) inhibitors. After a period when the treatment was no longer effective, the dose of ACE inhibitors was abruptly increased. Although this successfully reduced her blood pressure to 130/80 mm Hg, she complained that the medications now made her very dizzy. Reduced cerebral perfusion, resulting in dizziness, is most likely to be explained in this case by

   A. decreased brain angiotensin II levels
   B. decreased sympathetic tone
   C. inadequate blood flow autoregulation
   D. increased intracranial pressure
   E. increased parasympathetic tone

7. A 41-year-old woman has a routine physical examination as part of a well-woman initiative by her family physician. She is an office worker with a sedentary lifestyle and is concerned about being overweight, but reports no recent illness. Her blood pressure is 140/100 mm Hg, and her HR is 80 beats/min. The most likely reason for her increased systolic blood pressure is an increased

   A. baroreceptor sensitivity
   B. diastolic blood pressure
   C. HR
   D. SV
   E. vascular tone

8. A 40-year-old man with a history of rheumatic fever as a child is awaiting valve replacement surgery to treat chronic mitral valve stenosis. He is severely short of breath, with rales and crackles clearly audible over both lungs. There is pitting edema of the lower extremities and ascites in his abdomen. Which of the following changes in Starling's forces is the most likely cause of edema in this patient?

   A. Decreased capillary hydrostatic pressure
   B. Decreased capillary oncotic pressure
   C. Decreased interstitial hydrostatic pressure
   D. Decreased interstitial oncotic pressure
   E. Increased capillary hydrostatic pressure
   F. Increased capillary oncotic pressure

G. Increased interstitial hydrostatic pressure

H. Increased interstitial oncotic pressure

9. A 52-year-old man with a history of alcoholism has recently developed generalized edema. Abnormal liver function tests include increased serum levels of transaminase enzymes. His blood clotting time is increased, and he is unresponsive to vitamin K treatment. What is the most likely cause of edema in this patient?

A. Decreased capillary hydrostatic pressure

B. Decreased capillary oncotic pressure

C. Decreased interstitial hydrostatic pressure

D. Decreased interstitial oncotic pressure

E. Increased capillary hydrostatic pressure

F. Increased capillary oncotic pressure

G. Increased interstitial hydrostatic pressure

H. Increased interstitial oncotic pressure

10. A 14-year-old girl from the southern Caribbean was rescued after a major hurricane. She was initially treated for minor injuries and dehydration but was referred for further investigations due to a persistently low blood pressure (95/40 mm Hg). A continuous machinery-like murmur was heard upon auscultation of her chest. An ECG and an echocardiogram revealed left ventricular hypertrophy. Which of the following cardiac abnormalities is most likely to be present?

A. Aortic valve insufficiency

B. Aortic valve stenosis

C. Mitral valve prolapse

D. Mitral valve stenosis

E. Patent ductus arteriosus

Pulmonary Physiology

CHAPTER 5

Fundamentals

1. The primary function of the respiratory (pulmonary) system is to maintain systemic arterial blood gas levels within normal range.
   a. The rates of O_2 uptake and CO_2 excretion at the lungs must match the rates of O_2 use and CO_2 production by cellular respiration.
2. The main components of the respiratory system are the lungs, chest wall, and pulmonary blood vessels.
   a. Muscles of the chest wall power the movement of air into the lungs during inspiration.
   b. *The distribution of pulmonary blood flow and ventilation must match for proper gas exchange.*
3. The levels of systemic O_2 and CO_2 are monitored by **chemoreceptors,** allowing the pulmonary system to respond to changes in cellular respiration.
4. The blood-gas interface.
   a. Repeated dichotomous branching of the airways begins at the trachea and terminates in over 300 million closed air sacs called **alveoli,** with a collective surface area of 50–100 m^2.
   b. *Ventilation is the process whereby air enters the lungs and comes into contact with alveoli*, which are the sites of gas exchange.
   c. The blood-gas interface is less than 1 μm thick and consists of the following **four elements in series** (Figure 5-1):
      i. A thin layer of surface liquid.
      ii. Alveolar lining cells (**type 1 pneumocytes**).
      iii. A thin layer of interstitial fluid.
      iv. Pulmonary capillary endothelial cells.
5. Gas laws (Table 5-1).
   a. According to **Boyle's law,** the volume of a gas varies inversely with its pressure at a constant temperature. For example, a gas can be compressed to a smaller volume at higher pressure.
      i. Boyle's law explains air flow into the lung on inspiration—lung volume is first increased when contraction of the inspiratory muscles expands the chest, which reduces the alveolar pressure below atmospheric pressure and draws air into the lung.
   b. **Dalton's law** states that each gas in a mixture of gases exerts a **partial pressure** that is proportional to its concentration (Figure 5-2).
      i. The term "**gas tension**" is used interchangeably with partial pressure.
      ii. The sum of partial pressures equals the total pressure.

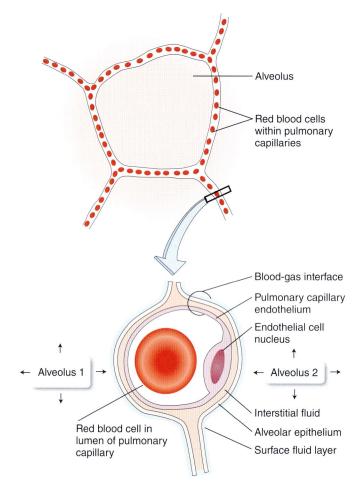

Figure 5-1. Alveolar blood-gas barrier.

Table 5-1. Gas Laws and Applications in Respiratory Physiology

Law	Formula	Application
Boyle's law	$P_1V_1 = P_2V_2$	• Basis of gas flow during ventilation: mechanical events change lung volume, resulting in pressure gradients that drive gas flow. • Derivation of residual volume using whole-body plethysmography.
Charles' law	$V_1/V_2 = T_1/T_2$	• Gas volume varies in proportion to temperature; air expands as it is warmed during inspiration.
Dalton's law	$P_{total} = \sum_{x=1}^{n} P_{gas(x)}$	• For atmospheric air: $P_B \approx P_{N_2} + P_{O_2}$ • Estimate of inspired O_2: $P_{IO_2} = P_B - P_{H_2O} - P_{N_2}$ *Or* $P_{IO_2} = (P_B - P_{H_2O}) \times F_{IO_2}$
Henry's law	$C_X = KP_X$	• Volume of dissolved gas is proportional to partial pressure. If arterial blood $P_{CO_2} = 40$ mm Hg and K (solubility constant) $= 0.06$ mL CO_2 per dL blood per mm Hg CO_2: $C_{CO_2} = 0.06 \times 40 = 2.4$ mL/dL (*note: total blood CO_2 content includes bicarbonate ions and carbamino compounds; this calculation is only for dissolved CO_2 molecules*).

C_X, gas content; P, pressure; T, temperature; V, volume.

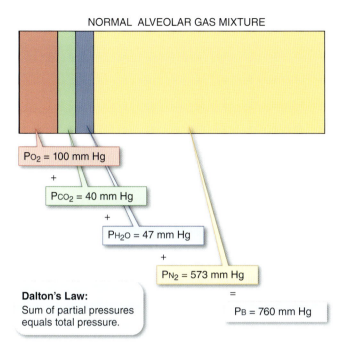

NORMAL ALVEOLAR GAS MIXTURE

P_{O_2} = 100 mm Hg

+

P_{CO_2} = 40 mm Hg

+

P_{H_2O} = 47 mm Hg

+

P_{N_2} = 573 mm Hg

=

P_B = 760 mm Hg

Dalton's Law:
Sum of partial pressures
equals total pressure.

Figure 5-2. Dalton's law of partial pressures applied to normal alveolar gas composition.

   c. **Henry's law** states that the volume of gas dissolved in a liquid is proportional to its partial pressure.

      i. In clinical medicine, partial pressures are reported for gases in blood as well as in air.

      ii. *Partial pressure in a liquid refers to gas molecules that are free in solution rather than bound to hemoglobin.*

      iii. At the alveolus, respiratory gases diffuse to equilibrium so that *the partial pressures of O_2 (P_{O_2}) and CO_2 (P_{CO_2}) are the same in alveolar air and in end-pulmonary capillary blood plasma.*

6. Units and terminology used in respiratory physiology (Table 5-2).

   a. Gas pressures are traditionally reported based on the height of a column of liquid; for example, mm Hg (also called **Torr**) or cm H_2O (1 mm Hg = 1.36 cm H_2O).

      i. The **Pascal** is the international unit of pressure: 1 kPa (kilopascal) = 7.5 mm Hg.

   b. **Barometric pressure (P_B)** is the total gas pressure in the atmosphere due to the weight of the Earth's atmosphere. P_B = 760 mm Hg at sea level; P_B decreases at higher altitudes and increases at greater depths.

      i. Individual gas quantities can be described as fractions: a **gas fraction** is partial pressure divided by total pressure.

      ii. Atmospheric gas is comprised of approximately 21% O_2 and 78% N_2 and very small quantities of other gases. Knowing that the fraction of O_2 in air is 21%, *the P_{O_2} in inspired air at sea level is 21% of 760 mm Hg = 160 mm Hg.*

7. Water vapor.

   a. *The composition of air is altered during inspiration because air is humidified in the upper respiratory tract.*

Table 5-2. Standard Notations Used for Gas Quantities and Locations

Symbol	Definition	Example
Px	Partial pressure of gas x	P_{CO_2}: partial pressure of carbon dioxide
Fx	Fractional volume or pressure $F_x = P_x / P_{total}$	F_{N_2}: nitrogen fraction of gas mixture
Sx	Saturation (usually of hemoglobin with O_2), expressed as decimal fraction or %	S_{O_2}: % saturation of hemoglobin with oxygen
Cx	Concentration (content) of gas; blood content for O_2 and CO_2 includes several forms of the gas (e.g., some O_2 is carried as dissolved molecules but most is bound to hemoglobin)	C_{O_2}: total oxygen content
Locations		
a	Arterial blood	Pa_{CO_2}: carbon dioxide partial pressure of arterial blood
v	Mixed venous blood	Pv_{CO_2}: carbon dioxide partial pressure of mixed venous blood
c	Pulmonary capillary blood	$C_c_{O_2}$: oxygen partial pressure of pulmonary capillary blood
A	Alveolar gas	Pa_{O_2}: alveolar oxygen partial pressure
I	Inspired air	F_{IO_2}: oxygen fraction of inspired gas
E	Mixed expired air	Pe_{CO_2}: carbon dioxide partial pressure in mixed expired air

    b. The water vapor pressure, or partial pressure of water (P_{H_2O}) in inspired air, is 47 mm Hg at 37°C.

    c. The addition of water vapor to inspired air reduces the partial pressure of other gases. For example, at sea level, inspired O_2 (P_{IO_2}) is reduced from 160 mm Hg to 150 mm Hg [$0.21 \times (760 - 47)$].

    d. When gas volume is reported clinically, the standard condition of **body temperature and pressure, saturated (BTPS)** is used and assumes a body temperature of 37°C (310°K), a barometric pressure of 760 mm Hg, and a water vapor pressure of 47 mm Hg.

Mechanics of Breathing

1. *Airflow in and out of the lungs requires pressure gradients between the mouth and the alveolus,* which are created by mechanical changes in lung volume.
2. Breathing becomes difficult if the lung or the chest wall is stiff (there is low compliance) or if the resistance to gas flow along the airway is high.
    a. **Resistance** is a dynamic property determined during gas flow.
    b. **Compliance** is an **elastic property** and is measured without gas flow.
3. Lung volumes.
    a. A **spirometer** is an instrument that is used during **pulmonary function testing** to measure lung volumes and gas flow rates. A patient breathes

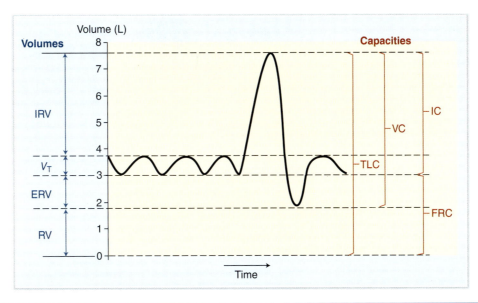

Primary Lung Volume	Definition
Tidal volume (V_T)	Volume of a quiet breath.
Inspiratory reserve volume (IRV)	Volume that can be inspired above V_T.
Expiratory reserve volume (ERV)	Volume that can be expired from the end of a tidal expiration.
Residual volume (RV)*	Volume remaining in the lung after maximal expiration.
Primary Lung Capacity	
Total lung capacity (TLC)*	(IRV + V_T + ERV + RV): Total volume of gas in the lung after maximal inspiration.
Vital capacity (VC)	(IRV + V_T + ERV): Volume of maximal expiration from a maximal inspiration.
Inspiratory capacity (IC)	(IRV + V_T): Maximal inspiration from the end of tidal expiration.
Functional residual capacity (FRC)*	(ERV + RV): Volume of gas in the lungs at the end of tidal expiration *(reflects equilibrium between lung and chest wall recoil forces).*

*These capacities cannot be measured directly by spirometry because they include residual volume.

Figure 5-3. Normal spirogram showing four primary lung volumes and four capacities.

normally for a period, and then inspires maximally before forcefully expiring as much air as possible (Figure 5-3).

  i. **Tidal volume (V_T)** is the amount breathed in and out during normal breathing.
 ii. **Vital capacity (VC)** is the maximum possible volume that can be expired following the largest breath inspired.
iii. **Residual volume (RV)** is the volume of gas remaining in the lung at the end of forceful expiration (and could not be expelled without collapsing the lung).
 iv. **Functional residual capacity (FRC)** is the resting lung volume at the end of quiet expiration.
  v. Normal FRC is approximately 40% of **total lung capacity (TLC)**. *Many variables are optimized at normal FRC, including work of breathing, vascular resistance, and ventilation/perfusion ($\dot{V}/\dot{Q}$) matching.* Mechanical ventilation of patients is often used to correct an abnormal FRC to help restore normal respiratory function.

4. Muscles of ventilation.
   a. *The **diaphragm** is the most important muscle of inspiration.* Its contraction increases the vertical height of the thoracic cavity due to flattening of the domes of the diaphragm.
   b. The **external intercostal muscles** slope downward and forward between adjacent ribs, which produces a "bucket-handle" movement of the ribs and increases the lateral and anteroposterior diameter of the chest.
   c. Expiration is passive during quiet breathing but becomes active during exercise.
      i. *The most important muscles of active expiration are those of the abdominal wall.*
      ii. The **internal intercostal muscles** are arranged at right angles to the external oblique muscles and assist expiration by pulling the ribs downward and inward.
   d. ▼ **Neuromuscular diseases** such as Guillain-Barré syndrome can affect respiratory function by causing respiratory muscle weakness. If there is severe muscle weakness, patients may require mechanical ventilation. ▼

5. Airway anatomy (Figure 5-4).
   a. As air is drawn into the lungs, it is distributed through a highly branched airway.
   b. The first 16–17 generations of airway division are the **conducting zone** (i.e., from the trachea through the various bronchi and bronchioles to the terminal bronchioles).
   c. Gas exchange occurs in the **respiratory zone** of the airway and begins distal to the terminal bronchioles.

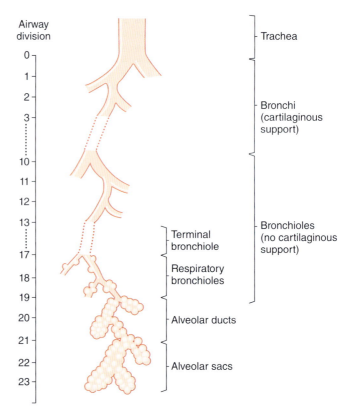

Figure 5-4. Airway divisions. The first 16–17 generations are conducting airways only. Gas exchange only occurs in the respiratory zone from generations 17 to 23. A lung acinus is formed from the divisions of a terminal bronchiole. A lung unit includes a lung acinus and associated blood vessels.

d. A **lung acinus** is a functional unit formed by the division of a terminal bronchiole into the respiratory bronchioles, alveolar ducts, and terminal alveoli.

e. *Gas moves by diffusion within lung acini because the cross-sectional area of the respiratory zone is so large that bulk gas flow approaches zero.*

f. ▼ The concept of a lung acinus is useful when describing certain lung pathologies. Alveolar damage in patients with **emphysema** is either centriacinar (most common) or panacinar.

   i. In centriacinar emphysema, the primary site of damage is the respiratory bronchioles, with sparing of the distal alveoli. *This type of emphysema is associated with smoking, and the most damage is seen in the apical regions of the upper lobes.*

   ii. In panacinar emphysema, the entire acinus is damaged. Panacinar emphysema is associated with α_1-**antitrypsin disease.**

     • α_1-Antitrypsin is a serum protein produced by the liver and combats damaging protease activity, particularly in the lung.

     • α_1-Antitrypsin disease is a genetic condition in which α_1-antitrypsin accumulates in the liver (resulting in cirrhosis), causing the protein to be systemically unavailable.

     • The panacinar emphysema that develops typically involves the entire lung, with the lung bases being most diseased. ▼

6. Lung and chest wall recoil.

a. The presence of subatmospheric pressure within the chest draws air into the airway during inspiration.

b. *Subatmospheric pressure in the intrapleural space is created by the opposing recoil of the lungs and chest wall.*

c. When all the respiratory muscles are relaxed, the lung is at its resting lung volume (FRC), and there is equilibrium between the recoil of the lung and the chest wall. *At this point, the lung tends to collapse and the chest wall tends to expand, with the two being held together by a thin layer of pleural fluid.*

d. If the chest wall is punctured, air will flow into the pleural space (**pneumothorax**) until intrapleural pressure (PIP) equals atmospheric pressure; the lung will then collapse and the chest wall will spring outward (Figure 5-5).

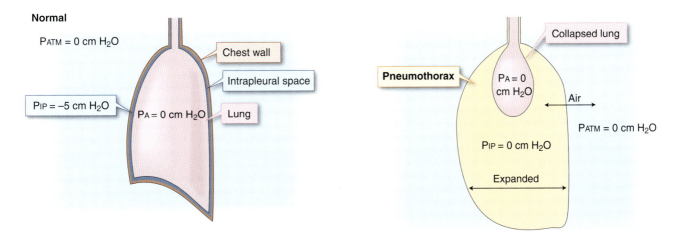

Figure 5-5. Effect of pneumothorax on lung volume and thoracic volume.

e. ▼ **Pneumothorax** can be spontaneous or traumatic in origin. Intrapleural air must be evacuated by connecting a chest tube to suction, which restores negative intrapleural pressures and expands the collapsed lung. ▼

f. The force acting across the wall of the lung to expand it is a transmural pressure called the **transpulmonary pressure** (P_{TP}). Transpulmonary pressure is calculated as the difference in pressure between the alveoli (P_A) and the intrapleural space (P_{IP}):

$$P_{TP} = P_A - P_{IP} \hspace{3cm} \textbf{Equation 5-1}$$

P_{TP} = Transpulmonary pressure
P_A = Alveolar pressure
P_{IP} = Intrapleural pressure

i. **Example.** When the respiratory muscles are relaxed, the alveolar pressure is the same as the atmospheric pressure (given a relative value of 0 cm H_2O), and the intrapleural pressure (P_{IP}) is about -5 cm H_2O:
At rest: $P_{TP} = 0 - (-5) = +5$ cm H_2O

ii. The force between the lung and the chest wall increases when the inspiratory muscles contract, causing P_{IP} to become more negative; for example, P_{IP} is -10 cm H_2O during normal quiet inspiration. The lung expands because P_{TP} is increased:
Inspiration: $P_{TP} = 0 - (-10) = +10$ cm H_2O

iii. Transmural pressure is calculated as the inside pressure minus the outside pressure. A positive value of transpulmonary pressure indicates a distending force (e.g., inspiration); a negative transpulmonary pressure is a compression force (e.g., forced expiration).

7. The ventilation cycle.
   a. *Air flows into or out of the lung when there is a difference in pressure along the airway between the mouth and alveoli.*
   b. Airflow is driven by changes in alveolar pressure, which in turn result from changes in intrapleural pressure.
   c. Contraction of the inspiratory muscles reduces P_{IP} and increases P_{TP}, providing a force for lung expansion.
   d. Increased lung volume decreases alveolar pressure, which drives inspiration.
   e. *Note: In Figure 5-6 airflow is in phase with alveolar pressure changes. As air flows into the lung to occupy the increased volume, alveolar pressure returns to atmospheric pressure, ending inspiration.*
   f. Passive recoil of the lung and chest wall during quiet expiration causes the lung volume to decrease. As a result, the alveolar pressure increases and gas flows out of the lung.

8. Pressure-volume relation of the lung.
   a. During the cycle of ventilation, several factors contribute to the **work of breathing,** including lung and chest wall compliance and resistance to gas flow.
   b. *Compliance is a pressure-volume relation,* and is defined as the transpulmonary pressure change that is required to produce a unit change in lung volume.

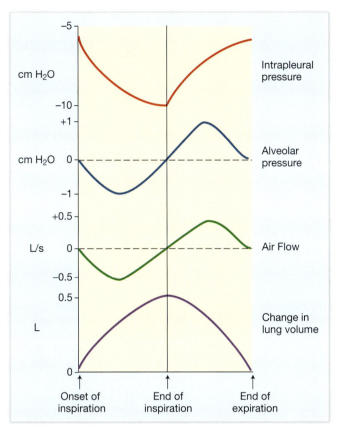

Figure 5-6. Ventilation cycle. Lung volume changes due to airflow into or out of the lung. Gas flow depends on a gradient of pressure from the mouth to the alveolus; alveolar pressure change occurs in response to altered intrapleural pressure.

   i. If measurements are recorded at the start and end of a tidal breath when gas flow has stopped, **static compliance** is determined as:

$$C_{STAT} = V_T / \Delta P_{TP} \qquad \textbf{Equation 5-2}$$

C_{STAT} = Static compliance (mL/cm H_2O)
  V_T = Tidal volume (mL)
  P_{TP} = Transpulmonary pressure (cm H_2O)

  ii. ▼ Patients with **pulmonary fibrosis** or **lung edema** have reduced lung compliance and, therefore, have increased work of breathing, which is sensed as dyspnea or shortness of breath. *These patients usually take small tidal breaths to minimize the change in transpulmonary pressure needed to inspire.* ▼

 iii. ▼ Patients with **pulmonary emphysema** have increased lung compliance. *They do not have difficulty breathing in but experience airway obstruction on expiration* (see Dynamic Airway Compression). ▼

  c. Figure 5-7 shows several important features of lung mechanics:

   i. *Lung compliance is reduced at both high and low lung volumes.* At high volume, lung tissue is already stretched and further distension requires more force. At low volume, many lung acini are collapsed and more force is needed to initiate inspiration.

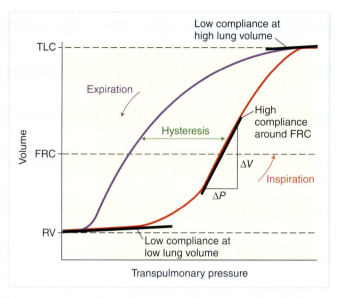

Figure 5-7. Pressure-volume (compliance) curve for a maximal breath. Compliance is low at both high and low lung volumes. Hysteresis is the phenomenon of the different path of the expiration curve compared to inspiration. FRC, functional residual capacity; RV, residual volume; TLC, total lung capacity.

  ii. The steepest part of the pressure-volume relation, where compliance is largest, is at the point of FRC. *This explains why it is easier for a person to breathe around FRC and uncomfortable to breathe at high or low lung volume.*
 d. The pressure-volume relation for expiration is positioned to the left of that of inspiration. This phenomenon is called **hysteresis** and is due to the action of **lung surfactants.**
   i. Surfactants are phospholipids, mainly dipalmitoyl phosphatidylcholine, secreted by **type 2 pneumocytes** in the alveolar walls.
  ii. As the lung volume decreases during expiration *surfactant molecules repel each other and resist the tendency of alveoli to become smaller, giving more time for gases to diffuse across the alveolar membranes.*
  iii. The left shift of the pressure-volume relation on expiration compared to inspiration (hysteresis) is explained by this action of surfactant to maintain alveoli open during expiration.
 e. Surfactants and surface tension.
   i. Surface tension acts at the air-liquid interface of alveoli and tends to reduce the area of the alveolus and to generate pressure within it.
  ii. *Surfactants are required to counteract surface tension, which is the main reason that the lung tends to collapse.*
  iii. Surfactant molecules at the air-liquid interface of the alveoli reduce surface tension, thereby maintaining normal lung compliance and preventing alveolar collapse.
  iv. ▼ **Atelectasis** is the name given to an area of collapsed lung, and is often considered the culprit that causes the mild fever that can occur within the first 24–48 hours after surgery. Atelectasis predisposes the patient to pneumonia, but can be reversed or prevented by having the patient cough or perform breathing exercises. ▼

v. The **law of Laplace** (Equation 5-3) predicts another problem caused by surface tension (as well as the collapse of alveoli)—alveoli with small radii (r) will have higher internal pressure (P) for a given surface tension (T) than will larger alveoli. As a consequence, small alveoli will empty into larger alveoli unless lung surfactants maintain a low surface tension.

$$P = \frac{2T}{r}$$
                                    Equation 5-3

P = Pressure
T = Surface tension
r = Radius of sphere

vi. ▼ **Respiratory distress syndrome (RDS) of the newborn (hyaline membrane disease)** is caused by a deficiency of surfactant and is associated with prematurity and with infants of diabetic mothers.
  - Without surfactant, the infant's lungs undergo widespread alveolar collapse, producing low lung compliance.
  - A collection of debris consisting of damaged cells, exudative necrosis, and proteins lines the alveoli and is referred to as the **hyaline membrane.**
  - Treating the mother with **corticosteroids** 48 hours prior to delivery increases surfactant production and decreases the incidence of RDS. ▼

9. Elastic properties of the lung and chest wall.
  a. Compliance is optimal around FRC; a normal FRC is associated with the smallest work of breathing.
  b. *FRC is controlled by the relative strength of the lung and the chest wall recoil forces.*
  c. There is opposition of the elastic forces of the lung and chest wall: The lung tends to collapse and the chest wall tends to expand.
  d. Figure 5-8 shows relaxation pressures in the airway if a patient is asked to take several breaths of different volume, and after each inspiration to then completely relax the respiratory muscles.
  e. When airway pressure is zero and all muscles are relaxed there is equilibrium between the lung and chest wall recoil and lung volume is at FRC.
  f. If the lung volume is increased or decreased away from this equilibrium position, effort must be applied by the respiratory muscles but the lung will return passively to FRC.
    i. *In normal quiet breathing, inspiration is active and expiration is passive.*
  g. Figure 5-8 shows how the individual elastic properties of the lung and chest wall compare to properties of the combined lung-chest wall unit (*note: individual lung and chest wall properties cannot be measured in a living person*).
  h. Lungs tend to collapse at all lung volumes from RV to TLC, shown by positive recoil pressures in the airway after the lung is inflated.
    i. *The tendency of the lung to collapse is due to surface tension and also to the elastic nature of lung tissue.*
  i. In contrast, the equilibrium position of the chest wall, where recoil pressure is zero, is at approximately 75% of TLC.

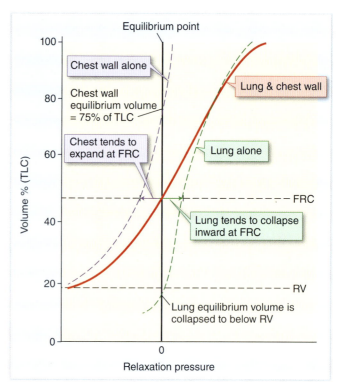

Figure 5-8. Control of functional residual capacity (FRC). Equilibrium between opposing lung and chest wall recoil forces determines FRC. In general, lungs tend to collapse and the chest wall tends to expand. RV, residual volume; TLC, total lung capacity.

Table 5-3. Causes and Effects of Low Thoracic Compliance

Cause	Effect
Pulmonary fibrosis	Lung tissue is difficult to distend; lung compliance is low.
Pulmonary edema	Lung is difficult to distend; lung compliance is low.
Pleural effusion	Increased fluid in pleural space resists lung expansion.
Thoracic musculoskeletal pain	Patient avoids deep inspiration due to pain.
Rib fracture	Example of musculoskeletal pain but with reflex spasm of intercostal muscles to produce rigid chest wall.
Morbid obesity	Especially in supine position, weight of tissue on chest wall and abdomen resists thoracic expansion.
Increased abdominal pressure (e.g., ascites, bowel distension)	The diaphragm is normally the most compliant part of the chest wall; pressure from below resists descent of the diaphragm during inspiration.

     i. At all volumes below 75% of TLC, recoil pressures are negative and the chest wall expands passively.

    ii. At thoracic volumes above 75% of TLC, both the lung and the chest wall passively decrease their volumes.

  j. When overall compliance of the lung-chest wall unit is reduced, greater force is needed for inspiration, increasing the work of breathing (Table 5-3).

  k. ▼ **Interstitial lung disease** is a general term used for many diseases that involve the lung parenchyma and cause the lung to be stiff and fibrotic with low compliance. Regardless of the cause, patients with interstitial lung disease typically present with similar manifestations of progressive exertional dyspnea, nonproductive cough, fatigue, and weight loss. ▼

10. Airway resistance.

   a. Mechanical work required for gas flow into and out of the lung requires overcoming airway resistance as well as the elastic properties of the lung and the chest wall.

   b. **Airway resistance** is referred to as a **dynamic property** because it is only apparent during gas flow. Airway resistance (R) determines the rate of gas flow ($\dot{V}$) for a given pressure gradient from the alveolus to the mouth (ΔP). According to **Ohm's law,**

$$\dot{V} = \Delta P / R \qquad\qquad \textbf{Equation 5-4}$$

$\dot{V}$ = Gas flow rate

ΔP = Pressure gradient from mouth to alveolus

  R = Airway resistance

   c. *Airway radius is the main component of airway resistance* (Figure 5-9).

     i. The upper airway offers significant fixed resistance.

     ii. Resistance rapidly decreases from the fifth through the tenth generation of airway division.

     iii. The respiratory zone of the lung has very low resistance because the collective cross-sectional area of lung acini is large.

     iv. Bronchi and **bronchioles** are sites of variable resistance and contain smooth muscle.

       • Parasympathetic nerves release acetylcholine and cause **bronchoconstriction.**

       • Catecholamines relax bronchial smooth muscle through β_2 receptors.

   d. ▼ **Asthma** is a classic obstructive lung disease whose key differentiating feature demonstrated on spirometry is *reversible bronchoconstriction following treatment with a β_2-agonist such as* **albuterol.**

     i. Asthma is characterized by inflammatory hyperreactive airways, and triggers can include allergens (most common), infections (often viral), exercise, cold air, and drugs such as aspirin.

     ii. When attempting to diagnose airway hyperreactivity, **methacholine** (a parasympathomimetic agent) can be given during pulmonary function testing to provoke bronchospasm. ▼

   e. **Lung volume** is an important determinant of airway resistance because the overall cross-sectional area of airways varies with lung volume, causing global changes in airway radius (Figure 5-10).

     i. At low lung volume, the cross-sectional area is reduced and airway resistance increases. For example, patients with pulmonary fibrosis have low lung compliance and low resting lung volume; high airway resistance contributes to their increased work of breathing.

     ii. ▼ **Idiopathic pulmonary fibrosis** is a specific type of interstitial lung disease. It is the most common cause of idiopathic interstitial pneumonia and has a poor prognosis. The histologic hallmark of idiopathic pulmonary fibrosis is alternating areas of a normal lung with

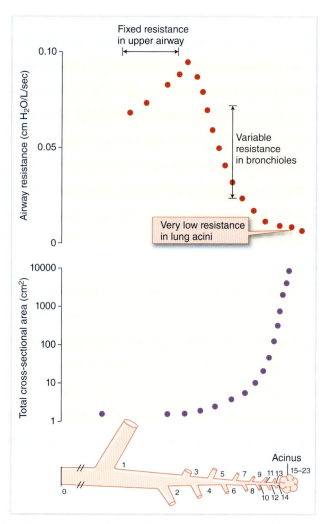

Figure 5-9. Location of airway resistance. The upper airway offers high fixed resistance. Bronchiolar resistance is variable and depends on smooth muscle tone. Resistance is very low in the respiratory zone due to the large total cross-sectional area of the airway at this location.

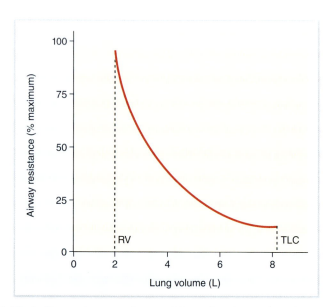

Figure 5-10. Effect of lung volume on airway resistance. Low lung volume increases airway resistance due to reduced airway diameter. RV, residual volume; TLC, total lung capacity.

Table 5-4. Breath Sounds

Breath Sound	Description	Occurrence
Wheezing	Prominent musical or whistling sound, typically during expiration, created by high-velocity airflow from restricted airways	Commonly occurs during bronchospasm (asthma), airway edema (allergic reaction/anaphylaxis), or airway partial obstruction (neoplasm, secretions, foreign object)
Rales (crackles, crepitus)	Typically inspiratory; described as fine (sounds similar to rubbing a strand of hair between the fingers) or coarse (sounds like Velcro), created by forceful opening of alveoli	Commonly occurs in pulmonary edema, atelectasis, and interstitial lung disease
Rhonchi	Low-pitched vibration (snoring), often rattling, occurring during inspiration and/or expiration; created by mucus-air interface	Commonly occurs in bronchitis or chronic obstructive pulmonary disease (COPD)
Stridor	Harsh high-pitched wheeze during inspiration created by severe upper-airway obstruction; often indicates a medical emergency	Commonly occurs in infants with croup (laryngotracheobronchitis), foreign body obstruction at the level of the larynx, epiglottis, or laryngeal tumor or edema

areas of inflammation and fibrosis with architectural changes known as **honeycombing.** These patients have a restrictive pattern of lung disease (see Clinical Spirometry). ▼

   f. **Turbulent gas flow** also increases airway resistance.

      i. Turbulent flow occurs in the larger central airways, where flow velocity is high, and at branch points along the conducting airways.

      ii. Disorganization of the gas stream requires more pressure to drive flow and effectively increases resistance.

      iii. Bronchoconstriction reduces the airway diameter and increases the velocity of flow. High velocity causes turbulent flow, which generates a **wheezing** sound (e.g., in asthma) (Table 5-4).

11. Dynamic airway compression.

   a. During forced expiration, contraction of the expiratory muscles increases the intrapleural pressure and alveolar pressure.

   b. Airway pressure declines from the alveolus to the mouth and air is expelled along this pressure gradient.

   c. *Airway resistance increases during forced expiration because the airways are compressed by the positive intrapleural pressure* (Figure 5-11).

      i. *The transmural pressure gradient compressing the airways is larger with increasing distance away from the alveolus* since the airway pressure is decreasing from the alveolus to the mouth.

      ii. The largest compression forces are applied to larger airways, which have cartilaginous support to resist collapse.

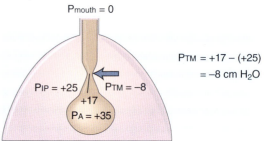

A. End-inspiration

$P_{mouth} = 0$

$P_{IP} = -10$

0 →

$P_{TM} = +10$

$P_A = 0$

$P_{TM} = 0 - (-10)$
$= +10$ cm H_2O

B. Forced expiration

$P_{mouth} = 0$

$P_{IP} = +25$

$P_{TM} = -8$

+17

$P_A = +35$

$P_{TM} = +17 - (+25)$
$= -8$ cm H_2O

Figure 5-11. Dynamic airway compression. At the end of deep inspiration (**A**), a positive transmural pressure maintains open airways. In the example of forced expiration shown in (**B**), 35 cm H_2O is added to both alveolar pressure and intrapleural pressure ($P_{IP} = -10 + 35 = +25$; $P_A = 0 + 35 = +35$). Airways are compressed by high intrapleural pressure. The transmural pressure compressing the airways increases with distance from the alveolus because pressure inside the airway decreases from the alveolus to the mouth. Small airways only have radial traction forces to prevent airway collapse.

    iii.   *The **distal bronchioles** are at risk of collapsing because they do not have cartilaginous support.*

    iv. Distal lung units partially resist collapse due to **radial traction forces**, created by structural connections between neighboring lung units.

  d. ▼ Dynamic airway compression is a problem in patients with **emphysema,** where destruction of the lung architecture weakens the radial traction forces. *Airway collapse occurs upon forced expiration, dramatically increasing airway resistance and trapping gas in the alveoli.* ▼

  e. ▼ **Air trapping** is a chronic problem for patients with emphysema. High lung compliance allows the chest wall to recoil outwards at rest, increasing the FRC and the RV.

    i. Clinical examination findings include increased anterior to posterior diameter, known as **barrel chest;** there is **hyperresonance** on percussion and decreased breath sounds on auscultation.

    ii. Chest radiography shows large hyperlucent lung fields and **flattened diaphragms** because the diaphragm is the most compliant part of the chest wall. ▼

  f. ▼ *Patients with emphysema usually take large, slow breaths and may exhale through **pursed lips** to reduce the work of breathing.*

i. Slow expiration requires less force so that intrapleural pressure is smaller, reducing the compression force on airways.

ii. Breathing out through pursed lips creates a positive pressure inside the airways to decrease airway collapse. ▼

12. Advanced Mechanics Concept 1: Expiratory flow limitation.

a. Maximal expiratory flow rate is achieved in normal lungs with only moderate expiratory effort due to dynamic airway compression.

b. Figure 5-12A shows plots of expiratory flow rate as a function of lung volume when a patient uses different degrees of effort to breathe out from TLC to RV.

i. In forced expiration from TLC, there is a rapid initial increase in flow rate to a peak and then a steady decline in flow rate as RV is approached.

A. Expiratory flow-volume curve

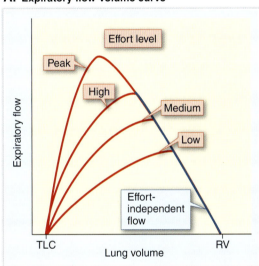

B. Isovolume pressure-flow curve

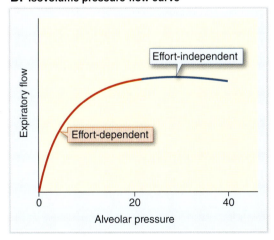

Figure 5-12. Expiratory flow limitation. A series of expirations from total lung capacity are measured with varying degrees of effort. Curves converge at mid and low lung volumes (**A**), showing that expiratory rate is independent of effort in this region. If alveolar pressure is measured as an index of effort (**B**), expiratory flow rate plateaus, demonstrating expiratory flow limitation. RV, residual volume; TLC, total lung capacity.

ii. Regardless of effort, the descending limb of the flow-volume loop follows the same curve (i.e., increased voluntary force does not increase expiratory flow rate).

iii. *Alveolar pressure increases with effort but the larger intrapleural pressure also compresses the airways.*

c. ▼ Patients with emphysema may experience expiratory flow limitation during normal quiet breathing; they attempt to breathe at even higher lung volumes, which usually lead to **dyspnea,** coughing, and discomfort. ▼

13. Advanced Mechanics Concept 2: Static and dynamic compliance.

a. *When patients are mechanically ventilated, positive pressure is used to push air into the lung.* If airway pressure is too high, there is a risk that the lung will rupture.

b. The peak airway pressure reached when a tidal volume is delivered includes the pressure required to overcome both elastic forces (**static compliance**) and airway resistance.

c. When static compliance is calculated, using Equation 5-2, pressure measurements are recorded at the beginning and end of inspiration, after gas flow has stopped.

d. If measurements are recorded during gas flow, an additional component of airway pressure is present due to air flowing through a resistance (Equation 5-4). **Dynamic compliance** includes the pressure component due to airway resistance.

e. Figure 5-13A shows a protocol to determine if development of high airway pressure in a mechanically ventilated patient is due to low static compliance (e.g., the patient has developed pulmonary edema) or to increased airway resistance (e.g., bronchoconstriction).

f. The respirator applies a **positive end-expiratory pressure (PEEP)** between breaths to help maintain open airways, which will reduce atelectasis in the mechanically ventilated patient.

g. A known tidal volume is pushed into the lung, and airway pressure is recorded. The highest pressure recorded is called **peak inspiratory pressure (PIP)** (*note: PIP is distinct from intrapleural pressure, which is notated by P_{IP}*).

h. The respirator then pauses for a short period but does not allow expiration. During this pause, airway pressure decreases to a stable **plateau pressure (P_{PLAT})**.

i. *Pressure decreases because gas flow has stopped, and the component of airway pressure caused by gas flow through resistance is no longer present.*

ii. P_{PLAT} only reflects the force needed to overcome elastic (static) properties of the lung and chest wall. Static compliance can be calculated as:

$$C_{STAT} = \frac{V_T}{P_{PLAT} - PEEP}$$ **Equation 5-5**

C_{STAT} = Static compliance

V_T = Tidal volume

P_{PLAT} = Plateau (pause) pressure

PEEP = Positive end-expiratory pressure

A. Normal response

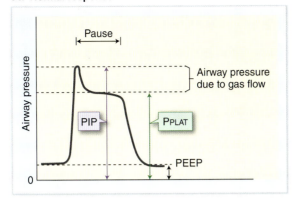

B. Low lung compliance

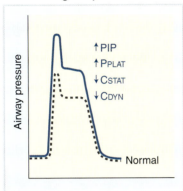

C. High airway resistance

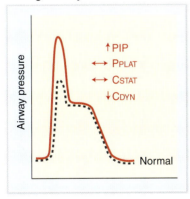

Figure 5-13. Measurement of static and dynamic compliance during mechanical ventilation. A tidal volume is delivered, causing a peak in airway pressure; dynamic compliance is calculated at the peak inspiratory pressure (PIP). A short pause is applied before expiration to eliminate airway pressure caused by gas flow, and airway pressure decreases to a plateau (P_{PLAT}). Static compliance is calculated during the plateau. **A.** Normal response. **B.** Low lung compliance causes a global increase in airway pressure and a decrease in both static and dynamic compliance. **C.** High airway resistance increases peak airway pressure but does not change the plateau pressure; dynamic compliance is decreased but static compliance is unchanged.

i. **Effective dynamic compliance (C_{DYN})** is then calculated, taking into account all components of airway pressure:

$$C_{DYN} = \frac{V_T}{PIP - PEEP}$$

Equation 5-6

C_{DYN} = Dynamic compliance
V_T = Tidal volume
PIP = Peak inspiratory pressure
PEEP = Positive end-expiratory pressure

j. **Example 1.** A patient receiving positive pressure mechanical ventilatory support has been stable for 24 hours. The following variables have been set by the ventilator: breathing frequency = 12 breaths/min, tidal volume (V_T) = 1000 mL, positive end-expiratory pressure (PEEP) = 5 cm H_2O, peak inspiratory airway pressure (PIP) = 25 cm H_2O, end-inspiratory plateau pressure (P_{PLAT}) = 20 cm H_2O (determined periodically).

Static compliance : $C_{STAT} = \dfrac{V_T}{P_{PLAT} - PEEP}$
$= 1000 / (20 - 5) \text{ mL} / \text{cm } H_2O$
$= 66.7 \text{ mL} / \text{cm } H_2O$

Dynamic compliance : $C_{DYN} = \dfrac{V_T}{PIP - PEEP}$
$= 1000 / (25 - 5) \text{ mL} / \text{cm } H_2O$
$= 50 \text{ mL} / \text{cm } H_2O$

k. Calculations of static and dynamic compliance are helpful to reveal the cause of high airway pressure in a mechanically ventilated patient. Compliance is inversely proportional to pressure; thus *increased airway pressures are associated with reduced compliance.*

l. **Example 2.** The patient in Example 1 has abruptly developed an increase in airway pressure due to bronchospasm. The results of his pulmonary function tests are: breathing frequency = 12 breaths/min (set by respirator), tidal volume (V_T) = 1000 mL (set by respirator), end-expiratory pressure (PEEP) = 5 cm H_2O (set by respirator), peak inspiratory airway pressure (PIP) = 45 cm H_2O, end-inspiratory plateau pressure (P_{PLAT}) = 20 cm H_2O.

Static compliance : $C_{STAT} = \dfrac{V_T}{P_{PLAT} - PEEP}$
$= 1000 / (20 - 5) \text{ mL} / \text{cm } H_2O$
$= 66.7 \text{ mL} / \text{cm } H_2O \textbf{ (unchanged)}$

Dynamic compliance : $C_{DYN} = \dfrac{V_T}{PIP - PEEP}$
$= 1000 / (45 - 5) \text{ mL} / \text{cm } H_2O$
$= 25 \text{ mL} / \text{cm } H_2O \textbf{ (reduced)}$

m. Figure 5-13B, C compares the two general causes of increased airway pressure in a mechanically ventilated patient.

      i. Figure 5-13B is an example of reduced static lung compliance in which both PIP and P_{PLAT} are increased (both static and dynamic compliance are reduced).

      ii. Figure 5-13C is an example of high airway resistance in which PIP increases but P_{PLAT} does not change (dynamic compliance is reduced but static compliance is unchanged).

      iii. In Example 2, the patient developed bronchospasms, the pattern shown in Figure 5-13C, and would benefit from treatment with a bronchodilator to reduce peak airway pressure when the respirator delivers a tidal breath.

14. Clinical spirometry.

  a. Figure 5-14A shows the results of a forced expiration test using a spirometer, in which the patient inspires and expires as hard and fast as possible.

      i. The volume expired in the first second is called the **forced expiratory volume (FEV) in 1 second ($FEV_{1.0}$).**

      ii. The total volume expired under maximum effort is the **forced vital capacity (FVC).**

      iii. $FEV_{1.0}$ is normally about 80% of FVC ($FEV_{1.0}$:FVC ratio $= 0.8$). $FEV_{1.0}$ represents forced expiration from high lung volume and is effort dependent.

      iv. Expiratory flow through the middle 50% of the expired breath (FEF_{25-75}) is also determined. *FEF_{25-75} is useful in patients who do not use maximal effort,* recalling that expiratory flow becomes effort independent at lower lung volumes (see Figure 5-12B).

  b. **Obstructive lung diseases** (e.g., emphysema, chronic bronchitis, and asthma) are characterized by difficulty in moving gas out of the lung due to high airway resistance (Figure 5-14B).

      i. *The $FEV_{1.0}$ and the $FEV_{1.0}$:FVC ratios are both reduced.*

  c. In **restrictive lung diseases** (e.g., pulmonary fibrosis), it is difficult to move gas into the lung due to low lung compliance (Figure 5-14C).

      i. All lung volumes, particularly TLC and FVC, are decreased.

      ii. Expiration is not impeded because lung recoil forces are increased. The absolute value of $FEV_{1.0}$ is low because inspired volume is initially low, *but the $FEV_{1.0}$:FVC ratio is either normal or increased.*

  d. Maximal expiratory **flow-volume curves** are also used during pulmonary function testing (Figure 5-15).

      i. Emphysema is used as an example of obstructive disease. The flow-volume loop is displaced to the left because weak lung recoil force causes hyperinflation of the lung. Although TLC is larger, peak expiratory flow is small due to dynamic airway collapse.

      ii. The loop is displaced to the right in restrictive disorders because patients have reduced TLC and RV. Peak expiratory flow is lower than normal because the patient is not able to reach high inspiratory volumes, where flow rate is effort dependent. The slope of the descending part of the curve may be steeper, reflecting higher lung recoil forces.

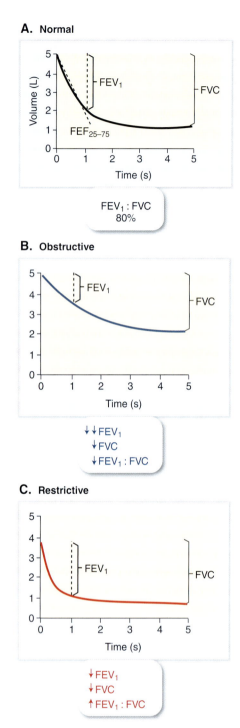

Figure 5-14. Spirograms showing a normal (**A**), obstructive (**B**), and restrictive (**C**) lung diseases. Obstructive and restrictive lung diseases are associated with smaller forced vital capacity (FVC) and forced expired volume in the first second ($FEV_{1.0}$). In obstructive lung disease, the $FEV_{1.0}$:FVC ratio is significantly decreased, whereas in restrictive lung disease, the $FEV_{1.0}$:FVC ratio is normal or increased.

    e. ▼ **Chronic obstructive pulmonary disease (COPD)** is a term that applies to patients with either emphysema or chronic bronchitis.

        i. Patients with emphysema are known as "**pink puffers**" because they are able to maintain adequate O_2 saturation by hyperventilating. The classic profile of a "pink puffer" is a thin person sitting in tripod position, breathing with pursed lips.

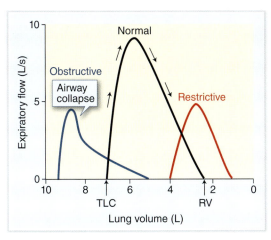

Figure 5-15. Flow-volume curves in obstructive and restrictive lung diseases. RV, residual volume ; TLC, total lung capacity.

    ii. Patients with chronic bronchitis are known as "**blue bloaters**" because they have a blunted respiratory response to high blood CO_2 (hypercarbia), which produces an inappropriately low respiratory drive that results in hypoxemia and cyanosis. Blue bloaters are typically overweight and have red faces due to polycythemia (increased hematocrit) secondary to chronic hypoxemia. They suffer from **cor pulmonale** (structural and functional changes in the right ventricle caused by chronic pulmonary hypertension). ▼

15. Work of breathing.
    a. Work of breathing has two major components: "**elastic work**," to overcome static compliance, and "**resistive work**," to overcome airway and tissue resistance.
    b. Patients usually adopt a pattern of breathing that minimizes work.
       i. In restrictive disease, small tidal breaths are taken more rapidly because a large amount of elastic work is needed to inflate the lungs.
       ii. Patients with obstructive lung disease often expire slowly, which reduces dynamic airway collapse and resistive work of breathing.

Ventilation and Carbon Dioxide Elimination

1. **Ventilation** can be defined as mechanical events producing gas movement in the lung, which results in CO_2 elimination from the body.
2. CO_2 diffuses readily from the pulmonary capillaries into the alveoli so that *CO_2 elimination depends solely on how well the alveoli are ventilated.*
3. Alveolar ventilation is reduced by the volume of dead space (wasted) ventilation.
    a. The conducting airways contribute fixed "anatomic" dead space.
    b. Alveoli that are ventilated but not perfused (**"alveolar" dead space**) further contribute to **total "physiologic" dead space**.
    c. In disease states, dead space can be large, resulting in inadequate CO_2 excretion.
4. *Hypoventilation is defined as inadequate CO_2 excretion, which results in an increase in arterial* P_{CO_2} (Table 5-5).

Table 5-5. Terminology Related to Ventilation

Term	Description
Apnea	No breathing; breathing frequency is zero.
Bradypnea	Low breathing frequency (<10 per minute).
Hypopnea	Slow and shallow breathing.
Eupnea	Normal breathing frequency (10–20 per minute).
Tachypnea	High breathing frequency (>20 per minute).
Hyperpnea	Fast and deep breathing.
Hypoventilation*	Functionally inadequate ventilation produces increased arterial P_{CO_2} (hypercarbia, hypercapnia) >45 mm Hg.
Hyperventilation*	Excessive ventilation produces decreased arterial P_{CO_2} (hypocarbia, hypocapnea) <35 mm Hg.
Dyspnea	Subjective sensation of shortness of breath or difficulty breathing; indicates physiologic demand for ventilation is greater than the patient's ability to respond.

*Note: Hypo- and hyperventilation should *not* be used to describe abnormal respiratory rate.

5. ▼ **Pulmonary embolism** is a potentially fatal condition that occurs when a thromboembolism lodges in a pulmonary artery, stopping all blood flow distal to the blockage. A pulmonary embolism is a classic example of a large, total "physiologic" dead space in which the affected lung segment continues to have alveolar ventilation but lacks blood flow. ▼

6. The alveolar ventilation equation.

   a. *The rate of alveolar ventilation is the sole determinant of the rate of CO_2 excretion.*

   b. Because entire CO_2 excretion is derived from alveolar gas, the relationship can be written as:

$$\dot{V}_{CO_2} = \dot{V}_A \times F_{ACO_2} \qquad \textbf{Equation 5-7}$$

   $\dot{V}_{CO_2}$ = Rate of CO_2 excretion
   $\dot{V}_A$ = Alveolar ventilation rate
   F_{ACO_2} = Fraction of alveolar CO_2

   c. The gas fraction is proportional to partial pressure, so F_{ACO_2} can be replaced by P_{ACO_2} multiplied by a constant (k) to produce the **alveolar ventilation equation**:

$$\dot{V}_{CO_2} = \dot{V}_A \times P_{ACO_2} \times k \qquad \textbf{Equation 5-8}$$

   $\dot{V}_{CO_2}$ = Rate of CO_2 elimination or production
   $\dot{V}_A$ = Alveolar ventilation rate
   P_{ACO_2} = Partial pressure of CO_2 in alveolar gas
   k = Constant

   d. The blood entering the left side of the heart has equilibrated with alveolar gas so that P_{ACO_2} can be replaced by P_{aCO_2}. In addition, if CO_2 production is understood to be constant, Equation 5-8 reduces to:

$$P_{A_{CO_2}} \propto \frac{1}{\dot{V}_A} \qquad\qquad \textbf{Equation 5-9}$$

$P_{A_{CO_2}}$ = Partial pressure of CO_2 in arterial blood
$\dot{V}_A$ = Alveolar ventilation rate

e. *Equation 5-9 demonstrates a fundamentally important concept that arterial P_{CO_2} varies inversely with alveolar ventilation; for example, if $\dot{V}_A$ is doubled, arterial P_{CO_2} is halved.*

f. Arterial P_{CO_2} is influenced by the balance between CO_2 production and excretion. However, changes in CO_2 production will only change arterial P_{CO_2} if pulmonary function is impaired and $\dot{V}_A$ cannot be adjusted appropriately.

   i. Patients with **acute respiratory depression** or those with COPD are at risk of having inadequate alveolar ventilation for the rate of CO_2 production, which results in increased arterial P_{CO_2}.

7. Ventilation of dead space.

   a. The alveolar ventilation rate is less than the expired ventilation rate because a proportion of each breath moves to areas of dead space.

   b. **Expired minute ventilation** is the product of tidal volume (V_T) and breathing frequency (f):

$$\dot{V}_E = V_T \times f \qquad\qquad \textbf{Equation 5-10}$$

$\dot{V}_E$ = Expired minute ventilation rate
V_T = Tidal volume
f = Breathing frequency

   c. For each breath, about 150 mL of air remains in the anatomic dead space; there is very little additional alveolar dead space in the lungs of a healthy person.

   d. $\dot{V}_E$ can be divided into two functional quantities, alveolar ventilation ($\dot{V}_A$) and dead space ventilation ($\dot{V}_D$):

$$\dot{V}_E = \dot{V}_A + \dot{V}_D \qquad\qquad \textbf{Equation 5-11}$$

$\dot{V}_E$ = Expired minute ventilation rate
$\dot{V}_A$ = Alveolar ventilation rate
$\dot{V}_D$ = Dead space ventilation rate

   e. Patients who have a large total physiologic dead space waste an excessive fraction of each tidal breath to regions of the lung that do not exchange gas. There are two possible outcomes: either the patient increases $\dot{V}_E$ to restore $\dot{V}_A$, or $\dot{V}_A$ is inadequate and arterial P_{CO_2} increases (hypoventilation).

   i. *Patients with severe COPD are unable to increase $\dot{V}_E$ sufficiently and often have a chronically elevated arterial P_{CO_2}.*

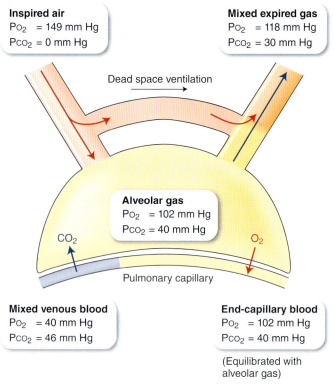

Inspired air
P_{O_2} = 149 mm Hg
P_{CO_2} = 0 mm Hg

Mixed expired gas
P_{O_2} = 118 mm Hg
P_{CO_2} = 30 mm Hg

Dead space ventilation

Alveolar gas
P_{O_2} = 102 mm Hg
P_{CO_2} = 40 mm Hg

CO_2

O_2

Pulmonary capillary

Mixed venous blood
P_{O_2} = 40 mm Hg
P_{CO_2} = 46 mm Hg

End-capillary blood
P_{O_2} = 102 mm Hg
P_{CO_2} = 40 mm Hg

(Equilibrated with alveolar gas)

Figure 5-16. Normal profile of P_{O_2} and P_{CO_2} in inspired air, mixed venous blood, alveolar gas, end-pulmonary capillary blood, and mixed expired gas. Alveolar gas composition is intermediate between inspired air and mixed venous blood, reflecting carbon dioxide (CO_2) excretion and oxygen (O_2) uptake. End-pulmonary capillary blood is in equilibrium with alveolar gas. Expired gas has a lower CO_2 and a higher O_2 than alveolar gas, because alveolar gas mixes with inspired air in anatomic dead space during expiration.

    f. ▼ Symptoms associated with **chronic hypercapnia** (elevated arterial P_{CO_2}) differ from those associated with **acute hypercapnia.**
      i. Clinical manifestations of the patient with chronic hypercapnia include sleep disturbance, daytime somnolence, myoclonic jerks, and asterixis (hand tremor when wrists are extended).
      ii. Conversely, clinical manifestations of acute hypercapnia include anxiety, dyspnea, confusion, psychosis, and coma. ▼

8. Quantifying dead space.
    a. Figure 5-16 shows P_{O_2} and P_{CO_2} in inspired air, in alveolar gas, and in mixed expired air.
    b. *The composition of alveolar gas is fairly constant throughout the ventilatory cycle*; there is a steady state between CO_2 diffusion from pulmonary capillary blood into the alveoli and from CO_2 removal by alveolar ventilation.
    c. On inspiration, the dead space is filled with inspired gas, which contains only a minimal amount of CO_2.
    d. The highest concentration of CO_2 is in the alveoli, which on expiration mixes with fresh air in the dead space, causing dilution of CO_2.
    e. Thus, the P_{CO_2} in mixed expired gas (P_{ECO_2}) is lower than the P_{CO_2} in alveolar gas (P_{ACO_2}).

f. *As dead space becomes larger, P_{ECO_2} is reduced.* The **Bohr equation** applies the idea that the difference between alveolar P_{CO_2} and expired P_{CO_2} is a function of the dead space volume:

$$\frac{V_D}{V_T} = \frac{P_{ACO_2} - P_{ECO_2}}{P_{ACO_2}} \qquad \textbf{Equation 5-12}$$

V_D/V_T = Ratio of dead space to tidal volume
P_{ACO_2} = Alveolar partial pressure of CO_2
P_{ECO_2} = Partial pressure of CO_2 in mixed expired air

   i. In clinical practice, P_{ACO_2} is estimated as P_{aCO_2}, and can be measured from an arterial blood sample. Equation 5-12 now becomes:

$$\frac{V_D}{V_T} = \frac{P_{aCO_2} - P_{ECO_2}}{P_{aCO_2}} \qquad \textbf{Equation 5-13}$$

   V_D/V_T = Ratio of dead space to tidal volume
   P_{aCO_2} = Partial pressure of CO_2 in arterial blood
   P_{ECO_2} = Partial pressure of CO_2 in mixed expired air

g. Dead space ventilation ($\dot{V}_D$) is the product of expired minute ventilation ($\dot{V}_E$) and the ratio of dead space to tidal volume $\left(\dfrac{V_D}{V_T}\right)$, and because $\dot{V}_D$ subtracted from $\dot{V}_E$ equals the alveolar ventilation ($\dot{V}_A$):

$$\dot{V}_A = \dot{V}_E - \left(\dot{V}_E \times \frac{V_D}{V_T} \right) \qquad \textbf{Equation 5-14}$$

   $\dot{V}_A$ = Alveolar ventilation rate
   $\dot{V}_E$ = Expired minute ventilation rate
   V_D/V_T = Ratio of dead space to tidal volume

h. **Example 1.** The following results of pulmonary function testing were obtained in a healthy man: tidal volume (V_T) = 600 mL, breathing frequency = 12 breaths/min, P_{aCO_2} (arterial) = 40 mm Hg, P_{ECO_2} (expired air) = 30 mm Hg.

$$\textbf{Minute ventilation}: \dot{V} = V_T \times f$$
$$= 600 \times 12$$
$$= \textbf{7200 mL / min}$$

$$\textbf{Dead space / tidal volume ratio}: \frac{V_D}{V_T} = \frac{P_{aCO_2} - P_{ECO_2}}{P_{aCO_2}}$$
$$\frac{V_D}{V_T} = \frac{40 - 30}{40}$$
$$= \textbf{0.25 (25\%)}$$

$$\textbf{Alveolar ventilation}: \dot{V}_A = \dot{V}_E - \left(\dot{V}_E \times \frac{V_D}{V_T} \right)$$

$$\dot{V}_A = 7200 - (7200 \times 0.25)$$
$$= \textbf{5400 mL / min}$$

i. **Example 2.** The following results of pulmonary function testing were obtained in a man with severe emphysema who had smoked two packs of cigarettes a day for 30 years: tidal volume (V_T) = 1400 mL, breathing frequency = 8 breaths/min, P_aCO_2 (arterial) = 60 mm Hg, P_ECO_2 (expired air) = 20 mm Hg.

$$\textbf{Minute ventilation}: \dot{V}_E = V_T \times f$$
$$= 1400 \times 8$$
$$= \textbf{11200 mL / min}$$

$$\textbf{Dead space / tidal volume ratio}: \frac{V_D}{V_T} = \frac{P_aCO_2 - P_{CEO_2}}{P_aCO_2}$$
$$\frac{V_D}{V_T} = \frac{60 - 20}{60}$$
$$= \textbf{0.67 (67\%)}$$

$$\textbf{Alveolar ventilation}: \dot{V}_A = \dot{V}_E - \left(\dot{V}_E \times \frac{V_D}{V_T} \right)$$

$$\dot{V}_A = 11200 - (11200 \times 0.67)$$
$$= \textbf{3733 mL / min}$$

j. *Despite a large expired minute ventilation rate, the patient has chronic hypercapnia (excess blood CO_2), resulting from the large dead space/tidal volume ratio of 0.67, which causes a low alveolar ventilation rate.*

9. CO_2 production.
   a. Blood-CO_2 concentration is determined by a balance between CO_2 production from cellular metabolism and excretion via alveolar ventilation.
   b. Metabolic rate is defined by O_2 consumption; CO_2 production is related to O_2 consumption by calculating the **respiratory quotient** using the following equation:

$$RQ = \frac{\dot{V}_{CO_2}}{\dot{V}_{O_2}} \qquad \textbf{Equation 5-15}$$

RQ = Respiratory quotient

$\dot{V}_{CO_2}$ = Rate of CO_2 production

$\dot{V}_{O_2}$ = Rate of O_2 consumption

   i. The respiratory quotient is determined by the nutrients that are metabolized: for carbohydrates (RQ = 1.0); for proteins (RQ = 0.8); and for lipids (RQ = 0.7).

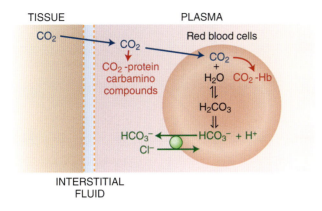

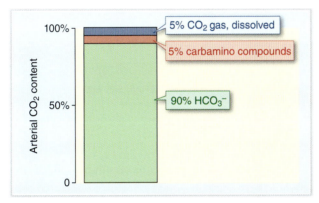

Figure 5-17. CO_2 transport in blood. CO_2 generated by tissues diffuses into blood. Most CO_2 is converted to HCO_3^- ions inside erythrocytes via carbonic anhydrase and is delivered into plasma via the Cl/HCO_3 exchange.

    ii. For example, more O_2 is required to metabolize lipids because fat molecules have less O_2 atoms than do carbohydrates, and more gaseous O_2 is needed to produce CO_2 and H_2O.

    iii. Under basal conditions, the average respiratory quotient is about 0.8 because less CO_2 is produced than O_2 is consumed.

    iv. ▼ *The respiratory quotient may change during trauma or infection, which in turn affects the rate of CO_2 production.* For example, in patients with **sepsis,** the respiratory quotient decreases due to increased fat oxidation. ▼

10. CO_2 transport in blood.

  a. Figure 5-17 illustrates how CO_2 diffuses as a dissolved gas along a gradient of partial pressure from cells to interstitium to systemic capillary blood plasma.

  b. CO_2 enters red blood cells and combines with H_2O to produce H_2CO_3 in a reaction catalyzed by **carbonic anhydrase.**

  c. H_2CO_3 dissociates to produce HCO_3^- ions inside red blood cells, which are delivered into plasma via the Cl/HCO_3 exchange (known as the "**chloride shift**").

  d. The total CO_2 content of arterial blood is about 48 mL of CO_2 per dL of blood. CO_2 is **carried in three forms:**

    i. 90% of CO_2 is carried as **HCO_3^- ions in plasma.**

    ii. 5% of CO_2 is carried as **dissolved CO_2 molecules.** CO_2 is 20 times more soluble than O_2 at body temperature, and about 2.4 mL of CO_2 is dissolved per liter of blood at a normal arterial P_{CO_2} of 40 mm Hg.

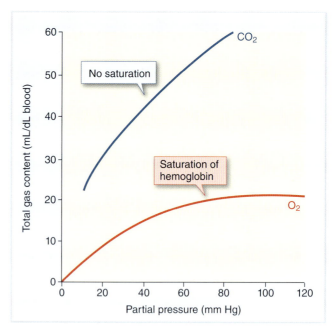

Figure 5-18. Carbon dioxide (CO_2) and oxygen (O_2) dissociation (content) curves. Hb, hemoglobin.

   iii.   5% of CO_2 is carried as **carbamino compounds,** which consist of CO_2 bound to plasma proteins or to hemoglobin within red blood cells.
   e.   Mixed venous blood contains about 52 mL of CO_2 per dL of blood, with approximately 88% HCO_3^-, 7% carbamino compounds, and 5% dissolved CO_2.
11. CO_2 content curve.
   a.   Figure 5-18 compares the CO_2 and O_2 content ("dissociation") curves, which describe the total amount of each gas present in blood as a function of its partial pressure.
   b.   The O_2 content curve (see Oxygenation) plateaus because hemoglobin becomes saturated with O_2. Further increases in arterial Po_2 have little effect on total O_2 content of blood.
   c.   In contrast, the CO_2 content curve is roughly linear. As a consequence, CO_2 excretion can continue to increase as a function of the alveolar ventilation rate.
      i.   This explains why a patient with a large area of lung that fails to excrete CO_2 can still have a normal arterial Pco_2. *Alveolar ventilation in other areas of the functional lung can increase to excrete more CO_2 and compensate for the dysfunctional areas.*
      ii.   The same cannot occur for O_2. If poorly oxygenated blood leaves a region of the lung, *other areas cannot take up more O_2 to compensate because blood from these areas is already saturated with O_2.*
   d.   ▼ **Pneumonia** is an infection of the airspaces and results in pus-filled alveoli, which effectively reduces alveolar ventilation in the affected areas. Other healthy areas of the lung can compensate to eliminate CO_2, but patients can become hypoxemic (low arterial Po_2) and require supplemental O_2. ▼
12.   The Haldane effect.
   a.   The Haldane effect refers to changes in the position of the CO_2 content curve that occur with oxygenation of the blood and which affect diffusion gradients for CO_2.

b. *The only form of CO_2 that can diffuse from cells to plasma at the tissues and from plasma to alveolar gas at the lung is free CO_2 molecules.*

c. Gases obey **Fick's law of diffusion** (see Chapter 1). The rate of diffusion is proportional to the surface area and inversely proportional to the thickness of the diffusion barrier, making the lung ideally suited for gas diffusion.

   i. The rate of diffusion is proportional to the diffusion constant. CO_2 has a high diffusion constant and diffuses about 20 times faster than O_2.

   ii. The diffusion rate is also proportional to the partial pressure gradient. CO_2 excretion at the lung occurs because PCO_2 is higher in mixed venous blood than in alveolar gas.

   iii. The partial pressure gradient is reversed in the tissues, where CO_2 is generated by cells and diffuses into the systemic capillary blood.

   iv. ▼ Diseases that increase the thickness of the diffusion barrier, such as **pulmonary fibrosis** or **pulmonary edema,** can affect O_2 uptake but *CO_2 diffusion is almost never a clinical concern.* ▼

d. The Haldane effect describes variations in plasma PCO_2 with oxygenation, which promote CO_2 diffusion at both the lung and tissues.

e. *The basis of the Haldane effect is redistribution of CO_2 between carbamino hemoglobin and dissolved CO_2.*

   i. In the pulmonary capillaries, O_2 binding to hemoglobin liberates free CO_2 from carbamino hemoglobin.

   ii. As a result, the pulmonary capillary partial pressure of CO_2 ($PCCO_2$) increases (shown by a right shift in the CO_2 dissociation curve) resulting in more CO_2 excretion (Figure 5-19).

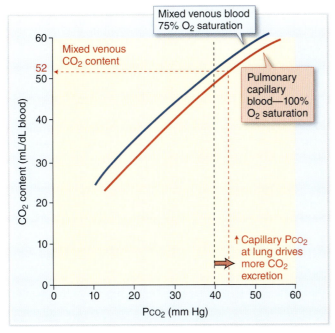

Figure 5-19. The Haldane effect. Formation of oxyhemoglobin in the pulmonary capillary blood reduces the affinity of hemoglobin for carbon dioxide (CO_2), thereby increasing the concentration of freely dissolved CO_2 (PCO_2). Increased PCO_2 in blood drives more CO_2 diffusion into the alveolus.

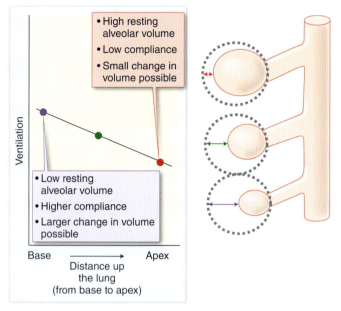

Figure 5-20. Gradient of ventilation in the lung when a person is standing. Gravity compresses alveoli at the base of the lung compared to the apex of the lung. Lung acini at the base have more optimal compliance and a larger range of volume change available during inspiration.

      iii. The reverse process occurs at the tissues—O_2 unloading from hemoglobin allows more carbamino hemoglobin to form.

      iv. This decreases the plasma P_{CO_2} in the systemic capillaries and increases the partial pressure gradient for CO_2 diffusion from tissues into blood.

13. Regional differences in ventilation.

   a. *As a result of gravity, ventilation is higher at the base of the lung than at the apex in a person who is standing* (Figure 5-20).

   b. Alveoli are smaller at the base of the upright lung than at the apex due to the weight of the lung compressing alveoli at the base.

   c. *When the lung is at FRC, the smaller alveoli at the base of the lung have optimal compliance and are more easily ventilated;* alveoli at the apex have a high resting volume and are more difficult to ventilate due to lower compliance.

   d. Basal alveoli also have a larger range of volume through which they can expand during inspiration.

Pulmonary Blood Flow

1. The pulmonary circulation receives the whole cardiac output from the right ventricle.

   a. Deoxygenated blood flows via pulmonary arteries through a network of vessels, which branch in concert with the airways.

   b. Alveoli are enveloped by dense interconnecting pulmonary capillaries.

   c. Oxygenated blood is returned to the left atrium via the pulmonary venous system.

2. Pulmonary blood pressure.

   a. Mean pulmonary artery pressure is only about 10 mm Hg, and systolic and diastolic pressures are about 25 and 8 mm Hg, respectively.

b. Outlet pressure from the pulmonary circulation into the left atrium is about 5 mm Hg.

c. Therefore, the driving pressure for blood flow through the pulmonary circulation is only about 10% that of the systemic circulation.

d. The lower blood pressure in the pulmonary circulation is reflected in the thin walls of the right ventricle and pulmonary arteries.

e. *A lower pressure blood circulation has the advantage of reducing workload on the right ventricle and also reduces the risk of excessive interstitial fluid formation, which would interfere with O_2 diffusion.*

f. ▼ **Cor pulmonale** is right ventricular failure due to excessively high pulmonary artery pressures that can arise from pulmonary emboli, pulmonary vascular disease (e.g., collagen vascular disease such as scleroderma), or parenchymal disease (e.g., COPD, pulmonary fibrosis). ▼

3. Pulmonary vascular resistance.

a. Low perfusion pressure is able to drive the entire cardiac output through the pulmonary circulation because pulmonary vascular resistance is very low.

b. In the systemic circulation, arterioles offer most vascular resistance. *In the pulmonary circulation, resistance is shared between arterioles, capillaries, and venules.*

c. The behavior of capillaries and larger vessels is different, giving rise to the concept of alveolar and extraalveolar vessels:

   i. Alveolar vessels are influenced by alveolar pressure and are compressed if the alveolar pressure increases above the vascular pressure.

   ii. *Extraalveolar vessels are affected most by lung volume.* As the lungs expand, increased radial traction forces causes the extraalveolar vessels to open, which reduces their resistance. When lung volume decreases, extraalveolar vessels are compressed.

d. The pulmonary circulation is forced to accommodate large increases in blood flow whenever cardiac output increases (e.g., exercise).

   i. Increased cardiac output through the pulmonary circulation can be accommodated because pulmonary vascular resistance decreases as cardiac output increases (Figure 5-21A).

   ii. *The decrease in pulmonary vascular resistance that is observed when cardiac output increases occurs because of the* **distention** *of the pulmonary capillaries and by* **recruitment** *of capillaries that were not perfused at rest.*

   iii. In contrast, most systemic vascular beds actively autoregulate blood flow in response to increased blood pressure.

e. Lung volume is an important passive determinant of pulmonary vascular resistance.

   i. Pulmonary vascular resistance is optimal around FRC (Figure 5-21B). *Vascular resistance increases at either high or low lung volume.*

   ii. At low lung volumes (patients with restrictive lung disease), compression of the extraalveolar vessels predominates to increase resistance.

   iii. At high lung volumes (e.g., patients with emphysema), the pulmonary capillaries are stretched resulting in reduced capillary diameter and increased pulmonary vascular resistance.

A.

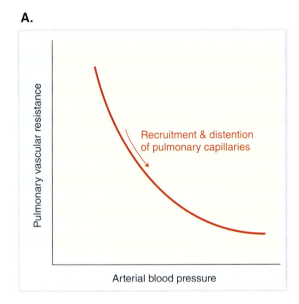

B.

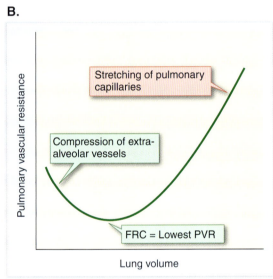

Figure 5-21. Effects of pulmonary arterial blood pressure (**A**) and lung volume (**B**) on pulmonary vascular resistance. FRC, functional residual capacity; PVR, pulmonary vascular resistance.

f. ▼ **Smoking** destroys the alveolar membranes and their corresponding pulmonary capillaries, significantly decreasing the pulmonary capillary cross-sectional area and therefore contributing to increased pulmonary artery pressure. ▼

g. Hypoxic pulmonary vasoconstriction.

    i. Active control of pulmonary vascular resistance occurs in response to **alveolar hypoxia** (low Po_2).

    ii. Figure 5-22 shows decreased pulmonary blood flow when the alveolar Po_2 decreases below 60 mm Hg.

    iii. A rapid ascent to a high altitude, where atmospheric Po_2 is low, causes pulmonary vasoconstriction and may cause **pulmonary hypertension.**

    iv. *This mechanism is the opposite response to most systemic vascular beds, which vasodilate in response to hypoxia.*

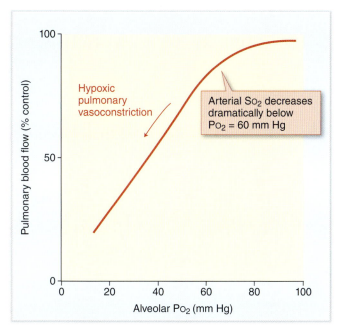

Figure 5-22. Hypoxic pulmonary vasoconstriction. Low alveolar P_{O_2} causes pulmonary vasoconstriction. The effect is marked at alveolar P_{O_2} lower than 60 mm Hg, where arterial SO_2 begins to sharply decrease on the oxyhemoglobin dissociation curve.

   v. Hypoxic pulmonary vasoconstriction has two important physiologic roles:
   - In **fetal life,** the lungs are not necessary for gas exchange. *Before a breath is taken, hypoxic pulmonary vasoconstriction shunts blood away from the lungs.* Immediately after birth, when the first inspiration occurs, the pulmonary arterioles dilate, pulmonary vascular resistance decreases, and normal lung perfusion is established.
   - After birth, hypoxic pulmonary vasoconstriction *shunts blood away from poorly ventilated regions of the lung, thereby improving ventilation-to-perfusion matching.*
   vi. ▼ **Nitric oxide** and phosphodiesterase type V inhibitors such as **sildenafil** are both substances that cause vasodilation in the lung and can be used to relieve **pulmonary hypertension.** ▼

4. Regional differences in perfusion.
   a. The distribution of pulmonary blood flow within the lungs is significantly affected by gravity, *which has a more marked effect on regional perfusion than on ventilation.*
   b. Blood flow is significantly greater at the base of the lung than at the apex. Within this gradient of perfusion, there are **three lung zones** based on interaction between alveolar and vascular pressure (Figure 5-23):
      i. **Zone 1.** Arterial and venous pressures are both less than alveolar pressure, resulting in compression of the pulmonary capillaries and no perfusion.
         - Pressure developed by the right ventricle is normally just large enough to prevent zone 1 from occurring at the apex of the lung.
         - Zone 1 is alveolar dead space, which is ventilated but not perfused.
         - *If blood pressure decreases (e.g., hemorrhage) or if alveolar pressure increases (e.g., mechanical ventilation), zone 1 may become a significant fraction of total perfusion.*

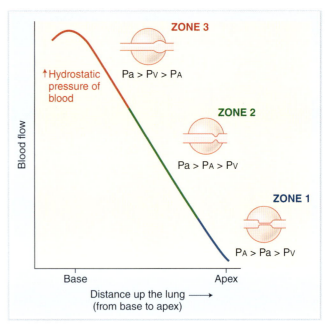

Figure 5-23. Gradient of perfusion in the lung when a person is standing. Perfusion is prevented if alveolar pressure exceeds arterial and venous pressure (zone 1). Blood flow is impeded when alveolar pressure exceeds venous pressure but not arterial pressure (zone 2) and perfusion depends on the arterial-to-alveolar pressure gradient. Blood flow is not impeded by alveolar pressure if both arterial and venous pressures are higher than alveolar pressure (zone 3). The base of the lung has the highest perfusion because gravity increases arterial and venous pressure, creating zone 3 perfusion.

    ii. **Zone 2.** Alveolar pressure is between arterial and venous pressure. The perfusion pressure in zone 2 is the difference between arterial and alveolar pressure. Vessels are partially constricted, and blood flow is more limited.

    iii. **Zone 3.** Arterial and venous pressures both exceed alveolar pressure. Perfusion pressure is the arterial-to-venous pressure difference. *Zone 3 represents the areas of the lung with the largest rate of blood flow (i.e., the base of the upright lung).*

    iv. ▼ A Swan Ganz catheter is used to obtain **pulmonary capillary wedge pressure,** an estimate of left atrial pressure and left ventricular end-diastolic pressure.

- The balloon-tipped catheter is inserted into a central vein and allowed to float along the path through the right atrium, the right ventricle, the pulmonary artery, and down to a pulmonary capillary.

- The inflated balloon will "wedge" into place, occluding the small pulmonary vessel. To estimate the left atrial and left ventricular pressures, the sensor on the tip of the catheter must have a continuous column of blood from the pulmonary capillary to the left atrium and ventricle.

- To achieve this, *the catheter must be placed in lung zone 3 because capillary collapse is present in zones 1 and 2, which prevents direct connection with the left atrium.* ▼

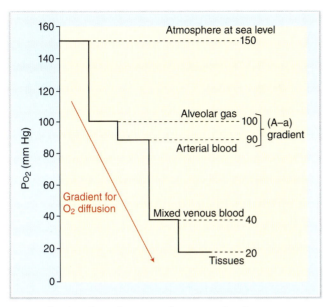

Figure 5-24. Cascade of P_{O_2} from the atmosphere at sea level to tissues.

Oxygenation

1. Delivery of O_2 from the atmosphere to cells involves several steps. Successful oxygenation requires:
   a. Ventilation of perfused alveoli with atmospheric O_2.
   b. Diffusion of O_2 across the blood-gas barrier and binding of O_2 to **hemoglobin** in the erythrocytes.
   c. Ventilation and perfusion matching to prevent desaturated venous blood from entering the systemic arterial circulation (i.e., **venous admixture**).
   d. Adequate blood flow to the tissues in relation to metabolic demand.
   e. Unloading of O_2 from hemoglobin at the tissues.
2. O_2 diffuses down a cascade of partial pressure from atmospheric gas (which has a P_{O_2} of about 150 mm Hg at sea level) to mitochondria (which can have a P_{O_2} of less than 5 mm Hg) (Figure 5-24).
   a. The gradient for O_2 diffusion along this cascade can be varied by the external conditions applied. For example, the P_{O_2} of inspired air for a patient at sea level on 100% O_2 is approximately 700 mm Hg, whereas the inspired P_{O_2} at the top of Mt. Everest is about 40 mm Hg!
3. Tissue O_2 delivery and consumption.
   a. *The body has very limited stores of O_2; therefore, interruptions to cardiac output or pulmonary oxygenation are fatal within a few minutes.*
   b. To avoid cellular hypoxia, matching between tissue O_2 consumption and O_2 delivery in arterial blood must be continuous. The rate of O_2 delivery is the product of cardiac output and arterial O_2 content:

$$D_{O_2} = \dot{Q}_T \times C_{aO_2} \times 10 \qquad \textbf{Equation 5-16A}$$

$D_{O_2} = O_2$ delivery (mL O_2/min)
$\dot{Q}_T =$ Cardiac output (L blood/min)
$C_{aO_2} = O_2$ content of arterial blood (mL O_2/dL blood)

c. The rate of O_2 consumption is the product of cardiac output and the arteriovenous difference in O_2 content:

$$\dot{V}_{O_2} = \dot{Q}_T \times (Ca_{O_2} - Cv_{O_2}) \times 10 \qquad \textbf{Equation 5-16B}$$

$\dot{V}_{O_2}$ = O_2 consumption (mL O_2/min)

$\dot{Q}_T$ = Cardiac output (L blood/min)

Ca_{O_2} = O_2 content of arterial blood (mL of O_2/dL of blood)

Cv_{O_2} = O_2 content of venous blood (mL of O_2/dL of blood)

d. Typical values for a resting adult are Q_T = 5 L/min, Ca_{O_2} = 20 mL/dL, and Cv_{O_2} = 15 mL/dL. From Equation 5-16, basal $\dot{V}_{O_2}$ = 250 mL/min.

e. ▼ V_{O_2} **max** is a measure of peak O_2 consumption at maximal aerobic exercise and is used as a measure of aerobic fitness. As such, it can vary from 20 mL/kg/min for a sedentary person, to 40 mL/kg/min for the average untrained person, to 90 mL/kg/min for an elite athlete. ▼

4. O_2 transport in blood.

  a. Despite the relatively low solubility of O_2 in plasma, the volume of gaseous O_2 per liter of blood is almost the same as that in air because red blood cells contain the O_2-binding protein **hemoglobin.**

    i. *Ninety-eight percent of O_2 in blood is carried bound to hemoglobin within red blood cells.* One gram of hemoglobin carries approximately 1.35 mL of O_2, when 100% saturated.

    ii. Only 2% of O_2 in arterial blood is present as dissolved O_2. At an arterial P_{O_2} of 100 mm Hg, only 0.3 mL of O_2 is dissolved in every 100 mL of blood.

  b. The **total O_2 content of arterial blood** is calculated as:

$$Ca_{O_2} = (1.35 \times [Hb] \times Sa_{O_2}) + (k_{O_2} \times Pa_{O_2}) \qquad \textbf{Equation 5-17}$$

Ca_{O_2} = O_2 content (mL O_2/dL blood)

$[Hb]$ = Hemoglobin concentration (g/dL)

Sa_{O_2} = O_2 saturation of hemoglobin (0–1.0)

k_{O_2} = O_2 solubility constant (0.0031 mL O_2/dL blood)

  c. The function of the pulmonary system is to provide an adequate arterial P_{O_2} for hemoglobin saturation.

  d. Low Sa_{O_2} results from hypoxemia (low arterial P_{O_2}). Potential causes of hypoxemia include inadequate ventilation, diffusion, and $\dot{V}/\dot{Q}$ matching.

  e. As illustrated by Equation 5-17, *O_2 content will also be inadequate if hemoglobin concentration is low (anemia).*

  f. ▼ When caring for a **critically ill patient** (e.g., shock from significant trauma) total arterial O_2 content must be maximized by assessment and correction of the hemoglobin concentration, arterial P_{O_2}, and Sa_{O_2}. ▼

5. The oxyhemoglobin dissociation curve.

  a. Figure 5-25 shows the normal relationship between percent hemoglobin saturation and P_{O_2}.

  b. Each hemoglobin molecule can bind four O_2 molecules. There is cooperative binding of O_2 so that each additional O_2 binds more easily, producing the **sigmoidal** shape of the O_2 dissociation curve.

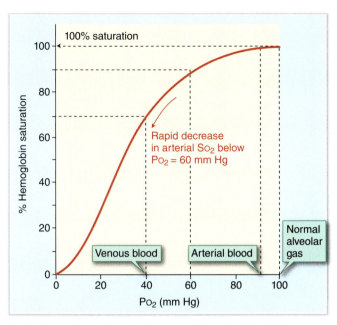

Figure 5-25. Oxyhemoglobin dissociation curve. Hemoglobin (Hb) is saturated at normal arterial Po_2 values at sea level. Arterial hypoxemia below 60 mm Hg threatens the arterial oxygen (O_2) content due to the loss of O_2-Hb saturation.

c. In healthy lungs with an alveolar partial pressure of O_2 of 100 mm Hg, pulmonary capillary blood is 100% saturated with O_2.

d. *When Po_2 decreases below 60 mm Hg, there is a rapid decline in hemoglobin saturation.*

   i. Mechanisms that control breathing strongly increase ventilation if arterial Po_2 decreases below 60 mm Hg.

   ii. A **general rule of thumb concerning oxygenation** is the "4-5-6:7-8-9" rule. An arterial Po_2 of 40, 50, or 60 mm Hg roughly corresponds to Sao_2 of 70%, 80%, or 90%, respectively.

   iii. *The therapeutic goals for oxygenation are arterial Po_2 >60 mm Hg (or Sao_2 >90%), which corresponds with the flat portion of the O_2 dissociation curve.*

e. The position of the O_2 dissociation curve can shift, affecting the ability to take up O_2 at the lung and altering the amount of O_2 unloaded from hemoglobin at the tissues (Figure 5-26).

f. The O_2 affinity of hemoglobin is described using a **P_{50} value** (the Po_2 resulting in 50% saturation).

   i. A normal P_{50} is about 27 mm Hg; lower P_{50} indicates an increase in O_2 affinity and a left shift in the dissociation curve; a higher P_{50} indicates a decrease in O_2 affinity and a right shift in the dissociation curve.

g. A left shift in the oxyhemoglobin dissociation curve causes hemoglobin to become saturated at lower Po_2.

   i. *Loading O_2 into blood at the lung is easier, but it is more difficult to unload O_2 at the tissues.*

   ii. The O_2 dissociation curve for **fetal hemoglobin** lies to the left of the curve for adult (maternal) hemoglobin; *higher O_2 affinity of fetal hemoglobin aids in O_2 transfer across the placenta.*

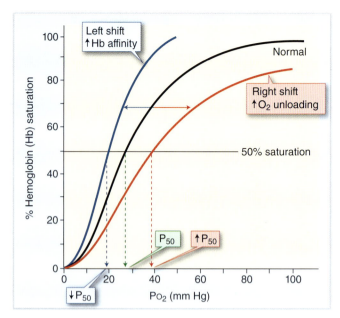

Figure 5-26. Effect of left and right shift of oxyhemoglobin dissociation curve on P_{50} values. A left shift increases S_aO_2 but reduces O_2 unloading at the tissues. A right shift has the opposite effect.

h. A right shift in the oxyhemoglobin dissociation curve causes hemoglobin to become saturated at higher Po_2.

   i. O_2 loading at the lungs is reduced and the proportion of hemoglobin saturated with O_2 (Sao_2) may be reduced, but O_2 is unloaded more readily at the tissues.

   ii. ▼ *In clinical management of acutely ill patients, it is preferable to retain some right shift in the curve to increase O_2 availability at the tissues.* This can be achieved by accepting a slightly lower blood pH because an acidic environment will cause a right shift, enhancing O_2 delivery to the tissues. ▼

i. Several factors cause a right shift in the O_2 dissociation curve:

   i. **Increased temperature** (e.g., exercise). Higher temperature increases O_2 unloading in working muscle.

   ii. **Increased CO_2.** High levels of CO_2 in metabolically active tissues indicate high O_2 demand, and more O_2 unloading is needed.

   iii. **Increased [H^+].** Buffering of H^+ by hemoglobin reduces its O_2 affinity (known as the **Bohr effect**). For example, anaerobic metabolism produces lactic acid, indicating that more O_2 delivery to tissue is needed.

   iv. **Increased concentration of 2,3-bisphosphoglycerate (BPG) in erythrocytes.** BPG is an end product of metabolism in erythrocytes. Hypoxemia increases BPG formation, causing more unloading of O_2 from hemoglobin.

j. ▼ If blood is stored in blood banks for a long period, BPG levels are reduced. *A **transfusion** with blood that has been stored for a long period causes an unwanted left shift in the O_2 dissociation curve.* ▼

k. ▼ **Carbon monoxide** (CO) is a product of incomplete combustion and is a colorless, odorless, tasteless, nonirritating gas that binds to hemoglobin with very high affinity to produce carboxyhemoglobin.

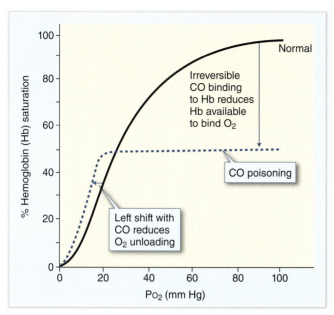

Figure 5-27. Effect of carbon monoxide (CO) poisoning on oxyhemoglobin dissociation curve. CO binds irreversibly to hemoglobin, decreasing the fraction of total hemoglobin available for oxygen (O_2) saturation. CO binding also causes a left shift in the curve, reducing O_2 unloading from the remaining oxyhemoglobin.

    i. In Figure 5-27, the amount of hemoglobin available to bind O_2 is reduced by 50%. *CO also causes a decrease in P_{50}, which reduces O_2 unloading at the tissues.* ▼

l. ▼ A **pulse oximeter** measures the ratio of deoxyhemoglobin to oxyhemoglobin (functional saturation) but is unable to detect **carboxyhemoglobin.**

    i. **CO poisoning** occurs when a person inspires toxic levels of CO, which can result in brain damage or even death.

    ii. Symptoms are very nonspecific and often mimic viral illness, with headache, malaise, nausea, vomiting, and drowsiness.

    iii. Classic findings associated with CO poisoning are cherry-red skin and bilateral necrosis of the basal ganglia, particularly the globus pallidus.

    iv. *Note: The **arterial P_{O_2} is normal in CO poisoning** unless there is separate pulmonary abnormality present that reduces the alveolar P_{O_2}.* ▼

6. Alveolar O_2 transfer.

  a. Before O_2 can bind to hemoglobin, it must first diffuse across the blood-gas barrier.

    i. Red blood cell transit time through a pulmonary capillary is about 0.75 seconds at rest, decreasing to about 0.25 seconds in extreme exercise.

    ii. In healthy persons, the equilibration of the partial pressure of O_2 occurs between alveolar gas and pulmonary capillary blood in this brief amount of time.

    iii. Patients with lung disease (e.g., pulmonary fibrosis) may have reduced diffusion capacity, and equilibration of O_2 across the alveolus may be incomplete.

    iv. *Diffusion defects are unmasked when the blood transit time is low (e.g., exercise) or if the driving force for O_2 diffusion is reduced (e.g., low inspired O_2 partial pressure at high altitude).*

A.

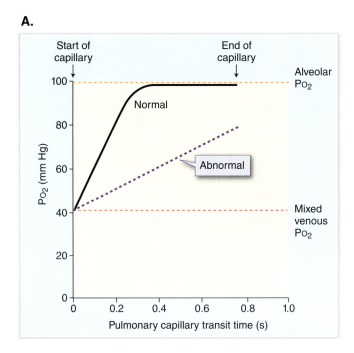

B.

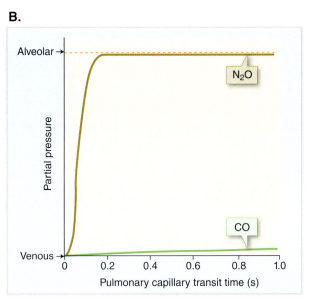

Figure 5-28. Gas uptake kinetics across the blood-gas barrier for oxygen (O_2) (**A**) compared to nitrous oxide (N_2O) and carbon monoxide (CO) (**B**). N_2O equilibrates almost immediately between blood and alveolar gas and uptake is perfusion limited. Alveolar P_{CO} never equilibrates with pulmonary capillary P_{CO} because blood has such a large capacity for the irreversible binding of CO to hemoglobin. CO uptake is diffusion limited.

b. Uptake of gas from the alveolus can be described as "**diffusion limited**" or "**perfusion limited**" (Figure 5-28).

   i. **Nitrous oxide** (N_2O) is a poorly soluble gas that does not bind to anything in blood. N_2O is perfusion limited because P_{N_2O} arrives at equilibrium very rapidly across the alveolus; N_2O uptake is only limited by the rate that blood arrives in pulmonary capillaries.

   ii. CO uptake is diffusion limited. P_{CO} does not equilibrate across the alveolus because almost all CO molecules that diffuse into the pulmonary capillaries bind to hemoglobin. As a result, the partial pressure of CO in the pulmonary capillaries remains at approximately zero.

c. *O_2 uptake is normally perfusion limited because blood equilibrates fully with alveolar Po_2 in transit through pulmonary capillaries.*

  i. There is a reserve for more O_2 uptake, demonstrated during exercise when perfusion increases and equilibration across the alveolus still occurs.

  ii. *O_2 uptake can become diffusion limited in lung disease (e.g., pulmonary fibrosis) when the partial pressure of O_2 is unable to equilibrate between the alveoli and the pulmonary capillary blood.*

  iii. In healthy individuals, diffusion limitation is also possible under extreme conditions such as heavy exercise at a high altitude.

d. Small nontoxic doses of CO can be administered to measure **lung diffusion capacity.** Even at low blood flow rates, the capacity for CO binding is so large that its uptake is only limited by the rate of diffusion:

$$D_L = \dot{V}_{CO} \div P_{ACO}$$ **Equation 5-18**

D_L = Lung diffusion capacity
$\dot{V}_{CO}$ = Rate of CO uptake
P_{ACO} = Alveolar partial pressure of CO

e. ▼ Diffusion capacity can be measured to assess for **diseases that impair the alveolar-capillary membrane.** Decreased diffusion capacity can be seen in interstitial lung disease, emphysema, and pulmonary vascular disease. (*Note: Diffusion capacity is normal in patients with asthma.*) ▼

7. Ventilation/perfusion matching.

a. *The most common cause of **hypoxemia** (low arterial O_2 partial pressure) is mismatch between the distribution of ventilation and pulmonary blood flow.*

b. Expired minute ventilation and cardiac output are both about 5–6 L/min at rest, yielding an overall $\dot{V}/\dot{Q}$ ratio of about 1.

c. Even when overall $\dot{V}/\dot{Q} = 1$, abnormalities in gas exchange result if there are regional differences in the distribution of ventilation and perfusion.

d. The two most extreme situations are **intrapulmonary shunt** ($\dot{V}/\dot{Q} = 0$), where lung units are perfused with blood but receive no ventilation (e.g., complete airway obstruction), and **dead space** ($\dot{V}/\dot{Q} = \infty$), where lung units are ventilated but not perfused (e.g., pulmonary embolism).

e. Figure 5-29 shows the spectrum of alveolar Po_2 and Pco_2 as $\dot{V}/\dot{Q}$ deviates from normal toward these extreme positions.

  i. *Perfusion without ventilation results in an alveolar gas composition in equilibrium with mixed venous blood.*

  ii. *Ventilation without perfusion results in alveoli containing inspired air.*

f. ▼ A $\dot{V}/\dot{Q}$ scan is a nuclear medicine study that can be used in the diagnosis of **pulmonary emboli** and illustrates the concept of matching ventilation to perfusion.

  i. Pulmonary emboli will show a reduced blood flow in an area of normal ventilation.

  ii. In cases of multiple pulmonary emboli, the perfusion scan can show a "moth-eaten" appearance in areas of normal ventilation. ▼

g. Characteristics of **high** $\dot{V}/\dot{Q}$.

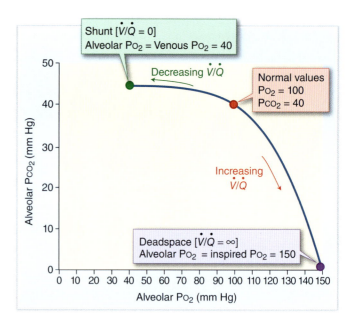

Figure 5-29. Spectrum of alveolar gas composition caused by $\dot{V}/\dot{Q}$ mismatch. Ventilation without perfusion represents pure inspired air only. In lung units with perfusion but no ventilation, alveolar gas equilibrates with mixed venous blood. Note the decrease in alveolar P_{O_2} as $\dot{V}/\dot{Q}$ decreases from normal toward zero, showing that low $\dot{V}/\dot{Q}$ areas will contribute to hypoxemia.

      i. Regions of the lung that are ventilated but not perfused contribute to physiologic dead space.

     ii. A patient with areas of high $\dot{V}/\dot{Q}$ will experience a decrease in useful alveolar ventilation unless total ventilation can be adequately increased.

    iii. This decrease results in less CO_2 excretion and a buildup of the arterial partial pressure of CO_2, a common finding in patients with COPD.

    iv. In many patients, loss of CO_2 excretion in a region of high $\dot{V}/\dot{Q}$ can be compensated by increasing ventilation of well-perfused lung units. *Oxygenation is not directly affected by high $\dot{V}/\dot{Q}$.*

     v. In acute situations when **hypoxemia** is present, the arterial P_{CO_2} is often normal or may even be reduced. This occurs because lung units that are well perfused can increase CO_2 excretion if their ventilation is increased.

  h. Intrapulmonary shunt.

      i. *Intrapulmonary (right-to-left) shunt mixes deoxygenated blood directly into arterial blood and, as a result, the arterial P_{O_2} may be dramatically reduced.*

     ii. Figure 5-30 shows an example where 50% of blood delivered to the left atrium is from a normal lung and 50% is shunted blood flow ($\dot{V}/\dot{Q} = 0$).

    iii. Pulmonary capillary blood from the normal lung has a partial pressure of O_2 ($P_{C_{O_2}}$) = 100 mm Hg, yielding a hemoglobin saturation of 100%.

    iv. Shunted blood is of the same composition as venous blood, in which the partial pressure of O_2 is about 40 mm Hg and hemoglobin saturation is about 75%.

     v. When equal volumes of oxygenated and deoxygenated blood are mixed, the resulting P_{O_2} is less than the average of the individual P_{O_2} values.

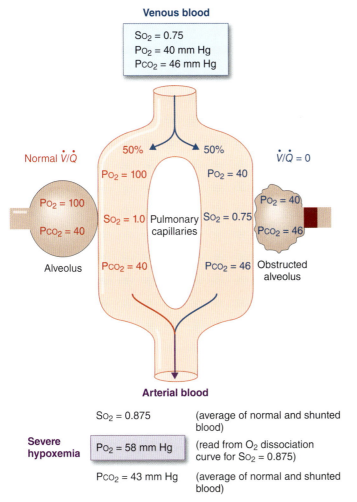

Figure 5-30. Effect of 50% intrapulmonary (right-to-left) shunt on arterial blood gases. Note the severe hypoxemia caused by mixing arterial and venous blood.

- Nonlinearity of the O_2 dissociation curve accounts for the low arterial O_2 partial pressure produced by shunt.
- The law of mass conservation allows the total O_2 content of two samples to be averaged; therefore, hemoglobin saturation can be averaged because the O_2 content is 98% oxyhemoglobin. Po_2 must then be read from the O_2 dissociation curve.

vi. In contrast to the effect of shunt to produce hypoxemia, there is little direct change in the arterial partial pressure of CO_2 because the venous CO_2 content is not much larger than the arterial CO_2 content.
- *When mixed venous blood is combined with oxygenated blood, the resulting arterial Pco_2 is only slightly increased* (Figure 5-30).
- In contrast to O_2, partial pressures of CO_2 can be averaged because the CO_2 dissociation curve is linear and differences in Pco_2 reflect differences in total CO_2 content.

vii. The physiologic response to the hypoxemia caused by intrapulmonary shunt is to increase ventilation. Increased ventilation would increase CO_2 excretion, but would not add more O_2 because pulmonary capillary blood leaving ventilated lung units is already saturated with O_2.

viii. ▼ *Treatment of hypoxemia caused by an intrapulmonary shunt is difficult because the hypoxemia is **refractory to supplemental O_2**.*

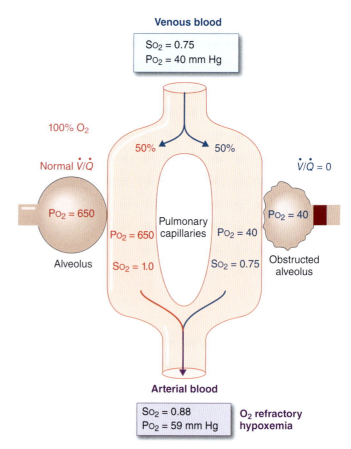

Venous blood

$So_2 = 0.75$
$Po_2 = 40$ mm Hg

100% O_2

50%   50%

Normal $\dot{V}/\dot{Q}$

$\dot{V}/\dot{Q} = 0$

$Po_2 = 650$

$Po_2 = 40$

$Po_2 = 650$ | Pulmonary capillaries | $Po_2 = 40$

Alveolus $So_2 = 1.0$ $So_2 = 0.75$ Obstructed alveolus

Arterial blood

$So_2 = 0.88$ O_2 refractory
$Po_2 = 59$ mm Hg   hypoxemia

Figure 5-31. Effect of breathing 100% O_2 in a patient with 50% intrapulmonary shunt. Note that supplemental O_2 does not reach unventilated regions and has almost no effect on arterial So_2 of mixed arterial blood. Very high Po_2 of blood exposed to 100% O_2 has little effect on total O_2 of blood, because hemoglobin is already saturated and dissolved O_2 is a minor component of total O_2.

- Figure 5-31 shows the effect of breathing 100% O_2 using an example of 50% shunt.
- Because nonventilated areas cannot receive supplemental O_2, they continue to deliver deoxygenated blood to the arterial circulation.
- There is a large increase in the alveolar and pulmonary capillary Po_2 in well-ventilated alveoli. However, the O_2 content of blood from these lung units increases only minimally because hemoglobin is already saturated with O_2.
- *Note that the amount of extra dissolved O_2 in pulmonary capillary blood is small, even at very high partial pressure of O_2.* ▼

ix. Calculation of the amount of right-to-left shunt, as a fraction of cardiac output, can be used clinically to determine the extent of right-to-left shunt in patients with arterial hypoxemia.

x. The total amount of O_2 delivered to the systemic circulation is the product of cardiac output and arterial O_2 content ($\dot{Q}_T \times Cao_2$). This amount must equal the sum of O_2 from shunted blood ($\dot{Q}_S \times Cvo_2$) and pulmonary capillary blood ($\dot{Q}_T - \dot{Q}_S) \times C_co_2$. Rearranging for the shunt fraction $\dot{Q}_S / \dot{Q}_T$:

$$\frac{\dot{Q}s}{\dot{Q}T} = \frac{C_co_2 - Cao_2}{C_co_2 - Cvo_2}$$ **Equation 5-19**

$\dot{Q}s$ = Shunt blood flow

$\dot{Q}T$ = Cardiac output

C_co_2 = Pulmonary capillary blood O_2 content

Cao_2 = Systemic arterial blood O_2 content

Cvo_2 = Mixed venous blood O_2 content

xi. **Example.** A 36-year-old man is admitted to the hospital with severe viral pneumonia. The results of his arterial blood gas analysis show hypoxemia with an arterial Po_2 of 58 mm Hg and hemoglobin saturation (Sao_2) of 88%: C_co_2 = 19.2 mL O_2/dL of blood, Cao_2 = 16.8 mL O_2/dL of blood, Cvo_2 = 15.0 mL O_2/dL of blood.

Shunt fraction $\dot{Q}s / \dot{Q}T = (19.2 - 16.8) / (19.2 - 15.0) = 0.57$

$= 57\% (normal\ 2–5\%)$

xii. ▼ A high shunt ratio ($\dot{Q}s / \dot{Q}T$) can result from either **intracardiac or intrapulmonary shunting.** Intracardiac shunting is an example of a cyanotic congenital heart disease caused by a ventriculoseptal defect, with pulmonary hypertension causing a right to left shunt (**Eisenmenger syndrome**). Intrapulmonary shunting can occur as a result of atelectasis, pulmonary edema, or pneumonia. ▼

8. Alveolar-arterial (A–a) Po_2 gradient.

a. Despite equilibration between alveolar gas and pulmonary capillary blood (alveolar Po_2 = pulmonary capillary Po_2), arterial Po_2 is always less than alveolar Po_2. *A person breathing atmospheric air at sea level has a normal $P(\text{A-a})o_2$ gradient of about 5–10 mm Hg* (Figure 5-32).

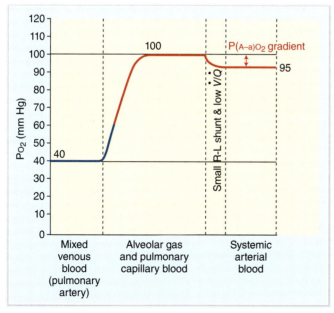

Figure 5-32. Normal A–a gradient.

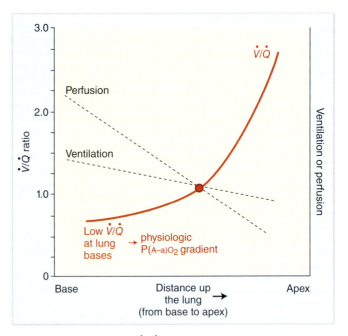

Figure 5-33. Ventilation/perfusion ($\dot{V}/\dot{Q}$) inequalities in the lung of a healthy person who is standing. High $\dot{V}/\dot{Q}$ areas at the lung apex excrete only a minimal amount of carbon dioxide (CO_2), but this is easily compensated by other areas of the lung. Slightly low $\dot{V}/\dot{Q}$ at the bases of the lung cannot be compensated by other areas and contributes to the normal $P(\text{A--a})O_2$ gradient.

   b. A small $P(\text{A-a})O_2$ gradient is normally present for two reasons:

   i. **Anatomic right-to-left shunting of blood.** Bronchial blood vessels from the systemic circulation deliver O_2 and nutrients to lung tissue. Some of the bronchial venous blood drains directly into the pulmonary vein. A small amount of coronary venous blood also drains directly into the left ventricle via the **thebesian veins**.

   ii. $\dot{V}/\dot{Q}$ **inequalities** exist in the lung of a person standing due to the effects of gravity.

   • There is both higher ventilation and perfusion at the base of the lung than at the apex; however, the gradient for perfusion is steeper than the gradient for ventilation (Figure 5-33).

   • *The $\dot{V}/\dot{Q}$ ratio is high at the apex of the lung and slightly low at the base of the lung.* Areas with low $\dot{V}/\dot{Q}$ at the base of the lung deliver blood that is not perfectly oxygenated.

   c. *The $P(\text{A-a})O_2$ gradient is calculated clinically to identify the cause of hypoxemia.* To calculate a $P(\text{A-a})O_2$ gradient, the alveolar PO_2 must first be calculated, using the **alveolar gas equation:**

$$P_{AO_2} = P_{IO_2} - \frac{P_{ACO_2}}{RQ}$$ **Equation 5-20**

P_{AO_2} = Alveolar O_2 partial pressure
P_{IO_2} = O_2 partial pressure of inspired gas
RQ = Respiratory quotient

9. Another form of the alveolar gas equation that is used clinically is:

$$P_{AO_2} = F_{IO_2}(P_B - P_{H_2O}) - \frac{P_{ACO_2}}{RQ}$$ **Equation 5-21**

P_{AO_2} = Alveolar O_2 partial pressure

F_{IO_2} = O_2 fraction of inspired gas

P_B = Barometric pressure

P_{H_2O} = Water vapor pressure of inspired gas

P_{aCO_2} = Arterial CO_2 partial pressure

RQ = Respiratory quotient

10. After alveolar P_{O_2} is calculated using Equation 5-21, and arterial P_{O_2} is measured in an arterial blood sample, the $P(_{A}\text{-}a)_{O_2}$ gradient then can be calculated:

$$P(_{A}\text{-}a)_{O_2} = P_{AO_2} - P_{aO_2} \qquad \text{Equation 5-22}$$

$P(_{A}\text{-}a)_{O_2}$ = Alveolar-arterial O_2 tension gradient

P_{AO_2} = Alveolar O_2 partial pressure

P_{aO_2} = Arterial O_2 partial pressure

11. ▼ When **breathing 100% O_2**, a healthy person has an alveolar-arterial O_2 tension gradient of up to 100 mm Hg. A larger $P(_{A}\text{-}a)_{O_2}$ gradient indicates oxygenation problems. ▼

12. **Example.** A patient with pneumonia was breathing 100% O_2 at sea level via a non-rebreather oxygen mask. This information, together with the results of an arterial blood gas analysis, provided the following data to calculate alveolar P_{O_2}: F_{IO_2} = 100% (1.0), P_B = 760 mm Hg, P_{H_2O} = 47 mm Hg, P_{aCO_2} = 36 mm Hg (measured from an arterial blood gas sample), RQ = 0.8 (standard respiratory quotient used clinically), P_{aO_2} = 168 mm Hg (measured from an arterial blood gas sample).

$$P_{AO_2} = F_{IO_2}(P_B - P_{H_2O}) - \frac{P_{aCO_2}}{RQ}$$

$$= 1.0(760 - 47) - (36 / 0.8)$$

$$= 668 \text{ mm Hg } (note: breathing\ 100\%\ O_2\ produces\ a\ very\ large\ alveolar\ P_{O_2})$$

$$P(_{A}\text{-}a)_{O_2} = P_{AO_2} - P_{aO_2}$$

$$= 668 - 168$$

$$= \textbf{500 mm Hg!}$$

a. *The presence of such a large difference between O_2 tension in alveoli compared to O_2 tension in arterial blood indicates a severe oxygenation defect.*

13. Causes of arterial hypoxemia (Table 5-6).

a. **Low P_{IO_2}** is an effect of high altitude but can also result from incorrect air mixtures used in scuba diving.

Table 5-6. Major Causes of Arterial Hypoxemia and Response to Supplemental Oxygen

Cause	$P_{(A\text{-}a)O_2}$ Gradient	Responds to Supplemental O_2
Low P_{IO_2}	Normal	Yes
Global hypoventilation	Normal	Yes
Diffusion abnormality	Increased	Yes
$\dot{V}/\dot{Q}$ mismatch (low $\dot{V}/\dot{Q}$)	Increased	Yes
Intrapulmonary shunt	Increased	No

     i. Low alveolar Po_2 is the cause of low arterial Po_2.

     ii. The $P(A-a)o_2$ gradient is normal, and the treatment is to restore alveolar Po_2 with supplemental O_2.

b. **Global hypoventilation** occurs when total minute ventilation is low. This condition may be due to defective central control of breathing, such as narcotic overdose or from paralysis of ventilatory muscles.

     i. High arterial Pco_2 is always present.

     ii. High alveolar Pco_2 develops because the venous blood Pco_2 is increased, and CO_2 diffuses readily into alveoli. CO_2 displaces O_2 in the alveolus, decreasing the alveolar Po_2.

     iii. The $P(A-a)o_2$ gradient is normal. Low arterial Po_2 responds to supplemental O_2; ventilatory support is needed to restore alveolar ventilation.

c. **Diffusion abnormality** (e.g., pulmonary fibrosis) is a rare cause of hypoxemia.

     i. Alveolar Po_2 is normal, but a $P(A-a)o_2$ gradient develops.

     ii. Supplemental O_2 is an effective treatment because it increases the driving force of O_2 diffusion.

d. **Regional $\dot{V}/\dot{Q}$ imbalance** (e.g., pneumonia) is the most common cause of hypoxemia.

     i. Unlike global hypoventilation, arterial Pco_2 is not increased because total alveolar ventilation is normal, or it may even be increased.

     ii. Regions of the lung with low $\dot{V}/\dot{Q}$ deliver poorly oxygenated blood and cause the development of a $P(A-a)o_2$ gradient.

     iii. Hypoxemia responds to supplemental O_2 because affected lung units have some ventilation that can be enriched with O_2.

e. **Intrapulmonary shunt** is the most dangerous cause of hypoxemia because no compensation is possible by normal lung units, even when 100% O_2 is given.

     i. The effect of shunt is magnified if venous desaturation (low Svo_2) develops.

     ii. The Svo_2 is determined by the balance between O_2 delivery and consumption. O_2 delivery is too low in conditions such as low cardiac output or severe anemia.

     iii. The causes of shunt and low Svo_2 must be addressed to treat these causes of hypoxemia (e.g., acute respiratory distress syndrome).

Control of Breathing

1. A **central pattern generator** in the medulla initiates the basic rhythmic pattern of breathing, which proceeds without the need for conscious control (e.g., during sleep). There are many inputs to the central pattern generator that influence breathing; for example:

a. Negative feedback responses to maintain the **arterial Pco_2 and Po_2 and pH.**

b. Sensory feedback relating to the **mechanical state of the lung and chest wall** to minimize work of breathing, to prevent overinflation of the lung, and to respond to irritants.

c. Sensory feedback from **receptors in the joints and muscles** to increase ventilation in response to exercise.

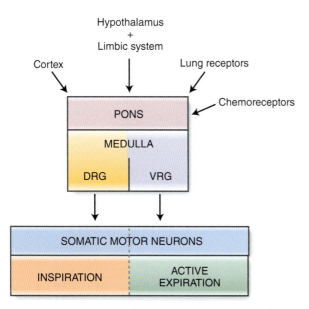

Figure 5-34. Components of the central nervous system controller for ventilation. DRG, dorsal respiratory group; VRG, ventral respiratory group.

    d. Integration with the **sympathetic nervous system** to increase ventilation during "fight or flight" responses, and with other stress responses such as a high body temperature or a low arterial blood pressure.

    e. Integration to allow **speech and swallowing**.

    f. **Conscious control** to allow hyperventilation or breath holding.

2. Central control of breathing (Figure 5-34).

    a. The basic rhythm of breathing is controlled by groups of neurons in the medulla.

        i. The medullary center has a **dorsal respiratory group** (DRG) of neurons in the nucleus of the tractus solitarius and a **ventral respiratory group** (VRG) in the nucleus ambiguus and nucleus retroambiguus.

        ii. *The DRG is thought to be the main integrator of **sensory information** and to have primarily inspiratory neurons.*

        iii. *The VRG is larger and has primarily **motor neurons** that mediate both inspiration and active expiration.*

          • The **pre-Bötzinger complex** is part of the VRG and thought to be an important part of the central pattern generator.

    b. Outflow from the medullary centers reaches the muscles of ventilation via somatic motor neurons; *control of the diaphragm via the **phrenic nerves** (spinal segments C3–C5) is most important.*

        i. ▼ **Hangman's fracture** results in a spinal cord injury at the level of C2. The fracture causes **apnea** (cessation of breathing) because the spinal cord is interrupted proximal to the origin of the phrenic nerve roots. In contrast, a spinal cord injury at the level of C4 will result in quadriplegia (motor dysfunction of the upper and lower extremities) and weakened ventilatory muscles because part of the phrenic nerve remains functional. ▼

    c. Activity of the medullary central pattern generator is modified by multiple inputs:

        i. Descending cortical inputs allow voluntary control of breathing.

        ii. Hypothalamic and limbic system inputs account for breathing patterns seen in emotional states such as rage or fear.

iii. Input from neural receptors in the lung and chest wall is conveyed to the central nervous system via the vagus nerves.
- **Pulmonary J receptors** surround blood vessels and initiate increased ventilation associated with edema in the lung.
- Stretch receptors in the airway initiate the **Hering-Breuer reflex,** which increases breathing frequency and prevents hyperinflation of the lungs.

iv. Ascending spinal inputs from neural receptors in working muscles and joints provide information about the workload of exercise.
- Ventilation is stimulated as a function of workload to match O_2 demand.
- Ventilation also matches increased cardiac output during exercise to ensure $\dot{V}/\dot{Q}$ matching and preservation of normal arterial blood gas tensions.

d. *Note: The traditional ideas of a dominant pontine* **apneustic center** *that promotes inspiration, and a pontine* **pneumotaxic center** *that inhibits inspiration are now thought to be incorrect.*

3. Negative feedback control of ventilation by CO_2, O_2, and pH.

a. *To help maintain normal arterial blood gases, ventilation is increased if the arterial P_{CO_2} increases or if the arterial P_{O_2} decreases.*

b. Under normal conditions, maintenance of arterial P_{CO_2} predominates.

c. Ventilation is also stimulated by **reduced arterial blood pH,** representing the pulmonary contribution to acid-base balance (see Chapter 6).

d. Figure 5-35 shows increased ventilation in response to high arterial P_{CO_2}, which represents a negative feedback response to increase CO_2 excretion and thereby to restore the arterial P_{CO_2} to normal.

e. The **predominance of arterial P_{CO_2}** in control of ventilation is indicated by the steepness of the curves shown in Figure 5-35.

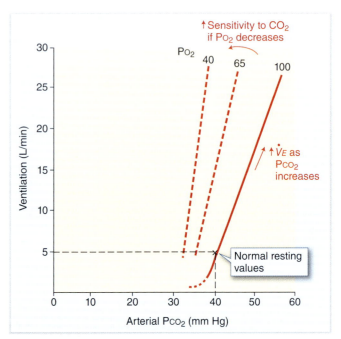

Figure 5-35. Regulation of ventilation by arterial P_{CO_2}. The steep increase in ventilation as arterial P_{CO_2} increases reflects dominant control of ventilation by carbon dioxide (CO_2). Low arterial P_{O_2} has a synergistic effect with high arterial P_{CO_2}.

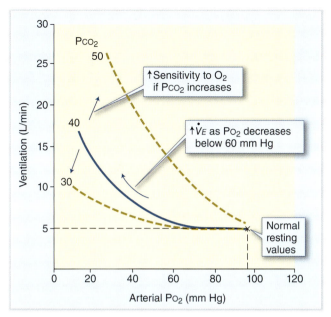

Figure 5-36. Regulation of ventilation by arterial P_{O_2}. Arterial P_{O_2} less than 60 mm Hg causes a large increase in ventilation. High arterial P_{CO_2} has a synergistic effect with low arterial P_{O_2}.

    i. The ventilatory response to hypercapnia is blunted by increased arterial P_{O_2} and stimulated by a coexisting hypoxemia.

  f. Figure 5-36 shows increased ventilation in response to reduced arterial P_{O_2}, which *accounts for a presentation of low arterial P_{CO_2} in patients with hypoxemia.*

    i. A marked increase in ventilation does not occur until arterial P_{O_2} is below 60 mm Hg, corresponding with the region of steep decline in oxyhemoglobin saturation on the O_2 dissociation curve.

    ii. The response to hypoxemia is blunted if arterial P_{CO_2} is reduced, but stimulated if arterial P_{CO_2} is increased.

  g. ▼ Many patients with COPD have hypercapnia; they often adapt to tolerate high arterial P_{CO_2} but rely on hypoxemia to drive ventilation. *Treatment with supplemental O_2 may cause these patients to stop breathing because arterial P_{O_2} is increased abruptly, removing their drive to breathe.* These patients have modified O_2 therapy guidelines and are closely monitored. ▼

  h. Patients with acidemia (e.g., lactic acidosis) usually have reduced arterial P_{CO_2} due to the stimulation of ventilation by low pH (Figure 5-37).

    i. The equilibrium $CO_2 + H_2O \leftrightarrow H_2CO_3 \leftrightarrow H^+ + HCO_3^-$ shifts to the left when the arterial P_{CO_2} is reduced, which reduces $[H^+]$ and moves pH back toward the normal range.

    ii. Ventilation is affected only slightly by alkalemia. If ventilation were to be reduced to return pH to normal, it would be at the cost of increased arterial P_{CO_2}, which is prevented by the powerful feedback control of arterial P_{CO_2}.

4. Chemoreceptors.

  a. Changes in ventilation due to altered blood gases and pH are initiated by chemoreceptors.

  b. **Central chemoreceptors** are located on the ventral surface of the medulla and respond to changes in arterial P_{CO_2}.

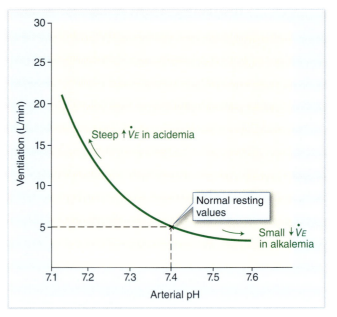

Figure 5-37. Regulation of ventilation by arterial pH. Increased ventilation due to acidemia reflects pulmonary compensation for metabolic acidosis. The response to alkalemia is weak because control of arterial P_{CO_2} prevents decreased ventilation.

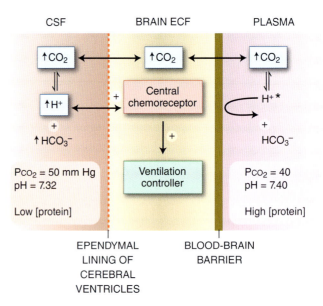

*No effect of plasma H+ on central receptor

Figure 5-38. Measurement of arterial CO_2 by central chemoreceptors. Central nervous system chemoreceptors sense [H+] in extracellular fluid (ECF) in the brain as an index of arterial P_{CO_2}. CO_2 diffuses readily across the blood-brain barrier. Levels of CO_2 in the brain reflect changes in arterial P_{CO_2} due to the high rate of blood flow in the brain. CO_2 is converted to $H^+ + HCO_3^-$ via carbonic anhydrase. The low buffering power of cerebrospinal fluid (CSF), due to low protein concentration, allows larger changes in [H+] in the CSF than occur in plasma. Central chemoreceptors are isolated from changes in blood [H+] by the blood-brain barrier.

    c. Altered arterial P_{CO_2} is sensed through changes in cerebrospinal fluid (CSF) pH (Figure 5-38):

        i. CO_2 diffuses readily across the blood-brain barrier.

        ii. **Cerebrospinal fluid pH** decreases because the CSF is poorly buffered due to its low protein content.

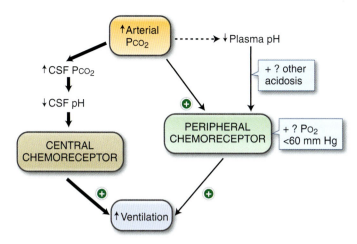

Figure 5-39. Integrated feedback control of ventilation by blood gases and pH. The carbon dioxide (CO_2) response of central chemoreceptors dominates control under normal circumstances. Central chemoreceptors are set to respond most strongly to an increase in arterial P_{CO_2}. Patients with metabolic acidosis or hypoxemia often have low arterial P_{CO_2} due to peripheral chemoreceptor activation. CSF, cerebrospinal fluid.

     iii. Decreased CSF pH (increased [H^+]) stimulates central chemoreceptors.

     iv. *Note: Changes in arterial blood pH are not sensed by the central chemoreceptors because the blood-brain barrier prevents H^+ from crossing into the brain.*

     v. Arterial P_{O_2} as well as arterial pH are not sensed by the brain and rely on input from peripheral chemoreceptors.

  d. **Peripheral chemoreceptors** are located in the carotid bodies at the bifurcation of the common carotid arteries and in the aortic bodies in the aortic arch.

     i. Glomus cells within the carotid body are able to sense changes in O_2, H^+, and CO_2, and relay signals to the central pattern generator via the glossopharyngeal and vagus nerves.

  e. *The control of ventilation by O_2 and pH is initiated in peripheral chemoreceptors. Control of ventilation by CO_2 is mainly through central chemoreceptors* (Figure 5-39).

Study Questions

Directions: Each numbered item is followed by lettered options. Some options may be partially correct, but there is only *ONE BEST* answer.

1. A 50-year-old man with a persistent cough and difficulty breathing is referred by his family physician for pulmonary function tests. The test results show that the forced vital capacity (FVC), forced expired volume in 1 s (FEV_1), and functional residual capacity (FRC) are all significantly below normal. Which of the following diagnosis is consistent with these pulmonary function test results?

    A. Asthma

    B. Chronic bronchitis

    C. Emphysema

    D. Pulmonary fibrosis

2. A 19-year-old man is taken to the emergency department after being stabbed in the right side of the chest. The entry of air through the wound resulted in a pneumothorax on the right side of his chest. What difference between the right and left sides of the chest would be apparent on a plain chest x-ray?

   A. The lung volume on the right would be larger
   B. The position of the diaphragm on the right would be higher
   C. The thoracic volume on the right would be larger
   D. There would be no differences in thoracic geometry

3. A 28-year-old man is involved in a high-speed motor vehicle accident in which he suffers multiple rib fractures. On arrival at the emergency department, he is conscious but in severe pain. His respiratory rate is 34 breaths/min, and his breathing is labored. His blood pressure is 110/95 mm Hg, and his pulse is 140 beats/min. His arterial P_{O_2} is 50 mm Hg, and he is unresponsive to supplemental O_2. His arterial P_{CO_2} is 28 mm Hg. What is the most likely cause of this patient's hypoxemia?

   A. Alveolar hypoventilation
   B. High ventilation/perfusion ($\dot{V}/\dot{Q}$) ratio
   C. Increased dead space ventilation
   D. Intrapulmonary shunt
   E. Low $\dot{V}/\dot{Q}$ ratio

4. A 16-year-old girl is found unconscious in the street. She has no visible injuries but is cold and is taking shallow breaths at a rate of 6–8 per minute. An arterial blood gas analysis recorded in the emergency department shows that her P_{O_2} is 55 mm Hg and her P_{CO_2} is 75 mm Hg. What is the most likely cause of hypoxemia in this patient?

   A. Alveolar hypoventilation
   B. High ventilation/perfusion ($\dot{V}/\dot{Q}$) ratio
   C. Increased dead space ventilation
   D. Intrapulmonary shunt
   E. Low $\dot{V}/\dot{Q}$ ratio

5. A 62-year-old man with a history of COPD is admitted to the hospital due to acute deterioration in lung function as a result of a viral chest infection. An analysis of arterial blood gases shows that his P_{O_2} is 60 mm Hg and his P_{CO_2} is 70 mm Hg. His exhaled minute ventilation rate is two times higher than that of a normal individual of the same age and body size. He has hypercapnea, despite having an increased exhaled minute ventilation rate because his

   A. alveolar ventilation is increased
   B. dead space ventilation is increased
   C. V_T is increased
   D. ventilation/perfusion ($\dot{V}/\dot{Q}$) ratio is decreased
   E. intrapulmonary shunt is increased

6. A 40-year-old woman presented with dyspnea, hematuria, and right flank pain. CT scans revealed a renal tumor, with an extensive venous thrombus that had

invaded the inferior vena cava. Fragments of the thrombus had entered the lungs and were blocking several major branches of the pulmonary arteries. Assuming that there was no change in V_T or respiratory rate, what effect would these pulmonary emboli have on arterial blood gases within the first few minutes of their occurrence?

A. Decreased P_{CO_2} and decreased P_{O_2}
B. Decreased P_{CO_2} and increased P_{O_2}
C. Increased P_{CO_2} and decreased P_{O_2}
D. Increased P_{CO_2} and increased P_{O_2}
E. No change in P_{CO_2} or P_{O_2}

7. A 9-year-old boy decided to find out for how long he could continue to breathe into and out of a paper bag. After approximately 2 minutes, his friends noticed that he was breathing very rapidly so they forced him to stop the experiment. What change in arterial blood gas composition was the most potent stimulus for this boy's hyperventilation?

A. Decreased P_{CO_2}
B. Decreased P_{O_2}
C. Decreased pH
D. Increased P_{CO_2}
E. Increased P_{O_2}
F. Increased pH

8. A 54-year-old woman with advanced emphysema due to many years of cigarette smoking is admitted to the hospital because of severe peripheral edema and shortness of breath. On physical examination, there is jugular venous distension and a widely split second heart sound with a loud pulmonic sound. A differential diagnosis of right heart failure and pulmonary hypertension is confirmed by cardiac catheterization. The results of her arterial blood gas analysis show $P_{O_2} = 55$ mm Hg, $P_{CO_2} = 75$ mm Hg, and pH $= 7.30$. What is the most likely cause of pulmonary hypertension in this patient?

A. Decreased alveolar P_{O_2}
B. Decreased lung compliance
C. Decreased parasympathetic neural tone
D. Increased alveolar P_{CO_2}
E. Increased thoracic volume
F. Increased sympathetic neural tone

9. A group of medical students is experimenting with a peak flow meter in the respiratory physiology laboratory. Two students decide to compete to see which of them can blow the hardest into the device. Which of the following muscles is most effective at producing a maximal expiratory effort such as this?

A. Diaphragm
B. External intercostal muscles
C. Internal intercostal muscles
D. Rectus abdominus
E. Sternocleidomastoid

10. A 22-year-old man was involved in a fight in which he received a severe blow to the head. On arrival at the emergency department, he was unconscious and initially received assisted ventilation via a manual bag-valve device. An analysis of his arterial blood gases shows:

$Po_2 = 45$ mm Hg

$Pco_2 = 80$ mm Hg

$pH = 7.05$

$HCO_3^- = 27$ mM

In what form was most CO_2 being transported in his arterial blood?

A. Bicarbonate ions

B. Carbaminohemoglobin compounds

C. Dissolved CO_2 molecules

Renal Physiology and Acid-Base Balance

CHAPTER

6

Anatomy of the Kidney

1. The paired kidneys are bean-shaped retroperitoneal organs, each about 12-cm long and located on the posterior abdominal wall.

2. The renal artery, the renal vein, and the renal pelvis pass through the renal hilus; the renal nerves and lymphatic vessels are associated with the renal blood vessels (Figure 6-1).

3. The cut surface of the kidney has a pale outer region, the **cortex,** and a darker inner region, the **medulla.**
   a. The medulla is divided into conical areas called **renal pyramids.**
   b. The apex of each pyramid tapers toward the renal pelvis, forming the **renal papillae.**
   c. The **renal pelvis** has a funnel-shaped upper end and is continuous with the **ureter** below it, which conveys urine to the bladder.

4. ▼ **Renal colic** is pain in the flank that radiates toward the groin. Colicky pain is usually severe and most commonly caused by **renal calculi** ("kidney stones"). The three common **sites of obstruction** leading to the clinical presentation of renal colic are:
   a. At the junction of the renal pelvis and ureter.
   b. At the site where the ureter passes over the pelvic brim.
   c. At the junction between the ureter and bladder. ▼

5. Structure of the nephron.
   a. The functional unit of the kidney is a nephron, a tube that consists of different transporting epithelia in sequence; each kidney has between 500,000 and 800,000 nephrons.

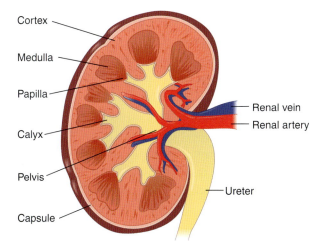

Figure 6-1. Gross anatomy of the kidney.

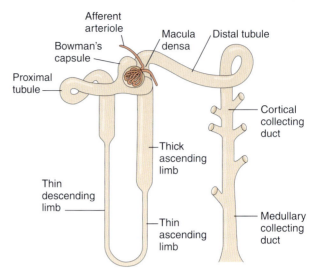

Figure 6-2. The nephron.

b. A nephron has several functionally and histologically distinct segments (Figure 6-2).

  i. The **glomerulus** is the site of primary urine formation where blood plasma is filtered into the nephron; the glomerular capillaries are enveloped by the blind-ended upper part of the nephron, known as **Bowman's capsule.**

  ii. Filtrate flows from Bowman's space into the **proximal tubule,** which consists of convoluted and straight portions.

  iii. The proximal tubule is continuous with the **loop of Henle,** which is a U-shaped tubule that descends into the medulla before turning back toward the cortex.

   • The loop of Henle has three functional parts: the **thin descending limb,** the **thin ascending limb,** and the **thick ascending limb (TAL).**

  iv. The **macula densa** is a short segment that passes close to the glomerulus and connects the TAL to the **distal tubule** in the cortex.

  v. Distal tubules from approximately six nephrons converge with a single **collecting duct.**

  vi. As the collecting ducts descend through the renal medulla, they converge to form the larger **ducts of Bellini,** which deliver final urine into the **renal calyces.**

  vii. Urine proceeds to the **renal pelvis** and then to the lower urinary tract.

c. There are two types of nephrons: about 85% are **cortical nephrons** and 15% are **juxtamedullary (JM) nephrons** (Figure 6-3).

  i. Glomeruli of cortical nephrons are located in the outer cortex and the loops of Henle are short.

  ii. JM nephrons have glomeruli located deep in the cortex and have long loops of Henle, many extending to the tip of the renal papilla.

   • *JM nephrons are "salt conserving" and are important for urine concentration.*

   • When effective circulating blood volume is reduced, a higher proportion of renal blood flow (RBF) is directed to JM nephrons, helping to conserve extracellular fluid (ECF) volume.

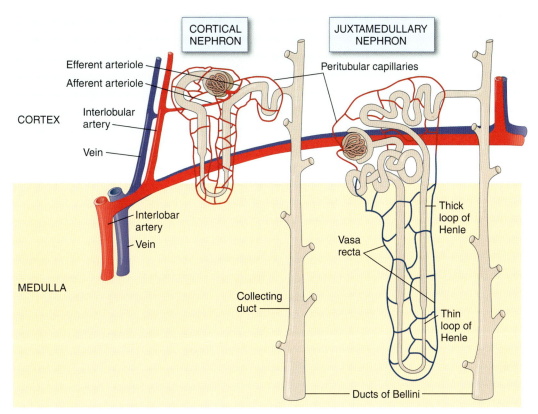

Figure 6-3. The cortical and juxtamedullary nephrons.

Principles of Urine Formation

1. The kidney is a homeostatic organ that varies the excretion of water, electrolytes, and other hydrophilic molecules to maintain constancy of ECF composition.

2. Urine formation begins with glomerular filtration of plasma at a rate of about 150–200 L/day.

3. *The **glomerular filtration rate (GFR)** is a controlled variable and in most circumstances is fairly constant.*

   a. ▼ **Renal insufficiency** occurs when GFR is low. A progressive decline in GFR indicates the **stages of chronic kidney disease** as mild (60–89 mL/min/1.73 m²), moderate (30–59 mL/min/1.73 m²), and severe (15–29 mL/min/1.73 m²). ▼

4. Glomerular filtrate is modified by epithelial transport as it flows along the nephron.

   a. For water and many solutes, 98–99% of the filtrate is reabsorbed back into the blood.

   b. *Variation of excretion rates in final urine usually reflects changes in renal tubular reabsorption.*

   c. The rate of reabsorption for most substances is highest in the proximal tubule.

   d. *Fine control of excretion usually occurs in the distal parts of the renal tubule, which receive a fairly constant fraction of the filtrate (about 10%).*

   e. The model of filtration-reabsorption applies to most substances. For others, such as K^+, H^+, and some organic molecules (e.g., penicillin), the rate of

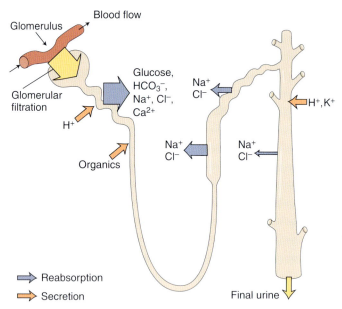

Figure 6-4. General principles of urine formation. Excretion of most solutes is determined by varying the amount that is reabsorbed from the glomerular filtrate. Reabsorption rates are high proximally and finely tuned in the distal segments. Excretion of some solutes (e.g., H⁺ and K⁺) is determined by secretion rather than reabsorption.

secretion into the urine across the nephron epithelia is the most important for determining the excretion rate (Figure 6-4).

5. Renal blood flow.

a. *The kidneys normally receive 20–25% of cardiac output; a very high rate of RBF is needed to supply enough plasma for glomerular filtration.*

b. All blood entering the kidney passes through larger branches of the renal artery to reach the glomerular capillaries in the renal cortex.

c. Renal perfusion is achieved with a typical systemic arterial perfusion pressure of about 90–100 mm Hg. *High rates of RBF are possible because renal vascular resistance is low.*

 i. The pressure decreases measured across the afferent and efferent arterioles demonstrate that vascular resistance is shared between the arterioles (Figure 6-5).

 ii. *Having an arteriolar resistance vessel at the distal end of the glomerular capillary instead of a venule creates a high capillary hydrostatic blood pressure to drive filtration.*

d. There are two other unique features of the renal microcirculation:

 i. The **peritubular capillary bed** receives water and solutes reabsorbed from the nephrons; being supplied from the efferent arterioles it is in series with the glomerular capillaries.

 • Filtration of protein-free fluid from the glomerular capillaries increases the osmolarity of blood entering the peritubular capillaries, which assists in water reabsorption from the nephron.

 • This promotes **glomerulotubular balance** in which the rate of proximal tubular absorption is proportional to the rate of filtration, providing consistent rates of fluid delivery to the distal nephron.

 ii. The **vasa recta** are long capillary loops, branching from peritubular capillaries, which travel with the loops of Henle.

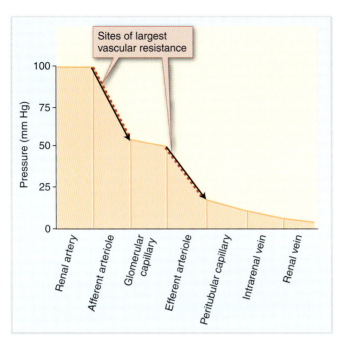

Figure 6-5. Vascular resistance is shared between the afferent and efferent arterioles. Glomerular capillary pressure is higher than in other systemic vascular beds due to the presence of an efferent arteriole at the glomerular outlet. Greater capillary pressure facilitates glomerular filtration.

- Less than 10% of RBF follows a course through the vasa recta to the renal medulla, and only about 1% reaches the renal papilla.
- *Low blood flow in the renal medulla helps to preserve the medullary hypertonicity necessary for the concentration of urine, but causes it to be susceptible to ischemia in the setting of hypotension or renal vasoconstriction.*

e. The normally high rates of perfusion provide an excess of O_2 for renal tissue metabolism. However, the kidney is readily injured in states of shock, where RBF decreases because renal tissue has a high rate of O_2 use. A s*ustained decrease in renal perfusion may result in* **acute renal failure (ARF).**

f. ▼ ARF is organized into the following three categories:

  i. **Prerenal ARF** is most common and is caused by any condition that results in renal hypoperfusion without impairing the renal parenchyma (e.g., hypovolemia).

  ii. **Renal ARF** describes diseases that directly result in damage to the renal parenchyma (e.g., glomerular nephritis). *(Note: Severe prerenal ARF can progress to renal ARF if hypoperfusion is severe enough to cause ischemic injury to the renal parenchyma. This results in* **acute tubular necrosis,** *which is the most common cause of renal ARF.)*

  iii. **Postrenal ARF** occurs in diseases that cause obstruction of the urinary tract (e.g., tumors or benign prostatic hyperplasia). ▼

Endocrine Functions of the Kidney

1. The kidney is a *target organ* for several hormones, including antidiuretic hormone (ADH), angiotensin II, aldosterone, atrial natriuretic peptide (ANP), and parathyroid hormone (PTH).

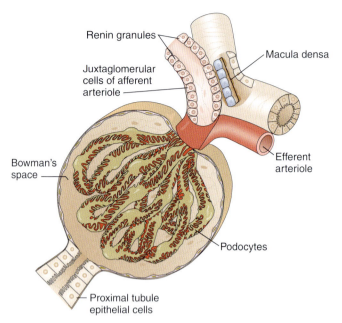

Figure 6-6. Juxtaglomerular apparatus. The juxtaglomerular apparatus comprises the granular renin-secreting cells in the wall of the afferent arteriole plus the macula densa segment of nephron. Paracrine signaling from the macula densa to the afferent arteriole influences glomerular filtration and renin secretion.

2. The kidney is also an *endocrine organ* that secretes **renin**, **erythropoietin**, and the active form of vitamin D, 1,25-dihydroxycholecalciferol (**1,25-(OH)$_2$ vitamin D**).

3. Renin secretion.

   a. *Renin is an enzyme released by the **juxtaglomerular apparatus** (JGA) of the kidney in response to a decrease in effective circulating blood volume.*

   b. The JGA is formed from the close association between the vascular and tubular structures where the distal nephron comes in contact with its own glomerulus (Figure 6-6).

   c. Renin is released from **juxtaglomerular cells** lining the afferent arterioles, which respond to reduced renal perfusion.

   d. Renin initiates a cascade of events that result in the production of the hormones angiotensin II and aldosterone (see Chapter 8). *The **renin-angiotensin-aldosterone system** is the most important endocrine axis in control of the ECF volume.*

   e. A second key regulatory function of the JGA is the feedback regulation of GFR (see Tubuloglomerular Feedback).

4. Erythropoietin secretion.

   a. Erythropoietin (EPO) is a glycoprotein hormone produced by **fibroblasts** in the renal interstitium.

   b. Local Po_2 in renal tissue is an indicator of the systemic arterial O_2 content; *EPO is released in response to low renal interstitial Po_2.*

   c. EPO stimulates red blood cell formation in the bone marrow to restore the O_2-carrying capacity of blood (Figure 6-7).

   d. About 80% of plasma EPO is produced in the kidney and the remainder is secreted by the liver.

   e. EPO production is controlled at the transcription level through **hypoxia-inducible factor (HIF).**

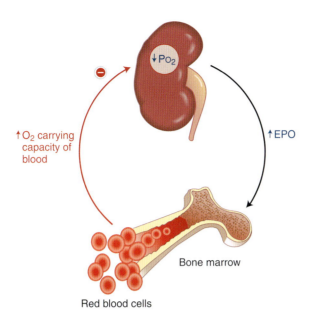

Figure 6-7. Negative feedback regulation of blood-O_2 content via erythropoietin (EPO) secretion.

   f. *Patients with chronic renal failure usually secrete insufficient EPO and develop anemia.*
   g. ▼ The main uses of EPO are related to treating **anemia** associated with chronic renal failure or cancer chemotherapy. However, EPO has also gained notoriety as a "**blood-doping**" agent that is used illegally by endurance athletes. In healthy individuals, injection of EPO will lead to increased red blood cells and consequently an increase in O_2-carrying capacity that boosts aerobic performance. ▼

5. Activation of vitamin D.
   a. Vitamin D is a steroid derived from precursors that are either ingested or produced by the action of ultraviolet light on the skin (see Chapter 8).
   b. The active form of vitamin D is 1,25-dihydroxycholecalciferol (1,25-$(OH)_2$ vitamin D), also known as **calcitriol.**
   c. The liver produces 25-hydroxycholecalciferol (25-OH vitamin D), which is converted to 1,25-$(OH)_2$ vitamin D in the kidney under the control of **parathyroid hormone.**
   d. *1,25-$(OH)_2$ vitamin D conserves Ca^{2+} in the body by increasing intestinal Ca^{2+} absorption, reducing urinary Ca^{2+} loss, and promoting bone formation (see Chapter 8) (Figure 6-8).*
   e. ▼ Manifestations of chronic renal failure plague many of the body's systems, including bone. **Osteitis fibrosa cystica (renal osteodystrophy)** is the classic bone disease related to chronic renal failure. The pathophysiologic cascade begins in the kidneys and ends in the bones:
      i. As the kidneys fail, there is inadequate phosphate excretion leading to increased plasma phosphate concentration; kidney failure also causes **vitamin D deficiency,** which results in low serum Ca^{2+} due to impaired dietary absorption.
      ii. A combination of high serum phosphate, low serum Ca^{2+}, and low vitamin D levels causes increase in PTH production (**secondary hyperparathyroidism**).

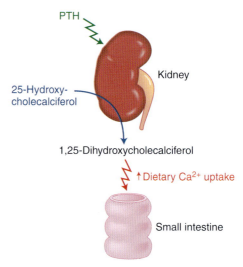

Figure 6-8. Renal activation of vitamin D. Parathyroid hormone (PTH) activates the mitochondrial enzyme 1α-hydroxylase in the proximal tubule to produce activated vitamin D$_3$ (1,25-dihydroxycholecalciferol).

    iii. PTH acts on bone to cause a high rate of bone turnover, which releases Ca^{2+} back into the serum.

    iv. The end result of this cascade is that near normal plasma Ca^{2+} concentration is maintained at the expense of chronic bone resorption resulting from hyperparathyroidism.

    v. *Osteitis fibrosa cystica is associated with increased risk of fracture.* ▼

Glomerular Filtration Rate (GFR)

1. *The adequacy of renal function is clinically defined by the GFR.*
2. Four key general principles related to GFR are:
   a. GFR is normally very large (approximately 200 L/day!), which provides the potential to excrete multiple solutes that may be present at low concentrations in plasma.
   b. *The glomerular filter should not allow passage of blood cells or plasma proteins.*
   c. **Starling's forces** are responsible for the net filtration pressure across the glomerular capillaries.
   d. GFR is generally stable due to autoregulation but can be varied by active changes in afferent and efferent arteriolar tone.
3. ▼ The term **glomerulonephritis** is used to denote glomerular injury. In virtually all cases, GFR is impaired and protein or blood cells can be seen in the urine. Diseases that affect the glomeruli can be classified according to the syndrome of symptoms produced.
   a. **Nephrotic syndrome** is characterized by severe proteinuria (>3.5 g/day), hypoalbuminemia (<3 g/L), generalized edema, and hyperlipidemia.
   b. **Nephritic syndrome** is characterized by hematuria, hypertension, oliguria (<400 mL/day of urine), and azotemia (increased blood urea nitrogen [BUN] and plasma creatinine concentration). ▼
4. The glomerular filtration barrier.
   a. Substances with a molecular weight of about 10 kDa are freely filtered; as molecular weight increases from 10 to 70 kDa, there is a roughly linear decline in the amount of solute filtered (Figure 6-9A).

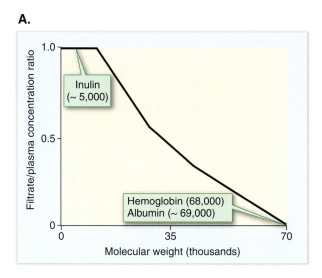

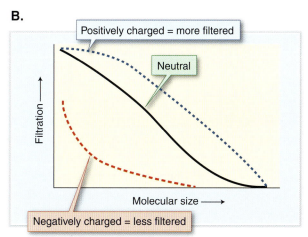

Figure 6-9. Properties of the glomerular filtration barrier. **A.** Effect of molecular size on the glomerular filtration of macromolecules: hemoglobin and albumin are just large enough to avoid filtration at normal glomeruli on the basis of their size. **B.** Effect of electrical charge on glomerular filtration of macromolecules: filtration of negatively charged macromolecules (but not small anions) is reduced.

      i. **Albumin,** with a molecular weight of 70 kDa, is almost small enough to be filtered. *It is essential that albumin is not lost in the urine because the plasma albumin concentration is the largest contributor to plasma oncotic pressure.*

  b. The electrical charge on a macromolecule also determines its filterability (Figure 6-9B).

      i. There is less filtration of negatively charged macromolecules compared to neutral molecules of the same size due to repulsion by fixed **negative charges** in the filtration membrane.

     ii. At a physiologic ECF pH of 7.4, proteins carry net negative charges, which reduce their filtration.

  c. During filtration, solutes pass through three anatomic structures (Figure 6-10):

      i. The **glomerular capillary endothelial cell layer.** The large fenestrations between glomerular capillary endothelial cells only exclude blood cells.

     ii. The **glomerular basement membrane** is a fiber meshwork that resists the sieving of macromolecules.

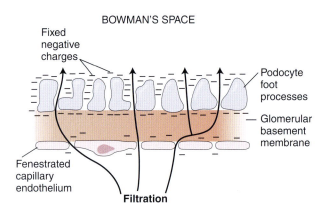

BOWMAN'S SPACE

Figure 6-10. The glomerular filtration membrane. Filtered water and solutes must pass through the glomerular capillary endothelium, through the glomerular basement membrane, and through the filtration slits between podocytes.

    iii. **Podocytes** are specialized epithelial cells that coat the glomerular capillaries and bear finger-like projections that interlock around the glomerular capillaries.
- *The membrane protein **nephrin** bridges the filtration slits and contributes significantly to the filtration barrier.*
- ▼ **Loss of nephrin,** such as that which occurs in **minimal change disease,** allows for selective loss of albumin resulting in a nephrotic syndrome. Minimal change disease (or nil disease) is most common in children. The name is derived from the lack of pathologic findings from a renal biopsy examined by light microscopy. ▼

5. Determinants of GFR.
  a. GFR is the product of the net driving pressure forcing fluid out of glomerular capillaries (P_{UF}) and the permeability of the filtration barrier (K_f):

$$\text{GFR} = P_{UF} \times K_f \qquad \textbf{Equation 6-1}$$

GFR = Glomerular filtration rate
P_{UF} = Net ultrafiltration pressure
K_f = Ultrafiltration coefficient (product of permeability and surface area)

  b. P_{UF} is determined by the balance of Starling's forces acting across the filtration membrane:

$$P_{UF} = (P_{GC} - P_{BS}) - \sigma(\pi_{GC} - \pi_{BS}) \qquad \textbf{Equation 6-2}$$

P_{GC} = Glomerular capillary hydrostatic pressure
P_{BS} = Hydrostatic pressure in Bowman's space
π_{GC} = Glomerular capillary oncotic pressure
π_{BS} = Oncotic pressure in Bowman's space
σ = Protein reflection coefficient

  c. Under normal circumstances, protein is not filtered, so π_{BS} is zero. Equation 6-2 simplifies to a more convenient form in which the sum of pressures that oppose filtration (P_{BS} and π_{GC}) are subtracted from P_{GC}:

$$P_{UF} = P_{GC} - (\pi_{GC} + P_{BS}) \qquad \textbf{Equation 6-3}$$

d. **Example.** Calculate the net pressure for glomerular filtration if the average hydrostatic pressure in the glomerular capillary is 58 mm Hg, the oncotic pressure in the glomerular capillary is 32 mm Hg, and the hydrostatic pressure in Bowman's space is 10 mm Hg.

   i. The net ultrafiltration pressure is:

$$P_{UF} = P_{GC} - (\pi_{GC} + P_{BS})$$

   ii. In this example, $P_{GC} = 58$ mm Hg, $\pi_{GC} = 32$ mm Hg, and $P_{BS} = 10$ mm Hg:

$$P_{UF} = 58 - (32 + 10)$$
$$= 58 - (32 + 10)$$
$$= 14 \text{ mm Hg}$$

e. The balance of **Starling's forces** changes as blood passes along the glomerular capillary from the afferent arteriole to the efferent arteriole (Figure 6-11).

   i. P_{GC} is high along the whole capillary because the efferent arteriole is a resistance vessel.

   ii. π_{GC} increases along the glomerular capillary because fluid is being filtered but protein remains in the blood.

   iii. π_{GC} may increase enough to prevent further filtration, at which point **filtration equilibrium** is reached.

   iv. The addition of π_{GC} and P_{BS} represents the sum of forces that oppose filtration; when subtracted from P_{GC}, this is the net ultrafiltration pressure, which is shown in gold in Figure 6-11.

f. *According to Equation 6-1, the rate of filtration produced in response to P_{UF} also depends on K_f (i.e., capillary permeability and surface area).*

   i. K_f is not a constant but can be regulated by **mesangial cells** interspersed between capillaries at the core of the glomerulus.

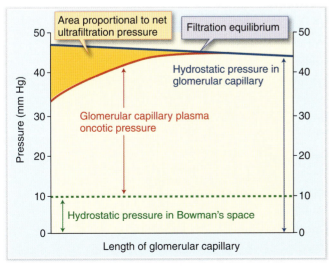

Figure 6-11. Starling's forces in glomerular filtration. The π_{GC} rises along the glomerular capillary due to filtration of protein-free fluid. Filtration stops if the sum of π_{GC} and P_{BS} increases to equal P_{GC} (filtration equilibrium).

Table 6-1. Effects of Changes in Afferent and Efferent Arteriolar Tone

Stimulus	RBF	P_{GC}	GFR	FF	End-Proximal Fluid Delivery
Afferent arteriole constriction (e.g., norepinephrine, NSAIDs)	↓	↓	↓	↔	↓
Efferent arteriole constriction (e.g., angiotensin II)	↓	↑	↑	↑	↔
Afferent arteriole dilation (e.g., prostaglandins)	↑	↑	↑	↔	↑
Efferent arteriole dilation (e.g., ACE inhibitors)	↑	↓	↓	↓	↔

ACE, angiotensin-converting enzyme; FF, filtration fraction; GFR, glomerular filtration rate; NSAID, nonsteroidal anti-inflammatory drug; P_{GC}, glomerular capillary hydrostatic pressure; RBF, renal blood flow.

      ii. Mesangial cells function as vascular smooth muscle cells and are targets for hormonal regulation; *contraction of mesangial cells decreases GFR by decreasing K_f.*

6. Afferent and efferent arteriolar resistance (Table 6-1).
   a. Constriction of either arteriole increases vascular resistance and reduces RBF.
   b. Afferent arteriolar constriction decreases blood flow into the glomerular capillary, decreasing P_{GC} and GFR.
   c. By contrast, efferent arteriolar constriction increases outflow resistance from the glomerular capillary, increasing P_{GC} and GFR.
   d. The **filtration fraction** is the proportion of RBF that is filtered and is normally about 20%.
      i. *Constriction of the afferent arteriole reduces both the RBF and GFR, leaving the filtration fraction unchanged.*
      ii. *Efferent arteriole constriction reduces RBF but conserves GFR, causing an increase in the filtration fraction.*
   e. **Norepinephrine,** released by the sympathetic nerves, preferentially constricts the afferent arteriole and reduces RBF, GFR, and Na^+ excretion.
   f. The hormone **angiotensin II** preferentially constricts the efferent arteriole, which reduces RBF but conserves GFR.
   g. ▼ **Angiotensin-converting enzyme (ACE) inhibitors** or **angiotensin II receptor blockers (ARBs)** have risks and benefits for patients with renal disease:
      i. They can prevent or slow the process of some renal diseases in part because they dilate the efferent arteriole and lower intraglomerular pressure.
      ii. However, lowering P_{GC} lowers GFR and risks inducing renal insufficiency (e.g., ACE inhibitors and ARBs would not be used in patients with narrowing of the renal arteries). ▼
   h. ▼ **Nonsteroidal anti-inflammatory drugs** (NSAIDs) such as ibuprofen can cause acute kidney injury. The mechanism involves decreased formation of **prostaglandins,** which are the primary endogenous vasodilators of the afferent arteriole. Vasoconstriction of the afferent arteriole and decreased

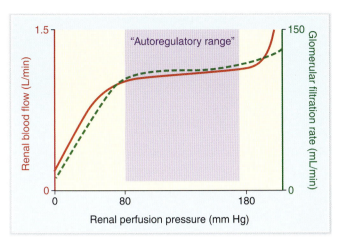

Figure 6-12. Autoregulation of renal blood flow (RBF) and the glomerular filtration rate (GFR).

GFR in response to NSAIDs increase the risk of renal insufficiency, particularly in volume-depleted patients. ▼

7. Autoregulation of RBF and GFR.
   a. Renal vascular resistance varies in proportion to renal arterial pressure so that RBF remains fairly constant across a range of blood pressures (i.e., RBF is autoregulated) (Figure 6-12).
   b. A **myogenic mechanism** operates such that increased blood pressure stretches the wall of the afferent arteriole, causing the vascular smooth muscle to contract, which increases vascular resistance and normalizes blood flow.
   c. The myogenic mechanism is assisted by **tubuloglomerular feedback** (Figure 6-13):
      i. The macula densa of each nephron senses changes in GFR by measuring the tubular fluid flow rate.
      ii. If the tubular fluid flow rate increases, the macula densa signals to the afferent arteriole by local release of adenosine.
      iii. Adenosine constricts the afferent arteriole, thereby reducing GFR and normalizing tubular fluid flow rate.
      iv. ▼ *The autoregulation mechanism can be overridden by strong sympathetic nervous system activation.* For example, a severe **hemorrhage** will reduce the mean arterial blood pressure, activating the sympathetic nervous system via the baroreceptor reflex (see Chapter 4). Renal sympathetic nerves constrict the afferent arteriole, decreasing GFR. ▼

Clearance

1. *Clearance is defined as the volume of plasma freed of a given substance per minute.* Clearance is calculated as the ratio of urinary excretion rate to plasma concentration:

$$C_x = (U_x \times \dot{V}) \div P_x \qquad \textbf{Equation 6-4}$$

C_x = Renal clearance of solute x
U_x = Urine concentration of solute x

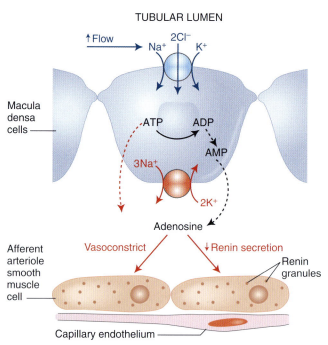

Figure 6-13. Tubuloglomerular feedback mechanism. The macula densa senses the glomerular filtration rate (GFR) through changes in fluid delivery to the distal nephron. Paracrine release of adenosine and adenosine triphosphate (ATP) by the macula densa is metabolically coupled to NaCl uptake. At the single nephron level, tubuloglomerular feedback (TGF) autoregulates GFR; global changes in GFR reflect altered circulating volume and are linked to changes in renin secretion. ADP, adenosine diphosphate; AMP, adenosine monophosphate.

$$\dot{V} = \text{Urine flow rate}$$
$$P_x = \text{Plasma concentration of solute x}$$

2. **Example.** If the plasma [urea] is 0.25 mg/mL, the urinary [urea] is 10 mg/mL, and the urine flow rate is 1 mL/min, calculate the excretion rate and the clearance of urea.

$$\begin{aligned} \text{Excretion} &= U_{\text{urea}} \times \dot{V} \\ &= 10\,\text{mg/mL} \times 1\,\text{mL/min} \\ &= 10\,\text{mg/min} \end{aligned}$$

$$\begin{aligned} \text{Clearance} &= 10\,\text{mg/min} \div 0.25\,\text{mg/mL} \\ &= 40\,\text{mL/min} \end{aligned}$$

a. Clearance is a volume of plasma "cleaned" per unit time (mL/min), *not* the amount of solute excreted in urine per unit time (mg/min).

b. A clearance of 40 mL/min means that 40 mL of plasma is required to supply the urea lost in urine every minute.

3. Clearance of the low-molecular-weight polysaccharide **inulin** is used in experimental studies as an ideal marker for GFR.

a. Inulin is freely filtered but is neither reabsorbed nor secreted by the nephron and it cannot be metabolized.

b. Therefore, *the rate of inulin filtration equals the rate of inulin excretion in the urine, so the volume of plasma cleared per minute equals GFR* (Figure 6-14).

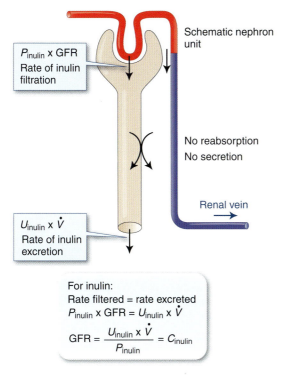

Schematic nephron unit

P_{inulin} x GFR
Rate of inulin filtration

No reabsorption
No secretion

Renal vein

U_{inulin} x $\dot{V}$
Rate of inulin excretion

For inulin:
Rate filtered = rate excreted
P_{inulin} x GFR = U_{inulin} x $\dot{V}$

$$GFR = \frac{U_{inulin} \times \dot{V}}{P_{inulin}} = C_{inulin}$$

Figure 6-14. Use of inulin clearance to measure the glomerular filtration rate (GFR).

4. **Creatinine** is a product of muscle metabolism and is a suitable endogenous alternative to inulin.
   a. The rate of creatinine production in the body is fairly constant because it is a function of muscle mass.
   b. Creatinine clearance overestimates GFR by about 10% because, in addition to free filtration, there is some secretion into the proximal tubule.
   c. Plasma [creatinine] is determined by the balance between the production rate and the excretion rate. Because the creatinine production rate is constant, and the excretion rate varies with GFR, plasma [creatinine] is a direct index of GFR. *When GFR is low, P_{creatinine} is increased.*
5. ▼ Calculation of GFR defines the stages of renal failure. A knowledge of GFR may be vital in determining the proper dosage of drugs that are excreted via the kidney, since the half-life of a drug can be significantly increased in the setting of renal failure. Creatinine clearance can be estimated clinically using different calculators, such as the **Cockcroft-Gault equation:**

$$C_{CR} = \frac{(140 - age) \times (W)}{(P_{CR}) \times (72)} (\times 0.85 \text{ for women}) \qquad \textbf{Equation 6-5}$$

C_{CR} = Creatinine clearance (mL/min)
W = Body weight (kg)
P_{CR} = Plasma [creatinine] (mg/dL) ▼

   a. ▼ **Cystatin C** is a protease increasingly used as a biomarker to estimate GFR. After filtration it is completely metabolized in the proximal tubule. When GFR decreases, serum cystatin C level increases proportionately.

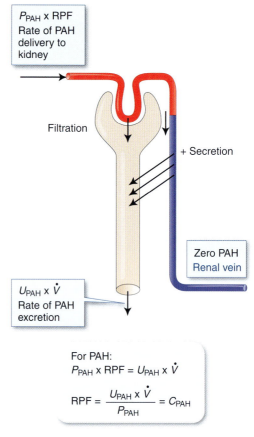

For PAH:
$$P_{PAH} \times RPF = U_{PAH} \times \dot{V}$$

$$RPF = \frac{U_{PAH} \times \dot{V}}{P_{PAH}} = C_{PAH}$$

Figure 6-15. Using para-aminohippuric acid (PAH) clearance to measure the renal plasma flow (RPF).

Advantages over creatinine include not being affected by gender, age, race, protein intake, or muscle mass. ▼

6. Using clearance to estimate RBF.
   a. The principle of clearance can be used to estimate the **renal plasma flow (RPF) rate** using the marker **para-aminohippuric acid (PAH),** which is a derivative of glycine.
   b. *PAH clearance provides an estimate of the RPF rate because all of the PAH entering the renal artery is excreted into the urine in a single pass through the kidney.*
   c. Approximately 20% of plasma PAH is filtered; at low plasma concentrations the remaining 80% entering the peritubular capillaries is secreted into the proximal tubule by organic anion transporters (Figure 6-15).
   d. The term **effective renal plasma flow (ERPF) rate** is sometimes used to describe PAH clearance, since the measurement relates to plasma flowing to functional nephron units.
   e. **RBF** can be calculated from the RPF rate if the hematocrit is known:

$$RBF = RPF \div (1 - Hct) \qquad \textbf{Equation 6-6}$$

RBF = Renal blood flow
RPF = Renal plasma flow
Hct = Hematocrit

Table 6-2. Formulae Used to Quantify Renal Tubular Function

Quantity	Expression	Calculation	Abbreviations
Filtered load (of solute z)	FL_z	$FL_z = GFR \times P_z$	GFR = glomerular filtration rate; P_z = plasma concentration of solute z
Excretion rate (of solute z)	E_z	$E_z = \dot{V} \times U_z$	$\dot{V}$ = urine flow rate; U_z = urine concentration of solute z
Fractional excretion (clearance ratio)	FE_z	$FE_z = \dfrac{(\dot{V} \times U_z)}{(GFR \times P_z)} \times 100$ OR $FE_z = \dfrac{(C_z)}{(C_{creatinine})} \times 100$ OR $^*FE_z = \dfrac{(U_z \times P_{creatinine})}{(U_{creatinine} \times P_z)} \times 100$	C = clearance
Fractional reabsorption	FR_z	$FR_z = 100 - FE_z$	

* This form of the fractional excretion equation is often used clinically because it applies values readily measured in the laboratory.

7. Quantifying tubular function.
   a. *The rate of urinary excretion of a substance can be affected by glomerular filtration, tubular reabsorption, and tubular secretion.*
   b. Calculations used to quantify tubular transport are summarized in Table 6-2 and are described as follows:
      i. The **filtered load** is the amount of a substance filtered per unit time.
      ii. The **excretion rate** is the amount excreted per unit time.
      iii. The rate of net tubular transport is the difference between the filtered load and the excretion rate.
         • When excretion is less than the filtered load, there is net tubular **reabsorption.**
         • When the excretion rate is more than the filtered load, there is net tubular **secretion.**
      iv. If there is net tubular reabsorption the solute clearance is less than GFR (i.e., less than C_{CR}).
      v. If there is net tubular secretion, solute clearance is greater than GFR.
      vi. **Fractional excretion (FE)** expresses solute excretion as a percentage of its filtered load. *FE is useful because changes reflect altered tubular transport rather than simply changes in GFR.* FE is also known as the **clearance ratio** because it can be calculated as the ratio of solute clearance to creatinine clearance.
   c. ▼ Calculating **FE_{Na}** can be useful in the setting of **acute renal failure** to help determine if ARF is due to prerenal (hypovolemia) versus renal (acute tubular necrosis) pathology.

      i. In the prerenal state, the FE_{Na} will be low (<1%) as the renal tubules attempt to maintain intravascular volume by maximally reabsorbing Na^+.

      ii. If ARF is caused by an intrinsic renal process (most commonly acute tubular necrosis), then FE_{Na} will be large (>2%) due to the reduced ability of the damaged renal tubules to reabsorb Na^+.

      iii. *Note: Diuretics interfere with tubular Na^+ reabsorption and therefore impair the ability to interpret FE_{Na}. In this setting, FE_{urea} can be used.* ▼

8. Relationships between clearance and plasma concentration.

  a. The clearance of a solute may change as a function of plasma concentration if a saturable transport process is involved in its renal handling.

  b. For inulin the filtered load and the excretion rate of inulin increase in parallel with plasma concentration because there are no tubular transport processes.

    i. Clearance is the ratio of excretion rate to plasma concentration; therefore, *inulin clearance remains constant at all plasma inulin concentrations.*

  c. PAH clearance decreases with increasing plasma PAH concentration (Figure 6-16).

    i. At low plasma PAH concentrations, all PAH is excreted and the PAH clearance represents the RPF rate.

    ii. As the plasma PAH concentration increases, the tubular secretion mechanism becomes saturated and some PAH remains in the plasma.

    iii. PAH clearance decreases because not all plasma is now being cleared of PAH.

    iv. PAH clearance never decreases below GFR because it is filtered but there are no tubular reabsorption mechanisms for PAH.

  d. At normal plasma glucose concentrations, glucose normally is not found in the urine because the filtered glucose load is completely reabsorbed.

    i. However, the glucose reabsorption mechanism can saturate if the plasma glucose concentration increases and the filtered load of glucose increases.

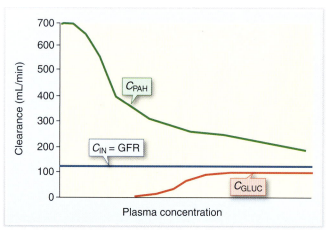

Figure 6-16. Relationships between clearance and plasma concentration. GFR, glomerular filtration rate.

   ii. *This explains why glucose is excreted in the urine of diabetic patients when there is poor glycemic control.*

   iii. Glucose clearance can never exceed the inulin clearance because there is no secretion mechanism for glucose.

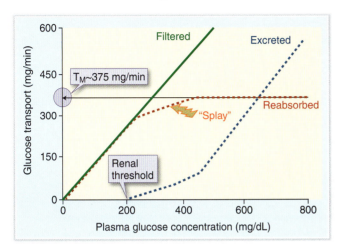

Figure 6-17. Renal titration curve for glucose. The renal threshold is the plasma glucose concentration at which glucose first appears in the urine. The plateau in the whole kidney reabsorption rate indicates the transport maximum (T_m) for glucose. The plateau is reached gradually as the filtered load increases (*splay*) due to differences in T_m between individual nephrons.

9. Renal titration curves (Figure 6-17).
   a. Renal titration curves can be used to determine the maximum rate of solute transport (**transport maximum, T_m**) for solutes with saturable transport.
   b. Construction of a titration curve requires calculation of the filtered solute load and urinary excretion rates for a range of plasma solute concentrations.
   c. Net tubular transport is calculated from the difference between the filtered load and the excretion rate.
      i. The plasma solute concentration at which the solute first appears in urine is called the **renal threshold.**
      ii. The glucose reabsorption curve levels off gradually rather than reaching the plateau abruptly. This phenomenon is called **splay** and is due to variability in the tubular transport maxima between nephrons.
      iii. The plateau of the glucose reabsorption rate is the T_m for glucose.
   d. ▼ Some of the presenting symptoms of hyperglycemia in the **untreated diabetic patient** can be explained by understanding the T_m for glucose as follows:
      i. **Polyuria.** When the T_m for glucose is surpassed, glucose (and water) remains in the urine causing an **osmotic diuresis.**
      ii. **Polydipsia.** The osmotic diuresis from the glucosuria results in free water loss, which increases serum osmolarity, activating osmoreceptors in the hypothalamus, and provoking the sensation of thirst.
      iii. **Hypovolemia.** Polyuria and urinary free water loss can cause significant hypovolemia. ▼

Renal Sodium Handling and Diuretics

1. The daily filtered load of Na^+ is far greater than the daily requirement for Na^+ excretion; Na^+ balance is achieved with a FE_{Na} of 1–2%.

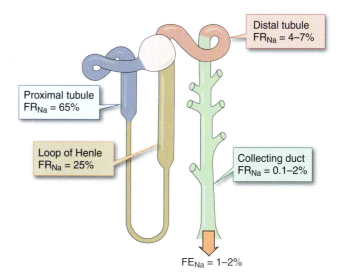

Figure 6-18. Overview of segmental sodium (Na^+) handling along the nephron. The fractional reabsorption (FR) is the percent of filtered Na^+ reabsorbed in each segment. The fractional excretion (FE) is the percent of filtered Na^+ excreted in final urine. FE_{Na}, fractional sodium excretion; FR_{Na}, fractional sodium reabsorption.

2. *Filtration and reabsorption are the only significant processes affecting NaCl and water excretion.*

3. If it is necessary to reduce the ECF volume in states such as **edema** or **hypertension, diuretic agents** can be given to increase urinary NaCl and water excretion. *Most diuretics inhibit tubular Na^+ reabsorption.*

4. Overview of segmental Na^+ handling (Figure 6-18).
    a. The proximal tubule reabsorbs approximately 65% of filtered Na^+.
    b. The loop of Henle reabsorbs 20–25% of the filtered load, with about 10% of filtered Na^+ consistently delivered to the distal tubule, independent of dietary salt intake.
    c. Final excretion of Na^+ is determined by variable reabsorption along the distal tubule and the collecting duct.
    d. **Active Na^+ reabsorption** is the key driving force behind NaCl reabsorption all along the nephron.
        i. Cl^- reabsorption is passive or occurs via secondary active transport, coupled to the movement of Na^+.
        ii. Water reabsorption is coupled to the reabsorption of NaCl and occurs by osmosis.

5. Proximal tubule.
    a. Na^+ reabsorption is coupled to the transport of several other solutes in the proximal tubule, including the absorption of nutrients and Cl^- and bicarbonate.
    b. In the **early proximal tubule,** Na^+ reabsorption is preferentially coupled to the recovery of filtered nutrients and HCO_3^-.
        i. This reabsorption accounts for the decline in the concentration of these solutes early in the proximal tubule, as shown in Figure 6-19A.
    c. In later portions of the proximal tubule, Na^+ reabsorption is coupled to Cl^- reabsorption.
    d. The osmolarity of tubular fluid does not change along the proximal tubule because the sum of all solute transport is **isosmotic** with plasma.

A.

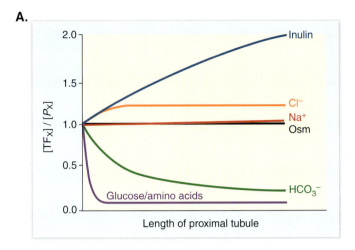

B.

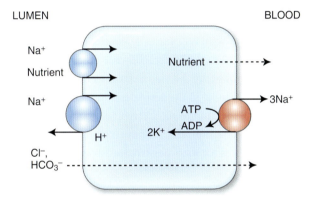

Figure 6-19. Na$^+$ reabsorption in the proximal tubule. **A.** Solute reabsorption profile along the proximal tubule. The tubular fluid:plasma (TF/P) concentration ratio of inulin is an index of water reabsorption. If TF/P_{solute} is less than TF/P_{inulin}, there is net solute reabsorption. Preferential reabsorption of nutrients and HCO$_3^-$ occurs in the early proximal tubule. **B.** Cellular mechanisms of Na$^+$ reabsorption in the proximal tubule. Most Na$^+$ is reabsorbed via the Na$^+$/H$^+$ exchange. ADP, adenosine diphosphate; ATP, adenosine triphosphate.

   e. The data in Figure 6-19A were obtained after the administration of inulin; the extent of water reabsorption is demonstrated by the large increase in inulin concentration, which becomes concentrated in the lumen as water is reabsorbed.

   f. Most Na$^+$ is reabsorbed via a **Na$^+$/H$^+$ exchanger** (NHE3). The H$^+$ secreted into the lumen is indirectly coupled to reabsorption of Cl$^-$ or HCO$_3^-$.

      i. Approximately one-third of Na$^+$ reabsorption in the proximal tubule occurs passively through the intercellular junctions via the paracellular pathway.

      ii. Glucose and amino acids are recovered from the glomerular filtrate via Na$^+$-linked cotransporters; nutrient uptake only requires a small proportion of filtered Na.

6. Loop of Henle.

   a. There is no active Na$^+$ transport in the thin limbs of the loop of Henle.

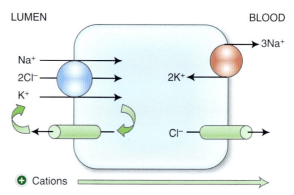

Figure 6-20. Na^+ reabsorption in the TAL. Na^+ uptake occurs via the $Na^+/K^+/2Cl^-$ cotransport. The combination of luminal K^+ channels and basolateral Cl^- channels creates a lumen-positive transepithelial potential difference, which drives paracellular cation reabsorption.

b. In contrast, the TAL is very metabolically active and Na^+ uptake occurs via cotransport with Cl^- and K^+ (Figure 6-20).

   i.   This uptake mechanism is electrically neutral, with 1 Na^+, 2 Cl^-, and 1 K^+ carried across the apical cell membrane during each transport cycle.

   ii. Na^+ is pumped out of the cell via the basolateral Na/K-ATPase. Cl^- leaves via a Cl^- channel in the basolateral membrane, and K^+ is recycled across the apical membrane via K^+ channels.

   iii. The conjunction of an apical K^+ conductance and basolateral Cl^- conductance creates a lumen-positive transepithelial electrical potential difference.

   • This voltage is important because it drives a significant paracellular flux of cations, particularly Ca^{2+} and Mg^{2+}.

   • *Loop diuretics (e.g., furosemide) induce natriuresis mainly by blocking the Na/2Cl/K cotransporter; the transepithelial voltage is also decreased resulting in the increased urinary loss of divalent cations.*

   iv. ▼ **Bartter's syndrome** is a salt-wasting disease caused by gene mutations in any of the Na/2Cl/K cotransporter, the luminal K^+ channel, or the basolateral Cl^- channel in the TAL. Very large urinary losses of NaCl reflect the high proportion of the filtered load normally reabsorbed at this site. Urinary wasting of Ca^{2+} and Mg^{2+} is observed due to the loss of the transepithelial voltage. ▼

7. Distal tubule and cortical collecting duct.

   a. *The distal tubule and the cortical collecting duct are important areas for fine regulation of Na^+ excretion.*

   b. In the early distal tubule, NaCl reabsorption is coupled via a **Na-Cl cotransporter** (Figure 6-21A). Na^+ exit at the basolateral membrane is via the Na/K-ATPase, and Cl^- exit is via the Cl^- channel.

   c. The cortical collecting duct has two distinct cell types. The **principal cells** are the most abundant cells and are associated with NaCl reabsorption; the **intercalated cells** are involved with acid-base balance.

   d. Na^+ uptake in the principal cells occurs through a Na^+ channel (Figure 6-21B). Na^+ reabsorption is associated with K^+ secretion through K^+ channels; Cl^- reabsorption occurs passively via the paracellular pathway.

   e. The late distal tubule is transitional between the distal convoluted tubule and the cortical collecting duct and expresses both Na-Cl cotransporters

A.

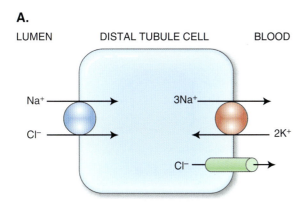

B.

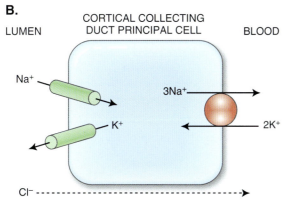

Figure 6-21. Mechanisms of Na⁺ reabsorption in the cortical collecting duct in the distal tubule.

and Na⁺ channels. **Na⁺/H⁺ exchange** also occurs all along the distal tubule and the cortical collecting duct and contributes to both Na⁺ uptake and acid excretion.

  f. **Aldosterone** increases the activity of all the Na⁺ transport proteins in this region to decrease renal Na⁺ excretion and maintain the ECF volume.

  g. *Thiazide diuretics block the Na-Cl cotransporter of the distal tubule (see Diuretics). Unlike loop diuretics, which cause urinary loss of Ca²⁺ by inhibiting Ca²⁺ reabsorption in the TAL, thiazides reduce urinary calcium loss by increasing Ca²⁺ reabsorption in the distal tubule.*

  h. ▼ **Gitelman's syndrome** is a salt-wasting condition caused by gene mutations in the distal tubule Na-Cl cotransporter. Salt wasting is less than occurs in Bartter's syndrome since the distal tubule reabsorbs less Na⁺ than the loop of Henle. *Hypocalciuria is a feature of Gitelman's syndrome and is the result of increased Ca²⁺ reabsorption in the distal nephron.* ▼

8. Diuretics (Figure 6-22).

  a. Diuresis is defined as an increase in the urine flow rate; diuretics are agents that induce diuresis.

  b. Most diuretics used clinically are **organic acids** and are efficiently **secreted by the proximal tubule;** they act by inhibiting various luminal membrane Na⁺ transport proteins (Table 6-3).

  c. **Loop diuretics** (e.g., furosemide) inhibit the Na/2Cl/K cotransporter in the TAL.

    i. Explosive increases in urine flow occur because this nephron segment normally reabsorbs 20–25% of filtered Na⁺.

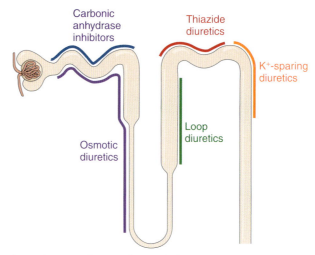

Figure 6-22. Sites of action of major classes of diuretics.

    ii. *Because of their powerful diuretic effect, loop diuretics are particularly useful when rapid diuresis is needed (e.g., **pulmonary edema**).*

  d. **Thiazide diuretics** (e.g., hydrochlorothiazide) inhibit Na-Cl cotransport in the distal tubule.

    i. Thiazides are less potent than loop diuretics since a lower proportion of the filtered NaCl load is reabsorbed in the distal tubule compared to the loop of Henle.

    ii. *Thiazides are considered first-line agents in the treatment of **hypertension,** but they can also be used in a variety of other conditions, including symptomatic relief of **edema** and **hypercalciuria.***

  e. Agents that act on the principal cells in the cortical collecting duct are called **K$^+$-sparing diuretics** because inhibition of Na$^+$ reabsorption at this site also inhibits K$^+$ secretion, lowering K$^+$ excretion rates.

    i. **Amiloride** is an example of this class of diuretic, which acts by blocking apical Na$^+$ channels in the principal cells.

Table 6-3. Sites of Diuretic Action and Clinical Uses

Class	Agents	Mechanism of Action	Examples of Use
Loop diuretics	Furosemide Bumetanide Torsemide	Inhibition of Na$^+$/K$^+$/2Cl$^-$ cotransport in the TAL	• Pulmonary edema • Hypertension • Heart failure
Thiazides	Hydrochlorothiazide	Inhibition of Na/Cl cotransport in the distal tubule	• Hypertension • Heart failure (supplement to loop diuretics)
K$^+$-sparing	Spironolactone Amiloride Triamterene	Aldosterone receptor antagonist Na$^+$ channel inhibition in the cortical collecting duct	• Hypertension due to hyperaldosteronism • Supplement to loop or thiazide diuretics to reduce K$^+$ wasting
Carbonic anhydrase inhibitors	Acetazolamide	Kidney: in the proximal tubule and other organs expressing carbonic anhydrase	• Rarely used to treat heart failure • Loss of HCO$_3$ in urine useful in acute mountain sickness and in metabolic alkalosis • Glaucoma (eye) • Epilepsy (central nervous system)

ii. **Aldosterone antagonists** (e.g., spironolactone) belong to the group of K^+-sparing diuretics and act by reducing the expression and activity of Na^+ transport proteins in the cortical collecting duct.

iii. **K^+-sparing agents** have a weak diuretic effect because less than 5% of filtered Na^+ is reabsorbed at this site.

iv. ▼ **Liddle's syndrome** is caused by a genetic mutation that increases the function of the apical Na^+ channels in the principal cells. Patients have aggressive sodium retention and are at risk of developing **salt-sensitive hypertension.** The affected Na^+ channels are the same ones blocked by amiloride, which makes it the drug of choice for treating Liddle's syndrome. ▼

v. ▼ **Primary hyperaldosteronism (Conn's syndrome)** most commonly occurs as a result of an aldosterone-secreting adenoma in the adrenal cortex (see Chapter 8). The classic clinical findings are hypertension, hypokalemia, and metabolic alkalosis. In addition to surgery, aldosterone antagonists (e.g., spironolactone) can be helpful in treating patients with Conn's syndrome. ▼

f. **Carbonic anhydrase inhibitors** (e.g., acetazolamide) dramatically reduce bicarbonate reabsorption in the early proximal tubule but are weak diuretics.

i. ▼ *Acetazolamide is commonly used in the treatment or prophylaxis of* ***altitude sickness*** *where urinary bicarbonate excretion is helpful to offset acute respiratory alkalosis; it is also used to reduce intraocular pressure associated with* ***glaucoma.*** ▼

g. **Osmotic diuretics** are nonreabsorbed solutes present in the tubule lumen; they cause water to remain in the lumen and to be passed into the urine.

i. An example of osmotic diuresis discussed previously is untreated diabetes mellitus, when the glucose T_m is exceeded and glucose remains in the tubule lumen.

ii. The proximal tubule and thin descending limb of the loop of Henle are the main sites of action because these areas have the highest membrane water permeability and are affected most by osmotic gradients.

iii. ▼ The inert sugar **mannitol** can be used to clinically induce an osmotic diuresis. *Mannitol can be helpful in the treatment of patients with* ***head injuries*** *to reduce intracranial pressure by producing a fluid shift out of the brain.* ▼

Urine Concentration and Dilution

1. Maintaining **plasma osmolarity** within narrow normal limits depends on the ability to vary **free water excretion** in response to changes in water and solute intake or loss.

a. An increase in plasma osmolarity results in the excretion of urine that is more concentrated than plasma; some solute-free water is thereby returned to the ECF, and plasma osmolarity is reduced toward normal.

b. A decrease in plasma osmolarity results in the excretion of urine that is more dilute than plasma; some **solute-free water** is excreted in the urine, thereby increasing the body fluid osmolarity toward normal.

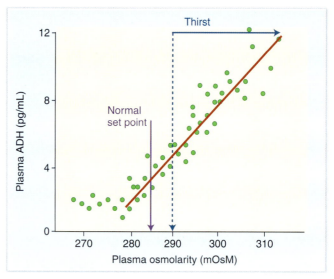

Figure 6-23. The relationship between plasma antidiuretic hormone (ADH) concentration and plasma osmolarity.

    c. These changes in urine osmolarity can occur without significant changes in GFR or total solute excretion. *Whether the kidney produces concentrated or dilute urine depends on ADH levels.*

2. Three general processes are required for the renal system to vary urine concentration:

    a. Adequate glomerular filtration is needed to deliver NaCl and water to the loop of Henle.

    b. Na$^+$ reabsorption without water reabsorption in the **ascending limb of the loop of Henle** dilutes tubular fluid, providing the potential to excrete dilute urine. At the same time, the medullary interstitial fluid becomes hypertonic, providing the potential to concentrate urine in the collecting ducts.

    c. Water permeability in the collecting duct must be variable.

3. Antidiuretic hormone (ADH; vasopressin).

    a. Plasma ADH concentration is closely correlated with plasma osmolarity (Figure 6-23).

        i. The normal set point for plasma osmolarity is 285–288 mOsm/L, which is associated with a low "resting" ADH concentration.

        ii. *ADH secretion is calibrated to defend against dehydration such that ADH secretion increases progressively as plasma osmolarity increases.*

    b. ADH secretion is highly sensitive to changes in plasma osmolarity; a 1% deviation of plasma osmolarity is enough to vary ADH secretion.

    c. ADH secretion becomes more sensitive to changes in plasma osmolarity if blood volume is decreased (typical in dehydrated patient) and less sensitive to osmolarity if blood volume is increased.

    d. *If blood volume decreases by more than 10%, low volume becomes the dominant stimulus to increase ADH secretion irrespective of plasma osmolarity.*

    e. Commonly ingested agents that affect ADH are **nicotine,** which increases secretion, and **ethanol,** which inhibits secretion.

    f. ADH is synthesized in the **supraoptic** and **paraventricular nuclei** of the hypothalamus and is secreted from nerve terminals in the posterior pituitary gland (see Chapter 8).

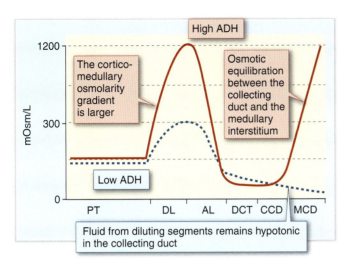

Figure 6-24. Effects of antidiuretic hormone (ADH) on tubular fluid osmolarity. AL, ascending limb of the loop of Henle; CCD, cortical collecting duct; DCT, distal convoluted tubule; DL, descending limb of the loop of Henle; MCD, medullary collecting duct; PT, proximal tubule.

   g. Neuronal **osmoreceptors** in the hypothalamus provide sensory input about osmolarity; **baroreceptors** in the carotid sinus, atria, and lungs provide sensory input about blood volume.

   h. ADH is also called **vasopressin** because it is a vasoconstrictor.

      i. *V_1 **receptors** mediate vasoconstriction.*

     ii. *V_2 **receptors** mediate renal water retention.*

4. Effects of ADH on the renal tubule (Figure 6-24).

   a. *Fluid in the proximal tubule always remains isosmotic with respect to plasma and makes no direct contribution to altering urine osmolarity.*

   b. In the descending thin limb of the loop of Henle, osmolarity reflects that of the surrounding medullary interstitium.

      i. There is always some degree of hypertonicity in the medullary interstitium, with a gradient of increasing osmolarity from the outer to the inner medulla.

     ii. *High ADH levels dramatically increase medullary osmolarity*, which is passively reflected by increasing osmolarity along the descending thin limb.

   c. The ascending limb of the loop of Henle is called the **diluting segment** because NaCl is reabsorbed without water. *By the time fluid leaves the loop of Henle, it is always hypotonic (dilute) relative to plasma.*

   d. When ADH levels are low, the water permeability of the distal nephron and collecting duct is low.

      i. Hypotonic fluid entering the distal nephron remains hypotonic during passage through the collecting duct so that **dilute urine** is produced.

     ii. The maximal diluting capacity of the renal system is about five- to tenfold (i.e., urine osmolarity of 30–60 mOsm/L).

   e. When ADH levels are high the water permeability in the distal tubule and collecting duct increases.

      i. *Osmotic water reabsorption from the collecting duct into the hypertonic medullary interstitium results in concentration of the urine.*

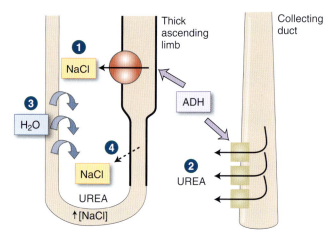

Figure 6-25. Countercurrent multiplication. Antidiuretic hormone (ADH) stimulates active NaCl reabsorption in the thick ascending limb (TAL) (*step 1*); passive countercurrent multiplication begins with ADH-stimulated reabsorption of urea from the medullary collecting duct (*step 2*). Water reabsorption in the descending limb (*step 3*) concentrates luminal NaCl and allows NaCl diffusion out of the thin ascending limb (*step 4*).

f.   Creation of a hypertonic medullary interstitium.
  i.   The ability to concentrate urine depends on the generation of a **corticomedullary gradient** of increasing interstitial osmolarity.
  ii.   Formation of the corticomedullary gradient relies on the countercurrent arrangement of the descending and ascending limbs of the loop of Henle and their differing transport properties (Figure 6-25).
  iii.   The thin descending limb is characterized by high water permeability and the lack of active transport. Osmolarity of the luminal fluid simply reflects that of the surrounding interstitium.
  iv.   The ascending limb has very low water permeability. Salt reabsorption into the interstitium occurs in the ascending limb by active transport in the TAL (see Figure 6-25, step 1) and by diffusion in the salt-permeable thin ascending limb (see below).
  v.   At any given horizontal level, the osmolarity of fluid in the descending limb and interstitium can be 200 mOsm/L greater than in the ascending limb. This is known as the **single osmotic effect** and is due to salt reabsorption from the ascending limb.
  vi.   Amplification of the single effect in the corticomedullary axis is called **countercurrent multiplication.**
  vii.   *About 40% of total osmolarity in the inner medulla is due to the presence of **urea**.* A high ADH level causes the expression of uniporters for urea transport in the collecting duct, accounting for high interstitial urea concentration (see Figure 6-25, step 2).
  viii.   High interstitial urea concentration draws water out of the descending limb by osmosis, concentrating NaCl in the tubular fluid (see Figure 6-25, step 3).
  ix.   NaCl moves out of the thin ascending limb into the interstitium down the concentration gradient (see Figure 6-25, step 4).
  x.   ▼ *The importance of urea is illustrated in patients with a **low protein intake** who have a reduced capacity to concentrate their urine because of lower urea levels. Children younger than 1 year of age have a reduced*

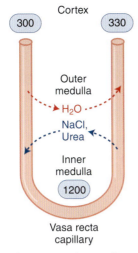

Cortex

300   330

Outer
medulla

H₂O

NaCl,
Urea

Inner
medulla

1200

Vasa recta
capillary

Figure 6-26. Countercurrent exchange. Numbers indicate typical osmolarity (mOsm/L) during maximal antidiuresis. Passive cycling of solutes from the ascending to the descending limbs of the vasa recta capillaries traps solutes in the medullary interstitium.

urine-concentrating ability because of lower urea levels; young children utilize proteins for rapid body growth and as a result do not produce much urea. ▼

5. Maintenance of a hypertonic medullary interstitium.
   a. In most organs interstitial fluid is similar to plasma (except for low protein concentration) due to free diffusion between the capillary blood and the interstitium.
   b. *In the kidney, the* **vasa recta capillary loops** *allow trapping of solutes in the medullary interstitium* (Figure 6-26).
   c. In the descending vasa recta, solutes diffuse into the plasma from the interstitium and water leaves by osmosis; blood reaching the renal papilla is highly concentrated.
   d. In the ascending vasa recta, solutes diffuse back out into the interstitium and water enters by osmosis.
   e. The net effect of retaining high solute concentration in the medulla is known as **countercurrent exchange.**
   f. The countercurrent exchange mechanism depends on low medullary blood flow. For example, *in states of low ADH, medullary blood flow increases causing washout of medullary hypertonicity that aids in the formation of dilute urine.*

6. Aquaporin 2 (AQP2).
   a. Whether final urine is dilute or concentrated depends on water reabsorption in the collecting duct.
   b. The change from a water-impermeable to a water-permeable epithelium is controlled by ADH and is due to the insertion of AQP2 water channels in the luminal cell membranes of the principal cells (Figure 6-27).
   c. *When ADH levels are high, the medullary interstitium is made very hypertonic and water is allowed to move out of the collecting duct via AQP2 to concentrate the urine.*
   d. When ADH levels are low, the hypotonic fluid entering the collecting duct remains in the tubule and final urine is dilute.

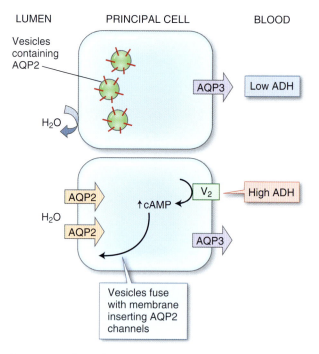

Figure 6-27. Aquaporin 2 (AQP2) water channel expression in the collecting duct. In the absence of antidiuretic hormone (ADH), the water permeability in the collecting duct is low because water channels are not present in the apical membranes. AQP3 channels are expressed continually in the basolateral membrane. Binding of ADH to the V_2 receptors on the basolateral membrane of the principal cells causes insertion of vesicles containing AQP2 water channels into the apical cell membrane, completing the pathway for water flux.

7. Diabetes insipidus.
   a. Patients with diabetes insipidus lack proper control of renal water flux by ADH.
   b. Water reabsorption under the control of ADH is called **facultative reabsorption,** and is about 20–25 L/day. Water reabsorption that occurs in the more proximal nephron segments not under ADH control is called **obligatory reabsorption.**
   c. *Patients with diabetes insipidus may excrete as much as 20–25 L/day and may require an equivalent water intake to maintain water balance.*
   d. ▼ There are two types of diabetes insipidus:
      i. **Central diabetes insipidus** is the inability of the posterior pituitary gland to adequately secrete ADH. This type of diabetes insipidus may occur in patients with pituitary tumors that interfere with ADH secretion, or it may occur as a complication following surgical removal of a pituitary tumor.
      ii. **Nephrogenic diabetes insipidus** is failure of the kidney to respond to ADH. It can be caused by drugs such as **lithium** or by rare genetic mutations in AQP2 or renal ADH receptors. ▼
   e. ▼ Pathologic oversecretion of ADH in a patient with normally functioning kidneys results in the **syndrome of inappropriate antidiuretic hormone** (SIADH).
      i. Continuous ADH secretion leads to retention of solute-free water and eventually to hyponatremia; *severe hyponatremia can be fatal.*
      ii. SIADH is caused by various clinical conditions, including small cell carcinoma of the lung (most common), pneumonia, or head injury.

     iii. Treatment of SIADH revolves around identifying and treating the underlying condition. ▼

  f. ▼ Severe changes in the hydration state manifest clinically as changes in mental status, and can result in seizures or coma. Altered CNS function results from osmotic water shifts into or out of neurons. Plasma Na^+ concentration is an indicator of water balance; dehydration causes **hypernatremia** and overhydration causes **hyponatremia.** ▼

8. Osmolar clearance and free water clearance.

  a. Free water clearance can be calculated to determine if the ADH endocrine axis and the renal concentrating mechanism are functioning properly; it is the volume of solute-free water excreted per minute.

  b. Osmolar clearance must be calculated to derive free water clearance. Osmolar clearance is the volume of plasma cleared of total solute per minute and is calculated from the general clearance equation:

$$C_{osm} = (U_{osm} \times \dot{V}) \div P_{osm} \qquad \textbf{Equation 6-7}$$

P_{osm} = Plasma osmolarity
U_{osm} = Urine osmolarity
$\dot{V}$ = Urine flow rate

  c. If urine and plasma osmolarity were equal ($U_{osm}/P_{osm} = 1$), Equation 6-7 would become ($C_{osm} = \dot{V}$) and urine flow rate would represent the volume of plasma cleared of total solute per minute. If the same amount of solute were excreted in dilute urine, a volume of water would be "added" during urine formation and is called **free water clearance** (C_{H_2O}):

$$\dot{V} = C_{osm} + C_{H_2O} \qquad \textbf{Equation 6-8}$$

  d. Free water clearance is therefore calculated by subtracting C_{osm} from $\dot{V}$.

     i. When urine is dilute C_{H_2O} is a positive number, whereas a negative free water clearance reflects concentration of the urine.

     ii. *Negative free water clearance should be present when a patient has elevated serum ADH levels; otherwise a renal defect is present.*

  e. **Example.** The following data were obtained over a period of several hours in a patient being monitored in the intensive care unit: urine flow rate = 0.1 L/h, urine osmolarity = 330 mOsm/L, plasma osmolarity = 310 mOsm/L. Calculate free water clearance using the above information and interpret the result, given further information that the patient had a normal increase in the plasma ADH concentration in the setting of this greater than normal plasma osmolarity.

     i. Osmolar clearance must first be calculated to proceed to calculate free water clearance:

$$C_{osm} = (U_{osm} \times \dot{V}) / P_{osm}$$
$$= (330 \times 0.1) / 310$$
$$= 0.1\,L/h$$

     ii. Free water clearance:

$$C_{H_2O} = \dot{V} - C_{osm}$$
$$= 0.10\,L/h - 0.11\,L/h$$
$$= -0.01\,L/h$$

iii. In the setting of increased plasma osmolarity and increased plasma ADH, the patient is expected to concentrate the urine and therefore to generate a significant negative free water clearance. In this case, free water clearance is near zero, indicating a failure of urine concentration and therefore renal dysfunction.

Regulation of ECF Volume

1. Long-term control of blood pressure requires maintenance of the normal ECF volume by the renal system.
2. The ECF volume is a function of the total amount of Na^+ in ECF. Regulation of water balance should ensure that increased Na^+ content results in increased water retention and an increase in ECF volume.
3. ▼ *Disorders of ECF volume (e.g., edema) reflect problems with Na^+ balance, whereas disorders of Na^+ concentration (i.e., **hypernatremia** or **hyponatremia**) indicate problems with water balance.* ▼
4. Effective circulating volume (ECV).
   a. Negative feedback control of ECF volume operates through control of the ECV, which is related to the volume of blood in the circulation and the pressure within specific parts of the circulation.
   b. *The kidney is the main ECV sensor* and is well-suited to this role because of the high rate of renal perfusion.
      i. The JGA measures changes in the afferent arteriolar wall tension as an index of renal perfusion.
      ii. If perfusion decreases, there is less stretch of the afferent arteriolar wall, triggering renin release, which in turn activates the **angiotensin-aldosterone axis** (see Chapter 8).
   c. Other sensors of ECV include arterial baroreceptors and low-pressure baroreceptors in the pulmonary system and the cardiac atria.
   d. Changes in ECV result in altered renal Na^+ excretion to produce a change in the ECF Na^+ content (Figure 6-28).

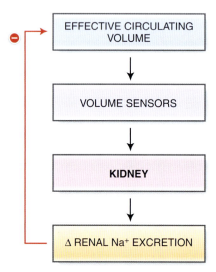

Figure 6-28. Feedback regulation of effective circulating volume (ECV). Changes in renal Na^+ excretion are linked to changes in ECV through altered extracellular fluid (ECF) osmolarity and resulting changes in water excretion. For example, increased Na^+ excretion reduces plasma osmolarity, which increases water excretion and reduces ECV.

e. *Coupling between changes in the ECF Na⁺ content and circulating volume occurs via changes in water excretion, which in turn are controlled by **ADH**.*

   i. For example, plasma osmolarity increases if more Na⁺ is retained, resulting in ADH release, water retention, and therefore in an increase in ECF volume.

f. ▼ Patients with **congestive heart failure** have low ECV because their cardiac performance is poor.

   i. *Na⁺ and ECF retention result, but ECV (i.e., RBF) does not improve due to cardiac failure.*

   ii. **Edema** results as venous and capillary hydrostatic pressures increase.

   iii. This demonstrates that the ECV is the controlled physiologic variable, not absolute ECF volume. ▼

5. Responses to low ECV.

  a. A decrease in the ECV is counteracted in four main ways (Figure 6-29):

    i. Activation of the **renin-angiotensin-aldosterone axis.**

    ii. Stimulation of the **sympathetic nervous system** via the baroreceptor reflex.

    iii. Increased **ADH secretion.**

    iv. Increased renal fluid retention via altered **Starling's forces** in the peritubular capillaries.

  b. The JGA secretes renin in response to reduced renal perfusion, triggering a cascade that increases the serum levels of angiotensin II and aldosterone.

    i. **Angiotensin II** increases Na⁺ reabsorption from the proximal tubule and causes generalized vasoconstriction to counter low blood pressure.

    ii. Angiotensin II supplements the stimulus from low-pressure baroreceptors to increase ADH secretion, which increases renal water conservation.

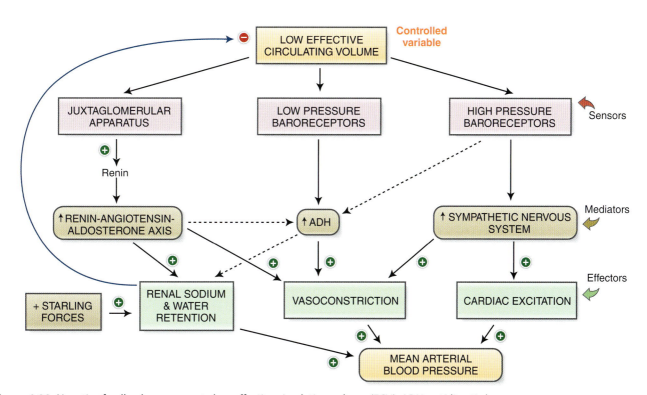

Figure 6-29. Negative feedback responses to low effective circulating volume (ECV). ADH, antidiuretic hormone.

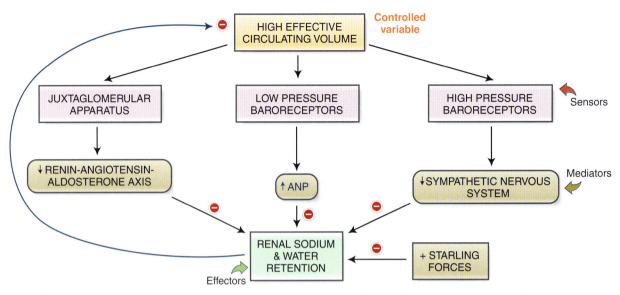

Figure 6-30. Negative feedback responses to high effective circulating volume (ECV). ANP, atrial natriuretic peptide.

    iii. Aldosterone from the adrenal cortex acts to increase Na^+ reabsorption throughout the distal nephron and the cortical collecting duct.

  c. If a decrease in the ECV is large enough to reduce the mean arterial blood pressure, the baroreceptor reflex activates the **sympathetic nervous system.**

    i. Cardiac output and blood pressure are supported by vasoconstriction and venoconstriction and by increased heart rate and myocardial contractility.

    ii. Renal sympathetic nerve activation constricts the afferent arterioles to decrease GFR, stimulates renin release via the β_1 **receptors,** and stimulates Na^+ reabsorption in the proximal tubule.

  d. Low ECV due to loss of NaCl and water concentrates the serum proteins while decreasing hydrostatic pressure, thereby changing **Starling's forces** at peritubular capillaries to promote fluid reabsorption from the nephron.

6. Responses to high ECV (Figure 6-30).

  a. In persons with normal ECV and osmolarity, the activity of renin, angiotensin, aldosterone, ADH, and the sympathetic nerves is generally low.

  b. This limits the scope for further suppression of these systems when the ECV increases, and their role is less important than it is during low ECV.

  c. Changes in Starling forces continue to be significant because volume loading increases capillary hydrostatic pressure and dilutes oncotic pressure. Reduced fluid reabsorption into the peritubular capillaries allows more fluid to be excreted by the renal tubule.

  d. A high ECV is also associated with secretion of the hormone **atrial natriuretic peptide,** which promotes the loss of Na^+ and water in urine.

    i. ANP is secreted from the cardiac atria in response to greater atrial stretch caused by increased venous blood volume.

    ii. ANP promotes natriuresis (Na^+ loss in urine) by increasing GFR and decreasing Na^+ reabsorption in the medullary collecting duct. ANP also inhibits the secretion of ADH, renin, and aldosterone.

  e. ▼ **Brain natriuretic peptide** (**BNP**) is named for the location where it was first isolated but was later found to be produced in the ventricles of the

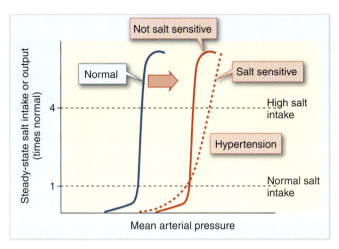

Figure 6-31. Pressure natriuresis. Acute increases in blood pressure induce renal Na$^+$ excretion (natriuresis). Chronically hypertensive patients regulate the mean arterial pressure (MAP) around a higher set point value. Salt-sensitive patients have a weaker pressure natriuresis response during salt loading, causing the MAP to increase further.

> heart. *BNP levels are increased in heart failure and serum levels are used as part of the clinical evaluation for heart failure.* BNP has similar physiological actions to ANP. ▼

7. Pressure natriuresis (Figure 6-31).
    a. Increased arterial blood pressure causes increased renal Na$^+$ excretion, known as pressure natriuresis.
    b. *Pressure natriuresis persists in the absence of hormones or renal nerves,* showing that there is also intrinsic renal control of Na$^+$ excretion, thought to involve an **intrarenal angiotensin II** system and local **nitric oxide** production.
    c. Pressure natriuresis occurs in concert with other mechanisms supporting Na$^+$ balance and provides another feedback mechanism to maintain normal blood pressure.
    d. ▼ *In patients with* **hypertension,** *the pressure natriuresis curve shifts rightward.*
        i. Hypertensive patients appear to have inadequate Na$^+$ excretion at normal blood pressure.
        ii. A subset of hypertensive patients are **salt sensitive,** shown by a pressure-natriuresis curve that has both a right shift and a reduced gradient; in these patients, higher salt intake further increases the blood pressure. ▼
8. Darrow-Yannet diagrams (Figure 6-32).
    a. Darrow-Yannet diagrams plot relative changes in the volume (*x*-axis) and osmolarity (*y*-axis) of ECF and ICF.
    b. *The contraction or the expansion of body fluid volume can occur with low, normal, or high osmolarity.*
    c. *Note: The osmolarities of ECF and ICF are always the same at steady state because water moves freely by osmosis between ECF and ICF.*
    d. **Secretory diarrhea (e.g., cholera)** and **hemorrhage** are examples of **isosmotic volume contraction.**
        i. The loss of NaCl from the ECF in an isosmotic solution causes a decrease in the ECF volume.

A. Volume contraction

Diarrhea

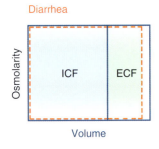

Sweating

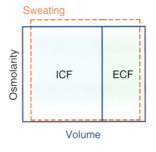

Adrenal failure

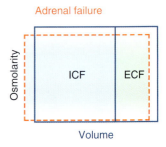

B. Volume expansion

0.9% saline

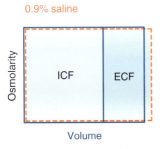

Salt intake

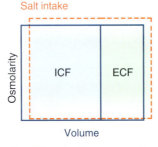

Drink water

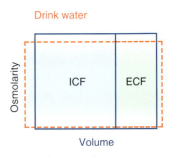

Figure 6-32. Darrow-Yannet diagrams. Volume contraction (**A**) and volume expansion (**B**) can be isosmotic (*left panels*), hyperosmotic (*center panels*), or hypoosmotic (*right panels*). ECF, extracellular fluid; ICF, intracellular fluid.

ii. There is no change in the osmolarity of ECF; therefore, there is no osmotic driving force to cause water exchange with ICF, and ICF volume is unchanged.

iii. The mechanisms for low ECV are activated, but salt and water ingestion or infusion are needed to restore normal conditions.

e. **Sweating** is an example of **hyperosmotic volume contraction.**

   i. NaCl is lost from ECF in a dilute solution, causing the ECF volume to decrease and the ECF osmolarity to increase.

   ii. Water shifts out of the ICF into the ECF by osmosis.

   iii. At steady state, fluid loss from sweating reduces both ECF and ICF volumes, and body fluids have higher osmolarity.

   iv. Mechanisms to correct low ECV are activated, particularly ADH secretion in response to high osmolarity.

f. **Adrenocortical insufficiency (e.g., Addison's disease)** is an example of **hypoosmotic volume contraction.**

   i. Chronic loss of aldosterone results in renal NaCl loss in excess of water loss. ECF volume and osmolarity are both reduced.

   ii. Net water flux from the ECF into the ICF is driven by osmosis. At steady state, ICF volume is increased, and ECF volume and body fluid osmolarity are reduced.

   iii. In this pathologic situation, restoration of the normal ECV is not possible due to the failure of aldosterone secretion.

   iv. Low ECV stimulates ADH secretion despite low osmolarity, but the ECV cannot be restored without renal Na^+ retention.

g. **Intravenous infusion of 0.9% saline** is an example of **isosmotic volume expansion** of ECF.

      i. There is no change in osmolarity, so there is no fluid shift from the ICF. Following infusion, the ECF volume is larger, and the ICF volume and the body fluid osmolarity are unchanged.

     ii. The mechanisms to counter high ECV will restore normal conditions by promoting renal excretion of the volume load.

  h. **Ingestion of salt** is an example of **hyperosmotic volume expansion.**

      i. Salt enters the ECF via the intestine, causing an increase in the ECF osmolarity. Water shifts from the ICF by osmosis.

     ii. After salt absorption, the ECF volume is larger, the ICF volume is smaller, and body fluids have a higher osmolarity.

    iii. Increased ADH secretion will result from high osmolarity and will initially cause further volume expansion due to water retention.

    iv. The mechanisms to counter high ECV will restore normal conditions by promoting renal Na^+ excretion.

  i. **SIADH** is an example of **hypoosmotic volume expansion.**

      i. Renal water retention delivers excess free water to the ECF, which is distributed throughout the total body water.

     ii. At steady state, both the ECF and ICF volumes are larger, and body fluid osmolarity is reduced.

    iii. The normal response (e.g., following water ingestion) would be to suppress ADH secretion. In this case, however, abnormal ADH secretion is the cause of hypoosmotic volume expansion and must be addressed to restore normal ECV.

Renal Urea Handling

1. Urea is the end product of **nitrogen metabolism;** it is water soluble and has low toxicity.
2. *Plasma urea concentration (BUN) ranges from 8 to 25 mg/dL and is not subject to homeostatic regulation.*
3. FE_{urea} varies with a urine flow rate from about 30% to 60%.

  a. Lower rates of urea excretion are found during antidiuresis because ADH stimulates urea reabsorption in the collecting duct (Figure 6-33).

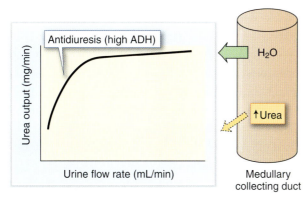

Figure 6-33. Dependence of urea excretion on urine flow rate. High plasma antidiuretic hormone (ADH) levels reduce urine flow rate. Urea excretion decreases during antidiuresis because urea reabsorption from the collecting duct increases. During antidiuresis, water reabsorption from the collecting duct concentrates urea in the lumen, creating a diffusion gradient for urea reabsorption. This mechanism accounts for increased blood urea nitrogen (BUN) in states of increased ADH.

    b. ADH-dependent water reabsorption causes luminal urea concentration to increase in the collecting duct, allowing passive urea absorption via uniporters.

4. ▼ **BUN** and plasma [creatinine] levels increase in patients with **renal insufficiency** because reduced filtered loads decrease their urinary excretion rates.

    a. *The BUN/creatinine concentration ratio can be used as a marker for prerenal ARF when the ratio is greater than 20:1.* More urea than creatinine accumulates in the plasma of these patients because hypovolemia stimulates ADH secretion, which increases tubular urea (but not creatinine) reabsorption. ▼

Renal Calcium Handling

1. Ca^{2+} homeostasis involves variable Ca^{2+} input from the gastrointestinal system and variable output by the renal system, plus exchanges of Ca^{2+} between the ECF and the bone matrix.

2. PTH and vitamin D are the major hormones controlling Ca^{2+} balance (see Chapter 8).

3. Calcium exists in three forms in plasma:

    a. Forty-five percent exists as **free ionized Ca^{2+}**. The plasma concentration of free ionized Ca^{2+} is tightly regulated in the range of 1.0–1.3 mmol/L (4.0–5.2 mg/dL).

    b. Forty-five percent is bound to anionic sites on plasma proteins. Protein-bound Ca^{2+} does not enter the interstitial fluid and is not filtered at the glomerulus.

    c. Ten percent is complexed with low-molecular-weight anions such as citrate and oxalate.

    d. ▼ *Acid-base disturbances can disrupt the distribution of Ca^{2+} in plasma.* For example, buffering of H^+ by albumin displaces bound Ca^{2+} resulting in increased serum free ionized Ca^{2+} that can cause symptoms of hypercalcemia in the presence of normal total plasma $[Ca^{2+}]$; by the same mechanism alkalosis causes reduction in serum free, ionized Ca^{2+}. ▼

4. Segmental Ca^{2+} handling.

    a. The filtered load of Ca^{2+} is the product of GFR and free plasma Ca^{2+} concentration.

    b. *The pattern of segmental Ca^{2+} reabsorption is similar to that of Na^+ and results in a typical FE_{Ca} of 1–2%;* a significant difference between Na^+ and Ca^{2+} is the absence of Ca^{2+} reabsorption in the collecting duct.

    c. In the TAL, the lumen-positive transepithelial potential difference drives paracellular Ca^{2+} reabsorption.

    d. In the distal tubule, Ca^{2+} enters the cells through Ca^{2+} channels. Ca^{2+}-binding proteins called **calbindins** keep the cytosolic Ca^{2+} concentration low; Ca^{2+} is transported across the basolateral membrane by active transport.

    e. The main sites of regulation are the TAL and distal tubule (Figure 6-34).

       i. Cells of the TAL can directly detect a decrease in plasma $[Ca^{2+}]$ through basolateral **extracellular Ca^{2+}-sensing receptors (CaRs)**, which increase the transepithelial voltage to stimulate Ca^{2+} reabsorption.

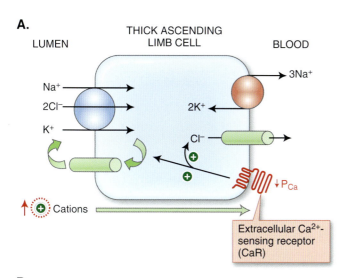

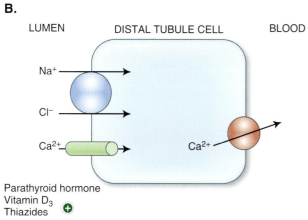

Figure 6-34. Sites of regulated Ca^{2+} reabsorption in the nephron. In the TAL (**A**), Ca^{2+} reabsorption depends on the size of a lumen-positive transepithelial potential difference. Stimulation of a Ca^{2+}-sensing receptor increases the voltage and Ca^{2+} reabsorption; loop diuretics reduce the voltage and Ca^{2+} reabsorption. In the distal tubule (**B**), Ca^{2+} uptake through the apical Ca^{2+} channel is stimulated by parathyroid hormone, vitamin D_3, and thiazide diuretics.

  ii. *In the distal tubule, PTH, vitamin D, and thiazide diuretics all stimulate*
   Ca^{2+} reabsorption.

5. ▼ **Urinary calculi** (stones) afflict many patients, causing painful renal
 colic. The most common chemical composition of the calculi is calcium
 oxalate.
 a. **Hypercalciuria** is the major risk factor for developing urinary calculi and is
  present in most patients who have calcium-based calculi.
 b. **Thiazide diuretics** can be used in the treatment of patients with
  hypercalciuria to reduce stone formation by increasing distal tubular
  calcium reabsorption and therefore decreasing the urinary calcium load.
  This prevents supersaturation of the urine with insoluble calcium oxalate
  crystals and, therefore, reduces stone formation.
 c. *Patients with kidney stone disease should maintain a high water intake so*
  urine volumes exceed 2.0–2.5 L/day to avoid high concentrations of calcium
  and oxalate in the urine. ▼

Magnesium Homeostasis

1. Mg^{2+} is an essential cofactor in many enzymatic reactions.
2. Only 1% of the total body Mg^{2+} is in the ECF and the remainder is in the **bone matrix** or ICF.
3. Dietary Mg^{2+} is absorbed via the paracellular pathway in the small intestine and via the Mg^{2+} channel TRPM6 in the cecum and colon.
4. The normal plasma $[Mg^{2+}]$ range is from 1.3 to 2.1 mEq/L; Mg is present in three forms in the plasma:
   a. Sixty percent of plasma Mg^{2+} is in the free ionized form.
   b. Twenty-five percent of plasma Mg^{2+} is bound to plasma protein.
   c. Fifteen percent of plasma Mg^{2+} is complexed to anions such as phosphate.
5. Plasma $[Mg^{2+}]$ is regulated by the balance between intestinal uptake and urinary excretion, with little exchange between ECF and bone.
6. *There are no major endocrine control mechanisms; the primary regulator of renal excretion is the plasma magnesium concentration itself.*
7. Mg^{2+} has an unusual profile of segmental handling along the nephron:
   a. Only 25% of filtered Mg^{2+} is reabsorbed in the proximal tubule.
   b. Fractional reabsorption is 65% in the **TAL**; Mg^{2+} is reabsorbed paracellularly via the tight junctional protein **paracellin-1** (a claudin 16/19 complex).
   c. One to five percent of filtered Mg^{2+} is reabsorbed in the distal tubule via the Mg^{2+} channel TRPM6/7.
8. ▼ *Loop diuretics cause urinary loss of divalent cations including Mg^{2+} and Ca^{2+} due to a decrease in the TAL lumen-positive transepithelial voltage. Thiazide diuretics and Gitelman syndrome are associated with increased renal Mg^{2+} excretion caused by decreased distal tubule Mg^{2+} reabsorption.* ▼

Renal Phosphate Handling

1. The concentration of inorganic phosphate in the ECF is influenced by intestinal uptake, renal excretion, and exchanges with bone.
2. Most phosphate is present in bone and ICF, with less than 1% in ECF.
3. Plasma phosphate concentration is regulated in the range of 0.8–1.5 mmol/L (2.5–4.5 mg/dL).
   a. Phosphate has two major forms in plasma: 80% is **alkaline phosphate** (HPO_4^{2-}) and 20% is **acid phosphate** ($H_2PO_4^-$).
4. Typical diets have excess phosphate, which is excreted from the kidney; normal $FE_{phosphate}$ is high, at approximately 20%.
   a. Mechanisms of phosphate recovery from the filtrate are mostly limited to **Na/phosphate cotransport** in the proximal tubule.
   b. *Phosphate excretion is dependent on GFR, and renal insufficiency results in inadequate phosphate excretion leading to increased plasma phosphate concentration.*
   c. **PTH** is the most important physiologic regulator of plasma phosphate concentration:
      i. Increased plasma phosphate concentration stimulates PTH secretion.
      ii. PTH inhibits Na/phosphate cotransport in the proximal tubule.
      iii. Increased urinary phosphate excretion restores normal plasma phosphate concentration.

5. ▼ **Hyperphosphatemia** is a persistent problem in patients with chronic renal failure due to decreased phosphate excretion. **Oral phosphate binders** (e.g., calcium salts) are used to decrease intestinal phosphate absorption, thereby reducing plasma phosphate concentration. ▼

Potassium Balance

1. Only 2% of total body K^+ is in the ECF but K^+ is exchangeable with the ICF. Plasma $[K^+]$ is controlled within the range of 3.5–5.5 mEq/L.
2. *Control of the ECF $[K^+]$ concentration is essential to prevent membrane potential disruption because K^+ conductance determines the resting membrane potential of most cells.*
3. Plasma $[K^+]$ is affected by shifts between the ICF and ECF (internal K^+ homeostasis) and by the balance between K^+ ingestion and excretion (external potassium homeostasis).
4. *Aldosterone is the central hormone controlling K^+ balance.*
    a. Increased ECF $[K^+]$ directly stimulates aldosterone secretion.
    b. Aldosterone increases cellular uptake of K^+ in skeletal muscle and increases renal K^+ excretion to restore normal plasma $[K^+]$.
5. Three other factors affect the internal distribution of K^+ between ECF and ICF: insulin, epinephrine, and acid-base status (Figure 6-35):
    a. **Insulin** stimulates K^+ movement from the ECF to the ICF.
        i. Sequestration of ingested K^+ into ICF is needed to prevent hyperkalemia after eating.
        ii. Insulin causes K^+ uptake by the liver and skeletal muscle in addition to its effects on glucose homeostasis (see Chapter 8).
    b. **Epinephrine** stimulates K^+ movement from the ECF to the ICF.
        i. An acute K^+ load is delivered into the ECF by exercising muscle due to K^+ efflux from active neurons and muscle fibers as they repolarize.
        ii. *Secretion of epinephrine during exercise stimulates K^+ reuptake into skeletal muscle cells through the activation of the β_2 receptors.*
    c. In **acidosis,** some H^+ is buffered by the ICF and this is associated with K^+ efflux from the cells, thereby increasing plasma K^+; the reverse occurs in **alkalosis.**

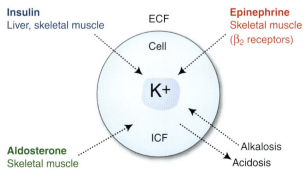

Figure 6-35. Factors affecting internal K^+ exchanges. Arrows indicate the net direction of K^+ flux between the ECF and the ICF in response to each stimulus.

A.

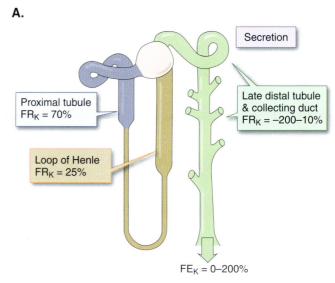

B.

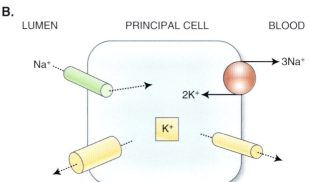

Figure 6-36. A. Segmental K⁺ handling. K⁺ excretion is mainly determined by secretion into the late distal tubule and the cortical collecting duct. **B.** Mechanism of K⁺ secretion by the principal cells in the cortical collecting duct. K⁺ enters the cell via the basolateral Na⁺/K⁺-ATPase and is secreted through K⁺ channels into the lumen. Increased Na⁺ reabsorption through Na⁺ channels depolarizes the apical membrane and increases K⁺ secretion.

6. Renal K⁺ handling (Figure 6-36A).
   a. K⁺ excretion varies with dietary K⁺ intake.
   b. To excrete the normal dietary K⁺ excess, the fractional K⁺ excretion (FE_K) is typically 10–20%, though *FE_K can be 0% in states of K⁺ deficiency, or it can reach 150–200% in states of severe K⁺ excess.*
   c. Seventy percent of filtered K⁺ is reabsorbed in the proximal tubule and an additional 25% is reabsorbed in the TAL; K⁺ reabsorption at these proximal sites is not physiologically regulated.
   d. *Secretion of K⁺ from the principal cells in the late distal tubule and the cortical collecting duct is the most important determinant of urinary K⁺ output.*
   e. K⁺ secretion occurs through K⁺ channels in the luminal cell membrane; the Na⁺/K⁺-ATPase in the basolateral membrane supplies K⁺ for secretion (Figure 6-36B).
   f. **Aldosterone** *stimulates the principal cells to secrete K⁺ while promoting Na⁺ uptake.* Aldosterone stimulates Na⁺ influx via the Na⁺ channels, causing depolarization of the luminal cell membrane and thereby increasing the driving force for K⁺ secretion.
   g. ▼ *An increase in Na⁺ delivery to the cortical collecting duct causes an increase in K⁺ secretion by the principal cells.* For example, **thiazide and loop**

    diuretics inhibit Na^+ reabsorption upstream from the cortical collecting duct, causing high Na^+ delivery to the cortical collecting duct, which drives further K^+ secretion by the principal cells. ▼

  h. The presence of **luminal fixed anions,** normally not present in the cortical collecting duct, also stimulates K^+ secretion; for example, the large bicarbonate load present in the tubule in **metabolic alkalosis** drives excess K^+ excretion.

  i. Net reabsorption of K^+ is possible in the collecting duct in the less usual state of **K^+ depletion**; α-intercalated cells reabsorb K^+ in exchange for H^+, via the **H/K-ATPase.**

7. Disturbances in plasma $[K^+]$ are a common clinical problem. For example:

  a. **Hypokalemia** is defined as plasma $[K^+]$ <3.5 mEq/L. The most common causes of hypokalemia are from gastrointestinal losses (e.g., diarrhea, vomiting, or gastric suctioning) or from a renal loss (e.g., caused by the use of a diuretic).

  b. **Hyperkalemia** is defined as a plasma $[K^+]$ >5.5 mEq/L.

  c. ▼ *In patients with chronic renal failure, hyperkalemia is an indication for hemodialysis treatment.* Acute hyperkalemia can be rapidly fatal as a result of **cardiac arrhythmia.** Medical treatment of hyperkalemia includes four approaches:

    i. **Calcium gluconate infusion.** Increased plasma Ca^{2+} stabilizes cardiac membrane potential, decreasing the immediate risk of arrhythmia.

    ii. **Insulin and glucose infusion.** Insulin infusion stimulates cellular K^+ uptake in the liver and skeletal muscles; concomitant glucose infusion prevents insulin-induced hypoglycemia.

    iii. **Oral sodium polystyrene sulfonate (Kayexalate).** This intestinal K^+ chelator reduces K^+ absorption and increases fecal K^+ elimination.

    iv. β_2-**agonists** (e.g., albuterol) stimulate cellular K^+ uptake in liver and skeletal muscle to provide a short-acting decrease in plasma $[K^+]$. ▼

Acid-Base Physiology

1. Normal plasma pH is maintained within the range of 7.35–7.45.

2. Regulation of pH occurs by varying CO_2 excretion from the lungs and by varying the rate of H^+ excretion and HCO_3^- production in the kidney.

3. In most clinical acid-base problems, *the primary variables considered are pH, arterial P_{CO_2}, and $[HCO_3^-]$; the normal values are 7.40, 40 mm Hg, and 24 mmol/L, respectively.*

4. Acids and bases.

  a. Acids are molecules that release H^+ in solution; bases are ions or molecules that can accept H^+.

  b. Strong acids rapidly dissociate releasing large amounts of H^+; weak acids partially dissociate releasing less H^+; strong bases react rapidly and strongly to neutralize H^+; weak bases bind less H^+. *Most acids and bases encountered physiologically are "weak."*

  c. The $[H^+]$ in ECF is only 0.00004 mmol/L = 40 nmol/L. The logarithmic pH scale is used to express these very small values:

$$pH = -\log_{10}[H^+]$$

                                           Equation 6-9

d. A tenfold H^+ concentration change represents a 1 unit pH change; a twofold H^+ concentration change represents approximately a 0.3 unit pH change. *The limits of ECF pH compatible with life are about 6.8–7.8.*

e. Daily metabolism produces about 15,000 mmol of CO_2 (**volatile acid**). Metabolism produces an additional 70 mmol of **fixed acids** (also called metabolic or nonvolatile acid), including organic acids and phosphoric and sulfuric acids.

5. Defense against pH disturbance has three components:

   a. **Buffers** resist pH change by neutralizing small amounts of added acid or base.

   b. Changes in ventilation and CO_2 excretion can occur over seconds to minutes to provide a rapid second line of defense against pH change.

   c. Renal system H^+ excretion and HCO_3^- synthesis are the final line of defense, acting over a period of hours to days to prevent sustained pH change.

6. Buffers.

   a. A buffer is a substance that can reversibly bind H^+; *the three major buffer systems are the carbonic acid/bicarbonate buffer system, the phosphate buffer system, and the protein (e.g., hemoglobin) buffer system.*

   b. **Buffering power** expresses the effectiveness of a buffer system and is defined as "moles of strong acid added to 1 liter of solution to reduce pH by 1 unit" or "moles of strong base added to 1 liter of solution to increase pH by 1 unit."

   c. *The bicarbonate buffer system is the most powerful system*; it is created by the reaction between water and CO_2 to form carbonic acid, which dissociates to H^+ and HCO_3^-. The pH resulting from this reaction is calculated from the **Henderson-Hasselbalch equation:**

$$pH = pK_a + \log(HCO_3 / s \cdot Pa_{CO_2}) \qquad \textbf{Equation 6-10}$$

$K_a =$ Dissociation constant for acid formation ($pK_a = 6.1$)
$s =$ Solubility of CO_2 ($s = 0.03$ mmol/mm Hg)

   d. **Example.** A healthy person in acid-base homeostasis has a plasma $[HCO_3^-]$ of 24 mmol/L, an arterial P_{CO_2} of 40 mm Hg, and a plasma pH of 7.4. Equation 6-9 correctly predicts this normal plasma pH:

$$pH = pK_a + \log(HCO_3 / s \cdot Pa_{CO_2})$$

$$pH = 6.1 + \log(24 / 0.03 \times 40)$$

$$pH = 7.40$$

   e. *The Henderson-Hasselbalch equation predicts that plasma pH is a simple function of the ratio of HCO_3 to Pa_{CO_2}.*

      i. If the pH increases, it could be due to an increase in HCO_3^- (**metabolic alkalosis**) or a decrease in arterial P_{CO_2} (**respiratory alkalosis**).

      ii. If the pH decreases, it could be due to a decrease in HCO_3^- (**metabolic acidosis**) or an increase in arterial P_{CO_2} (**respiratory acidosis**).

   f. *The buffering power of bicarbonate system is very large because it is an open system* in which each of the major reactants can be both synthesized and excreted.

7. Respiratory contribution to acid-base balance.
   a. *Normal pulmonary function balances CO₂ excretion with metabolic CO₂ production.*
   b. Arterial P_{CO_2} is monitored primarily by central chemoreceptors (see Chapter 5); alveolar ventilation increases to excrete more CO_2 when the arterial P_{CO_2} increases and decreases when the arterial P_{CO_2} decreases.
   c. Pulmonary pathology may result in defects in respiratory performance or control that cause acid-base disturbances. Hypoventilation results in high arterial P_{CO_2} (**respiratory acidosis**); hyperventilation results in low arterial P_{CO_2} (**respiratory alkalosis**).
   d. Changes in CO_2 excretion can help to **compensate** for metabolic acid-base disturbances (Figure 6-37).

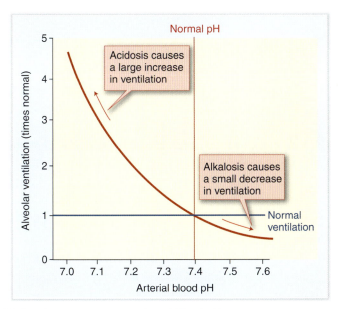

Figure 6-37. Respiratory response to altered blood pH.

   i. Low plasma pH increases alveolar ventilation, a response that is mediated through peripheral chemoreceptors (see Chapter 5). The resulting decrease in arterial P_{CO_2} increases the plasma pH back toward normal.
   ii. An increase in plasma pH causes a smaller change in alveolar ventilation because correction for increased pH would require low ventilation rates, which compromise oxygenation of the blood.
8. Renal regulation of acid-base balance.
   a. The kidney has two major functions related to acid-base homeostasis:
      i. Net excretion of **metabolic acids** including recovery of filtered bicarbonate and secretion of H^+.
      ii. Regulation of **plasma [HCO₃⁻]** in the range of 22–28 mmol/L. *Although the kidneys can excrete an excess of bicarbonate, most of the time they must continuously add bicarbonate to the blood to neutralize net acid production from metabolism.*

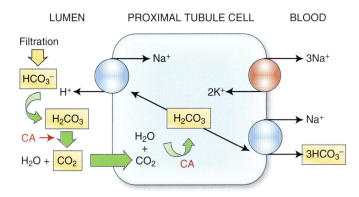

Figure 6-38. Mechanism of the proximal tubule HCO_3 recovery. The pathway taken by filtered HCO_3^- is highlighted in yellow. The enzyme carbonic anhydrase (CA) catalyzes conversions of HCO_3^- to CO_2 via carbonic acid. Inhibition of CA by the diuretic acetazolamide causes bicarbonaturia.

   b. Most bicarbonate reabsorption occurs in the early proximal tubule (Figure 6-38).

      i. H^+ is secreted into the lumen via the Na/H exchange, where it combines with filtered bicarbonate to form carbonic acid.

      ii. The enzyme **carbonic anhydrase** is anchored to the brush border membrane of the proximal tubular cells, where it generates CO_2 from carbonic acid.

      iii. CO_2 diffuses into the proximal tubule cells, where carbonic anhydrase facilitates carbonic acid formation in the cytoplasm.

      iv. H^+ and bicarbonate are produced inside the cell from dissociation of carbonic acid.

      v. H^+ is secreted into the lumen; bicarbonate enters ECF via a Na/HCO_3 cotransporter in the basolateral membrane.

      vi. ▼ The proximal tubular mechanism of bicarbonate recovery is disrupted in **renal tubular acidosis (RTA) type 2** (aka proximal RTA), resulting in urinary bicarbonate loss in the setting of systemic acidosis. RTA type 2 is associated with conditions that injure the proximal tubule (e.g., excretion of immunoglobulin light chains), use of carbonic anhydrase inhibitors (e.g., acetazolamide), or isolated transporter mutations (e.g., the Na/HCO_3 cotransporter, NBC). ▼

   c. *Acid in the urine is mainly in the form of ammonium ions (NH_4^+) or phosphoric acid ($H_2PO_4^-$).*

   d. **Renal ammonia production** accounts for approximately 75% of H^+ excretion as well as bicarbonate synthesis, as follows (Figure 6-39A):

      i. The proximal and distal tubules produce ammonia (NH_3) from glutamine.

      ii. NH_3 consumes free H^+ and is converted to NH_4^+.

      iii. NH_4^+ is secreted as an alternate substrate to H^+ via the Na/H exchangers in the luminal membrane.

      iv. Deamination of glutamate also produces two bicarbonate ions, which are transported into the ECF across the basolateral membrane.

      v. *The net effect of this process is excretion of acid in urine, plus generation of new bicarbonate to replenish that consumed by buffering of metabolic acids in the ECF.*

A.

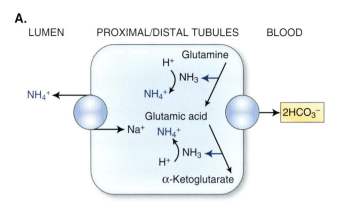

B.

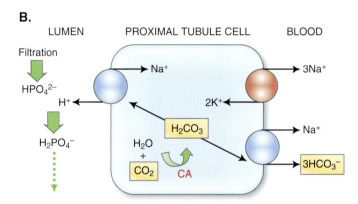

Figure 6-39. Mechanisms of H^+ excretion and HCO_3^- generation. **A.** Renal ammoniagenesis results in the formation of NH_4^+ within cells because NH_3 readily combines with H^+ at physiologic pH. NH_4^+ is secreted via the Na/H exchangers. **B.** Titratable acid excretion as $H_2PO_4^-$ occurs when secreted H^+ combines with filtered HPO_4^{2-}. CA, carbonic anhydrase.

   e. Acid-excreted phosphate ions are referred to as "**titratable acid**" because titration of urine to the plasma pH of 7.4 does not involve H^+ associated with NH_4^+, since it has a pK_a of 9.25.

      i. When H^+ is secreted into the tubule lumen, it may be buffered by HPO_4^{2-} to produce $H_2PO_4^-$, some of which is excreted in the urine (Figure 6-39B).

     ii. The H^+ secreted by the proximal tubule was derived from carbonic acid.

    iii. *The net effect is urinary excretion of H^+, plus generation of new HCO_3^- for the ECF.*

   f. *Acidification of urine occurs along the entire renal tubule.*

      i. The proximal tubule secretes the most H^+, but the proximal tubular fluid pH usually does not decrease below 6.8 due to the large amount of bicarbonate and phosphate buffers present in the glomerular filtrate.

     ii. Cells in the loop of Henle and the distal tubule and the principal cells in the cortical collecting duct all secrete H^+ via the **Na/H exchange.**

    iii. The α-intercalated cells in the collecting duct use primary active H^+ secretion via the **H^+-ATPase** and **H/K-ATPase.**

   g. ▼ Na/H exchange in the distal tubule and the principal cells of the cortical collecting duct is stimulated by aldosterone; ***hyperaldosteronism** can cause metabolic alkalosis as a result of excessive H^+ secretion into the urine.* ▼

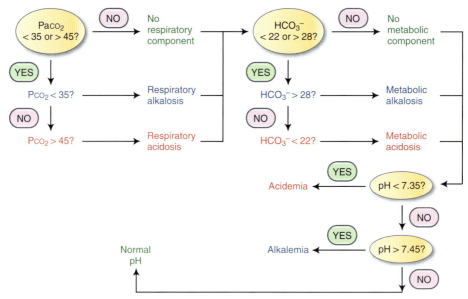

Figure 6-40. Algorithm used to describe acid-base disorders. $Paco_2$ defines the presence of respiratory disorders; plasma $[HCO_3^-]$ defines the presence of metabolic disorders.

9. Describing acid-base disorders (Figure 6-40).
   a. **Respiratory disorders** are defined based on arterial Pco_2:
      i. *$Paco_2$ >45 mm Hg defines respiratory acidosis.*
      ii. *$Paco_2$ <35 mm Hg defines respiratory alkalosis.*
   b. **Metabolic disorders** can be defined based on plasma HCO_3^- concentration:
      i. *P_{HCO_3} <22 mEq/L defines metabolic acidosis.*
      ii. *P_{HCO_3} >28 mEq/L defines metabolic alkalosis.*
   c. **Base excess** (BE) is a calculated value that estimates the size of a metabolic disturbance independent of Pco_2 that is sometimes used to define metabolic acidosis or alkalosis.
      i. BE is defined as the amount of strong acid (or base), in mmol/L, needed to titrate the pH of 100% oxygenated blood to 7.4 at 37°C and at a Pco_2 of 40 mm Hg:
      ii. *BE >2 mmol/L defines metabolic alkalosis.*
      iii. *A negative BE (a base deficit) >2 mmol/L defines metabolic acidosis.*
   d. *The most common clinical presentation is two opposing acid-base disorders in which a primary disorder is compensated by a secondary disorder.*
   e. **Compensation** refers to responses that normalize plasma pH (Table 6-4).
10. **Metabolic acidosis** can be caused by excess production or ingestion of fixed acids or by loss of bicarbonate. Common examples include:
   a. Accumulation of **ketoacids** in diabetic patients.
   b. Accumulation of **lactic acid** during hypoxia.
   c. Failure of the kidney to excrete metabolic acid in patients with **chronic renal failure.**
   d. Ingestion of poisons such as **methanol** and **ethylene glycol** or excessive ingestion of **aspirin,** which results in the generation of excess fixed acids.
   e. In all cases the excess H^+ is buffered by plasma bicarbonate, causing a decrease in plasma $[HCO_3^-]$, which defines metabolic acidosis.
   f. Increased plasma H^+ stimulates ventilation via peripheral chemoreceptors. ***Compensatory respiratory alkalosis** is usually present, which reduces the arterial Pco_2 and increases the pH toward normal.*

Table 6-4. Simple Acid-Base Disorders and Compensation

Disorder	Expected Respiratory Compensation	Expected Renal Compensation	[H⁺]	[HCO₃⁻]	Arterial Pco₂
Metabolic acidosis	Hyperventilation (2° respiratory alkalosis)		↑	↓	↓
Metabolic alkalosis	Hypoventilation (2° respiratory acidosis)		↓	↑	↑
Respiratory acidosis		↑ H⁺ excretion ↑ Bicarbonate generation (2° metabolic alkalosis)	↑	↑	↑
Respiratory alkalosis		↓ H⁺ excretion ↓ Bicarbonate generation (2° metabolic acidosis)	↓	↓	↓

Red arrow, primary disorder; blue arrow, compensation; 2°, secondary.

g. The resolution of metabolic acidosis without treatment requires increased renal generation of new bicarbonate and increased H⁺ excretion via NH_3 production and titratable acid excretion.

h. The most common example of metabolic acidosis caused by loss of bicarbonate is gastrointestinal fluid loss due to **diarrhea.**

i. Renal bicarbonate losses are also possible and may occur, for example, in patients with **renal tubular acidosis.**

j. *Calculation of the serum anion gap is used to help differentiate between metabolic acidosis caused by the addition of acid or the loss of bicarbonate:*

   i. **Anion gap** is calculated by subtracting the sum of serum Cl⁻ and bicarbonate concentrations from serum Na⁺ concentration:

$$\text{Anion Gap} = [\text{Na}^+] - ([\text{Cl}^-] + [\text{HCO}_3^-]) \qquad \textbf{Equation 6-11}$$

   ii. ECF is an electroneutral solution in which the total number of anions and cations must be equal.

   iii. *Anion gap is normally in the range of 8–16 mEq/L and indicates the concentration of **unmeasured anions** such as protein, phosphate, sulfate, and citrate.*

   iv. The addition of a metabolic acid consumes bicarbonate and replaces it with a conjugate base anion (e.g., lactate ions in the case of lactic acidosis). This adds to the unmeasured anions, which increases the calculated anion gap.

   v. *When metabolic acidosis is caused by a loss of bicarbonate, there is an increase in Cl⁻ (**hyperchloremic metabolic acidosis**) rather than the addition of other unmeasured anions, and the calculated anion gap is normal.*

k. ▼ The most common causes of **metabolic acidosis with *an increased anion gap*** are as follows: **M**ethanol ingestion, **U**remia, **L**actic acidosis, **E**thylene glycol ingestion, **P**araldehyde ingestion, **A**spirin overdose, **K**etoacidosis (*note: MULEPAK can be a helpful mnemonic*). ▼

l. ▼ The most common causes of **metabolic acidosis *without* an increased anion gap** are as follows: diarrhea, carbonic anhydrase inhibitors, RTA, hyperalimentation (intravenous feeding). ▼

m. **Example.** A 16-year-old girl with diabetes mellitus was found unconscious and unresponsive. The results of arterial blood gas analysis showed the following abnormalities: $Po_2 = 90$ mm Hg, $Pco_2 = 36$ mm Hg, $[HCO_3^-] = 7$ mEq/L (normal $= 22–28$ mEq/L), pH $= 6.91$ (normal $= 7.35–7.45$), plasma $[Na^+] = 145$ mEq/L, plasma $[Cl^-] = 110$ mEq/L.

i. The acid-base disorder described in the algorithm in Figure 6-40 is metabolic acidosis (low $[HCO_3^-]$) with no respiratory component (normal arterial Pco_2), which is producing a severe acidemia (low plasma pH). The anion gap is calculated as follows:

$$\text{Anion Gap} = [Na^+] - ([Cl^-] + [HCO_3^-])$$

$$= [145] - ([110] + [7])$$

$$= 28 \, \text{mEq} / \text{L (normal } 8 - 16 \, \text{mEq/L)}$$

ii. **Comment.** The patient has **diabetic ketoacidosis,** which produces an increased anion gap. A metabolic acidosis is present with no respiratory compensation, resulting in a severe life-threatening acidemia.

11. **Metabolic alkalosis** usually has a gastrointestinal or renal cause:
    a. The most common cause is a loss of gastric H^+ due to **vomiting,** resulting in excess bicarbonate in the blood.
    b. *Hyperaldosteronism causes renal bicarbonate retention and excess H^+ excretion;* an example is "**contraction alkalosis,**" when bicarbonate retention can occur as a side-effect of responses to low ECV.
    c. *Increased arterial blood pH (alkalemia) usually results in some* ***compensatory respiratory acidosis.***
        i. Arterial Pco_2 increases as a result of reduced alveolar ventilation and decreases the pH toward normal.
        ii. Physiologic correction of metabolic alkalosis requires increased renal excretion of bicarbonate, with reduced rates of acid excretion and bicarbonate synthesis.
    d. ▼ *Metabolic alkalosis may be either chloride sensitive or chloride resistant.* The presence of high plasma $[HCO_3^-]$ in metabolic alkalosis "displaces" Cl^- from the plasma. Patients with metabolic alkalosis are given intravenous saline (NaCl):
        i. If the administered Cl^- is retained in the plasma, the $[HCO_3^-]$ is reduced and the metabolic alkalosis is Cl^- sensitive. Examples of Cl^--sensitive metabolic alkalosis include contraction alkalosis and vomiting or gastric suction.
        ii. Cl^--resistant metabolic alkalosis occurs if urinary Cl^- excretion is persistently large; this occurs, for example, during active use of loop or thiazide diuretics or in tubular NaCl reabsorption disorders such as Bartter's or Gitelman's syndromes. ▼
    e. **Example.** A 2-year-old child who is lethargic and dehydrated has a 3-day history of vomiting. The results of arterial blood gas analysis show the following abnormalities: $Po_2 = 90$ mm Hg, $Pco_2 = 44$ mm Hg, $[HCO_3^-] = 37$ mEq/L (normal $= 22–28$ mEq/L), pH $= 7.56$ (normal $= 7.35–7.45$).
        i. The acid-base disorder described in the algorithm in Figure 6-40 is metabolic alkalosis (high $[HCO_3^-]$) with no respiratory component (normal arterial Pco_2), which is producing an alkalemia (high plasma pH).

Treatment of the patient with saline infusion and an antiemetic agent will restore acid-base homeostasis.

    ii. Metabolic alkalosis in this child was caused by a loss of HCl in gastric fluids. The alkalosis was Cl^- sensitive because fluid loss was stopped and the renal system was able to retain Cl^- and excrete HCO_3^-.

12. ***Respiratory acidosis** is caused by inadequate alveolar ventilation that results in CO_2 retention.*

   a. Inadequate ventilation may result from neuromuscular disorders, pulmonary disease, airway obstruction, or ingestion of agents that suppress breathing (e.g., narcotics).

   b. An increase in arterial P_{CO_2} defines respiratory acidosis, which increases H^+ through the Henderson-Hasselbalch equilibrium reaction.

   c. If respiratory acidosis occurs acutely, there is inadequate time for renal compensation.

   d. In chronic respiratory acidosis, the renal system normalizes the pH by excreting more acid and synthesizing bicarbonate.

   e. **Example.** A 24-year-old man who is a known heroin addict was found unresponsive with a hypodermic needle in his arm. The results of arterial blood gas analysis showed the following abnormalities: P_{O_2} = 50 mm Hg (normal = 80–100 mm Hg), P_{CO_2} = 80 mm Hg, $[HCO_3^-]$ = 23 mEq/L (normal = 22–28 mEq/L), pH = 7.08 (normal = 7.35–7.45).

     i. The acid-base disorder described in the algorithm in Figure 6-40 is respiratory acidosis (high arterial P_{CO_2}) with no metabolic component (normal $[HCO_3^-]$), which is producing a severe acidemia (low plasma pH).

    ii. **Comment.** The patient overdosed on a narcotic that caused respiratory depression, alveolar hypoventilation, and respiratory acidosis.

13. ***Respiratory alkalosis** is caused by excessive alveolar ventilation, resulting in greater CO_2 loss than production.*

   a. Increased ventilation is most commonly a response to hypoxemia (e.g., ascent to high altitude; pulmonary embolism); another common acute cause is psychogenic hyperventilation.

   b. A low arterial P_{CO_2} decreases the plasma [bicarbonate] and $[H^+]$.

   c. If respiratory alkalosis occurs acutely, there is no time for renal compensation.

   d. In chronic respiratory alkalosis, the renal system normalizes the pH by excreting less acid and producing less bicarbonate.

   e. **Example.** A 56-year-old man suffered a panic attack while awaiting surgery. The results of arterial blood gas analysis showed the following abnormalities: P_{O_2} = 112 mm Hg (normal 80–100 mm Hg), P_{CO_2} = 24 mm Hg, $[HCO_3^-]$ = 23 mEq/L (normal = 22–28 mEq/L), pH = 7.60 (normal = 7.35–7.45).

     i. The acid-base disorder described in the algorithm in Figure 6-40 is respiratory alkalosis (low arterial P_{CO_2}) with no metabolic component (normal plasma $[HCO_3^-]$), which is producing an alkalemia (high plasma pH).

    ii. **Comment.** The patient's panic attack resulted in acute hyperventilation and respiratory alkalosis. The acid-base abnormality will be readily corrected when breathing returns to normal.

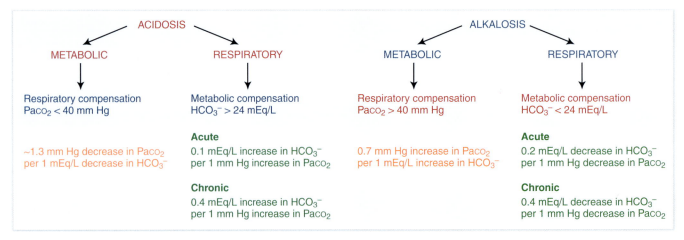

Figure 6-41. Compensatory acid-base changes. Primary acid-base disorders are usually consistent with plasma pH unless there is complete compensation. The expected degree of compensation for each primary disorder is shown.

14. Compensation of primary acid-base disorders (Figure 6-41).
    a. *Compensation refers to responses that normalize plasma pH.*
    b. Compensation usually is not complete, which allows the primary acid-base disorder to be recognized as the disorder that is consistent with plasma pH.
    c. For example, *if both alkalosis and acidosis are present and the plasma pH is acidic, the acidosis must be considered the **primary disorder**, partially compensated by the alkalosis.*
    d. When $[H^+]$, $[HCO_3^-]$, and arterial P_{CO_2} differ from the expected compensatory range, the patient has a **complex (or mixed) acid-base disorder.**
        i. This can arise if more than one acid-base disturbance is present with independent causes such as a trauma patient in shock and respiratory failure. This can then result in primary lactic acidosis and a primary respiratory acidosis. Prior clinical interventions such as intravenous infusion with fluids containing buffers also commonly produce complex acid-base disorders.
    e. ▼ **Excessive aspirin ingestion** is an example causing a mixed acid-base disorder.
        i. Aspirin uncouples oxidative phosphorylation, resulting in a primary metabolic lactic acidosis.
        ii. Additionally, the direct effects of aspirin on the respiratory centers in the medulla cause the central chemoreceptors to be more sensitive to arterial P_{CO_2} levels, which results in a primary respiratory alkalosis. ▼
    f. **Example.** A 42-year-old man in chronic renal failure is being treated with hemodialysis. The results of arterial blood gas analysis showed the following abnormalities: $P_{O_2} = 87$ mm Hg, $P_{CO_2} = 28$ mm Hg (normal $= 35–45$ mmHg), $[HCO_3^-] = 15$ mEq/L (normal $= 22–28$ mEq/L), pH $= 7.35$, anion gap $= 20$ mEq/L.
        i. The acid-base disorder described in the algorithm in Figure 6-40 is metabolic acidosis (low $[HCO_3^-]$) with a respiratory alkalosis (normal arterial P_{CO_2}) and a normal pH.

ii. **Comment.** The primary acid-base disorder is a chronic metabolic acidosis produced by renal failure and loss of urinary H^+ excretion.

iii. The expected respiratory compensation (see Figure 6-41) is approximately a 1.3 mm Hg decrease in arterial P_{CO_2} for every 1 mEq/L decrease in $[HCO_3^-]$.

iv. In this case $[HCO_3^-]$ is $24 - 15 = 9$ mEq/L below normal. The expected decrease in arterial P_{CO_2} is $9 \times 1.3 = 11.7$, which corresponds with the observed data (28 mm Hg is 12 mm Hg less than a normal average arterial P_{CO_2} of 40).

v. The respiratory compensation is complete because pH is in the normal range. (*Note: This is not a primary chronic respiratory alkalosis compensated by metabolic acidosis because the plasma pH is 7.35 and compensation never overshoots the normal pH of 7.40.*)

vi. The same conclusion is indicated by the observation that the decrease in plasma $[HCO_3^-]$ in this patient differs significantly from that expected for compensation of a chronic respiratory alkalosis. An arterial P_{CO_2} of 28 mm Hg is $40 - 28 = 12$ mm Hg less than normal, giving an expected decrease in $[HCO_3^-]$ of only 4–5 mEq/L (see Figure 6-41), whereas the actual decrease in $[HCO_3^-]$ is 9 mEq/L.

Study Questions

Directions: Each numbered item is followed by lettered options. Some options may be partially correct, but there is only *ONE BEST* answer.

1. A 67-year-old woman involved in a motor vehicle accident lost 1 L of blood because of an open fracture of her left femur. Paramedics were able to prevent further bleeding. What changes to her intracellular fluid (ICF) and extracellular fluid (ECF) volumes would be observed 15 minutes after this blood loss?

   A. ECF volume smaller; ICF volume unchanged
   B. ECF volume smaller; ICF volume smaller
   C. ECF volume unchanged; ICF volume unchanged
   D. ECF volume unchanged; ICF volume smaller

2. The following pressure measurements were obtained from within the glomerulus of an experimental animal:

   Glomerular capillary hydrostatic pressure = 50 mm Hg
   Glomerular capillary oncotic pressure = 26 mm Hg
   Bowman's space hydrostatic pressure = 8 mm Hg
   Bowman's space oncotic pressure = 0 mm Hg

   Calculate the glomerular net ultrafiltration pressure (positive pressure favors filtration; negative pressure opposes filtration).

   A. +16 mm Hg
   B. +68 mm Hg
   C. +84 mm Hg
   D. 0 mm Hg
   E. −16 mm Hg
   F. −68 mm Hg
   G. −84 mm Hg

3. A novel drug aimed at treating heart failure was tested in experimental animals. The drug was rejected for testing in humans because it caused an unacceptable decrease in the glomerular filtration rate (GFR). Further analysis showed that the drug caused no change in mean arterial blood pressure but renal blood flow (RBF) was increased. The filtration fraction was decreased. What mechanism is most likely to explain the observed decrease in GFR?

A. Afferent arteriole constriction
B. Afferent arteriole dilation
C. Efferent arteriole constriction
D. Efferent arteriole dilation

4. A healthy 25-year-old woman was a subject in an approved research study. Her average urinary urea excretion rate was 12 mg/min, measured over a 24-hour period. Her average plasma urea concentration during the same period was 0.25 mg/mL. What is her calculated urea clearance?

A. 0.25 mL/min
B. 3 mL/min
C. 48 mL/min
D. 288 mL/min

5. A 54-year-old woman received a life-saving kidney transplant 6 months ago and had been well until the past few days. She now reports severe fatigue and dizziness upon standing. Urinalysis is positive for glucose, and there is excessive excretion of HCO_3^- and phosphate. In which segment of the nephron is function most likely to be abnormal?

A. Proximal tubule
B. Loop of Henle
C. Distal tubule
D. Collecting duct

6. A resident in internal medicine was called to the hospital room of an 85-year-old patient in the middle of night. The man was sitting up in bed coughing, and was severely short of breath. Crackles heard in both lungs suggested pulmonary edema. Which diuretic is most appropriate for this patient?

A. Carbonic anhydrase inhibitor
B. Loop diuretic
C. Thiazide diuretic
D. Potassium-sparing diuretic

7. A 46-year-old woman visited her family physician because she was urinating many times a day and was constantly thirsty. She was evaluated in the hospital to find out the cause of her severe polydipsia and polyuria. She was not given any fluids for 6 hours before testing, and no change in urine osmolarity was measured during this period. A nonpressor ADH agonist was then given, which produced a rapid increase in urine osmolarity. Which diagnosis is most likely to account for this patient's polydipsia and polyuria?

A. Central diabetes insipidus
B. Compulsive overconsumption of water

C. Nephrogenic diabetes insipidus

D. Type 1 diabetes mellitus

E. Type 2 diabetes mellitus

8. A 61-year-old woman with moderate renal insufficiency ate a large amount of prunes in an effort to treat chronic constipation. She was unaware that prunes have high potassium content and the meal caused her serum potassium concentration to double. Which of the following short-term intravenous infusions would be most effective at reducing her serum potassium concentration?

A. α-Adrenoceptor agonist

B. Aldosterone antagonist

C. Dilute hydrochloric acid

D. Insulin/glucose

E. Parathyroid hormone

9. A 3-month-old infant presented with persistent vomiting and was lethargic. Arterial blood gas analysis showed the following results:

$Pao_2 = 88$ mm Hg

$Paco_2 = 44$ mm Hg

pH $= 7.60$

$[HCO_3^-] = 36$ mEq/L

Base excess $= +12$ mEq/L

Which of the following primary acid-base disturbances is present?

A. Respiratory alkalosis

B. Respiratory acidosis

C. Metabolic alkalosis

D. Metabolic acidosis

10. The results of an arterial blood gas analysis of a 56-year-old man with a history of heavy smoking are as follows:

$Pao_2 = 60$ mm Hg

$Paco_2 = 60$ mm Hg

pH $= 7.33$

$[HCO_3^-] = 32$ mEq/L

Base excess $= +8$ mEq/L

The patient has a partially compensated

A. respiratory alkalosis

B. respiratory acidosis

C. metabolic alkalosis

D. metabolic acidosis

CHAPTER 7

The Gastrointestinal System

Overview

1. The gastrointestinal (GI) system consists of the GI tract and the accessory exocrine glands.
   a. The **GI tract** includes the mouth, the esophagus, the stomach, the small intestine, and the large intestine.
   b. The major **accessory glands** are the salivary glands, the liver, the gallbladder, and the pancreas.
2. The GI system is traditionally two functions:
   a. **Assimilation of nutrients.**
   b. **Excretion of waste products** via the biliary system.
3. *Mucosal immunology is a third major function of the GI system.*
   a. The GI system is the largest immunological compartment in the body reflecting the need to protect against microbial pathogens but also allow immunological tolerance to antigenic substances in the diet.
   b. The **mucosa-associated lymphoid tissue (MALT)** are lymphoid aggregates in the intestine known as **Peyer's patches:**
      i. Specialized cells in the overlying epithelium called **microfold or M-cells** take up antigens from the lumen.
      ii. Peyer's patches contain T and B lymphocytes.
      iii. CD4 T-cells recognize extracellular antigens (e.g., pathogenic microorganisms).
      iv. CD8 T-cells recognize intracellular antigens (e.g., tumors and viruses).
      v. *B-cells in MALT mostly secrete **immunoglobulin A.***
4. Assimilation of nutrients from food occurs in the following sequence (Figure 7-1):
   a. **Chewing** (mastication) breaks food down to create a bolus for swallowing. **Saliva** lubricates food and provides enzymes for digestion. It takes about 10 seconds for swallowed food to travel down the esophagus to the stomach.
   b. Food remains in the **stomach** for 1–4 hours. Stomach motility mixes and grinds food into small particles suitable for delivery to the small intestine via the pyloric sphincter. Exocrine secretions from the stomach mucosa help to dilute and dissolve food; **gastric acid** assists in dissolving and denaturing the components of food.
   c. Entry of food into the small intestine is coordinated with the delivery of major **exocrine secretions** from the **biliary system** and the **pancreas.**
      i. *Pancreatic enzymes are essential for digestion.* The pancreas also secretes HCO_3^-, which neutralizes acid from the stomach.

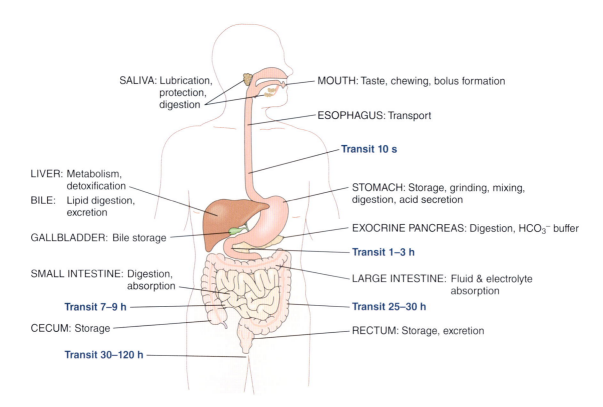

Figure 7-1. Functions of the GI organs. Transit times shown are the length of time it takes food to reach each indicated point after ingestion.

ii. Contractions of the **gallbladder** deliver stored **bile** to the intestine. *Bile acids are the major organic component of bile and are important for lipid assimilation.*

d. Food moves through the **small intestine** within 7–10 hours. Motility patterns in the fed state mix food with digestive enzymes and distribute nutrients over the absorptive surface. *All significant absorption of nutrients occurs in the small intestine.*

e. Transit through the **large intestine,** from the **cecum** to the **sigmoid colon,** usually occurs over a period of 12–24 hours.

i. Functions include fluid and electrolyte transport and fermentation of undigested carbohydrates (e.g., cellulose).

ii. Storage of fecal waste occurs in the distal large intestine; elimination of fecal waste typically occurs within 1–3 days after ingestion of a meal.

Structural Features of the GI Tract

1. There are four major histologic layers in the GI tract, starting from the gut lumen and moving outward: **mucosa, submucosa, muscularis externa,** and **serosa** (Figure 7-2).

a. The **mucosa** is variable but consists of an epithelium, which is a single cell layer from the stomach to the anus. The epithelium:

i. Is often folded to increase its surface area.

LUMEN

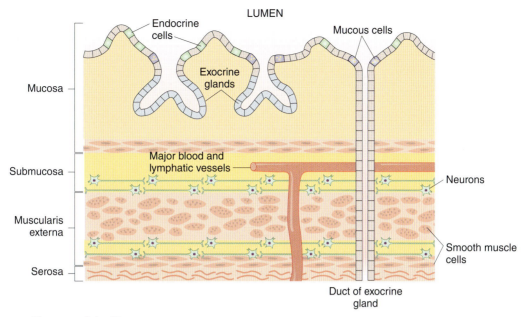

Figure 7-2. Structural features of the GI tract.

    ii. Is invaginated to form the tubular exocrine glands (e.g., secreting mucus, electrolytes, water, and digestive enzymes).

    iii. Is supported by a connective tissue lamina propria containing capillaries and nerve endings, and by a thin smooth muscle layer, the **muscularis mucosae.**

    iv. Has endocrine cells scattered among the epithelial cells that release **GI hormones** into the blood in response to changes in the luminal environment.

  b. The **submucosa** is a layer of connective tissue that contains the major blood and lymphatic vessels that serve the GI tract. This area also contains numerous ganglion cells organized to form the **submucosal (Meissner) nerve plexus.**

  c. The **muscularis externa** contains inner circular and outer longitudinal smooth muscle layers responsible for mixing and moving food along the GI tract. The **myenteric (Auerbach) nerve plexus** lies between the two layers of muscle.

  d. The **serosa** is a thin connective tissue layer, which is continuous with the peritoneal mesentery in most locations. Several major structures enter and leave through the serosa, including blood vessels, extrinsic nerves, and the ducts of the large accessory exocrine glands.

Control Mechanisms

1. GI control integrates neural, endocrine, and paracrine mechanisms.
2. The major regulated processes (effectors) are:
  a. Gut motility.
  b. Epithelial secretion.
  c. Blood flow.

3. Enteric nervous system (ENS).

   a. The ENS is a division of the autonomic nervous system located within the wall of the GI tract.

   b. *The ENS is responsible for much of the moment-to-moment control of gut motility and secretion.*

   c. The ENS is arranged as myenteric and submucosal nerve plexuses (Figure 7-3A):

      i. The **myenteric plexus** is mainly involved with control of gut motility and innervates the inner circular and outer longitudinal smooth muscle layers.

      ii. The **submucosal plexus** coordinates intestinal absorption and secretion through its innervation of the glandular epithelium, intestinal endocrine cells, and submucosal blood vessels.

   d. ▼ **Hirschsprung's disease** is a congenital absence of the myenteric plexus, usually involving a portion of the distal colon.

      i. The pathologic aganglionic section lacks peristalsis and undergoes continuous spasm, leading to functional obstruction.

A.

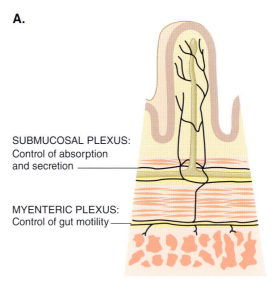

SUBMUCOSAL PLEXUS:
Control of absorption
and secretion

MYENTERIC PLEXUS:
Control of gut motility

B.

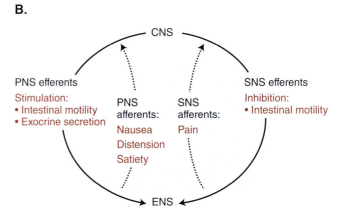

Figure 7-3. A. Organization of the enteric nervous system (ENS). The ENS is functionally organized as the submucosal plexus and the myenteric plexus. **B.** The gut-brain axis. The ENS is linked to the central nervous system (CNS) via the sensory and motor nerves of the parasympathetic nervous system (PNS) and the sympathetic nervous system (SNS).

ii. The normally innervated proximal bowel dilates; sustained obstruction can lead to "**toxic megacolon!**" ▼

e. The ENS utilizes many **neurotransmitters,** including acetylcholine, adenosine triphosphate (ATP), nitric oxide, and numerous peptides.

i. *Acetylcholine is the primary neurotransmitter involved in the stimulation of secretion and motility.* Drugs that interact with cholinergic systems often have GI side effects as a result.

ii. *ATP* and *nitric oxide function as inhibitory neurotransmitters.*

iii. Numerous peptide neurotransmitters are found in both the ENS and the CNS and are referred to as **gut-brain peptides.** An example of a peptide neurotransmitter is **vasoactive intestinal polypeptide (VIP),** *which is a potent stimulator of intestinal fluid and electrolyte secretion but inhibits motility.*

f. Gut-brain axis.

i. The ENS is linked with the CNS via parasympathetic and sympathetic nerves, giving rise to the concept of a **gut-brain neural axis** (Figure 7-3B).

ii. **Parasympathetic innervation** to the GI system is via the **vagus nerve** and the **sacral (S2–S4) spinal outflow.**

• *Efferent innervation generally causes* **excitation** *(more secretion, more propulsive motility).* Vagal efferents stimulate upper GI tract motility, gastric secretion, pancreatic secretion, and contraction of the gallbladder.

• *Visceral afferents within the parasympathetic distribution convey nonpainful distension and nausea.*

• **Vagovagal reflexes** are responses in which the afferent and efferent signals are confined to the vagus nerve; for example, distension of the stomach during a meal gives rise to an afferent signal, which results in stimulation of gastric acid secretion via the vagal efferents.

iii. *Postganglionic efferent* **sympathetic fibers** *are inhibitory through vasoconstriction and decreased motility.*

iv. *Visceral afferents within the sympathetic distribution convey the sensations of pain and nausea to the CNS.*

g. *The immune system is part of the gut-brain axis.* For example: **mast cells** respond to sensory information from the gut lumen and to neurotransmitters, and are linked to GI responses through the release of histamine.

4. GI hormones (Table 7-1).

a. **Enteroendocrine cells** within the mucosa have microvilli-bearing receptors that "taste" the gut lumen, allowing the cells to secrete hormone at the appropriate time.

b. GI hormones are secreted into the capillary blood in the GI tract and must pass through the portal venous system and the liver before entering the systemic circulation, a process known as **first-pass metabolism.**

i. ▼ First-pass metabolism is an important concept in pharmacology. Orally administered drugs that are absorbed in the GI tract may be significantly metabolized by the liver enzymes, which reduces the amount of drug that is "**bioavailable**" to other areas of the body. ▼

Table 7-1. Major Examples of GI Peptide Hormones

Hormone	Source	Stimulus for Secretion	Target Organ	Actions
Gastrin	G cells, antrum of stomach	• Amino acids in stomach • Distention of stomach • Vagus nerve (gastrin-releasing peptide)	Stomach	↑ H^+ secretion ↑ Stomach motility
Cholecystokinin	I cells, duodenum, and jejunum	Fat and protein digestion products in small intestine	Gallbladder Pancreas Stomach	↑ Contraction ↑ Enzyme secretion ↓ Gastric emptying
Secretin	S cells, duodenum	H^+ in small intestine	Pancreas Stomach	↑ Pancreatic HCO_3^- secretion ↓ Gastric H^+ secretion
Ghrelin	X cells, body of stomach	Hypoglycemia	CNS	↑ Food intake ↑ Growth hormone secretion
Motilin	M cells, duodenum, and jejunum	ENS "clock" in fasted state	Stomach Duodenum	↑ Contraction (migrating motor complex)
Guanylin	Crypt and goblet cells, small and large intestine	High salt meal	Small intestine Kidney	↓ Intestinal Na^+ absorption ↑ Urinary Na^+ excretion
Glucagon-like peptide-1	L cells, jejunum, and ileum	Glucose in small intestine	Pancreas	↑ Insulin secretion

5. Paracrine control.
   a. Paracrine control occurs when a hormone diffuses locally to affect target cells.
   b. Three major examples of paracrine mediators in GI physiology are serotonin, somatostatin, and histamine.
   c. **Serotonin** is secreted by **enterochromaffin (EC) cells** in response to distension of the gut wall. It exerts most of its effects indirectly through interactions with the ENS. *The effects of serotonin are generally excitatory and result in increased intestinal motility and secretion.*
      i. ▼ **Carcinoid tumors** arise from EC cells and most commonly secrete serotonin.
         • Systemic release of serotonin results in **carcinoid syndrome** with clinical manifestations of flushing, diarrhea, bronchospasm, and cardiac valvular disease.
         • When carcinoid tumors arise in the GI tract the serotonin is secreted into the hepatic portal circulation and is rapidly metabolized in the liver, resulting in very little systemic serotonin.
         • *Carcinoid syndrome will manifest once the tumor has metastasized to the liver and can release serotonin directly into the systemic circulation.* ▼
   d. *Somatostatin is a peptide produced by D cells and is a potent inhibitor substance in the GI system.* It may be an endocrine or paracrine mediator.
      i. Somatostatin inhibits pancreatic and gastric secretion, relaxes the stomach and gallbladder, and decreases nutrient absorption in the small intestine. These actions result partly from inhibition of several other stimulatory gut hormones.

ii. ▼ *Somatostatin is a potent GI vasoconstrictor* and analogues such as octreotide can be used to reduce bleeding such as occurs in patients with **ruptured esophageal varices.** ▼

e. **Histamine** is released by **enterochromaffin-like (ECL) cells** in the stomach and acts on neighboring oxyntic cells to stimulate H^+ secretion.

  i. ▼ **Histamine (H_2) receptors blockers** are an over-the-counter antacid medication that block stimulation of gastric acid secretion from parietal (oxyntic) cells. ▼

The Mouth and Esophagus

1. Mastication (chewing):
    a. Reduces the particle size of food.
    b. Distributes food around the mouth to stimulate taste receptors.
    c. Increases food exposure to saliva.
2. Saliva.
    a. Saliva is a composite secretion from the submandibular (70%), parotid (25%), and sublingual (5%) glands. It is mildly alkaline and secreted at a rate of approximately 1.5 L/day.
    b. The **salivon** is the functional unit of a salivary gland and consists of clusters of acinar cells that drain via a duct system (Figure 7-4).
    c. Acinar cells secrete enzymes in an isotonic electrolyte solution; duct cells modify the primary saliva by absorbing NaCl.

A.

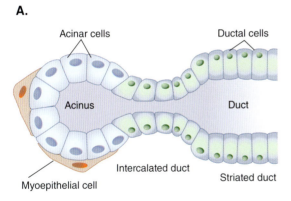

B.

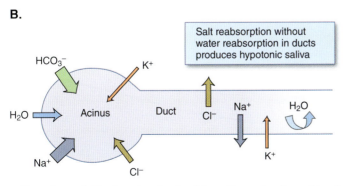

Figure 7-4. The salivon. **A.** The functional unit of the salivary gland consists of acinar cells, which secrete primary saliva into a duct system. **B.** Primary saliva secreted by the acinus is an isotonic solution resembling interstitial fluid; the duct reabsorbs NaCl (but not water), causing saliva to become hypotonic.

d. The functions of saliva are:
  i. **Lubrication** to facilitate swallowing, taste, and speech.
  ii. **Protection** against oral bacteria through washing the mouth and neutralizing bacterial acids, and secretion of agents that reduce bacterial growth (e.g., **lysozyme, lactoferrin, immunoglobin A binding protein**).
  iii. **Digestion** of starches and fats via the enzymes **salivary amylase** and **lingual lipase** respectively.

e. ▼ **Sjögren's syndrome** is an autoimmune disease that destroys exocrine glands and most commonly affects tear and saliva production. Classical presentation is dry eyes and dry mouth, known as **sicca symptoms.** Patients with **xerostomia** (dry mouth) typically have dental caries and halitosis due to bacterial overgrowth and have difficulty speaking or swallowing solid food due to inadequate lubrication. ▼

f. Mechanism of saliva secretion.
  i. Salivary acini secrete an isotonic primary solution.
  ii. Contraction of myoepithelial cells moves fluid into striated ducts via short intercalated ducts.
  iii. *Saliva becomes hypotonic because the striated duct cells reabsorb NaCl, but not water* (Figure 7-5).
  iv. Saliva is K^+ rich because it is secreted by both acini and ducts.

g. *Salivation is mainly controlled by stimulation from **acetylcholine,** which is released from parasympathetic neurons and acts mainly via **M3 muscarinic receptors.***
  i. Stimuli for salivation include the thought, smell, or taste of food, conditioned reflexes, and nausea.
  ii. Inhibitors of salivation include sleep, dehydration, fatigue, and fear.
  iii. Sympathetic nervous system activation also weakly stimulates salivation.
  iv. The only hormonal effect on saliva secretion is from **aldosterone,** which increases ductal Na^+ absorption and K^+ secretion.

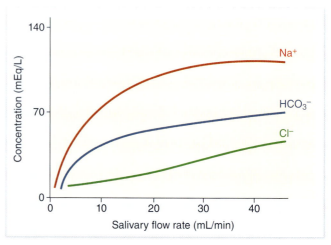

Figure 7-5. Salivary flow rate curves. The salivary ducts reabsorb NaCl without water, causing saliva to become hypotonic. Saliva is more hypotonic at slow flow rates because ducts have more time to reabsorb NaCl; at high flow rates saliva resembles the primary isotonic solution produced by the acini.

3. Swallowing (deglutition).
   a. Swallowing carries food from the pharynx into the esophagus and has two phases:
      i. In the **voluntary stage** food is shaped into a bolus. *The tongue is raised against the hard palate to create a pressure gradient that forces the bolus into the pharynx and beyond.*
      ii. After food enters the pharynx the events of the involuntary stage (**swallowing reflex**) occur:
         • The nasopharynx is closed by the **soft palate.**
         • Food is prevented from entering the airway by the **epiglottis.**
         • The **upper esophageal sphincter** relaxes to allow the bolus to enter the esophagus.
         • Breathing is inhibited until food is in the esophagus.
         • The upper esophageal sphincter quickly regains tone to prevent aspiration of the esophageal contents into the airway.
   b. ▼ The oral and pharyngeal component of swallowing can be adversely affected by a **stroke** because this phase is controlled solely by extrinsic nerves. ▼
4. Esophagus.
   a. The function of the esophagus is to move food and liquids to the stomach and to keep them there.
   b. The esophagus has **three functional zones:**
      i. The **upper zone** (6–8 cm) is closely related to the pharyngeal musculature and consists of striated muscle.
      ii. The **middle zone** (main body, 12–14 cm) consists of smooth muscle.
      iii. The **lower zone** (3–4 cm) consists of smooth muscle and corresponds with the **lower esophageal sphincter.**
   c. The area of the esophagus between the upper and lower esophageal sphincters remains quiescent until called upon to transport gas, fluids, or solids.
   d. Swallowing induces a wave of peristalsis in the esophagus known as **primary peristalsis.** If this wave is insufficient to move a bolus all the way to the stomach, distension of the esophageal wall by a remaining bolus induces **secondary peristalsis,** which is repeated until the bolus enters the stomach.
   e. The technique of **esophageal manometry,** in which pressures are simultaneously measured at several locations along the esophagus, is used to assess swallowing and esophageal function (Figure 7-6).
   f. Notable features of luminal pressure in the **resting esophagus** include:
      i. High pressure at the **upper and lower esophageal sphincters** because both sphincters exhibit continuous resting smooth muscle tone.
      ii. Subatmospheric pressure in the body of the esophagus above the diaphragm because it is passing through the intrathoracic space.
   g. Notable events upon swallowing a bolus include:
      i. Brief relaxation of the **upper esophageal sphincter** allowing the food bolus to pass into the esophagus.
      ii. A **contractile (peristaltic) wave** that sweeps down the esophagus.
      iii. Relaxation of the **lower esophageal sphincter** and the **proximal stomach** to allow the bolus to enter the stomach.

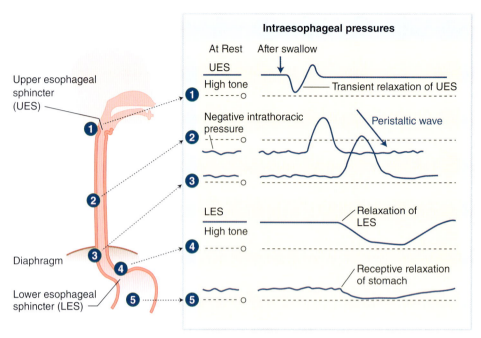

Figure 7-6. Esophageal manometry. Pressure sensors are located at each numbered location. Intraesophageal pressures are shown by solid lines; dashed lines indicate atmospheric (zero) pressure. The arrow indicates the moment at which a solid bolus was swallowed.

h. ▼ **Gastroesophageal reflux disease (GERD)** occurs when the lower esophageal sphincter is incompetent, allowing the flow of gastric juices and contents back into the esophagus.

   i. Factors that reduce the lower esophageal sphincter tone and predispose to GERD include smoking, obesity, pregnancy, hiatal hernia, and smooth muscle relaxants (e.g., nitroglycerin, β blockers, and calcium channel blockers).

   ii. GERD presents clinically as "**heartburn**" (substernal chest pain) and a sour taste in the mouth. However, reflux of acid is a common trigger for cough and asthma-like symptoms or is more rarely a cause of aspiration pneumonitis.

   iii. Recurrent reflux of gastric acids damages the esophageal mucosa causing esophagitis, esophageal ulcers, and strictures.

   iv. *Barrett's esophagus is a GI metaplasia of the lower esophagus that results from chronic GERD-induced esophagitis. The transformation from squamous epithelium to intestinal epithelium (metaplasia) is the main risk factor for adenocarcinoma of the lower esophagus.* (*Note: carcinoma of the upper esophagus is typically squamous cell carcinoma and is related to smoking and alcohol consumption.*) ▼

i. The **control of swallowing** and esophageal peristalsis involves interaction between the extrinsic nerves and the ENS.

   i. The **upper esophageal sphincter** is part of the pharyngeal musculature and is controlled by the extrinsic cranial nerves.

   ii. The **peristaltic wave** is coordinated by the ENS and involves a wave of relaxation preceding a wave of contraction. *Relaxation is mediated*

*by the neurotransmitter nitric oxide, and contraction is mediated by the
release of acetylcholine.*

   iii. Relaxation of the **lower esophageal sphincter** requires an intact ENS.

j. ▼ Patients with **achalasia** have a defect in the esophageal ENS.

    i. *Esophageal manometry shows disruption of esophageal peristalsis and
sustained high pressure at the lower esophageal sphincter because the
sphincter fails to relax.*

   ii. Upper esophageal function is normal in patients with achalasia because
it is controlled by the extrinsic nerves, not by the ENS.

  iii. Swallowed food is retained in the esophagus, leading to dilation of the
esophageal body and eventually to a reduction in peristalsis. ▼

The Stomach

1. The main anatomic areas of the stomach are:

  a. The **cardia**—the area where the esophagus enters the stomach.

  b. The **fundus**—the rounded area above the cardiac area.

  c. The **body of the stomach**—the area below the cardiac region.

  d. The **gastric antrum**—the distal part of the stomach.

  e. The **pyloric sphincter**—a smooth muscle sphincter between the stomach
and duodenum.

2. There are two functional regions of the stomach (Figure 7-7):

  a. The **oxyntic (parietal) gland area** that delivers exocrine secretions and
comprises the proximal 80% of the stomach.

  b. The **pyloric gland area** that is the major source of gastric hormones and
comprises the distal 20% of the stomach.

3. The stomach mucosa consists of **gastric pits** and **gastric glands.**

  a. The surface mucosa and pits are lined by mucous cells.

  b. The gastric glands in the oxyntic area mainly consist of the **oxyntic
(parietal) cells,** which secrete **hydrochloric acid (HCl)** and **intrinsic
factor,** and the **peptic (chief) cells,** which secrete **pepsinogen** and gastric
lipase.

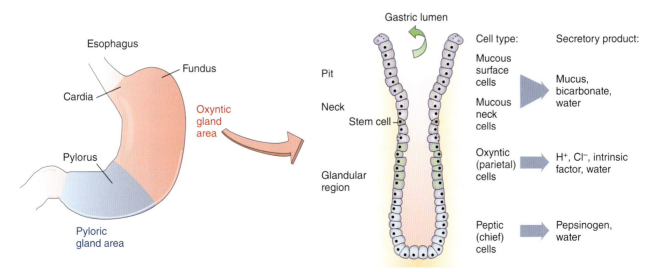

Figure 7-7. Anatomy and microanatomy of the stomach.

    c. Gastric glands in the antrum and pyloric area consist of endocrine cells, which secrete **gastrin** and **somatostatin.**

4. ▼ **Gastritis** (inflammation of the gastric mucosa) is most commonly caused by an infection by the bacteria *Helicobacter pylori.* Other common causes include smoking, use of alcohol and nonsteroidal anti-inflammatory drugs (NSAIDs), and chronic stress.

    a. **Restitution** is the process of rapid regrowth of the surface epithelium after injury, from stem cells located at the neck of the gastric gland. ▼

5. Overview of gastric functions.

    a. The **motor (motility) functions** of the stomach are to:

        i. Act as a reservoir for ingested food.

        ii. Mix and grind food.

        iii. Regulate delivery of food into the duodenum.

    b. The five main **exocrine secretions** of the stomach are:

        i. **Water,** to dissolve and dilute ingested food.

        ii. **Acid** (HCl), to denature dietary proteins and to kill ingested microorganisms.

        iii. **Enzymes (pepsin and gastric lipase),** to contribute to protein and fat digestion.

        iv. **Intrinsic factor,** a glycoprotein that is necessary for vitamin B_{12} absorption in the ileum.

        v. **Mucous and bicarbonate,** to protect the mucosal surface against the corrosive properties of gastric juice.

        vi. ▼ **Autoimmune atrophic gastritis** is an antibody-mediated destruction of gastric oxyntic (parietal) cells, which causes **hypochlorhydria** (insufficient acid secretion) and a deficiency of intrinsic factor. *The loss of intrinsic factor results in vitamin B_{12} malabsorption and **pernicious anemia.*** ▼

    c. Endocrine functions of the stomach include the secretion of the hormones gastrin, somatostatin, and ghrelin.

        i. **Gastrin** and **somatostatin** are produced in the gastric antrum and regulate gastric acid secretion.

        ii. **Ghrelin** is produced in the body of the stomach and is a factor involved in the regulation of hunger, and in growth hormone secretion (see Chapter 8).

6. Gastric motility (Figure 7-8).

    a. In the **fasted state** the stomach is relaxed except for bursts of peristalsis occurring every 90 minutes called the **migrating motor complex (MMC)** that flush the stomach and small intestine.

    b. **Receptive relaxation** is the transient relaxation of the proximal stomach with the arrival of each bolus of food.

    c. **Accommodation** is the gradual relaxation and dilation of the entire stomach during eating, which allows storage of a large meal without increasing intragastric pressure.

    d. *Vagovagal reflexes mediate both receptive relaxation and accommodation.*

    e. Once food is ingested, the proximal stomach exhibits **tonic contractions** that gradually press food into the distal stomach. *Tonic contraction of the proximal stomach determines intragastric pressure, which is the main determinant of gastric emptying of liquids.*

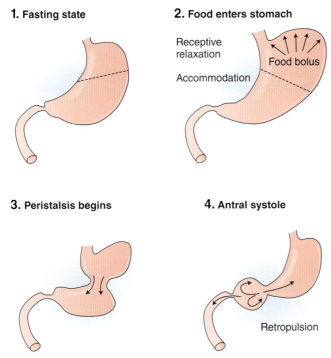

1. Fasting state

2. Food enters stomach

Receptive
relaxation

Food bolus

Accommodation

3. Peristalsis begins

4. Antral systole

Retropulsion

Figure 7-8. Gastric motility. **1.** The stomach is quiescent most of the time between meals. **2.** Receptive relaxation of the proximal stomach facilitates the entry of food from the esophagus after swallowing. Accommodation is progressive relaxation of the entire stomach as it fills to prevent increased intragastric pressure during a meal. **3.** Peristalsis begins in the midstomach. **4.** Antral systole is the vigorous peristaltic rhythm in the distal stomach. Retropulsion is forceful reflection of food off the closed pyloric sphincter.

    f. **Antral systole** describes rhythmic contraction of the distal stomach to mix food with gastric juice and reduce the particle size.

    g. The meal becomes a suspension of partially dissolved particles called **chyme.**

    h. Peristaltic waves occur at a rate of 3–4 per minute in the distal stomach during antral systole. Each peristaltic wave pushes about 1 mL of chyme through the pyloric sphincter, which at this stage of digestion only allows small particles (about 0.5–2 mm) to pass through.

    i. **Retropulsion** describes the forceful reflection of most of the food back from the pyloric sphincter into the stomach with each antral systolic wave and is important in mixing and grinding the food.

7. Gastric acid secretion (Figure 7-9).

    a. The oxyntic cells produce and secrete acid, described as follows:

      i. H^+ is generated through the action of **carbonic anhydrase,** which produces carbonic acid from CO_2 and H_2O.

      ii. H^+ is pumped from the cytoplasm to the stomach lumen by the **H^+/ K^+-ATPase;** K^+ used in this exchange process is available from food or saliva, but it is also secreted via a luminal membrane K^+ channel.

      iii. Cl^- is secreted into the lumen via a **Cl^- channel**, which also results in the generation of a large lumen-negative transepithelial potential difference across the stomach mucosa.

      iv. Cl^- supply into oxyntic cells from the extracellular fluid occurs via **Cl^-/ HCO_3^- exchange** at the basolateral cell membrane. *HCO_3^- exits the cell*

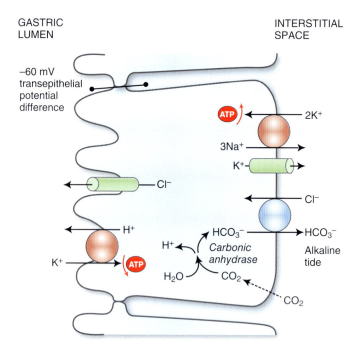

GASTRIC
LUMEN

INTERSTITIAL
SPACE

−60 mV
transepithelial
potential
difference

Figure 7-9. The cellular mechanism of gastric acid secretion. H^+ and HCO_3^- are generated inside the parietal cell by the action of carbonic anhydrase. H^+ is pumped across the luminal membrane by H^+/K^+-ATPase. HCO_3^- exits the basolateral membrane; the alkaline tide is the resulting alkalinity of gastric venous blood that is created during gastric stimulation. ATP, adenosine triphosphate.

in such a large quantity that the gastric venous blood becomes alkaline; this is known as the **postprandial alkaline tide.**

v. ▼ **Proton pump inhibitors** (e.g., omeprazole) are the most effective inhibitors of gastric acid secretion. Omeprazole binds irreversibly to the H^+/K^+-ATPase pump, thereby inhibiting H^+ secretion until new H^+/K^+-ATPase protein is synthesized. ▼

b. Stimulation of gastric acid production (Figure 7-10).

i. Gastric acid secretion is stimulated by acetylcholine from the **vagus nerves,** by endocrine stimulation from **gastrin,** and by paracrine stimulation from **histamine.**

ii. There is strong cooperativity (potentiation) between acetylcholine or gastrin and histamine at the oxyntic cell due to convergence of their different second messenger pathways:

iii. **Gastrin** and **acetylcholine** stimulate secretion via an increase in intracellular Ca^{2+}.

iv. **Histamine** stimulates secretion via an increase in cyclic adenosine monophosphate (cAMP).

v. ▼ A large proportion of gastrin's effect on H^+ secretion is mediated by its stimulation of histamine release from ECL cells. *This explains why histamine H2 blockers are effective antacids.* **Prostaglandin E$_2$**, which is produced locally in the stomach, is a physiologic antagonist of histamine at the oxyntic cell and acts by inhibiting the production of cAMP. **NSAIDs** *inhibit prostaglandin formation and increase gastric acid secretion as a side effect.* ▼

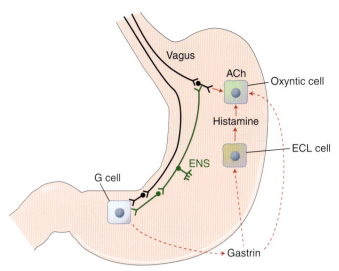

Figure 7-10. Stimulation of gastric acid secretion. Efferent vagal nerve fibers and local enteric nervous system (ENS) stretch reflexes stimulate oxyntic (parietal) cells directly and stimulate antral G cells to secrete gastrin. Gastrin stimulates the oxyntic cells directly and stimulates histamine release from the enterochromaffin-like (ECL) cells. Histamine stimulates acid secretion by the oxyntic cells. ACh, acetylcholine.

c. Phases of the GI response.
  i. The **cephalic phase** describes events occurring in response to the anticipation and the sight, smell, and taste of food.
  ii. The **gastric and intestinal phases** overlap and refer to the period when food is present in the stomach and intestines respectively.
  iii. *Stimulation of gastric secretion occurs during the cephalic and gastric phases, whereas there is inhibition of secretion in the stomach during the intestinal phase.*
  iv. The period between meals is referred to as the **interdigestive phase** when there is a small volume of very acidic gastric juice.
  v. During the cephalic phase, post-ganglionic vagal neurons stimulate H^+ secretion:
    • Directly through **acetylcholine** release at the oxyntic cells.
    • Indirectly through release of the neurotransmitter **gastrin-releasing peptide (GRP)** on the antral G cells.
  vi. G-cells are stimulated by:
    • Distension of the stomach, which triggers vagovagal and ENS reflexes.
    • Amino acids from protein breakdown.
d. Negative feedback **autoregulation** of gastric acid secretion.
  i. Gastric acidity inhibits gastrin secretion in two ways:
    • Direct inhibition of G cells by H^+ ions when pH <3.0.
    • Paracrine inhibition of G cells by **somatostatin** because D cells are stimulated to secrete somatostatin by low gastric pH.
  ii. Conversely, increasing gastric pH stimulates gastrin secretion. This occurs upon eating because buffers present in food remove free H^+, which removes inhibition of G-cells.
  iii. ▼ **Zollinger-Ellison syndrome** is caused by a gastrin-producing tumor (gastrinoma) that is usually located in the pancreas. *Since the*

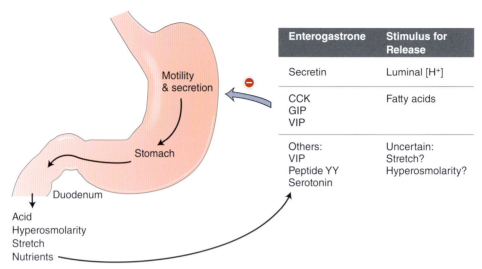

Enterogastrone	Stimulus for Release
Secretin	Luminal [H+]
CCK GIP VIP	Fatty acids
Others: VIP Peptide YY Serotonin	Uncertain: Stretch? Hyperosmolarity?

Figure 7-11. Negative feedback inhibition of gastric emptying by enterogastrones. The duodenum senses acidity, osmolarity, distension, and nutrient composition of the luminal contents to gauge the rate of gastric emptying. An increase in these variables stimulates the release of the hormones shown, resulting in feedback inhibition of gastric motility and secretion. This mechanism ensures that the rate of gastric emptying is not excessive. CCK, cholecystokinin; GIP, glucose-dependent insulinotropic polypeptide; VIP, vasoactive intestinal polypeptide.

tumor is located outside the stomach it is not exposed to paracrine regulation from somatostatin. Gastrinoma causes overgrowth of the stomach mucosa and ulceration distal to the duodenal bulb due to excess gastric acids. ▼

iv. Feedback inhibition of gastric H^+ secretion by the small intestine occurs due to hormones that are collectively known as **enterogastrones** (Figure 7-11).

- The luminal factors that trigger the release of enterogastrones include H^+, fatty acids, and hypertonicity.
- *Secretin is the primary enterogastrone and is released in response to the low pH in the duodenum.*

8. **Pepsins.**
   a. Pepsins are proteolytic enzymes that attack the internal peptide bonds in proteins. Pepsins are secreted as inactive precursors (**pepsinogens**).
   b. Conversion of pepsinogen to pepsin occurs spontaneously when the pH is below 5.
   c. Active pepsin further autocatalyzes the conversion of pepsinogen to pepsin in a **positive feedback** manner.
   d. Pepsinogen secretion is stimulated by two main mechanisms:
      i. Release of acetylcholine from the vagus nerves.
      ii. Stimulation of the ENS by a local **acid-sensitive reflex** that ensures pepsinogen is released when H^+ is available for its conversion to pepsin.

9. Gastric mucosal protection.
   a. A layer of **mucus** serves as a barrier against acid erosion of the mucosa. *This layer is effective in neutralizing acid because HCO_3^- secreted from the surface cells is trapped in the mucus* (Figure 7-12).
   b. There is no mucous layer inside the gastric glands to protect cells in this area from high levels of luminal acidity. The oxyntic cells have a thick plasma

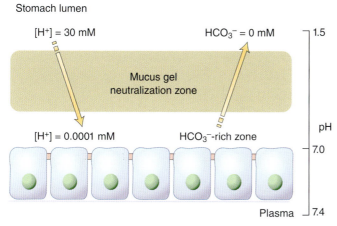

Stomach lumen

$[H^+] = 30$ mM $HCO_3^- = 0$ mM   1.5

Mucus gel
neutralization zone

$[H^+] = 0.0001$ mM HCO_3^--rich zone

pH

7.0

Plasma   7.4

Figure 7-12. The mucous-bicarbonate barrier for gastric mucosal protection. Surface epithelial cells secrete HCO_3 ions, which become trapped in a layer of mucus at the mucosal surface. H^+ is neutralized by HCO_3^- as it diffuses through the surface mucus.

membrane for protection, and the tight junctions between oxyntic cells have a very high resistance to prevent H^+ back-diffusion into the submucosa.

c.   ▼ **Erosive gastritis** can occur as a result of chronic use of NSAIDs. The mechanism by which NSAIDs cause gastritis involves the inhibition of prostaglandin synthesis in the stomach. *Prostaglandins normally maintain the physicochemical barrier on the gastroduodenal mucosal surface by stimulating the secretion of mucus and bicarbonate.* ▼

The Pancreas

1. The two main functions of the exocrine pancreas are to secrete:
    a. Digestive enzymes. (*Note: pancreatic enzymes are essential for digestion.*)
    b. A bicarbonate-rich fluid to neutralize the acidic chyme entering the small intestine from the stomach. *This fluid is necessary because pancreatic enzymes have a neutral pH optimum.*
2. The pancreas has a separate endocrine function to secrete the hormones insulin and glucagon (see Chapter 8).
3. Functional anatomy of the exocrine pancreas.
    a. Pancreatic **acini** produce a low-volume, enzyme-rich fluid that drains via a series of ducts into the main pancreatic duct.
    b. Pancreatic **duct** epithelial cells produce a **HCO_3^--rich fluid,** which is added to the acinar secretion.
    c. The main pancreatic duct joins the common bile duct to form a common excretory duct, which is guarded by the **Sphincter of Oddi.**
    d. About 1–2 L of pancreatic juice, consisting of a mixture of secretions from the acini and ducts, is secreted daily (Figure 7-13).
4. Acinar cell secretion.
    a. Acinar cells produce hydrolytic enzymes to digest fats, proteins, carbohydrates, and nucleic acids (Figure 7-14).
    b. *There are two pathways that stimulate pancreatic enzyme secretion:*
        i. *The neurotransmitter **acetylcholine**, released from vagal efferents, acts via the **M_3 muscarinic receptor.***
        ii. *The hormone **cholecystokinin (CCK) acts via the CCK-A** receptor.*

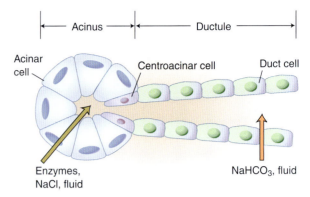

Figure 7-13. Schematic of the pancreatic structure. Pancreatic juice is a composite of two secretions; acinar cells produce enzymes in an isotonic NaCl solution, and pancreatic ducts secrete an isotonic NaHCO$_3$ solution.

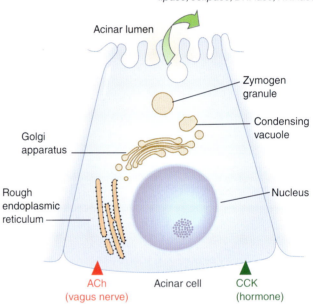

Figure 7-14. Enzyme synthesis and secretion by the pancreatic acinar cells. Enzymes are synthesized and stored in zymogen granules in the apical region of the cell. Acetylcholine (ACh) and cholecystokinin (CCK) are secretagogues that stimulate exocytosis of zymogens into the acinar lumen.

5. Pancreatic autodigestion is prevented by several features:
   a. Most pancreatic enzymes are produced as inactive precursors called **zymogens.**
   b. Enzymes are packaged in **membrane-limited vesicles** until release by exocytosis.
   c. Activation of zymogens occurs outside the pancreas in the small intestine:
      i. Trypsinogen is converted to the active proteolytic enzyme trypsin by the enzyme **enterokinase.**
      ii. Enterokinase is only found outside the pancreas bound to the apical cell membranes of enterocytes.
      iii. *Once trypsin is activated, it cleaves and activates all other zymogens.*
   d. The pancreas also produces a specific **trypsin inhibitor.**

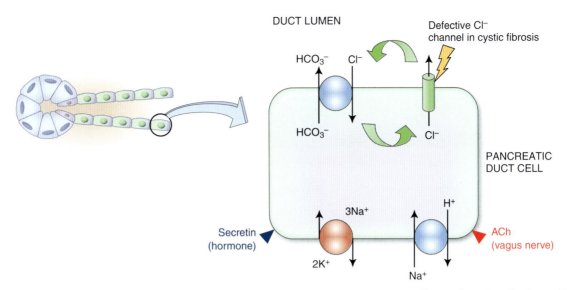

Figure 7-15. Simplified cellular model of pancreatic duct cell secretion. HCO_3^- secretion requires Cl^- recycling via a Cl^- channel in the apical cell membrane. The channel is missing or defective in patients with cystic fibrosis, causing failure of $NaHCO_3$ and fluid secretion by the pancreatic ducts. ACh, acetylcholine.

6. ▼ **Pancreatitis** occurs when pancreatic enzymes are activated within the pancreas, resulting in autodigestion of the tissues.
   a. *The most common causes of pancreatitis are gender specific and include gallstones in women and alcohol use in men.*
   b. Pancreatitis is a painful condition, classically described as an epigastric pain radiating from the epigastrium to the back that is *often relieved by leaning forward.*
   c. Underlying mechanisms that increase the risk of pancreatitis include defective zymogen processing in acinar cells and overstimulation of the gland (e.g., by acetylcholine). ▼

7. Pancreatic ducts.
   a. The mechanism of Na^+ and HCO_3^- secretion by the pancreatic duct cells occurs via the following steps (Figure 7-15):
      i. HCO_3^- secretion across the luminal cell membrane occurs via Cl^-/HCO_3^- exchange.
      ii. Cl^- is recycled from the cell into the lumen via the **cystic fibrosis transmembrane conductance regulator (CFTR)** Cl^- channel.
      iii. Na^+ is secreted into the duct lumen following HCO_3^- secretion; water follows by osmosis to produce fluid secretion.
   b. ▼ Patients with **cystic fibrosis** who lack a functional CFTR Cl^- channel have defective duct cell secretion.
      i. The ducts become blocked with precipitated enzymes and mucus, and the pancreas undergoes fibrosis (hence the name "cystic fibrosis").
      ii. Blocked ducts impair secretion of needed pancreatic enzymes for digestion of nutrients, resulting in **malabsorption.** *Treatment of this type of malabsorption includes oral pancreatic enzyme supplements taken with each meal.* ▼

8. Control of pancreatic secretion.
   a. During the interdigestive state, there is minimal secretion of pancreatic juice.

b. Stimulation of pancreatic secretion during the **cephalic phase** is mediated via the **vagus nerve** and the release of acetylcholine.

c. There is minimal additional stimulation of the pancreas during the gastric phase.

d. *Most pancreatic stimulation occurs in the* **intestinal phase** *so that secretion is coordinated when chyme enters the small intestine.*

    i. **CCK** *stimulates acinar enzyme secretion;* the secretion of cholecystokinin is stimulated by long chain fatty acids and protein digestive products in the small intestine.

    ii. **Secretin** *stimulates ductal* HCO_3^- *secretion;* acid entering the duodenum from the stomach stimulates the secretion of secretin. *Secretin increases cAMP and activates the CFTR channel.*

e. As food moves beyond the duodenum, the stimuli for pancreatic secretion gradually decrease and the pancreas returns to its resting condition.

The Liver

1. The microanatomy of the liver is classically organized in **hepatic lobules** (Figure 7-16).

a. **Portal triads** are found at the periphery of lobules and consist of a branch of the portal vein, hepatic artery, and bile duct.

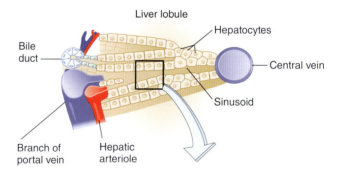

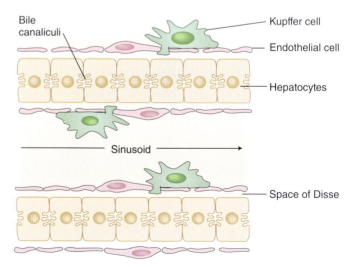

Figure 7-16. Microanatomy of hepatic lobules. Sinusoids are wide, permeable capillaries containing a mixture of blood from the hepatic artery and the portal vein. Sinusoidal blood flows toward the central vein. Bile secreted by the hepatocytes flows in the opposite direction toward bile ductules at the periphery of the lobule.

b. *Approximately 75% of hepatic blood flow is delivered by the hepatic portal vein and 25% is from the hepatic artery.*

c. Blood from both the portal vein and the hepatic artery is mixed in the wide capillaries called sinusoids, which are separated by chains of hepatocytes and are lined by highly permeable fenestrated endothelia.

d. The space of Disse lies between the hepatocytes and endothelia and contains interstitial fluid.

e. The sinusoids of a single lobule drain into a **central vein.**

f. The central veins of neighboring lobules unite to form the **hepatic veins,** which drain into the **inferior vena cava.**

g. ▼ **Kupffer cells** are macrophages interspersed between endothelial cells. **Stellate (Ito) cells** are pericytes located in the space of Disse. Resting stellate cells are antigen-presenting cells and store **vitamin A;** *activated stellate cells are myofibroblasts that orchestrate* **liver fibrosis.** ▼

2. The **portal lobule** is an alternative description of a functional unit and is the mass of hepatocytes from neighboring hepatic lobules that all drain into a single bile duct.

3. *The* **liver acinus** *is the usually regarded as the true functional unit of the liver* and consists of those hepatocytes that all receive a blood supply from the same hepatic arteriole and portal venule. Within a liver acinus there are functional zones based on oxygen tension:

a. **Zone I** is closest to the arteriole, where cells receive the greatest delivery of oxygen and nutrients. *Cells in zone I preferentially undertake oxidative metabolism, ureagenesis, and bile acid production.*

b. **Zone II** is a transitional zone between zones I and III.

c. **Zone III** is furthest away from the arteriole, where the concentration of oxygen and nutrients is the lowest. *Zone III cells undertake glycolysis, ketogenesis, and detoxification reactions.*

4. The digestive functions of the liver relate to the secretion of bile (see Biliary System) but the liver has many other integrative functions, summarized below.

5. Carbohydrate metabolism.

a. *The liver is a key effector in the control of blood glucose concentration because it can either consume glucose or add glucose to the blood.*

   i. Glycogen synthesis, glycolysis, oxidative metabolism, and fat synthesis all consume blood glucose.

   ii. Glycogenolysis and gluconeogenesis add glucose to the blood.

b. ▼ *A key pathogenic mechanism in* **diabetes mellitus** *is an inappropriately high output of hepatic glucose.* The antidiabetic drug **metformin** reduces hepatic glucose output. ▼

6. Lipid metabolism.

a. When the blood glucose concentration is low, the liver oxidizes fatty acids for energy and synthesizes **ketones** for export into the blood to be metabolized by other tissues.

b. When the blood glucose or amino acids concentrations are high, the liver converts them to fatty acids and triglycerides, which are exported for storage in adipose tissue.

   c. Lipids must be transported in the circulation as lipoprotein complexes.

      i. Lipoproteins have a hydrophobic core containing triglycerides and cholesteryl esters, and are coated by an envelope of phospholipid, free cholesterol, and **apolipoproteins.**

      ii. Apolipoproteins are needed for assembly and secretion of the lipoprotein particle and maintenance of structural integrity; they *regulate enzymes such as lipoprotein lipases and act as binding sites for receptors.*

   d. The liver and intestine are major sources of lipoprotein complexes. There are five major classes of lipoprotein classified in order of decreasing size (i.e., increasing density). Larger particles have a higher triglyceride and lower cholesterol content:

      i. *Chylomicrons are generated in intestinal cells and deliver dietary lipids to the circulation.*

         • Chylomicrons are partially broken down by the enzyme **endothelial lipoprotein lipase.**

         • The fatty acids that are released enter the adipose and muscle cells; remnant chylomicrons are taken up by the liver.

      ii. **Very low-density lipoproteins (VLDLs)** are generated by the liver to *deliver endogenous triglycerides to the tissues.* Remnant VLDLs are taken up by the liver.

      iii. **Intermediate-density lipoproteins (IDLs)** are generated within the liver from remnant VLDLs.

      iv. **Low-density lipoproteins (LDLs)** are generated within the circulation and liver from VLDLs and IDLs; *LDLs have the highest cholesterol content and function to deliver cholesterol to the tissues.*

      v. **High-density lipoproteins (HDLs)** are generated by the liver and intestine and perform *reverse cholesterol transport, delivering cholesterol from the tissues to the liver for elimination in the bile.*

      vi. Lipoproteins in each classification express different mixtures of apolipoproteins that direct their metabolic fate. For example:

         • LDLs express **ApoB100,** which allows binding and uptake by cells expressing the LDL receptor; *ApoB100 is measured clinically to assess how many LDL particles there are in the blood.*

   e. ▼ *High levels of LDL ("bad cholesterol") and low levels of HDL ("good cholesterol"), as well as high levels of total cholesterol and triglyceride, are major risk factors for development of* **coronary artery disease.** ▼

  7. Cholesterol homeostasis.

   a. Cholesterol is an important cell membrane component in all cells and is the precursor molecule for synthesis of steroid hormones and bile acids.

   b. *The liver balances cholesterol inputs and outputs from the circulation.*

   c. Cholesterol is derived either from the diet or from cellular synthesis; *the liver is the main site of cholesterol synthesis.*

      i. ▼ The **statins** are widely used cholesterol-lowering drugs that work by inhibiting the enzyme 3-hydroxy-3-methyl-glutaryl-coenzyme A reductase (**HMG-CoA reductase**, **HMGCR**), which is the rate-limiting enzyme in the cholesterol synthesis pathway. ▼

   d. The most important pathway for **elimination of cholesterol** is via the bile, mostly through conversion to bile acids, some of which are lost in feces.

8. Protein metabolism.
   a. The liver can synthesize nonessential amino acids or it can remove excess amino acids by converting them to glucose or lipids.
   b. *When amino acids are broken down,* **urea** *is formed in the liver as the final breakdown product and is excreted in the urine.*
   c. The liver consumes amino acids for synthesis of serum proteins (e.g., **albumin, clotting factors,** and **hormone-binding proteins**).
   d. ▼ *Patients with liver failure show decreased serum albumin and are at risk for* **edema** *formation due to low plasma oncotic pressure. Hemostasis may also be impaired due to loss of clotting factors and thrombopoietin.* ▼

9. Storage functions.
   a. *The liver is the main storage site for the fat-soluble vitamins A, D, E, and K, and for vitamin B$_{12}$, iron, and copper.*

10. Detoxification and biotransformation functions.
    a. *Removal of the bioactivity of many organic molecules, including steroids and hydrophobic drugs, occurs in the liver,* generally in three phases:
       i. **Phase I biotransformation** involves cytochrome P-450 enzymes located in the endoplasmic reticulum, which mainly catalyze hydroxylation reactions.
       ii. **Phase II biotransformation** involves conjugation to generate products that are more soluble for excretion. *Conjugation reactions involve the addition of glucuronate, sulfate, or glutathione to the parent molecule.*
       iii. **Phase III** refers to transport of the substrate either into the bile or into the blood to allow subsequent urinary excretion.
    b. Many organic substances needing elimination interact with nuclear receptors such as the **steroid and xenobiotic receptor** to upregulate the enzymes and transporters in the elimination pathway.
    c. ▼ In the setting of **liver failure,** accumulating toxins can cause a myriad of clinical signs and symptoms. For example, accumulation of **estrogen** is thought to be responsible for gynecomastia, testicular atrophy, spider hemangiomas, and palmar erythema. ▼

11. Immune function.
    a. *Kupffer cells in the liver are the largest group of fixed macrophages in the body.*
    b. Kupffer cells filter the blood, ingesting old red cells and foreign bodies entering the blood via the GI tract.

12. The liver has several endocrine functions. For example, it:
    a. Is the main source of circulating **insulin-like growth factor-1 (IGF-1)** and is under the control of growth hormone.
    b. Secretes the iron-regulating hormone **hepcidin.**
    c. Contributes to activation of **vitamin D** through 25-hydroxylation, prior to final activation in the kidney via 1-hydroxylation.
    d. Is a major site for deiodination of thyroxine (T$_4$) to yield the more active thyroid hormone **tri-iodothyronine (T$_3$).**

13. ▼ The biochemical assessment of the liver includes measuring serum markers of liver cell injury and a series of indicators of liver cell function.
    a. Serum markers of **liver cell injury:**
       i. **Alanine aminotransferase (ALT)** and **aspartate aminotransferase (AST)** are markers of hepatocellular injury.

    ii. **Alkaline phosphatase (AP)** and **gamma-glutamyl transferase (γGT)** are nonspecific markers of biliary duct injury.

  b. Serum markers and tests of liver cell function include:

    i. **Bilirubin** levels to assess the function of the hemoglobin breakdown and excretion pathway.

    ii. **Albumin/total protein** levels to provide a rough assessment of overall synthetic function.

    iii. **Prothrombin time** to assess the extrinsic clotting pathway, which relies on liver-derived clotting factors (see Chapter 3).

    iv. **Ammonia** levels to assess detoxification functions. ▼

14. Overview of bile and the biliary system.

  a. The three general functions of bile are to:

    i. Aid in dietary lipid assimilation through secretion of bile acids.

    ii. Contribute to the neutralization of acid chyme in the duodenum by secreting bicarbonate ions.

    iii. Provide an excretion pathway for hydrophobic molecules via the feces.

  b. The **biliary tract** consists of a series of ducts that convey bile from the liver to the duodenum (Figure 7-17).

    i. Hepatocytes secrete bile into the **canaliculi,** which are small 1-μm spaces bounded by neighboring hepatocytes.

    ii. Canaliculi transport bile toward the portal triads. (*Note: bile flows in the opposite direction to sinusoidal blood within a hepatic lobule.*)

    iii. Bile moves through a sequence of progressively larger ducts in each lobe of the liver and emerges in a **hepatic duct.**

    iv. The hepatic ducts from each lobe join outside the liver to form the **common hepatic duct.**

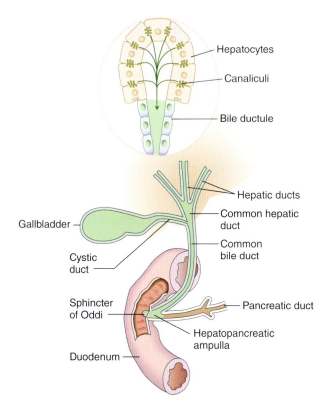

Figure 7-17. The biliary tract ("biliary tree").

v. The **cystic duct** from the gallbladder joins the common hepatic duct to form the **common bile duct.**

vi. The common bile duct usually joins with the **main pancreatic duct** to form the **hepatopancreatic ampulla.**

vii. The opening of the ampulla into the duodenum is guarded by the **sphincter of Oddi.**

15. Contributions to bile formation.

a. Bile exiting the liver in the hepatic ducts is called **hepatic bile** and is a combination of **canalicular bile** and **ductular bile.**

b. *Hepatocytes secrete canalicular bile, which is an isotonic fluid containing NaCl, together with organic molecules that include bile salts, cholesterol, phospholipids, and bile pigments.*

i. The organic molecules secreted into bile are either synthesized by hepatocytes or are transported from the sinusoidal blood.

c. Canalicular bile flows into the biliary tree, where ductular bile is added by epithelial cells called **cholangiocytes,** which line the biliary ducts.

i. *Cholangiocytes resemble pancreatic duct cells and produce a HCO_3^--rich fluid in response to the hormone* **secretin.**

16. Bile acids (Figure 7-18).

a. Approximately 70% of the organic molecules in bile are bile acids.

b. Hepatocytes synthesize and secrete the **primary bile acids** cholic acid and chenodeoxycholic acid.

i. Primary bile acids are conjugated with glycine or taurine to produce **glycocholate** and **taurocholate.**

ii. *Conjugation with amino acids makes bile acids ionize more readily into bile salts, which are more soluble in water.*

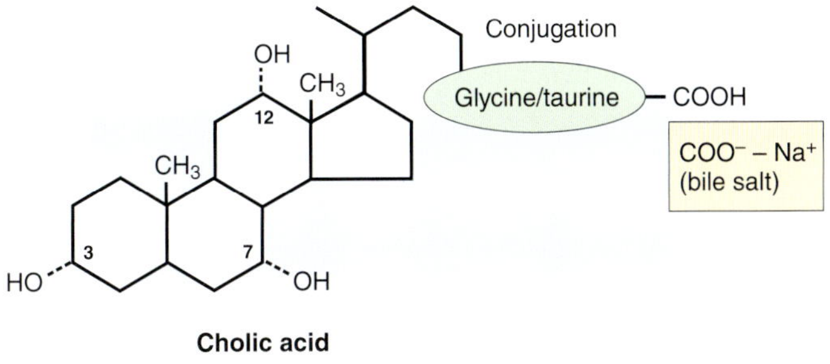

	Group at Position			% in Bile
	3	7	12	
Cholic acid	OH	OH	OH	50
Chenodeoxycholic acid	OH	OH	H	30
Deoxycholic acid	OH	H	OH	15
Lithocholic acid	OH	H	H	5

Figure 7-18. Bile acids and bile salts. Cholic acid and chenodeoxycholic acid are the primary bile acids produced by the liver. Conjugation with glycine and taurine favors ionization of bile acids to form more soluble bile salts. Dehydroxylation of the primary bile acids by intestinal bacteria produces the secondary bile acids deoxycholic acid and lithocholic acid.

c. **Secondary bile acids** (cholic → deoxycholic acid; chenodeoxycholic acid → lithocholic acid) are produced when intestinal bacteria dehydroxylate primary bile acids.

d. When the bile acid concentration exceeds a "critical micellar concentration," bile salts interact to form aggregates known as **micelles.**

e. The micelle provides a polar outer shell, which interacts with water, and a hydrophobic inner region. *Long chain fatty acids, cholesterol, and other hydrophobic molecules readily dissolve inside the micelles.*

17. Approximately 20% of the organic molecules secreted by hepatocytes into the bile are **phospholipids.**

a. Phospholipid molecules align with bile salts to form **mixed micelles,** which are better at dissolving hydrophobic molecules than pure bile salt micelles.

18. **Cholesterol** constitutes about 4% of the organic molecules in bile. *Cholesterol is very hydrophobic and must be at the center of a micelle to be dissolved.*

19. ▼ There are two types of **gallstones:**

a. *Cholesterol gallstones are the most common.* The main risk factor for cholesterol gallstone formation is excessive excretion of cholesterol, which is *common in obese patients.*

b. **Pigment gallstones** are mainly composed of calcium bilirubinate. *Patients with chronic hemolytic diseases are most at risk of developing this type of gallstone due to the high levels of bilirubin excretion. The presence of calcium causes the radiopacity of pigment gallstones.* ▼

20. The **enterohepatic circulation** (Figure 7-19).

a. Molecules in the enterohepatic circulation are:

   i. Secreted into bile by hepatocytes.

   ii. Delivered to the small intestine via the biliary tract.

   iii. Reabsorbed from the small intestine.

   iv. Returned to the liver via the portal venous system to become available again for uptake and secretion by hepatocytes.

b. ▼ *Many hydrophobic drugs (e.g., acetaminophen) are deactivated by the liver and excreted into bile; enterohepatic recycling frequently occurs, slowing the rate of drug elimination.* ▼

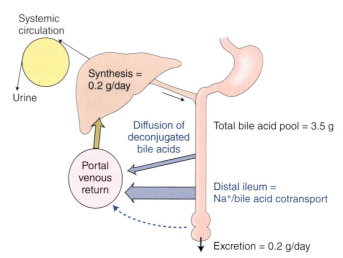

Figure 7-19. Enterohepatic circulation of bile acids. Most bile acids are reabsorbed in the distal ileum and are returned to the liver, via the portal vein, for recycling.

   c. The **bile acid pool** is limited such that bile acids/salts are recycled approximately two for during each meal eaten (i.e., six to eight times each day). About 95% of the bile salts that arrive in the intestine are reabsorbed:

      i. Bile salts that become deconjugated by intestinal bacteria and revert to bile acids are returned to the liver after absorption by simple diffusion in the jejunum.

      ii. *Most bile salts are reabsorbed via* Na^+*-bile salt cotransport when they reach the* **distal ileum**.

      iii. A small amount of bile acid (mostly as lithocholic acid) is lost in fecal excretion each day.

      iv. The rate of bile acid loss in feces is matched by the rate of hepatic bile acid synthesis.

      v. The **bile acid receptor FXR** is a nuclear receptor that senses bile acid levels to regulate the rates of hepatic bile acid synthesis and of bile acid absorption in the ileum.

   d. ▼ The enterohepatic circulation of bile acids can be disrupted as a treatment for high blood cholesterol levels (**hypercholesterolemia**).

      i. **Bile-binding resins** (e.g., cholestyramine) prevent bile acid reabsorption in the distal ileum, thereby causing bile acid excretion in feces.

      ii. When bile acids fail to return to the liver, the hepatic synthesis of new primary bile acids is stimulated, which requires an increased supply of LDL cholesterol from the blood. ▼

21. Choleresis (Figure 7-20).

   a. Choleresis describes the secretion of bile; **choleretics** are substances that stimulate choleresis.

   b. Water secretion into canalicular bile occurs by osmosis, driven by the secretion of solutes:

      i. Bile salts are the most important choleretics and produce **bile salt-dependent flow.**

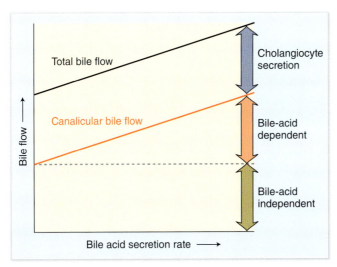

Figure 7-20. Determinants of biliary fluid secretion. Total bile flow is the sum of canalicular and ductular bile secretion. Canalicular bile flow is driven by secretion of bile acids and other solutes, which are grouped together as non-bile acids.

    ii. ▼ Bile secretion can be *stimulated pharmacologically by administering exogenous bile salts (e.g., ursodiol).* ▼

    iii. Solutes other than bile acids drive a smaller more constant fluid secretion, described as the **non–bile salt-dependent fraction**.

  c. **Ductular bile** secreted by cholangiocytes lining the biliary tract is driven by active $NaHCO_3$ secretion and is added to canalicular bile to produce hepatic bile.

22. The gallbladder.

  a. The gallbladder is a blind outpouching of the biliary tree with a capacity of only 20–50 mL.

  b. *It functions to store and concentrate bile between meals and to eject bile into the duodenum during the digestion of a meal.*

  c. During the interdigestive phase, the gallbladder is relaxed and the sphincter of Oddi is contracted, promoting storage of hepatic bile in the gallbladder.

  d. During the cephalic phase, there is gradual rhythmic contraction of the gallbladder, mediated by the **cholinergic vagal neurons.**

  e. During the intestinal phase when the meal enters the small intestine, CCK and secretin levels increase:

    i. *CCK mediates gallbladder contraction and relaxation of the sphincter of Oddi, allowing biliary and pancreatic secretions to enter the duodenum* (Figure 7-21A).

    ii. **Secretin** stimulates cholangiocyte secretion, providing additional HCO_3^- to neutralize acidic chyme.

  f. The rate of bile secretion between meals far exceeds the volume of the gallbladder.

    i. Gallbladder epithelium absorbs NaCl and fluid to concentrate the bile; *concentrated bile is more effective for promoting fat digestion* (Figure 7-21B).

    ii. The surface epithelium secretes mucins and H^+ for protection against the alkaline bile in the gallbladder lumen.

  g. ▼ **Gallbladder disease** is common and occurs in several forms, ranging from asymptomatic cholelithiasis (gallstones) to biliary colic (painful blockage of the cystic duct). Different areas of the biliary tract can be involved:

    i. **Cholecystitis** is the blockage of the cystic duct with associated inflammation of the gallbladder.

    ii. **Choledocholithiasis** is the blockage of the common bile duct.

    iii. **Ascending cholangitis** is the blockage of the common bile duct with associated inflammation of the bile ducts.

    iv. **Gallstone pancreatitis** occurs if the hepatopancreatic ampulla becomes blocked. ▼

23. Bile pigments.

  a. The major bile pigment is **bilirubin,** which is a breakdown product of hemoglobin. (*Note: bile pigments have no digestive function.*)

  b. The bile pigment elimination pathway is complex and is responsible for the normal coloration of both feces and urine (Figure 7-22):

    i. *Old red blood cells are ingested by macrophages.* **Heme oxygenase** is the key enzyme in macrophages that breaks down the heme moiety from hemoglobin; **bilirubin** is the end-product of this pathway.

A.

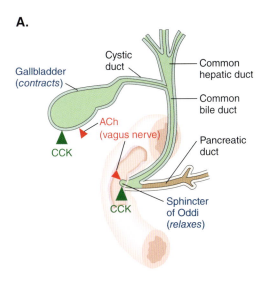

B.

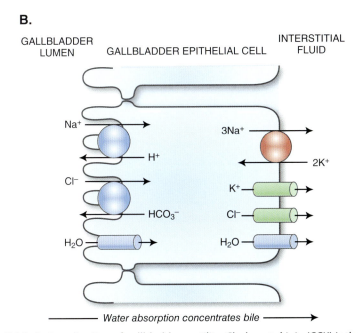

Figure 7-21. A. Coordination of gallbladder motility. Cholecystokinin (CCK) is the main agent causing contraction of the gallbladder and simultaneous relaxation of the sphincter of Oddi. **B.** Mechanism of isotonic NaCl and fluid reabsorption by the gallbladder epithelium. ACh, acetylcholine.

ii. *Bilirubin is released from macrophages and binds to albumin in the plasma because of its low solubility in water.*

iii. *The protein-bound form of bilirubin is referred to as* **unconjugated, free,** *or* **indirect bilirubin.**

iv. *Hepatocytes take up unconjugated bilirubin from plasma and convert it to* **bilirubin diglucuronide** *via the enzyme* **uridine 5'-diphospho-glucuronosyltransferase** *(UDP-glucuronosyltransferase, "UGT").*

v. *Bilirubin diglucuronide is called* **conjugated or direct bilirubin** *and is water soluble.*

vi. *Hepatocytes secrete conjugated bilirubin into bile canaliculi via the* **multidrug resistance protein-2 (MRP-2).**

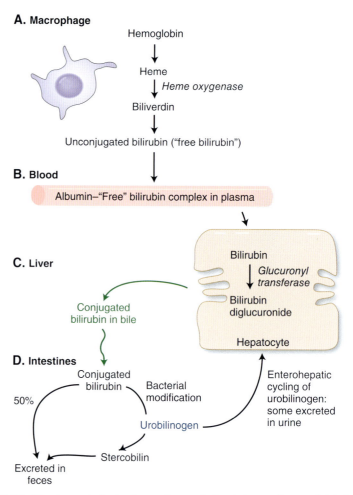

A. Macrophage

Hemoglobin
↓
Heme
↓ *Heme oxygenase*
Biliverdin
↓
Unconjugated bilirubin ("free bilirubin")
↓

B. Blood

Albumin–"Free" bilirubin complex in plasma
↓

C. Liver

Bilirubin
↓ *Glucuronyl transferase*
Bilirubin diglucuronide

Hepatocyte

Conjugated bilirubin in bile

D. Intestines

Conjugated bilirubin
Bacterial modification
50%
Urobilinogen

Enterohepatic cycling of urobilinogen: some excreted in urine

Stercobilin

Excreted in feces

Figure 7-22. Bile pigment elimination pathway. **A.** Breakdown of hemoglobin in macrophages produces bilirubin. **B.** Carriage of free bilirubin in plasma. **C.** Conjugation of bilirubin by hepatocytes. **D.** Excretion of bilirubin.

    vii. About half the conjugated bilirubin delivered to the intestine is excreted unaltered in feces and half is converted by intestinal bacteria to the colorless molecule **urobilinogen.**
- Eighty percent of urobilinogen passes to the colon, where it is metabolized by bacteria and colors feces with the brown pigment **stercobilin.**
- Twenty percent of intestinal urobilinogen enters the enterohepatic recycling pathway; some enters the systemic blood circulation and is excreted in urine as the yellow pigment **urobilin.**

  c. ▼ *Jaundice is a disease that manifests with yellowing of the sclera, the mucous membranes, and the skin, and occurs when plasma bilirubin concentration (unconjugated or conjugated) exceeds about 2 mg/dL.*

    i. Excess production of bilirubin, or a failure of the hepatocytes to take up or conjugate bilirubin, results in an accumulation of the unconjugated form in blood.

    ii. Inadequate bilirubin secretion by hepatocytes, or blockage of the bile duct, causes accumulation of conjugated bilirubin in the blood. ▼

Table 7-2. Causes of Unconjugated (Indirect) versus Conjugated (Direct) Hyperbilirubinemias

Type of Hyperbilirubinemia	Unconjugated (Indirect) Bilirubinemia	Conjugated (Direct) Bilirubinemia
Prehepatic	**Hemolytic anemias** • Sickle cell disease • Hereditary spherocytosis **Ineffective hematopoiesis** • Thalassemia	
Hepatic	**Physiologic jaundice** (low UGT activity) • Neonates **Hereditary** (UGT mutations) • Crigler-Najjar syndrome (type 1 and 2) • Gilbert's syndrome	**Hereditary** (MRP-2 mutations) • Dubin-Johnson syndrome • Rotor's syndrome **Liver disease** • Hepatitis (viral, toxin) • Cirrhosis
Posthepatic		**Biliary tract disease** • Gallstones • Tumors (bile duct, gallbladder, or pancreas) • Primary biliary cirrhosis • Primary sclerosing cholangitis

d. ▼ The terms prehepatic, hepatic, and posthepatic are used to categorize causes of jaundice (Table 7-2).

   i. **Prehepatic** is caused by conditions that present an excessive bilirubin load to the liver.

   ii. **Hepatic** jaundice results from an inability to take up, metabolize, or excrete bilirubin.

   iii. **Posthepatic (obstructive) jaundice** is caused by an obstruction to the biliary tract. Suppressed bile flow results in **acholic (light or clay-colored) stool,** whereas reabsorbed bile is excreted in urine, causing **dark urine (bilirubinuria).** ▼

The Small Intestine

1. The small intestine extends from the pyloric sphincter of the stomach to the junction with the large intestine at the ileocecal sphincter; from proximal to distal it consists of the **duodenum,** the **jejunum,** and the **ileum.**

2. Several anatomic features amplify the surface area for absorption (Figure 7-23A):

   a. **Plicae circulares** (transverse folds in the mucosa).

   b. Arrangement of the mucosa into **villi.**

   c. A **microvillous brush border** on the apical cell membrane of enterocytes.

3. *The **villous** is the functional unit of the intestine.*

   a. The villous epithelium consists of **enterocytes,** mucous-secreting goblet cells, and endocrine cells.

   b. The three regions of a villous form a functional continuum: the crypt, the maturation zone, and the villous tip (Figure 7-23B).

A. Plicae circulares

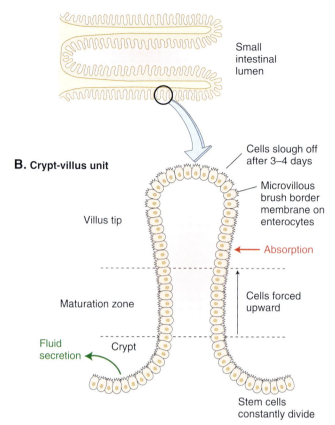

Small intestinal lumen

B. Crypt-villus unit

Cells slough off after 3–4 days

Microvillous brush border membrane on enterocytes

Villus tip

Absorption

Maturation zone

Cells forced upward

Fluid secretion

Crypt

Stem cells constantly divide

Figure 7-23. A. Amplification of the absorptive area of the small intestine. Plicae circulares are transverse folds of intestinal mucosa. **B.** The crypt-villous unit. The surface area is greatly increased by villi and microvilli on the apical membrane of the enterocytes. The crypt-villous unit is the functional unit of the small intestine. Stem cell division produces immature cells in crypts, which secrete fluid; mature cells at the villous tip absorb nutrients, electrolytes, and fluid.

    c. The **crypt** contains rapidly dividing **stem cells** that force migration of cells up the side of a villous.
       i. Crypt cells are immature and do not express enzymes or membrane transporters for nutrient absorption. *Crypt cells are the source of intestinal fluid secretion.*
    d. In the **maturation zone** cells are beginning to expresses enzymes and absorptive membrane transport proteins.
    e. At the **villous tip,** enterocytes are fully differentiated and undertake the **absorption** of nutrients, electrolytes, and fluid.
       i. *After 3–4 days, the cells are sloughed off the villous tip as a defense mechanism against insults from the luminal contents.*
    f. ▼ **Celiac sprue** is a malabsorption syndrome caused by hypersensitivity to wheat **gluten** and **gliadin,** resulting in immune-mediated destruction of villi. ▼

4. **Motility.**
    a. The three functions of small intestinal motility during the fed state are:
       i. **Mixing** of foodstuffs with digestive secretions.
      ii. **Distribution** of the luminal contents around the mucosa for absorption.
     iii. **Propulsion** of the luminal contents.

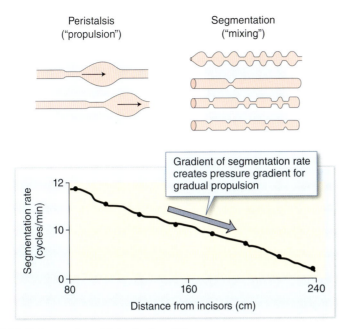

Figure 7-24. Patterns of small intestinal motility.

b. There are two major types of motility that occur in the small intestine during the fed state (Figure 7-24):

  i. **Segmentation** contractions produce a string of segments that constantly form and reform. *The main function of segmentation contractions is mixing of the luminal contents.*

  ii. **Peristalsis** consists of a wave of contractions that moves a bolus aborally. *The function of peristalsis is propulsion of luminal material.*

   • Peristalsis is a reflex. Moderate distension of the gut wall leads to contraction of circular muscle upstream and **receptive relaxation** of the circular muscle downstream.

c. There is overlap in the function between peristaltic and segmenting contractions:

  i. *Most peristaltic contractions travel less than 2 cm and thus contribute to mixing.*

  ii. Segmentations have a higher frequency in the proximal small intestine than more distally; *this **gradient of segmentation rate** creates a pressure gradient that assists aboral propulsion.*

d. An alternative functional classification of intestinal movements used clinically defines three variations:

  i. **Tonic contraction** of sphincters.

  ii. **Rhythmic phasic contractions** (small peristaltic contractions and segmentation).

  iii. **Giant migrating contractions** (powerful peristaltic contractions).

5. Fluid absorption.

a. A typical daily fluid load to the jejunum is 7–10 L/day, consisting of about 1–2 L each of dietary water, saliva, gastric juice, pancreatic juice, and intestinal secretion, and about 0.5 L of bile.

b. The small intestine reabsorbs about 6–8 L/day of fluid by **isosmotic transport,** with a maximum possible absorption rate of approximately 12 L/day.

c. *The rate of absorption of small intestinal fluid is not regulated by the mechanisms that govern the extracellular fluid volume (e.g., renin-angiotensin-aldosterone system).*

d. There is rapid **osmotic equilibration** between the duodenal chyme and plasma.

   i. If food has a high water content and is hypotonic to plasma, there is rapid water uptake.

   ii. *More frequently, a meal is hypertonic and water initially enters the small intestine from the extracellular fluid by osmosis.*

   iii. ▼ **Dumping syndrome** occurs when food moves too quickly from the stomach to the intestines (e.g., after gastrectomy). *Rapid fluid shifts into the intestine may result in symptoms of acute extracellular fluid (ECF) volume depletion such as dizziness and tachycardia, and symptoms of GI distress such as nausea, vomiting, abdominal pain, and bloating.* ▼

e. Absorption of fluid depends on the active transport of nutrients and electrolytes (Figure 7-25).

   i. Fluid absorption in the upper small intestine is mainly coupled to **Na⁺/nutrient uptake.**

   ii. *By the time the food reaches the ileum, most nutrients have been absorbed and fluid absorption is more dependent on active NaCl reabsorption.*

f. Approximately 2 L of fluid per day is delivered to the large intestine, which is roughly the initial dietary fluid load.

   i. The colon absorbs approximately 1.9 L, leaving about 0.1 L/day in feces.

   ii. The maximum absorptive capacity of the colon is approximately 5 L/day; *diarrhea results if the total fluid delivery to the colon exceeds 5 L/day.*

6. Fluid secretion.

a. Both the small intestine and the large intestine secrete fluid from the crypt cells. Fluid secretion has four functions:

   i. **Washout of pathogens;** *intestinal secretion is activated by several bacterial enterotoxins that cause secretory diarrhea.*

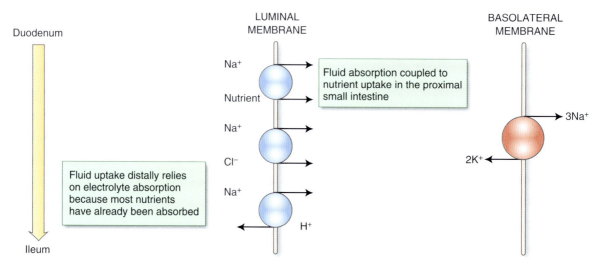

Figure 7-25. Mechanisms of fluid reabsorption along the small intestine. Different luminal entry mechanisms of Na⁺ exist at different locations along the GI tract. The gradient for passive Na⁺ uptake into the enterocytes is maintained by active Na⁺ extrusion across the basolateral cell membranes. Water reabsorption occurs by osmosis, secondary to Na⁺ absorption.

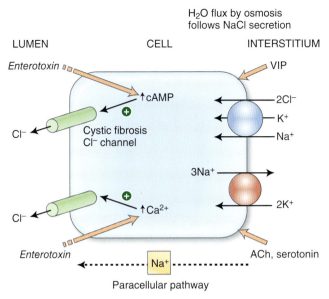

H₂O flux by osmosis
follows NaCl secretion

LUMEN   CELL   INTERSTITIUM

Figure 7-26. Mechanism of intestinal fluid secretion. Opening the luminal membrane Cl⁻ channels initiates secretion. Na⁺ secretion follows passively via the paracellular pathway, and water secretion occurs by osmosis. Secretagogues, including bacterial enterotoxins, can activate fluid secretion via cyclic adenosine monophosphate (cAMP) or increased intracellular Ca²⁺ concentration. VIP, vasoactive intestinal polypeptide; ACh, acetylcholine.

     ii. **Lubrication,** as evidenced by the increased incidence of obstruction when secretion is impaired (e.g., **cystic fibrosis**).

    iii. To provide a **source of Na⁺** for coupling to nutrient absorption if a meal contains insufficient Na⁺ for sugar and amino acid uptake.

    iv. To provide a **vehicle for antibodies** secreted in the area of the intestinal crypts to reach the gut lumen.

  b. The mechanism of intestinal fluid secretion centers on the opening of Cl⁻ channels in the luminal cell membrane (Figure 7-26). There are two types of Cl⁻ channels present:

    i. **cAMP-activated CFTR Cl⁻ channels,** stimulated via the ENS neurotransmitter **VIP.**

    ii. Ca²⁺-activated Cl⁻ channels, stimulated via **acetylcholine** from ENS neurons and **serotonin** from the EC cells.

  c. ▼ **Enterotoxic Escherichia coli** (traveler's diarrhea due to *E. coli*) and **Vibrio cholera** (cholera due to *V. cholera*) both produce enterotoxins that utilize cAMP to induce **secretory diarrhea.** ▼

    i. Cholera, irreversibly activates **adenylyl cyclase,** causing continuous production of cAMP and a severe Cl⁻-rich watery diarrhea. There can be a significant fluid loss, and death can occur if there is a delay in rehydration and electrolyte replacement.

7. Intestinal Ca²⁺ absorption.

  a. Ca²⁺ is reabsorbed in the **duodenum** and upper jejunum; 30–80% of dietary Ca²⁺ typically is absorbed.

  b. About one-third of the net Ca²⁺ uptake occurs passively via the paracellular route across the tight junctions. The remaining fraction occurs actively through **regulated Ca²⁺ transport pathways** in the enterocytes (Figure 7-27):

    i. Ca²⁺ enters the enterocytes via **Ca²⁺ channels.**

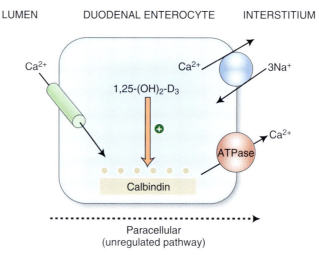

LUMEN   DUODENAL ENTEROCYTE   INTERSTITIUM

Ca²⁺

Ca²⁺

1,25-(OH)₂-D₃

3Na⁺

Ca²⁺

ATPase

Calbindin

Paracellular
(unregulated pathway)

Figure 7-27. Mechanism of intestinal calcium absorption. Vitamin D₃ stimulates intestinal Ca²⁺ uptake by stimulating calbindin expression, as well as activating Ca²⁺ transport proteins.

    ii. Ca²⁺ binds to the protein **calbindin** within the cytoplasm.

    iii. Extrusion of Ca²⁺ from the cells occurs by active transport via **Ca²⁺-ATPases** and **3Na⁺/Ca²⁺** exchangers.

    iv. *The cellular Ca²⁺ transport mechanism is stimulated by **vitamin D**.*

8. Iron homeostasis.

  a. *The regulation of iron homeostasis centers on the control of dietary uptake rather than on renal excretion.*

  b. About 70% of total body iron is associated with **hemoglobin,** and an additional 3% is associated with the muscle oxygen-binding protein **myoglobin.** Most of the remainder of total body iron is in a tissue storage form bound to the protein **ferritin.**

  c. Iron is transported in blood plasma using a binding protein called **transferrin.**

  d. The iron bound to transferrin is in equilibrium with the very small amounts of free Fe²⁺ in the extracellular fluid and with iron that is bound to ferritin in the tissues.

  e. The total amount of iron in the body is subject to negative feedback regulation (Figure 7-28A):

    i. When the iron ferritin store in the liver is full, the liver releases the iron regulatory factor **hepcidin.**

    ii. Hepcidin inhibits Fe²⁺ uptake by the intestinal enterocytes, preventing iron overload.

  f. Normal daily losses of iron are small, with only 0.6 mg/day in men and about double this amount in women (due to variable menstrual loss).

  g. ▼ In the Western diet iron intake usually exceeds daily losses but *in the developing world, dietary iron deficiency is the most common cause of anemia.* ▼

  h. Intestinal iron absorption occurs through several mechanisms (Figure 7-28B):

    i. In a nonvegetarian diet, most dietary iron is absorbed via carrier-mediated **heme uptake;** iron is released by the action of **heme oxygenase** within the enterocyte.

A.

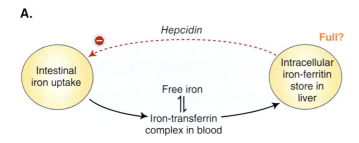

B.

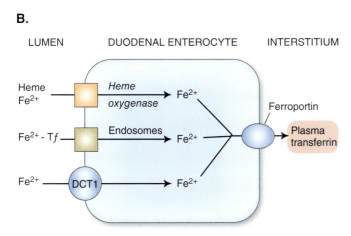

Figure 7-28. A. Overview of iron homeostasis. **B.** Mechanisms of intestinal iron uptake. DCT, divalent cation transporter-1.

    ii. Other sources of **dietary iron** become available following exposure to the low pH gastric environment. This accounts for the *high incidence of iron deficiency anemia in patients who have had a **gastrectomy.***

    iii. Most free dietary iron is presented in the **Fe³⁺** form and must be converted to Fe^{2+} prior to uptake via the enzyme **Fe³⁺ reductase** in the brush border membrane.

    iv. Most Fe^{2+} absorption occurs via a **divalent cation transporter (DCT1).**

    v. Uptake of Fe^{2+} can also occur by endocytosis of **transferrin,** which is secreted by enterocytes into the intestinal lumen, where it binds free Fe^{2+}.

    vi. Iron is transported from the cytoplasm into the ECF via the transport protein **ferroportin.**

  i. ▼ **Hemochromatosis** is an autosomal recessive disease caused by mutations in a gene referred to as **HFE** (short for High iron Fe).

    i. *The abnormal HFE gene is unable to regulate iron absorption, resulting in toxic iron overload.*

    ii. The hepcidin system becomes less effective, which results in loss of negative feedback to stop excess iron absorption.

    iii. The most common tissues affected by the **iron toxicity** are the liver (cirrhosis), the skin (bronze discoloration), and the pancreas (diabetes). Therefore, *hemochromatosis is said to cause "**bronze diabetes.**"* ▼

9. Nutrient digestion and absorption.

  a. Digestion is the chemical **breakdown of food by enzymes** and can occur at three sites (Figure 7-29A):

    i. In the lumen of the GI tract mediated by enzymes from the salivary glands, the stomach, and the pancreas.

A.

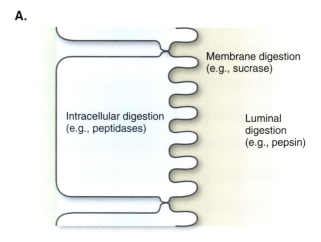

B.

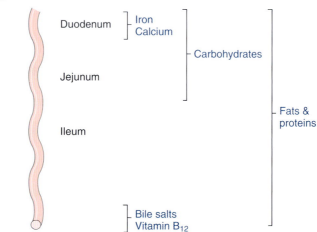

Figure 7-29. A. Sites of digestive enzyme action. **B.** Overview of nutrient absorption in the small intestine.

    ii. By the action of enzymes fixed to the brush border membrane of enterocytes.

    iii. By cytoplasmic enzymes within enterocytes.

  b. Nutrient absorption occurs in the small intestine (Figure 7-29B):

    i. *The proximal small intestine absorbs almost all of the* **iron** *and* **Ca²⁺** *that is assimilated from food.*

    ii. **Carbohydrates** can be absorbed along all parts of the small intestine, but their absorption is usually completed in the proximal small intestine.

    iii. Absorption of **protein, fat, salts,** and **water** is spread more uniformly along the small intestine.

    iv. *Bile acids and vitamin B₁₂ are absorbed specifically in the distal ileum.*

  c. Carbohydrate digestion (Figure 7-30A).

    i. Carbohydrates are the major source of calories in the Western diet, with about 400 g/day consumed. Approximately 60% is starch, about 30% is sucrose, and about 10% is lactose.

    ii. *Digestion reduces carbohydrates to their component* **monosaccharides:** *glucose, galactose, and fructose.*

A.

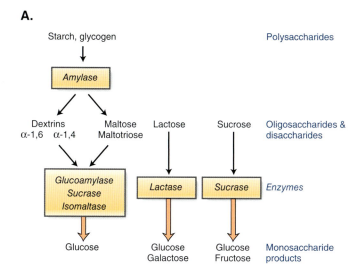

B.

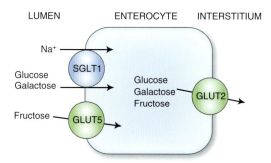

Figure 7-30. A. Major dietary forms of carbohydrates and their digestion. **B.** Absorption mechanisms for glucose, galactose, and fructose. SGLT-1 is a Na$^+$/glucose cotransporter; GLUT2 and GLUT5 are uniporters for facilitated diffusion.

  iii. Starch is a polymer of glucose; its luminal digestion with **salivary amylase** and **pancreatic amylase** produces oligosaccharides known as **dextrins**.
  iv. Oligosaccharide and disaccharide digestion occurs by membrane digestion:
  - **Glucoamylase** and **isomaltase** break down oligosaccharides.
  - The disaccharides sucrose, lactose, and maltose are broken down by sucrase, lactase, and maltase, respectively.
  v. ▼ *Lactase deficiency is common in adults from nonwhite populations and results in milk intolerance, with manifestations of osmotic diarrhea and bloating due to fermentation of lactose in the colon.* ▼
 d. Carbohydrate absorption (Figure 7-30B).
  i. *Sugars are all absorbed as* **monosaccharides**:
  - **Glucose and galactose** uptake from the gut lumen occurs via the Na$^+$-coupled cotransporter **SGLT-1.**
  - **Fructose** uptake occurs by facilitated diffusion via **GLUT5.**
  - Fructose, glucose, and galactose all exit enterocytes in the ECF via the facilitated diffusion carrier **GLUT2.**

ii. ▼ *Oral rehydration therapy is effective at restoring body fluid volume because the ingested fluid contains Na^+ and glucose, and their uptake drives fluid absorption.* ▼

e. Protein digestion.

i. Dietary protein is assimilated either as amino acids or small peptides.

ii. A combination of luminal digestion, membrane digestion, and intracellular digestion is used to break down proteins.

iii. Luminal digestion begins with **pepsin** in the stomach.

iv. The partially digested proteins that enter the small intestine are hydrolyzed by three pancreatic **endopeptidases** (acting on internal peptide bonds): **elastase, chymotrypsin,** and **trypsin.**

v. The oligopeptides produced by endopeptidases are further broken down by **ectopeptidases,** which act from the carboxy terminus of a peptide to remove one amino acid at a time.

- *Carboxypeptidase A digests the products produced by the actions of chymotrypsin and elastase.*
- *Carboxypeptidase B acts on the products of trypsin digestion.*

vi. The enzyme **aminooligopeptidase** is anchored to the enterocyte brush border membrane and acts at the amino terminus of short peptides to release amino acids.

f. Amino acid and peptide absorption (Figure 7-31).

i. Amino acid uptake mostly occurs via Na^+-coupled cotransporters.

ii. Uptake of di- and tripeptides occurs via H^+-coupled cotransporters.

g. Fat digestion.

i. *Triglycerides are the most abundant dietary form of lipid.*

ii. Other lipids include phospholipids, sphingolipids, sterols, and the fat-soluble vitamins A, D, E, and K.

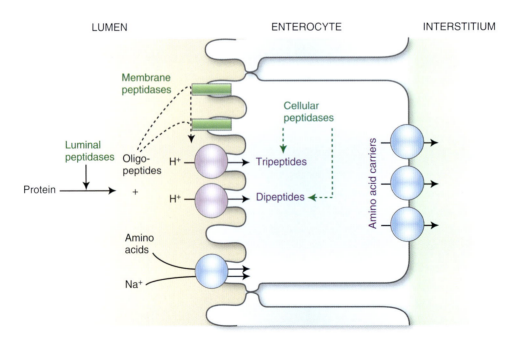

Figure 7-31. Protein digestion and absorption. Protein digestion includes the luminal, membrane, and intracellular digestion sites. Products of enzyme digestion include amino acids and small peptides, which are absorbed by a range of facilitated or Na^+-linked amino acid carriers as well as by H^+-linked dipeptide and tripeptide carriers.

   iii. Nondietary sources of lipids present in the small intestine include cholesterol from bile, sloughed enterocytes, and microbes.

   iv. The **mechanical phase** of lipid digestion includes chewing and grinding peristalsis in the stomach to create an **emulsion.**

   v. Addition of **bile** in the small intestine produces a micellar solution of lipids.

   vi. The **chemical phase** of fat digestion occurs when **lipases** remove fatty acids from the triglyceride molecules.

   vii. **Lingual lipase** from the salivary glands and **gastric lipase** from the fundus of the stomach are **acid lipases** with a pH optimum between 3.5 and 5.5.
- *In adults, acid lipases account for about 20% of total lipolysis, but in neonates this can be over 50% of the total lipolytic activity.*

   viii. **Alkaline lipase** is secreted by the pancreas and has a pH optimum between 6 and 8. The action of pancreatic lipase on triglycerides produces a monoglyceride and two free fatty acids.
- Pancreatic lipase requires **colipase** to effectively hydrolyze fats. Colipase is secreted by the pancreas and acts at the surface of a micelle by displacing a bile salt molecule, thereby providing a binding site for pancreatic lipase.

   ix. *Long chain fatty acids produced by the action of pancreatic lipase are insoluble in water and must enter the core of a micelle to be dissolved.*

   x. Other lipases include **phospholipase A$_2$**, which degrades lecithins and other phospholipids, and **carboxyl ester lipase (nonspecific lipase).**

h. Fat absorption.

   i. *Medium chain fatty acids (i.e., 6–12 carbons) are able to freely diffuse from the intestinal lumen into the blood without modification.*

   ii. Most triglyceride digestion produces **long chain fatty acids** (i.e., 13–21 carbons), which are absorbed via the following steps (Figure 7-32):
- Long chain fatty acids dissolve in micelles, which are able to diffuse through an **unstirred fluid layer** at the intestinal surface.
- Micelles destabilize within the unstirred fluid layer because it has a lower pH than the neutralized chyme.
- Long chain fatty acids escape the micelle and enter the enterocyte via **fatty acid transport proteins** and diffusion through the plasma membrane.
- *Enterocytes convert long chain fatty acids back into triglycerides within the smooth endoplasmic reticulum.*
- Triglycerides are complexed with **apoproteins** within the smooth endoplasmic reticulum and Golgi apparatus to form **chylomicrons,** which are transported across the basolateral membrane by exocytosis.
- *Chylomicrons are too large to pass across the capillary endothelia and instead enter the lymphatic **lacteals.***
- Chylomicrons enter the systemic blood when lymph drains into the venous system.

i. ▼ Fat malabsorption results in increased levels of fecal fat excretion. **Steatorrhea** is the presence of more than 7 g/day of fatty acids in the stool and has many potential **causes:**

   i. Fat emulsification is poor in patients who have had a **gastrectomy** and who experience rapid dumping of ingested food into the small intestine.

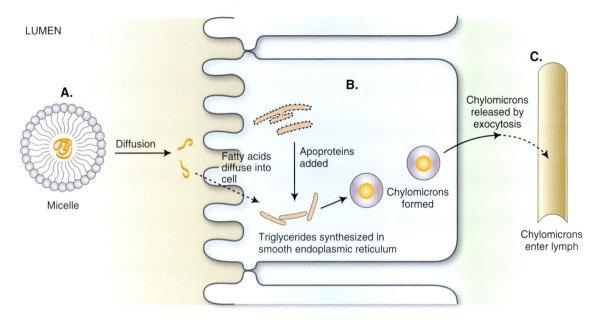

Figure 7-32. Absorption and intracellular processing of fatty acids. **A.** Diffusion of micelles through the unstirred surface fluid layer. **B.** Intracellular synthesis of triglyceride and formation of chylomicrons. **C.** Exocytosis of chylomicrons to lymphatic vessels.

      ii. Patients with **hypersecretion of gastric acid** (e.g., Zollinger-Ellison syndrome) may have an acidic duodenal environment that inhibits pancreatic lipase.

      iii. **Biliary obstruction** or **cholecystectomy** (removal of the gallbladder) reduces the availability of bile.

      iv. **Pancreatic insufficiency** (e.g., gallstone disease, alcoholism, cystic fibrosis) causes inadequate pancreatic lipase secretion.

      v. **Abetalipoproteinemia** is a rare condition in which the assembly of chylomicrons is defective.

      vi. **Small bowel disease** including having a short bowel or inflammatory diseases such as celiac sprue can reduce the absorptive surface area. ▼

10. Vitamin absorption.

    a. Vitamins are organic molecules that are required for metabolism but cannot be synthesized in the body. Therefore, *vitamins must be present in the diet* (Table 7-3).

    b. **Vitamins A, D, E,** and **K** are **fat soluble;** a meal must contain fat if these vitamins are to be assimilated from food.

      i. Fat-soluble vitamins enter micelles and are absorbed into enterocytes by membrane transporters or simple diffusion.

      ii. Fat-soluble vitamins diffuse into the smooth endoplasmic reticulum and are incorporated into chylomicrons.

    c. ▼ *Fat malabsorption is associated with a deficiency of fat-soluble vitamins because the vitamins are excreted along with excess fecal fat.* ▼

    d. The **water-soluble group** of vitamins includes the **B vitamins and vitamin C.**

      i. Intestinal absorption of water-soluble molecules mostly occurs via carrier-mediated membrane transporters (e.g., Na^+/ascorbate and H^+/folate cotransporters).

    e. **Vitamin B$_{12}$** uptake involves the following steps (Figure 7-33):

      i. When vitamin B$_{12}$ is **ingested,** it is bound to the proteins in food and must be released in the stomach by the action of pepsin.

Table 7-3. Functions of Vitamins and the Effects of Deficiencies

Vitamin	Function	Deficiency
A (β-carotene)	Pigment in retina	Night blindness
		Hyperkeratosis
B₁ (thiamine)	Coenzyme in pyruvate and α-ketoacid metabolism	Beriberi
B₂ (riboflavin)	Coenzyme in mitochondrial oxidative metabolism	Normocytic anemia
B₃ (niacin)	Coenzyme in mitochondrial oxidative metabolism	Pellagra
B₅ (biotin)	Coenzyme for carboxylation reactions	Neurologic signs
B₆ (pyridoxine)	Coenzyme in amino acid synthesis	Normocytic anemia
B₇ (pantothenic acid)	Coenzyme A: needed for metabolism of carbohydrate and fat via acetyl-coenzyme A and amino acid synthesis	Neurologic and GI signs
B₉ (folic acid)	Purine synthesis	Megaloblastic anemia
B₁₂ (cobalamin)	Facilitates formation of erythrocytes and neuronal myelin sheath	Megaloblastic ("pernicious") anemia
C (ascorbic acid)	Coenzyme in hydroxyproline formation, used in collagen synthesis	Scurvy
D (cholecalciferol)	Increased Ca²⁺ absorption	Rickets (childhood deficiency)
E (α-tocopherol)	Antioxidant	Peripheral neuropathy
K₁ (phylloquinone)	Blood clotting: needed for synthesis of factors VII, IX, X, and prothrombin	Hemorrhage

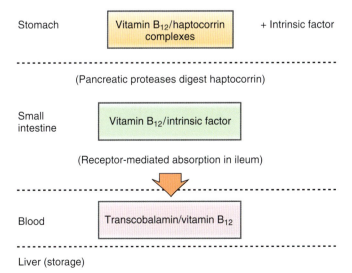

Figure 7-33. Vitamin B₁₂ assimilation. Haptocorrin binds vitamin B₁₂ in the stomach. Intrinsic factor secreted by the stomach is required for intestinal uptake of vitamin B₁₂. Binding of vitamin B₁₂ to intrinsic factor occurs in the small intestine.

        ii. Vitamin B_{12} forms a complex with a glycoprotein called **haptocorrin (R-protein),** which is secreted into the saliva and gastric juice.

        iii. Pancreatic proteases hydrolyze haptocorrin to free vitamin B_{12}, which then binds to **intrinsic factor** within the small intestine.

        iv. The vitamin B_{12}-intrinsic factor complex is absorbed via **receptor-mediated endocytosis** in the distal ileum.

        v. Vitamin B_{12} uses the binding protein **transcobalamin** in blood, which carries it to the liver for storage.

  f. ▼ The mechanism for assimilation of vitamin B_{12} requires normal function in several GI organs. As a result, there are multiple etiologies that lead to **vitamin B_{12} deficiency,** including:

        i. Dietary deficiency.

        ii. Lack of intrinsic factor (known as **pernicious anemia**), which may be caused, for example, by autoimmune destruction of the oxyntic cells or by gastric atrophy.

        iii. Pancreatic insufficiency (enzymes are needed to break down R-protein).

        iv. Surgical resection of the ileum or terminal ileum disease (e.g., Crohn's disease), which remove the site of vitamin B_{12} absorption.

        v. Intestinal microorganisms. ▼

  g. ▼ Clinical signs and symptoms of vitamin B_{12} deficiency may take months to manifest due to extensive storage in the liver.

        i. Vitamin B_{12} deficiency results in **megaloblastic anemia** and neurologic degeneration caused by **demyelination.**

        ii. *Treatment of vitamin B_{12} deficiency with only supplemental folic acid should never be attempted; the folic acid will resolve the anemia but without vitamin B_{12} replacement, the patient will have irreversible neurologic dysfunction.* ▼

The Large Intestine

1. The large intestine is wider than the small intestine and begins beyond the ileocecal sphincter and ends at the anus; it consists of the **cecum, ascending colon, transverse colon, descending colon, sigmoid colon, rectum,** and **anal canal.**

  a. The longitudinal layer of smooth muscle is arranged in three discrete strips called **teniae coli.**

  b. Contractions of this discontinuous muscle layer cause the wall of the large intestine to form bulges known as **haustra.**

  c. The colon is lined with transporting epithelial cells called **colonocytes,** which absorb fluid and transport electrolytes but do not express digestive enzymes.

2. Functions of the large intestine (Figure 7-34).

  a. *Nutrient absorption should be completed by the time the luminal contents reach the large intestine.*

  b. The main functions of the large intestine are completion of **fluid absorption** and the storage and elimination of **fecal waste.**

  c. Most water absorption occurs in the **right colon** (the cecum, the ascending colon, and the first half of the transverse colon).

  d. Prior to defecation, fecal waste is stored in the **left colon** (the distal half of the transverse colon, the descending colon, and the sigmoid colon).

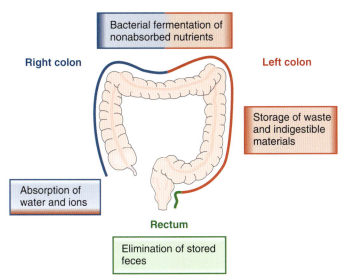

Figure 7-34. Areas and functions of the large intestine. The right colon includes the cecum, the ascending colon, and the proximal half of the transverse colon; the left colon includes the distal half of the transverse colon, the descending colon, the sigmoid colon, and the rectum.

    e. By the time fecal material reaches the rectum, it consists of a small volume of **K⁺-rich fluid** containing **undigested plant fibers,** bacteria, and inorganic material.

3. Colonic motility (Figure 7-35).

    a. Both **segmentation** and **peristalsis** facilitate fluid and electrolyte absorption and allow the storage and orderly evacuation of feces.

    b. *Segmenting contractions are more rapid in the left colon than in the right colon, which tends to slow the movement of feces toward the rectum, allowing more time to complete fluid absorption.*

    c. Peristaltic contractions are infrequent and are giant migrating-type contractions called **mass movements** that propel feces into the rectum.

4. Colonic fluid transport.

    a. Colonic fluid absorption reduces the 2 L/day of fluid that enters from the small intestine to about 0.1 L of fluid excretion in feces.

    b. The mechanisms for Na^+ absorption are as follows (Figure 7-36):

       i. In the ileum and right (proximal) colon, most NaCl absorption occurs via the parallel operation of Na^+/H^+ and Cl^-/HCO_3^- exchangers.

         • ▼ *Mutations in the colonic Cl^-/HCO_3^- exchanger cause diarrhea with high fecal [Cl^-] known as* **congenital chloride diarrhea.** ▼

      ii. In the left (distal) colon, Na^+ absorption occurs via a Na^+ channel, and K^+ secretion occurs at the same time via K^+ channels.

        • The transport model in the distal colon resembles that of the cortical collecting duct in the kidney (see Chapter 6). In both locations, the hormone *aldosterone stimulates Na^+ absorption and K^+ secretion.*

5. Diarrhea.

    a. *Diarrhea is defined as excretion of more than 200 mL of stool water within 24 hours.*

    b. Diarrhea may result from the delivery of more fluid to the colon than it can absorb, or it may result if feces move too rapidly through the colon.

A.

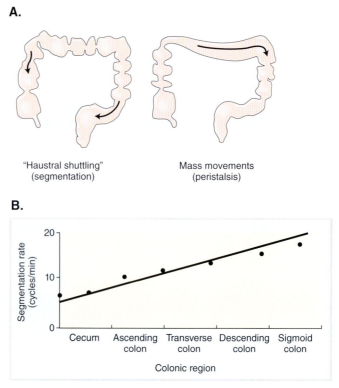

"Haustral shuttling"
(segmentation)

Mass movements
(peristalsis)

B.

Figure 7-35. **A.** Colonic motility patterns. **B.** The gradient of segmentation rates along the colon. A more rapid segmentation distally slows the aboral movement of the feces. Propulsion is achieved by giant migrating peristaltic contractions (mass movements).

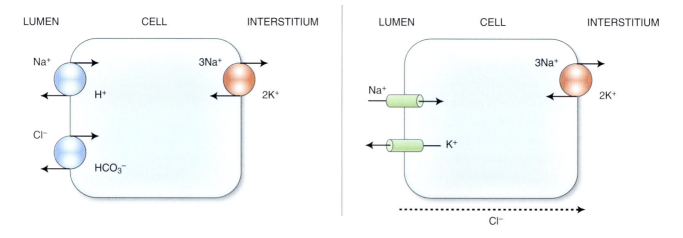

Figure 7-36. (A) Colonic electrolyte transport mechanisms in the proximal (right) colon and (B) in the distal (left) colon.

c. The general causes of diarrhea are:
  i. **Osmotic diarrhea,** when there is an agent in the intestine that causes water to be retained in the lumen. The agent may be a malabsorbed nutrient or an exogenous agent such as saline laxatives.
  ii. **Secretory diarrhea,** when there is excess endogenous fluid secretion by enterocytes and colonocytes.

- Bacterial **food poisoning** is a common cause of secretory diarrhea (e.g., traveler's diarrhea caused by enterotoxic *E. coli*).
- Rare causes of secretory diarrhea include hormone-secreting tumors that release secretagogues such as VIP or serotonin.

   iii. **Rapid intestinal motility,** when transit times are too brief to complete fluid and electrolyte absorption.

   iv. **Inflammation** of the bowel, causing diarrhea as a result of increased fluid secretion and motility (e.g., inflammatory bowel disease).

d. *Acute diarrhea is likely to cause hypovolemia due to fluid loss and in addition may cause excessive loss of K^+ and HCO_3^- in feces, resulting in* **hypokalemia** *and* **metabolic acidosis.**

   i. The mechanism of increased HCO_3^- loss in the stool is increased Cl^-/HCO_3^- exchange, as well as loss of organic anions.

   ii. The mechanism of increased K^+ loss in the stool is increased K^+ secretion via apical K^+ channels in distal colon; increased Na^+ entry via Na^+ channels leads to increased K^+ secretion in response to membrane depolarization.

e. ▼ In addition to tests for infectious and inflammatory causes of diarrhea, **physiological testing** can help to identify the cause of diarrhea. For example:

   i. **Xylose** is a sugar that is absorbed in the intestine but is not metabolized; the appearance of xylose in the blood and urine after an oral load gives an index of absorptive capacity.

   ii. **Hydrogen breath test** upon lactose administration. Fermentation of undigested lactose yields hydrogen that can be detected in the breath, which indicates *lactose intolerance.*

   iii. **The fecal osmolal gap** can be used to determine whether diarrhea is secretory or osmotic.

$$FOG = Stool\ Osm - 2x(stool\,[Na] + stool\,[K]) \qquad \textbf{Equation 7-1}$$

FOG = Fecal osmolal gap (mOsm/kg H_2O)
Stool Osm = Stool water osmolality (mOsm/kg H_2O)
Stool [Na], [K] = Stool water ion concentrations (mEq/L)

- *If the measured stool osmolality is predicted by the total ionic content of stool water then the diarrhea originates from excess ion secretion.*
- An osmolal gap is identified when other nonionic solutes (e.g., nutrient molecules) are present. Osmotic diarrhea is indicated when the osmolal gap >50 mOsm. ▼

6. Dietary fiber.

a. The main undigested material in feces is **nonstarch polysaccharides,** including cellulose, hemicellulose, lignin, pectin, gums, and algal polysaccharides, which are collectively called **dietary fiber.**

b. ▼ *High intakes of dietary fiber lower the risk for developing coronary heart disease, stroke, hypertension, diabetes, obesity, and several GI diseases. Increased fiber intake lowers blood pressure, serum cholesterol and improves control of blood glucose concentration in type 2 diabetes and in nondiabetic patients.* ▼

c. Dietary fiber undergoes fermentation by bacteria in the colon, which produces the **short chain fatty acids** acetate, propionate, and butyrate.

    i. Short chain fatty acids create a more acidic colonic fluid, which prevents bacterial overgrowth.

    ii. Fermentation reactions also produce gases (e.g., hydrogen, methane, carbon dioxide, and hydrogen sulfide), which are excreted as **flatus.**

Enteric Motility

1. The general functions of enteric motility include **propulsion** (i.e., aboral movement of luminal material), **mixing** of luminal contents, or the creation of reservoirs for temporary **storage** of material (e.g., distal colon).

2. The sphincters along the GI tract separate the gut into functional segments (Table 7-4).

    a. Sphincters are characterized as zones of high resting pressure that relax in response to an appropriate stimulus.

    b. Distention of the gut segment immediately distal to a sphincter causes it to contract, preventing retrograde flow.

3. **A basic electrical rhythm** (slow waves) in the GI smooth muscle are spontaneous oscillations in the membrane potential that underlie many of the phasic contractions of the GI tract (Figure 7-37).

    a. **Spike potentials** are triggered if the peak of a slow wave depolarizes the membrane to a threshold potential. *Spike potentials are slow action potentials mediated by the opening of Ca^{2+} channels.*

    b. **Ca^{2+} entry** into smooth muscle cells occurs during spike potentials and triggers **muscle contraction;** *this explains why the amount of force developed by muscle contraction correlates with the appearance of spike potentials.*

    c. If spike potentials occur with every slow wave, a rhythmic contraction would occur with the same frequency as the slow wave. *The maximum frequency of rhythmic contraction in a given region of the gut is therefore set by the local rate of slow wave generation.*

    d. The observed pattern of gut motility (e.g., segmentation) is programmed by the **ENS,** which determines when slow waves will produce spike potentials and give rise to a contraction.

        i. **Excitatory transmitters** often cause nonselective cation channels in the smooth muscle cells to open; the resting membrane potential is depolarized and more slow waves cross the threshold for the generation of a spike potential.

Table 7-4. Sphincters in the GI Tract

Sphincter	Segments Separated
Upper esophageal sphincter	Mouth and pharynx
Lower esophageal sphincter	Esophagus and stomach
Sphincter of Oddi	Common bile duct and duodenum
Pyloric sphincter	Stomach and duodenum
Ileocecal sphincter	Ileum and cecum
Anal sphincter	Rectum and external environment

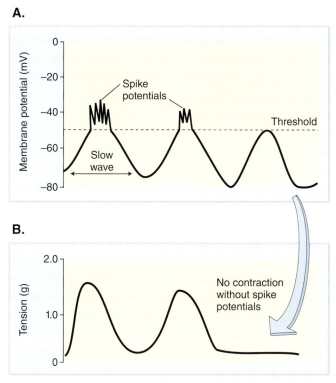

Figure 7-37. A. Basic electrical rhythm (slow waves) in GI smooth muscle. **B.** Correlation of muscle contraction to the spike potentials. Spike potentials are Ca^{2+}-mediated action potentials triggered when slow waves cross a threshold potential.

ii. **Inhibitory transmitters** often act by opening the K^+ channels in smooth muscle cells, hyperpolarizing the membrane potential and preventing the slow waves from reaching threshold.

4. **Interstitial cells of Cajal.**
   a. *The origin of the basic electrical rhythm is a network of fibroblast-like cells called the interstitial cells of Cajal,* which are positioned between the longitudinal and the circular smooth muscle layers.
   b. The interstitial cells of Cajal have multiple processes, many of which are electrically coupled to the smooth muscle cells via gap junctions and conduct the **pacemaker currents** to smooth muscle cells.
   c. Slow waves propagate down the GI tract for variable distances via the extensive network of cell-to-cell contacts between adjacent interstitial cells of Cajal.

5. Esophagus and stomach.
   a. There are no slow waves in the esophagus, which remains quiescent unless stimulated by swallowing or by the presence of a bolus in the lumen.
   b. The proximal stomach does not produce slow waves but has a steady tone that pushes the contents toward the pylorus.
   c. *Slow waves are first encountered in the distal stomach from a pacemaker in the **greater curvature.*** Slow waves occur at about 3–4 per minute and underlie the rhythmic contractions of **antral systole** that are observed when food is present.

6. Small intestinal motility.
   a. The rate of pacemaker activity declines along the small bowel from about 12 cycles per minute in the duodenum to about 6–8 cycles per minute in the ileum.

b. The gradient of segmenting contraction rates promotes gradual aboral movement of food along the intestine.

c. If nutrients reach the terminal ileum, this reflects inadequate absorption and triggers negative feedback inhibition of motility at more proximal sites:

    i. The **ileal brake** is an endocrine feedback pathway in which nutrients in the distal ileum trigger release of the hormones **glucagon-like peptide-1** and **peptide YY.**

    ii. The **ileogastric reflex** describes a neural pathway involving the ENS and extrinsic nerves when there is distension of the terminal ileum.

d. ▼ *If the distal ileum is surgically removed, a common side-effect is severely disrupted small intestinal motility.* ▼

e. As a signal that colonic material has entered the small intestine, the distal ileum also reacts to **short chain fatty acids** by increasing peristalsis and quickly returning material to the colon.

7. Large intestinal motility.

a. *Most contractions of the large intestine are segmenting contractions that continually mix the fecal contents.*

b. Occasional giant migrating contractions (**mass movements**) propel fecal material into the rectum.

c. Mass movements are increased in frequency and intensity by the **gastrocolic reflex,** which is triggered by the entry of food into the stomach and duodenum. The neuronal pathway includes both the ENS and the autonomic nerves.

d. *Fecal continence is maintained by the action of several anal sphincters.*

    i. The **internal anal sphincter** is a thickening of smooth muscle around the anal canal and is controlled by autonomic nerves.

    ii. The **external anal sphincter** is distal to the internal sphincter and is composed of skeletal muscle around the anal canal.

    iii. The **pelvic diaphragm** is also important in the maintenance of fecal continence and is a sling of skeletal muscle, originating from the bony pelvis that forms the **acute anorectal angle.**

e. **Defecation** has voluntary and involuntary components.

    i. Mass movements propel feces into the rectum.

    ii. Rectal distension initiates the **rectosphincteric reflex,** in which the internal anal sphincter initially relaxes and the intraluminal pressure recorded in the anal canal decreases (Figure 7-38).

    iii. As fecal material moves down into the upper part of the anal canal, it initiates the urge to defecate.

    iv. Voluntary contraction of the external anal sphincter can override the rectosphincteric reflex, causing the internal sphincter to regain tone. In this situation, the rectal wall relaxes to reduce rectal pressure, and feces are temporarily **accommodated** in the rectum.

    v. If the defecation reflex is allowed to continue, the internal and external anal sphincters both relax. Coordinated voluntary acts of straining occur in conjunction with propulsive involuntary contractions of the left colon and rectum to expel the feces.

8. Migrating motor complex (MMC) (Figure 7-39).

a. The MMC is a pattern of motility that occurs about every 90 minutes between meals; the start of an **interdigestive period** is defined by the first MMC that occurs after the last meal.

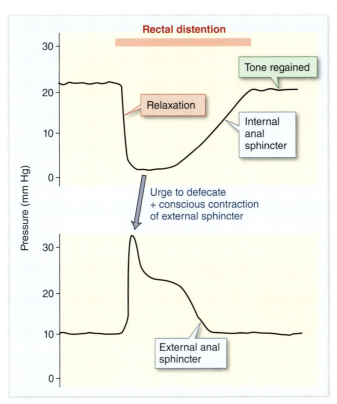

Figure 7-38. The rectosphincteric reflex. Pressure recordings within the internal and the external anal sphincters are shown during sustained rectal distension. Pressure at the internal sphincter decreases, indicating relaxation of the sphincter muscle. Increased pressure in the external anal sphincter reflects conscious contraction and causes the internal sphincter to regain its tone. The rectum relaxes to accommodate and store feces until an appropriate time for defecation.

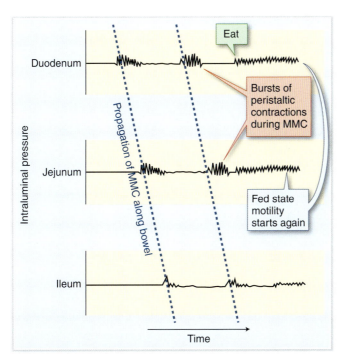

Figure 7-39. The migrating motor complex (MMC). Intraluminal pressure is measured at several sites along the small intestine. Isolated clusters of pressure spikes indicate the presence of the MMC at a given location. Dashed lines follow propagation of the MMC along the small intestine.

    b. The MMC involves intervals of strong propulsive contractions, which pass down the distal stomach and small intestine.

    c. *The functions of MMCs are to sweep the stomach and small intestine of indigestible materials and to prevent* **bacterial colonization** *of the upper intestine.*

    d. ▼ The appearance of MMCs in infants indicates the developmental maturity of the intestines and can be absent in **premature neonates.** ▼

    e. MMCs are an ENS-controlled motor program. *The ENS stimulates secretion of the hormone* **motilin,** *which stimulates propulsive contractions of the intestine.*

    f. ▼ **GI distress** (i.e., nausea, vomiting, and diarrhea) is the most common adverse effect of **erythromycin,** a macrolide antibiotic. Erythromycin binds to motilin receptors, causing increased GI motility, which is responsible for the unfavorable adverse effects of this drug. ▼

9. **Vomiting.**

    a. Vomiting removes noxious or harmful irritants from the GI tract and can be initiated by several mechanisms, including:

       i. Noxious stimuli in the **gut lumen** (e.g., infected food), which stimulate sensory receptors in the gut wall, resulting in the subjective sensation of nausea carried by autonomic nerves to the CNS.

      ii. **Higher brain centers** can induce nausea and vomiting in the absence of noxious stimuli in the gut; for example, as a result of seeing a disturbing image, smelling a nauseating odor, or by motion sickness.

     iii. Chemicals in the circulation can induce vomiting by acting on a region of the area postrema on the lateral wall of the fourth ventricle, called the **chemoreceptor trigger zone (CTZ).**

        • ▼ *Examples of CTZ activation include opioids, some cancer chemotherapeutics, and the altered hormonal milieu of early pregnancy.* ▼

    b. The CNS **vomiting center** integrates stimuli and coordinates the act of vomiting, which involves reverse peristalsis in the small intestine and stomach, together with sequential relaxation of the pyloric, the lower esophageal, and the upper esophageal sphincters.

       i. ▼ Serotonin (5-HT) and dopamine (D) are important transmitters in the central vomiting pathway; antagonists at the 5-HT_3 (e.g., ondansetron) and the D_2 receptors (e.g. prochlorperazine) are effective **antiemetics.** ▼

Splanchnic Circulation

1. *The splanchnic circulation is the largest regional circulation at rest and receives about 30% of the cardiac output.*

2. The splanchnic circulation is also the largest reservoir of blood that can be redirected to other vascular beds (e.g., during exercise).

3. Most of the blood in the splanchnic circulation is distributed to the GI organs via the celiac and superior mesenteric arteries. Most of the venous drainage from the digestive system passes to the liver via the hepatic portal vein.

4. *The* **sympathetic nervous system** *is a dominant effector that controls splanchnic vascular resistance.*

a. The release of norepinephrine by the postganglionic nerves causes **vasoconstriction** and **venoconstriction.**

b. Norepinephrine is responsible for the decrease in splanchnic blood flow associated with the general cardiovascular stressors that activate the sympathetic nervous system, including reduced blood pressure, reduced blood volume, and fear and pain.

c. *The GI system is vulnerable to low blood flow and ischemia in states of **shock,** which can result in the release of toxins or the entry of pathogens.*

5. ▼ **Mesenteric ischemia** results from low blood flow to the bowel.

a. The most common cause of this disorder is due to the rupture of an **atheroma** (plaque in the arterial wall) with associated blockage of blood vessels.

b. This condition is most common in elderly people and presents as unremitting abdominal pain that is out of proportion to physical findings and is associated with bloody diarrhea.

c. Bacterial migration across the injured bowel wall quickly results in **potentially fatal peritonitis.** ▼

6. The period of increased splanchnic blood flow after a meal is called **postprandial hyperemia.**

a. Splanchnic vasodilation results from several factors, including the hormonal environment (e.g., high levels of cholecystokinin) and the action of enteric nerves (e.g., VIPergic neurons).

b. The increase in parasympathetic nerve activity after a meal stimulates GI secretion and motility, which also *indirectly increases splanchnic blood flow as a result of increased local metabolism* (see Chapter 4).

Study Questions

Directions: Each numbered item is followed by lettered options. Some options may be partially correct, but there is only *ONE BEST* answer.

1. A healthy 28-year-old woman participated in a study of gastrointestinal function. She ingested a single nutritionally balanced meal containing small inert plastic beads, which could be visualized using medical imaging techniques. What is the most likely location of the beads 8 hours after ingestion of the meal?

   A. Arrested at lower esophageal sphincter
   B. Arrested at the pyloric sphincter
   C. Duodenum
   D. Ileum
   E. Sigmoid colon
   F. Excreted in feces

2. A 9-year-old boy awoke in the night complaining of abdominal pain that was dull and poorly localized. Which of the following pathways conveys these sensations of pain to consciousness?

   A. Myenteric plexus
   B. Sacral parasympathetic nerves
   C. Splanchnic sympathetic nerves
   D. Submucosal plexus
   E. Vagus nerve

3. A 49-year-old university professor volunteered to be the subject in a clinical demonstration in which a pressure sensor was passed an unknown distance into his esophagus via the nasopharynx. At one moment, the sensor was located in a region of tonically high resting pressure. When he was asked to swallow, there was an immediate decrease in pressure, followed by a rapid increase in the pressure at this location. Where was the pressure sensor located?

   A. Upper esophageal sphincter
   B. Thoracic esophageal body
   C. Abdominal esophageal body
   D. Lower esophageal sphincter
   E. Fundus of stomach

4. A 61-year-old man saw his physician with a complaint of progressive difficulty swallowing solid food. He reported a weight loss of about 18 kg (40 lb) despite trying to eat. He was frequently aspirating his food. The results of a radiology series and esophageal manometry suggested a diagnosis of achalasia. Which element of esophageal function would be LEAST affected in this patient?

   A. Relaxation of the upper esophageal sphincter
   B. Peristalsis in the upper esophageal body
   C. Peristalsis in the lower esophageal body
   D. Relaxation of the lower esophageal sphincter

5. Experiments were conducted using an in vitro stomach preparation to determine individual dose-response relationships for the stimulation of gastric acid production by histamine, gastrin, and acetylcholine. The dose corresponding to 50% stimulation was selected for each agonist. Which combination of agonists at this dose would produce the greatest stimulation of acid production?

   A. Histamine alone
   B. Gastrin alone
   C. Acetylcholine alone
   D. Gastrin + acetylcholine
   E. Histamine + gastrin
   F. Histamine + acetylcholine
   G. Histamine + gastrin + acetylcholine

6. A 17-year-old girl with cystic fibrosis has a history of recurrent lung infections. Until recently, she has reported few gastrointestinal symptoms. Due to recent weight loss and problems with bloating and discomfort, her pancreatic function is now being assessed using a secretin stimulation test. Which of the following abnormal responses to intravenous injection of secretin would be observed in this patient when compared with a normal subject?

   A. Increased secretion of pancreatic enzymes
   B. Increased pancreatic bicarbonate secretion
   C. Reduced gastric acid secretion
   D. Reduced volume of pancreatic juice

7. A 41-year-old woman with a history of biliary colic and gallstone disease was taken to the emergency department because of severe acute pain in the epigastric region. The patient also reports pain in the right shoulder area. Physical

examination revealed generalized yellowing of skin and scleral membranes. Which profile of bile pigments would be expected in this patient?

	Free Plasma Bilirubin	Conjugated Plasma Bilirubin	Plasma Urobilinogen
A.	High	High	Normal
B.	High	Normal	High
C.	High	High	Low
D.	Normal	Normal	High
E.	Normal	High	Normal

8. A 22-year-old woman who has Crohn's disease underwent surgical removal of the distal ileum. Without supportive therapy, this patient is most likely to develop which of the following conditions within 1 year?

   A. Anemia
   B. Calcium deficiency
   C. Caloric malnutrition
   D. Iron deficiency
   E. Lactase deficiency

9. A 52-year-old man visited his physician because of persistent epigastric pain. The patient reported defecating at least five times a day and had lost weight despite trying to eat more. A 24-hour fecal sample revealed high rates of fat excretion. Which of the following differential diagnoses should be considered?

   A. Hypersecretion of gastric acid
   B. Inflammatory bowel disease
   C. Obstructive gallstone disease
   D. Pancreatic insufficiency
   E. All of the above

10. A 4-week-old boy was brought to the emergency department in a semiconscious state. He was severely dehydrated and an electrocardiogram showed abnormal waveforms. The boy's parents reported that he had severe acute diarrhea that had worsened over the past 24 hours. No vomiting had occurred. They had tried to treat the child with fluids orally. Serum analysis revealed a potassium concentration of 1.9 mM. Which mechanism accounts for severe hypokalemia in this case?

   A. Excess secretion of potassium in the small intestine
   B. Excess secretion of potassium in the large intestine
   C. Failure to absorb potassium in the small intestine
   D. Failure to absorb potassium in the large intestine

Endocrine Physiology

CHAPTER 8

General Principles of Endocrinology

1. A **hormone** is a chemical produced by the body that has a specific regulatory effect on a target cell or organ.
2. Chemical signaling can occur in three modes (Figure 8-1).
   a. **Endocrine**: The hormone is carried a large distance via the blood.
   b. **Paracrine**: The hormone only diffuses in local extracellular fluid.
   c. **Autocrine**: The hormone acts at receptors on the cell that secreted it (e.g., growth factors made by cancer cells).

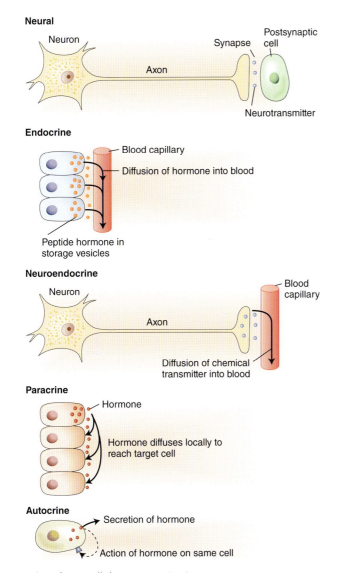

Figure 8-1. Modes of intercellular communication.

3. The seven classical endocrine glands are the pituitary, adrenal, thyroid, parathyroid, pancreas, testis, and ovary (Table 8-1).
4. Other organs also secrete hormones (e.g., hypothalamus, heart, kidney, gastrointestinal tract, liver, adipose tissue, bone).
5. Endocrine diseases may be caused by **excess** or **deficiency** of a hormone or by defects in hormone receptors or downstream intracellular signaling.
6. Certain neoplasms (e.g., small cell lung cancer) may secrete hormones, causing **paraneoplastic syndromes.**

Table 8-1. Summary of Hormones Produced by the Major Endocrine Organs

Endocrine Gland	Hormone(s) Produced	Chemical Structure	Overview: Major Function(s)
Hypothalamus	Corticotropin-releasing hormone (CRH)	Peptide	• Stimulates adrenocorticotropic hormone (ACTH)
	Growth hormone-releasing hormone (GHRH)	Peptide	• Stimulates growth hormone (GH) release
	Growth hormone inhibitory hormone (GHIH; also known as somatostatin)	Peptide	• Inhibits GH release
	Gonadotropin-releasing hormone (GnRH)	Peptide	• Stimulates luteinizing hormone (LH) and follicle-stimulating hormone (FSH) release
	Prolactin-inhibiting factor (PIF; also known as dopamine)	Peptide	• Inhibits prolactin release
	Thyrotropin-releasing hormone (TRH)	Peptide	• Stimulates thyroid-stimulating hormone (TSH) and prolactin release
Anterior pituitary	ACTH	Peptide	• Trophic to adrenal cortex • Stimulates synthesis and secretion of cortisol, aldosterone, and androgens
	FSH	Peptide	• Promotes sperm maturation via Sertoli cells in testes • Stimulates ovarian follicle development
	GH	Peptide	• Acute metabolic effects oppose insulin • Chronic growth-promoting effect via insulin-like growth factor 1 (IGF-1)
	LH	Peptide	• Stimulates Leydig cells of testes to secrete testosterone • LH surge important for ovulation and formation of corpus luteum
	Prolactin	Peptide	• Required in lactation for mammary growth, initiation of milk secretion, and maintenance of milk production
	TSH	Peptide	• Stimulates synthesis and secretion of thyroid hormones
Posterior pituitary	Antidiuretic hormone (ADH) (also called arginine vasopressin, or AVP)	Peptide	• Increases water retention at kidney • Vasoconstricts arterioles
	Oxytocin	Peptide	• Stimulates uterine contractions during labor • Milk ejection in lactation
Thyroid	Triiodothyronine (T_3) and thyroxine (T_4)	Amine	• Increase metabolic rate • Required for normal growth and development
Adrenal cortex	Aldosterone	Steroid	• Decreases urinary Na^+ excretion • Increases urinary K^+ and H^+ excretion
	Cortisol	Steroid	• Released in response to stress • Multiple metabolic actions

Table 8-1. Summary of Hormones Produced by the Major Endocrine Organs (*continued*)

Endocrine Gland	Hormone(s) Produced	Chemical Structure	Overview: Major Function(s)
Adrenal medulla	Epinephrine and norepinephrine	Amine	• Produces effects similar to actions of the sympathetic nervous system
Pancreas	Insulin (β cell)	Peptide	• Promotes storage of glucose as glycogen in liver and muscle • Promotes uptake of glucose and storage as triglyceride in adipose tissue and liver
	Glucagon (α cell)	Peptide	• Increases blood glucose by promoting glycogenolysis, gluconeogenesis, and ketogenesis in liver
Parathyroid	Parathyroid hormone (PTH)	Peptide	• Regulates serum $[Ca^{2+}]$ • Increases Ca^{2+} resorption from bone • Increases renal and intestinal Ca^{2+} absorption • Increases renal phosphate excretion
Testes	Testosterone	Steroid	• Required for male puberty; development and maintenance of male reproductive organs and secondary sex characteristics
Ovaries	Estrogens	Steroid	• Required for female puberty; development and maintenance of female reproductive organs and secondary sex characteristics
	Progesterone	Steroid	• Supports secretory phase of endometrial cycle • Important in maintenance of pregnancy
Other Endocrine Organs			
Placenta	Human chorionic gonadotropin (hCG)	Peptide	• Maintains corpus luteum early in pregnancy
	Human chorionic somatomammotropin (hCS) (also called human placental lactogen, or hPL)	Peptide	• Supports breast development in pregnancy • Regulates fuel metabolism of fetoplacental unit
Stomach	Gastrin	Peptide	• Stimulates HCl secretion by parietal cells of gastric mucosa
Small intestine	Cholecystokinin (CCK)	Peptide	• Stimulates release of pancreatic enzymes • Contracts gallbladder • Relaxes sphincter of Oddi • Inhibits stomach motility • Acts as satiety signal
	Secretin	Peptide	• Increases fluid and HCO_3^- secretion by pancreatic duct • Feedback inhibition of gastric H^+ secretion
Kidney	Renin	Peptide	• Cleaves circulating angiotensinogen to angiotensin I • Rate-limiting step in renin-angiotensin II-aldosterone axis
	1-25-Dihydroxycholecalciferol (1,25-$(OH)_2D_3$)	Steroid	• Stimulates gastrointestinal Ca^{2+} and phosphate absorption
	Erythropoietin (EPO)	Peptide	• Stimulates red blood cell production
Heart	Atrial natriuretic peptide (ANP)	Peptide	• Increases renal Na^+ excretion
Adipose tissue	Leptin	Peptide	• Decreases appetite • Initiation of puberty
Liver	Insulin-like growth factor 1 (IGF-1)	Peptide	• Secreted in response to GH; stimulates linear growth
	Hepcidin	Peptide	• Actions decrease plasma iron concentration

Classes of Hormones

1. Most hormones belong to one of three major groups (Table 8-2):
   a. **Peptides**; many examples such as pancreatic, pituitary, parathyroid, gastrointestinal etc.
   b. **Steroids** (cholesterol-based); aldosterone, cortisol, estradiol, progesterone, testosterone, vitamin D.
   c. **Amines** (tyrosine-based):
      i. Catecholamines (dopamine, epinephrine, norepinephrine).
      ii. Thyroid hormones (thyroxine, T_4, triiodothyronine, T_3).
2. Other small molecule hormones include:
   a. Serotonin, derived from the amino acid tryptophan.
   b. Gaseous transmitters (e.g., nitric oxide).
   c. Nucleotides (e.g., adenosine).
   d. Ions (e.g., Ca^{2+}).

Table 8-2. Typical Properties of Peptide and Steroid Hormones

Hormone Characteristic	Peptide Hormone*	Steroid Hormone
Water soluble	Yes	No
Uses carrier protein in plasma	No	Yes
Is stored in vesicles prior to secretion	Yes	No
Receptor location at target cell	Plasma membrane	Intracellular
Mechanism of action	Mainly second messengers	Mainly altered gene expression
Speed and duration of action	Usually fast onset but short-acting responses	Usually slow onset but long-lasting responses

*The amine class has variable characteristics; catecholamines have properties more like peptides, whereas thyroid hormones share many of the characteristics of steroids.

Plasma Hormone Concentration

1. The magnitude of a response to a hormone depends on how many receptors are occupied at the target cell, which in turn depends on the free hormone concentration in the extracellular fluid.
2. The plasma **free hormone concentration** is affected by:
   a. The rate of hormone **secretion.**
   b. The rate of hormone **elimination.**
   c. The extent of hormone **binding to plasma proteins.**
3. The rate of hormone secretion is usually under **negative feedback control** (Figure 8-2).
   a. Simple negative feedback: A hormone inhibits further secretion of itself.
   b. Complex (**hierarchical**) negative feedback: Hormone secretion from a primary target gland (e.g., thyroid) inhibits upstream pituitary/hypothalamic factors.
4. Based on the hierarchical control scheme, endocrine disorders can be classified as primary, secondary, or tertiary.
   a. A **primary disorder** is an excess or deficiency of secretion by the target gland.

A. Simple negative feedback

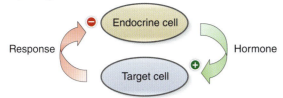

B. Complex negative feedback

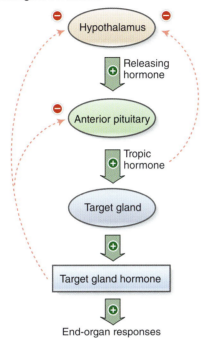

Figure 8-2. Negative feedback control of hormone secretion. **A.** Simple negative feedback in which a hormone, or a response to the hormone, inhibits further hormone secretion. **B.** Complex (hierarchical) negative feedback in which a hormone secreted from a primary target gland exerts negative feedback on the hypothalamus and pituitary gland.

 b. A **secondary disorder** is an excess or deficiency of secretion by the pituitary gland.

 c. A **tertiary disorder** is an excess or deficiency of secretion by the hypothalamus.

5. Positive feedback and feedforward control are less commonly observed control systems.

 a. **Positive feedback:** The effects of the hormone result in further hormone secretion. Examples include:

  i. LH surge stimulated by estrogen to produce ovulation.

  ii. Oxytocin release caused by cervical stretching to stimulate uterine contraction during childbirth.

 b. **Feedforward control** describes an anticipatory mechanism:

  i. Example: Glucagon-like peptide-1 secretion from enteroendocrine cells in the small intestine is triggered by glucose in the gut lumen and acts as a feedforward signal to insulin secretion before the ingested glucose is absorbed into the blood.

6. Assessment of plasma hormone concentration requires knowledge of any rhythmic patterns of secretion. For example:

 a. Cortisol has a **circadian** (day/night) pattern of secretion, with the highest hormone concentration in the early morning hours.

b. **Dynamic tests** to measure *changes* in hormone levels are often more useful than single blood samples (e.g., ACTH-stimulation test to assess cortisol secretion).

7. Hormone elimination strongly influences plasma hormone concentration. Hormones can be removed from plasma by:

   a. Metabolism.

   b. Binding in the tissues.

   c. Hepatic excretion.

   d. Renal excretion.

8. Useful terms to know:

   a. **Half-life** is the time it takes to reduce the plasma hormone concentration by one half.

   b. **Metabolic clearance rate** is the *volume* of plasma cleared of a hormone per minute, calculated by dividing the rate of hormone removal from plasma by the plasma hormone concentration.

9. Hormone binding to proteins influences plasma hormone concentration.

   a. Only free hormone molecules can diffuse out of capillaries and bind to their receptors at the target cell.

   b. Binding of a hormone to plasma proteins reduces the free concentration available.

   c. Steroids and thyroid hormones, and some peptides such as IGF-1, are highly protein bound.

   d. Protein binding increases half-life and provides a more stable reservoir of the hormone in plasma.

10. Hormones are effective at very low concentrations, in the 10^{-9}–10^{-12} molar range and must be measured using **immunoassay** techniques (Figure 8-3).

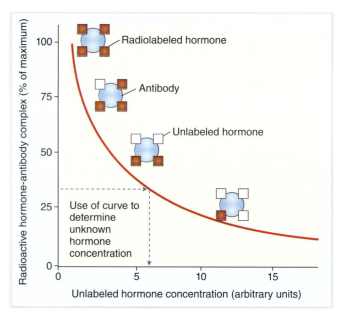

Figure 8-3. Radioimmunoassay standard curve used to measure hormone concentrations. A specific antibody to the hormone is incubated with radiolabeled hormone. A standard curve is created by introducing known concentrations of unlabeled hormone to displace radiolabeled hormone. The amount of radioactivity remaining is a function of unlabeled hormone concentration. When unknown samples are used, the measurement of the radioactivity remaining allows the hormone concentration to be read from the standard curve.

Hormone Receptors and Intracellular Signaling

1. *A response is seen only in cells with specific receptors for a hormone.*
2. There are four major types of receptors:
   a. Ligand-gated ion channels ("ionotropic receptors"). For example, nicotinic acetylcholine receptor.
   b. G-protein coupled receptors.
   c. Catalytic receptors.
   d. Intracellular receptors.
3. Hormone binding to a receptor can lead to changes in cellular function through:
   a. Altered membrane voltage.
   b. Phosphorylation/dephosphorylation of target proteins.
   c. Altered gene expression.
4. The functions of intracellular second messengers are to:
   a. Connect the process of hormone-receptor binding to changes in cell function.
   b. Amplify the hormone signal.
   c. Provide integration of simultaneous hormone signals.
5. **G-proteins** exist in many combinations of different α, β, and γ subunits and can control several second messenger systems.
   a. G-proteins work via an activation cycle:
      i. A hormone binds to G-protein coupled receptor.
         - The **Gα subunit** exchanges GDP for GTP and dissociates from $\beta\gamma$ subunit.
         - The Gα subunit regulates downstream effector proteins.
         - The Gα subunit terminates the signal by hydrolyzing ATP.
      ii. There are many Gα families. Major examples you should know:
         - Gα_s stimulates adenylyl cyclase (activated by **cholera toxin**).
         - Gα_i inhibits adenylyl cyclase (inhibited by whooping cough agent **pertussis toxin**).
         - Gα_q activates Ca^{2+} signal via phospholipase C.
6. There are several second messenger pathways controlled via heterotrimeric G-proteins (Figure 8-4):
   a. Adenylyl cyclase $\rightarrow$ **cAMP** $\rightarrow$ **protein kinase A** (PKA).
   b. **Phospholipase C** $\rightarrow$ **inositol 1,4,5 trisphosphate (IP$_3$)** $\rightarrow$ Ca^{2+} signaling $\rightarrow$ calmodulin-dependent protein kinase; **diacylglycerol (DAG)** $\rightarrow$ **protein kinase C (PKC).**
   c. **Phospholipase A$_2$** $\rightarrow$ **arachidonic acid (AA)** $\rightarrow$ **eicosanoids**
      i. There are three major eicosanoid synthesis pathways:
         - **Cyclooxygenase pathway** produces thromboxanes, prostaglandins, and prostacyclins.
         - **Lipoxygenase pathway** produces leukotrienes.
         - **Epoxygenase pathway** produces hydroxyeicosatetraenoic acid (HETE) and cis-epoxyeicosatrienoic acid (EET) compounds.
      ii. Eicosanoids are hormones released as paracrine/autocrine agents.
      iii. Eicosanoids act via G-protein coupled **prostanoid receptors** to activate many intracellular signaling pathways.

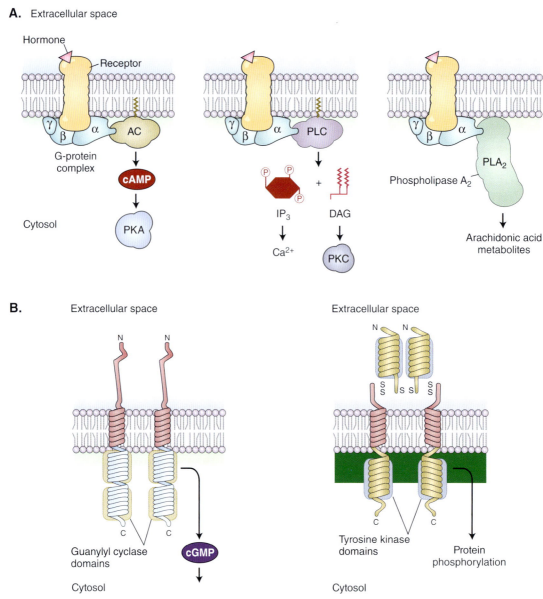

Figure 8-4. Generation of second messengers via heterotrimeric G-proteins. **A.** Coupling of the hormone-receptor complex to generation of intracellular second messengers by heterotrimeric G proteins. **B.** Hormone receptors that do not interact with G proteins. For example, some hormone receptors express enzyme activity when the hormone binds, including receptor guanylyl cyclases and receptor tyrosine kinases. AC, adenylyl cyclase; cAMP, cyclic adenosine monophosphate; PKA, protein kinase A; PLC, phospholipase C; IP_3, inositol 1,4,5-triphosphate; DAG, diacylglycerol; PKC, protein kinase C; cGMP, cyclic guanosine monophosphate.

    iv. ▼ Several anti-inflammatory drugs inhibit the synthesis or actions of eicosanoids. For example, corticosteroids inhibit arachidonic acid production, nonsteroidal anti-inflammatory drugs inhibit cyclooxygenase, and "lukast" drugs inhibit lipoxygenase (Figure 8-5). ▼

7. Hormone binding to **catalytic receptors** stimulates enzyme activity on the cytoplasmic side of the membrane. Major examples include:

  a. **Receptor tyrosine kinases** (e.g., insulin receptor) and **receptor-associated tyrosine kinases** (e.g., growth hormone receptor).

    i. Phosphorylated tyrosine motifs → kinase cascades (e.g., mitogen-activated protein kinase [**MAPK**] pathway).

    ii. Small GTP-binding proteins (e.g., Raf, Ras) are activated.

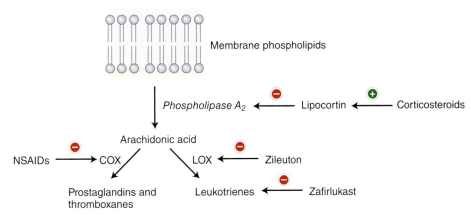

Figure 8-5. Pharmacologic interventions affecting the synthesis or actions of eicosanoids. Arachidonic acid is the precursor of eicosanoids, including prostaglandins, thromboxanes, and leukotrienes. Corticosteroids inhibit arachidonic acid production by inducing lipocortins, which block phospholipase A₂. Nonsteroidal anti-inflammatory drugs (NSAIDs) reversibly inhibit cyclooxygenase (COX), which decreases the formation of prostaglandins and thromboxanes (*note: acetylsalicylic acid [aspirin] irreversibly inhibits COX*). Zileuton inhibits lipoxygenase (LOX), which decreases leukotriene production. Zafirlukast (and other "lukast" drugs) block leukotriene receptors and are used in the treatment of asthma.

    b. **Receptor guanylyl cyclase** (e.g., natriuretic peptide receptors) → **cGMP** → cGMP-dependent kinase (**PKG**).
        i. Some cells express a soluble guanylyl cyclase activated by **nitric oxide (NO).**
       ii. ▼ Nitroglycerin is an NO donor that dilates coronary arterioles to treat symptoms of **angina pectoris.** Phosphodiesterases (PDEs) break down cAMP and cGMP; **sildenafil,** a PDE5 inhibitor, is a vasodilator used to treat erectile dysfunction and pulmonary hypertension. ▼
    c. **Receptor serine/threonine kinases** (e.g., transforming growth factor-β [TGF-β] receptor); TGF-β is involved in pathology of **organ fibrosis.**
  8. **Phosphatases** reverse the action of kinases.
    a. Serine/threonine kinases (e.g., PKA, PKC) are opposed by phosphoprotein phosphatases (PPs).
    b. Tyrosine kinases are opposed by phosphotyrosine phosphatases (PTPs).
  9. **Intracellular (nuclear) receptors.**
    a. Major examples include receptors for steroids, thyroid hormones, vitamin D, and retinoic acid.
    b. The mechanism of hormone action is as follows: Hormone enters cell → binds to receptor → receptors dimerize → become activated transcription factors → alter gene expression (Figure 8-6).

The Hypothalamus and Pituitary Gland

  1. The pituitary gland has two major lobes:
    a. The anterior pituitary is derived in the embryo from the endoderm of Rathke's pouch and consists of glandular tissue.
    b. The posterior pituitary is a part of the nervous system and consists of non-myelinated axons and nerve terminals from neurons in the hypothalamus.

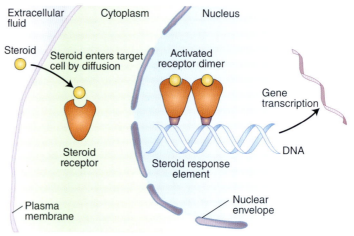

Figure 8-6. Mechanism of steroid hormone action. Steroids bind to intracellular receptors, usually located in the cytoplasm (as shown). Steroids enter target cells by diffusion. Receptors with a bound steroid molecule are chaperoned to the nucleus. Steroid-bound receptors form dimers and bind to steroid response elements in DNA to direct gene transcription.

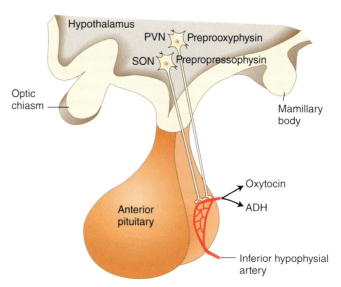

Figure 8-7. Posterior pituitary gland. The neurohormones antidiuretic hormone (ADH) and oxytocin are synthesized in neurons located in the hypothalamic paraventricular and supraoptic nuclei from the precursor peptides prepropressophysin and preprooxyphysin, respectively. ADH and oxytocin are secreted into the systemic blood from axon terminals in the posterior pituitary gland. PVN, paraventricular nucleus; SON, supraoptic nucleus.

2. Posterior pituitary gland (Figure 8-7).
   a. The posterior pituitary gland secretes **antidiuretic hormone (ADH; aka vasopressin)** and **oxytocin.**
   b. ADH and oxytocin are peptides produced in neurons that originate in the **paraventricular nucleus** and the **supraoptic nucleus** of the hypothalamus.

   c. The nerve tracts run through the pituitary stalk and terminate in the posterior pituitary.

   d. ADH and oxytocin are synthesized in the neuron cell bodies from the larger precursor molecules preprooxyphysin and prepropressophysin.

   e. Cleavage produces the active hormone plus a **neurophysin** that is co-secreted with the hormone.

      i. Neurophysins are carrier proteins that assist in the axonal transport to the axon terminals in the posterior pituitary gland.

         • Neurophysin I—Oxytocin

         • Neurophysin II—ADH; mutations can cause central diabetes insipidus (see Chapter 6).

   f. **Oxytocin** has 3 main functions:

      i. Stimulates uterine contractions during **parturition.**

      ii. Stimulates milk let down and ejection from the lactating breast.

      iii. Promotes maternal and social bonding behavior.

   g. ▼ *Oxytocin agonists are used for **labor induction** and as a uterotonic to decrease post-partum hemorrhage.* ▼

   h. ADH is the main hormone controlling water balance in the body.

      i. *The two main stimuli for ADH secretion are increased ECF osmolarity and decreased blood volume.*

      ii. ADH combats dehydration and hypovolemia by:

         • Vasoconstriction, via V_1 receptors on vascular smooth muscle cells, to increase blood pressure.

         • Increased urine concentration, via V_2 receptors in the kidney.

      iii. Thirst is stimulated to promote drinking and restore fluid balance.

      iv. Failure of ADH secretion results in **central diabetes insipidus** in which there is formation of copious amounts of dilute urine (see Chapter 6).

3. Anterior pituitary gland.

   a. With the exception of prolactin, the anterior pituitary hormones are all **tropins,** which control the release of another hormone from a target gland.

   b. The anterior pituitary gland secretes the following six major peptide hormones:

      i. Growth hormone (GH)

      ii. Thyroid-stimulating hormone (TSH)

      iii. Adrenocorticotropic hormone (ACTH)

      iv. Follicle-stimulating hormone (FSH)

      v. Luteinizing hormone (LH)

      vi. Prolactin

   c. The following five major cell types are present in the anterior pituitary gland:

      i. **Somatotropes** secrete GH.

      ii. **Thyrotropes** secrete TSH.

      iii. **Corticotropes** secrete ACTH.

      iv. **Gonadotropes** secrete both LH and FSH.

      v. **Lactotropes** secrete prolactin.

   d. Hypothalamic neurohormones control the release of anterior pituitary hormones and are delivered via the **hypophyseal portal** blood supply (Figure 8-8).

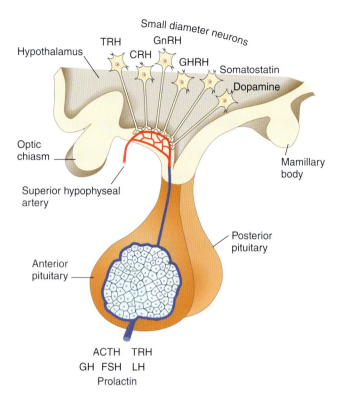

Figure 8-8. Relationship between hypothalamus and anterior pituitary gland. Hypothalamic neurohormones reach the anterior pituitary gland via the hypothalamic-hypophysial portal venous system. TRH, thyrotropin-releasing hormone; CRH, corticotropin-releasing hormone; GnRH, gonadotropin-releasing hormone; GHRH, growth hormone-releasing hormone; ACTH, adrenocorticotropic hormone; TRH, thyrotropin; GH, growth hormone; FSH, follicle-stimulating hormone; LH, luteinizing hormone.

   e. *Except for prolactin, the release of anterior pituitary hormones is under the dominant control of stimulatory hypothalamic release factors.*
      i. Secretion of TSH is stimulated by **thyrotropin-releasing hormone** (TRH).
      ii. Secretion of ACTH is stimulated by **corticotropin-releasing hormone** (CRH).
      iii. Secretion of FSH and LH is stimulated by **gonadotropin-releasing hormone** (GnRH).
      iv. Secretion of GH is controlled by a balance between the stimulatory factor **growth hormone-releasing hormone** (GHRH) and the inhibitory factor **somatostatin.** *GHRH control is dominant, because severing the pituitary stalk decreases GH secretion.*
   f. ▼ Secretion of prolactin is under negative control by **dopamine.**
      i. Severing the pituitary stalk increases prolactin secretion due to loss of dopamine inhibition,
      ii. Prolactinomas are the most common pituitary adenoma.
      iii. Hyperprolactinemia often presents with galactorrhea (milky nipple discharge).
      iv. *Prolactin hypersecretion is treated with dopamine agonists.* ▼

g. All hormones in the hypothalamic-pituitary axis exhibit **pulsatile release,** reflecting the bursting patterns of nerve impulses.

h. ▼ *Pulsatile release is needed to prevent receptor downregulation and loss of sensitivity to hypothalamic release hormones.* For example: Constant doses of GnRH agonists (e.g., **leuprolide**) suppress LH and FSH secretion through down-regulation of the gonadotropin receptors, an approach used to treat hormone-dependent **prostate cancer.** ▼

4. The GH axis (Figure 8-9).

a. GH has two types of effect:

i. Stimulation of growth in children and maintenance of lean body mass in adults.

A.

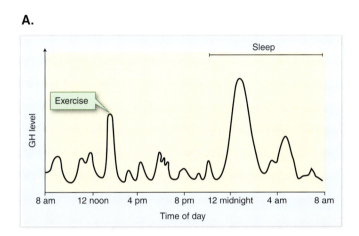

B.

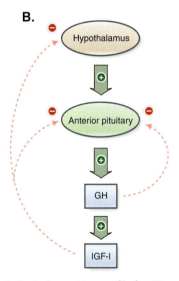

Figure 8-9. Typical secretion profile for GH and major negative feedback control via IGF-1. **A.** Circadian rhythm of GH secretion, with the greatest secretion in the early hours of sleep. GH secretion in response to acute stress is superimposed on the circadian rhythm. **B.** Hierarchical (complex) negative feedback of GH secretion. Insulin-like growth factor-I (IGF-1) secretion is stimulated by GH, and both hormones contribute to negative feedback control. GHRH, growth hormone-releasing hormone; GH, growth hormone.

ii. Acute **anti-insulin** metabolic effects (i.e., increased lipolysis in adipose tissue, increased hepatic gluconeogenesis, and decreased glucose uptake in muscle).

b. Stimulation of growth occurs indirectly through stimulation of **insulin-like growth factor-1 (IGF-1)** secretion.

c. Acute metabolic stimuli for GH secretion include:

i. Hypoglycemia.

ii. Increased serum arginine concentration.

iii. Hunger signal from the GI peptide hormone **ghrelin.**

d. Starvation strongly stimulates GH secretion, promoting increased use of fat stores for energy to preserve body protein.

5. **Insulin-like growth factor-I (IGF-1).**

a. IGF-1 is a peptide hormone that acts via the IGF-1 tyrosine kinase receptor.

b. GH stimulates the secretion of IGF-1 in many tissues; *the liver is the largest source of circulating IGF-1.*

c. IGF-1 is greater than 90% protein bound.

i. *IGF binding protein 3 (IGFBP3) is the main binding protein.*

ii. *IGFBP3 is secreted by the liver in response to GH.*

6. ▼ *Dynamic testing is needed to assess GH secretion.*

a. GH stimulation can be tested using GHRH, arginine infusion, or induced hypoglycemia.

b. GH suppression can be tested in response to a glucose load.

c. *Levels of IGF-1 and IGFBP3 are measured in growth deficiency because they are stable and reflect average GH secretion over time.* ▼

7. **Growth and growth defects.**

a. The GHRH-GH-IGF-1 axis is the most important for the growth of cartilage, bone, and muscle during linear growth.

b. Other endocrine systems, including the thyroid hormones, sex steroids, insulin, adrenal steroids, and growth factors, all contribute to growth.

c. **Gigantism** results from GH secreting tumor before closure of the epiphyseal growth plates (Figure 8-10).

d. Excess secretion of GH after puberty results in **acromegaly** (Figure 8-11).

e. ▼ *GH excess is associated with hyperglycemia and may cause **diabetes mellitus** due to the anti-insulin actions of GH.* Cardiomegaly leading to congestive heart failure is the most common cause of death in acromegaly due to continued growth of internal organs. ▼

f. Short stature has four major causes:

i. **Pituitary dwarfism** caused by deficiency of GHRH, GH, or IGF-1.

ii. **Laron dwarfism** caused by unresponsive GH receptors.

iii. **Cretinism** caused by hypothyroidism.

iv. **Acondroplasia** caused by defect in the fibroblast growth factor receptor.

g. Prolactin is structurally related to GH and is discussed in Chapter 9. Other anterior pituitary hormones are discussed below together with their target glands.

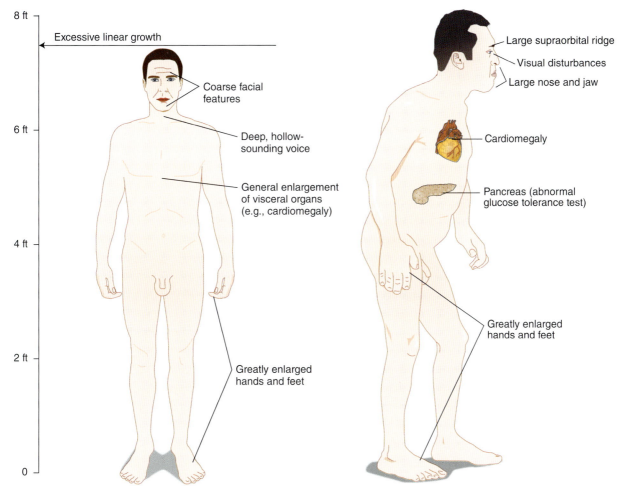

Figure 8-10. Characteristic features of gigantism caused by a pituitary tumor. The patient is a 14-year-old boy; his linear height is 7 feet 5 inches.

Figure 8-11. Characteristic features of acromegaly.

The Thyroid Axis

1. The thyroid gland (Figure 8-12):
   a. Is palpable in the anterior neck in front of the trachea.
   b. Has right and left lobes connected by the isthmus.
   c. Consists of **thyroid follicles** containing **thyroid colloid.**

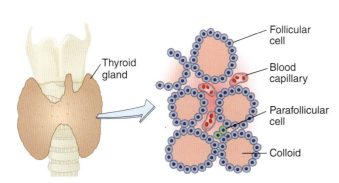

Figure 8-12. The location and histologic features of the thyroid gland.

2. Follicular cells produce the thyroid hormones **thyroxine (T₄)** and **triiodothyronine (T₃)**.

3. Thyroid hormones consist of two coupled iodinated tyrosine derivatives with four possible iodination sites (Figure 8-13). The following **patterns of iodination** occur naturally:
   a. Complete iodination at all four sites produces **T₄**.
   b. Iodination at three sites produces either **T₃** or **reverse T₃ (rT₃)**, depending on which sites are iodinated.
   c. *T₃ is the most biologically active thyroid hormone, whereas rT₃ is inactive.*

4. There are five steps in the synthesis and secretion by follicular cells of thyroid hormones (Figure 8-14):
   a. Step 1: **Iodide trapping** is uptake of I⁻ ions from the blood via a **Na⁺/I⁻ cotransporter.**
   b. Step 2: **Thyroglobulin** is synthesized and secreted into the colloid by exocytosis. This large protein contains tyrosyl groups, which will be iodinated.
   c. Step 3: Iodination and conjugation of tyrosyl residues on thyroglobulin, catalyzed by **thyroid peroxidase.**
   d. Step 4: **Endocytosis** of thyroid colloid into the follicular cells and release within the lysosomal pathway of T₄, T₃. Incompletely iodinated residues diiodothyronine (DIT) and monoiodothyronine (MIT) are recycled.
   e. Step 5: Secretion by exocytosis into the extracellular fluid of T₄ and T₃. *Ninety percent of secreted hormone is T₄, and the remaining 10% is T₃.*

5. T₄ and T₃ are >99% bound in plasma to either **thyroid-binding globulin, transthyretin,** or **albumin**. Protein binding provides a large reservoir of thyroid hormones in the plasma and produces a long half-life (>2 days).

6. *T₄ is the prohormone for T₃, which has much greater biologic activity.*

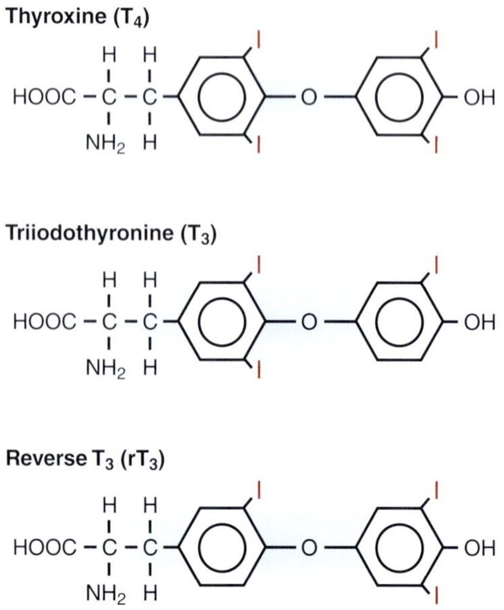

Thyroxine (T₄)

Triiodothyronine (T₃)

Reverse T₃ (rT₃)

Figure 8-13. Iodination sites for thyroid hormones. Thyroid hormones are tyrosine derivatives, with four potential iodination sites. Iodination of all four sites produces thyroxine (T₄), the major hormone secreted by the thyroid gland. The enzyme 5′-deiodinase converts T₄ to the more active hormone triiodothyronine (T₃) in the peripheral tissues. The enzyme 5-deiodinase converts T₄ to the inactive hormone reverse triiodothyronine (rT₃).

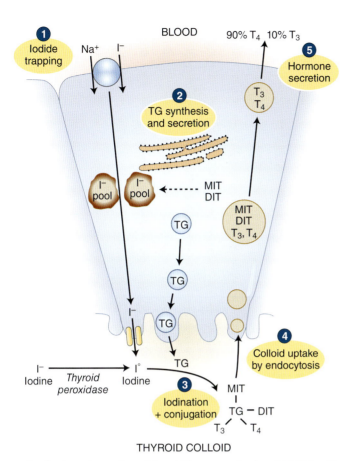

Figure 8-14. Synthesis and secretion of thyroid hormones by thyroid follicles. Steps 1–5 are fully described in the text. **1,** Iodine trapping; **2,** thyroglobulin secretion into the thyroid colloid; **3,** iodination and conjugation of thyroglobulin; **4,** endocytosis of colloid; **5,** secretion of thyroid hormones into extracellular fluid by exocytosis. DIT, diiodothyronine; MIT, monoiodothyronine; T_3, triiodothyronine; T_4, thyroxine; TG, thyroglobulin.

7. One of three **deiodinase** enzymes can activate or inactive thyroid hormones:
   a. Type 1 deiodinase can either activate or inactivate thyroid hormones and is the major activating enzyme in the periphery of **hyperthyroid patients.**
   b. *Type 2 deiodinase is the major activating enzyme (removes outer ring iodine to convert T_4 to T_3) in* **euthyroid patients.**
   c. Type 3 deiodinase is the major inactivating enzyme (removes inner ring iodine to convert T_4 to rT_3 or T_3 to T_2).
8. Thyroid hormones mainly act via nuclear receptors expressed in all body tissues, with the following major effects:
   a. *Increases basal metabolic rate* by simultaneously stimulating anabolic and catabolic processes to produce heat.
   b. Increases Na-K-ATPase activity.
   c. *Increases expression of β-adrenergic receptors.*
9. Control of the synthesis and secretion of thyroid hormones occurs via the hypothalamic-pituitary-thyroid axis (Figure 8-15).
10. TSH has a trophic effect on the thyroid gland; a sustained excess of TSH in plasma causes growth of the thyroid gland (i.e., **goiter** formation). *Measurement of TSH is typically used to screen thyroid function.* Low TSH indicates hyperthyroidism; high TSH indicates hypothyroidism.

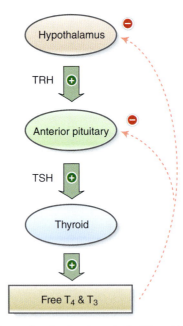

Figure 8-15. Hierarchical negative feedback control of thyroid hormone secretion. TRH, thyrotropin-releasing hormone; TSH, thyroid-stimulating hormone; T$_4$, thyroxine; T$_3$, triiodothyronine.

11. *Hypothyroidism is a common endocrine disorder, and affects about 1% of the adult population at some time.*
    a. Primary hypothyroidism is most common and with low plasma concentrations of thyroid hormones but high levels of TSH due to a lack of negative feedback (Figure 8-16A).
    b. Secondary hypothyroidism is rare and characterized by low levels of TSH, resulting in low levels of thyroid hormones (Figure 8-16B).
12. ▼ The **symptoms of hypothyroidism** may include: **Fatigue, weight gain,** and **cold intolerance** due to the reduction in the metabolic rate, **bradycardia** due to reduced β-adrenergic receptor expression, **constipation and depression.** Chronic hypothyroidism may cause **myxedema,** which is a syndrome with clinical manifestations of thick coarse skin and peripheral edema. ▼
13. ▼ The two most common causes of **primary hypothyroidism** are:
    a. **Hashimoto's autoimmune thyroiditis.** Autoantibodies against **thyroid peroxidase** (anti-TPO antibodies) and **antithyroglobulin antibodies** are commonly found in the serum of patients with Hashimoto's thyroiditis.
    b. **Dietary iodide deficiency.** Sustained high plasma concentrations of TSH often cause the development of a painless **goiter** (swelling in the anterior neck due to enlargement of the thyroid gland), reflecting the trophic effect of TSH on the thyroid gland. ▼
14. Thyroid hormones are essential for normal postnatal growth and development. *Thyroid deficiency after birth causes **cretinism,** associated with irreversible mental retardation and short stature.*
15. **Hyperthyroidism** (excess secretion of thyroid hormones) can result from primary or secondary causes (Figure 8-17):

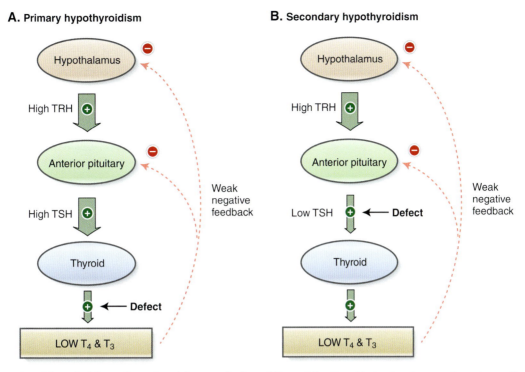

Figure 8-16. Hypothyroidism. **A.** Primary hypothyroidism results from failure of the thyroid gland and causes low plasma thyroid hormone levels. There is loss of negative feedback on thyrotropin-releasing hormone (TRH) and thyroid-stimulating hormone (TSH) secretion. **B.** Secondary hypothyroidism results from the failure of the anterior pituitary to secrete TSH and causes a lack of stimulation of thyroid hormone secretion. High TRH levels result from loss of negative feedback on the hypothalamus. T_3, triiodothyronine; T_4, thyroxine.

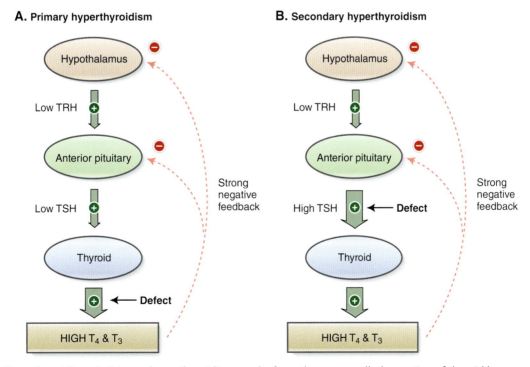

Figure 8-17. Hyperthyroidism. **A.** Primary hyperthyroidism results from the uncontrolled secretion of thyroid hormones by the thyroid gland, which exerts strong negative feedback on thyrotropin-releasing hormone (TRH) and thyroid-stimulating hormone (TSH) secretion. **B.** Secondary hyperthyroidism results from the uncontrolled secretion of TSH from the anterior pituitary, which drives thyroid hormone secretion. TRH levels are strongly suppressed. T_3, triiodothyronine; T_4, thyroxine.

a. Primary hyperthyroidism is characterized by increased thyroid hormones and decreased TSH.

b. Secondary hyperthyroidism has increased levels of both TSH and thyroid hormones.

16. ▼ Thyroid hormone excess increases metabolic rate with symptoms that include **weight loss, heat intolerance, sweating, muscle weakness, tachycardia,** and **tremor** due to over expression of β-adrenergic receptors.

    a. Catabolism is greater than anabolism so that patients may experience:

        i. Muscle wasting.

        ii. Loss of fat stores.

        iii. Increased glucose production by gluconeogenesis but with *normal blood glucose concentrations unless insulin production is abnormal.* ▼

17. ▼ The most common cause of thyroid hormone excess is **Graves' disease** in which **thyroid-stimulating immunoglobulins** activate the TSH receptor, causing hypersecretion of thyroid hormones and goiter formation (Figure 8-18). ▼

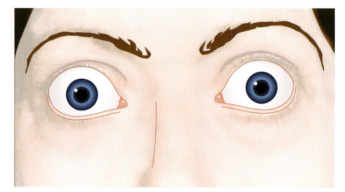

Figure 8-18. Characteristic wide-eyed appearance of exophthalmos in a woman with Graves' disease.

The Adrenal Glands

1. Each kidney has an adrenal (suprarenal) gland located above its upper pole.

2. An adrenal gland consists of an outer cortex and an inner medulla (Figure 8-19).

3. The adrenal cortex secretes steroid hormones from three zones:

    a. The **glomerulosa layer** is the outermost zone and secretes **aldosterone.**

    b. The **fasciculata layer** is the middle zone and secretes **cortisol** and **androgens.**

    c. The **reticularis layer** is the inner zone and continues from the fasciculata layer to the corticomedullary boundary. The reticularis layer secretes cortisol and androgens.

4. The adrenal medulla consists of **chromaffin cells,** which are embryologically derived from neuronal precursor (neural crest) cells.

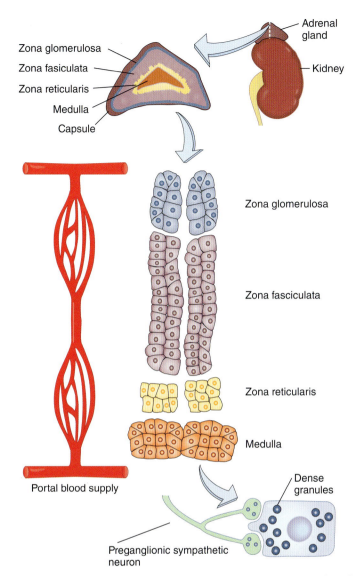

Figure 8-19. Structure of the adrenal gland. The adrenal cortex and the adrenal medulla are distinct structures visible in a cross-section of the adrenal gland. The adrenal cortex has three cellular layers, the *zona glomerulosa,* the *zona fasciculata,* and the *zona reticularis.* The adrenal medulla is composed of chromaffin cells, which receive a rich preganglionic sympathetic innervation and a portal blood supply from the adrenal cortex.

  a. *Chromaffin cells mainly secrete epinephrine plus a small amount of norepinephrine in response to preganglionic sympathetic stimulation.*
  b. Chromaffin cells are equivalent to the postganglionic neurons of the sympathetic nervous system.
  c. The chromaffin cells directly receive cortisol via a portal venous blood supply that is rich in cortisol from the adrenal cortex; high concentrations of cortisol stimulate epinephrine synthesis.
5. Synthesis and secretion of adrenocortical hormones (Figure 8-20).
  a. The three functional categories of steroid hormone are:
     i. The **mineralocorticoids** (aldosterone) that regulate electrolyte balance, mainly via the kidney.

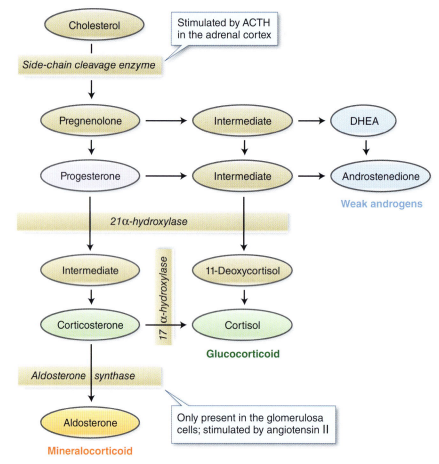

Figure 8-20. Synthesis of adrenocortical steroids.

    ii. The **glucocorticoids** (cortisol), so named because a primary function is to increase the blood glucose concentration.

    iii. The **weak androgens** androstenedione and dehydroepiandrosterone (**DHEA**).

  b. Steroid synthesis begins with cholesterol.

  c. All steroid-producing tissues (except the placenta) can synthesize cholesterol from acetate but they also utilize circulating cholesterol.

  d. Trophic hormones act on their particular steroidogenic cells (e.g., ACTH→zona fasciculata, angiotensin II→zona glomerulosa) to increase expression of the **steroidogenic acute regulatory protein (StAR)**, which translocates cholesterol from the outer to inner mitochondrial membrane.

  e. The rate-limiting step in steroid synthesis is conversion of cholesterol to **pregnenolone,** which occurs in mitochondria via the **side-chain cleavage enzyme** (also called **cholesterol 20, 22 desmolase, P450scc, or CYP11A1**).

  f. The identity of the final steroid hormone synthesized depends on which other enzymes are expressed.

    i. **Aldosterone** is only produced in the *glomerulosa* cells because these cells are the only ones that express the enzyme **aldosterone synthase.**

    ii. **Cortisol** is produced by the *fasciculata* and *reticularis* cells because these cells are the primary source of the required enzyme **17α-hydroxylase.**

    iii. **Weak androgens** are the sex steroids produced by the adrenal glands because these cells lack the enzymes needed to produce testosterone and estrogens.

    iv. Progesterone is produced as an intermediate but is normally used in the synthesis of cortisol and aldosterone rather than being secreted by the adrenal gland.

6. Actions of cortisol.

  a. *Cortisol is secreted in response to virtually all forms of stress, including trauma, infection, illness, temperature change, and mental stress; in the absence of cortisol, even minor illnesses can be fatal.*

  b. The major actions of cortisol are:

    i. Anti-insulin metabolic effects to mobilize glucose and fatty acids.

    ii. Maintain vascular responsiveness to pressor effect of catecholamines.

    iii. Anti-inflammatory immune functions.

      • ▼ Synthetic corticosteroids (e.g., prednisone) are used to control chronic inflammatory conditions such as arthritis, chronic obstructive pulmonary disease, and inflammatory bowel disease. ▼

7. Metabolism of cortisol.

  a. Circulating cortisol is ~90% bound to the **corticosteroid-binding protein (transcortin)** and a further 5% is bound to albumin.

  b. *Cortisol is metabolized by the liver and kidney to 17-hydroxycorticosteroids, which are measured in 24-hour urine samples to assess cortisol secretion.*

8. Control of cortisol secretion.

  a. The **hypothalamic-pituitary-adrenal axis** (Figure 8-21A):

    i. Hypothalamic **CRH** stimulates the release of **ACTH** from the anterior pituitary.

    ii. ACTH stimulates cortisol release from the adrenal cortex.

    iii. Cortisol exerts negative feedback by inhibiting the secretion of both CRH and ACTH.

  b. Cortisol secretion has a circadian variation, with hormone levels highest in the early morning hours (Figure 8-21B).

    i. *The circadian rhythm of cortisol helps the body in becoming active and alert in the morning and in reducing activity prior to sleep.*

  c. In addition to the circadian rhythm, CRH is under the control of higher brain centers, demonstrated by peaks of CRH (and ACTH) release in response to stress.

9. Pro-opiomelanocortin (POMC)-derived hormones.

  a. **POMC** is a prohormone produced by anterior pituitary corticotropes as well as other cells including certain CNS neurons (Figure 8-22).

  b. POMC is cleaved to produce several different hormones or neurotransmitters.

    i. ACTH (main product in pituitary corticotropes).

    ii. β-lipotropin.

    iii. β-endorphin—An endogenous opioid.

    iv. **Melanocyte-stimulating hormone (MSH).**

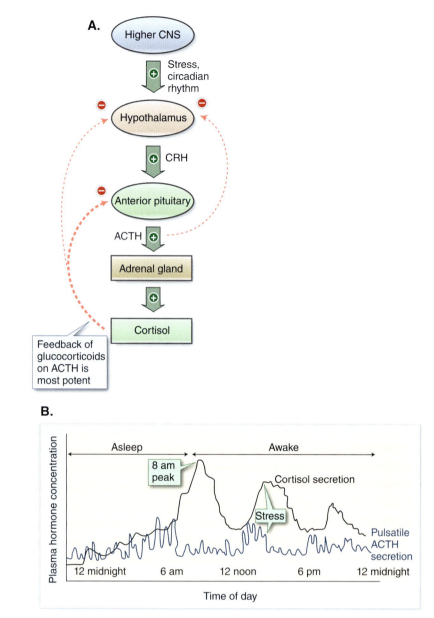

Figure 8-21. A. The hypothalamic-pituitary-adrenal axis. **B.** Pattern of daily ACTH and cortisol release. Cortisol secretion is driven by pulsatile adrenocorticotropic hormone (ACTH) secretion and has a circadian rhythm, with the greatest secretion in the early morning. ACTH secretion is driven by corticotropin-releasing hormone (CRH) from the hypothalamus. Other peaks of cortisol concentration occur in response to stress, when higher parts of the central nervous system drive greater CRH secretion.

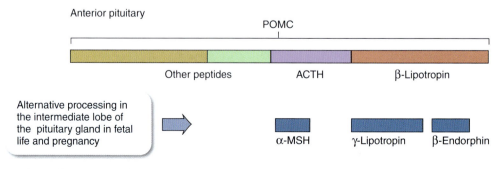

Figure 8-22. Post-translational processing of pro-opiomelanocortin (POMC) to produce various peptide hormones. ACTH, adrenocorticotropic hormone; MSH, melanocyte-stimulating hormone.

- MSH was named because in large doses it stimulates the production of the dark skin pigment, **melanin,** by melanocytes in skin.
  - *MSH is also released as a neurotransmitter by neurons of the hypothalamus causing a decrease in the appetite.*
  c. ACTH and MSH effects occur via one of five **melanocortin receptors (MCRs),** key examples include:
    i. MCR1 mediates increased melanin production in the skin.
    ii. MCR2 mediates ACTH stimulation of cortisol production.
    iii. MCR4 mediates appetite suppression of MSH in the hypothalamus.
10. Actions of ACTH.
  a. Cortisol secretion is stimulated in the fasciculata and reticularis layers because these are the sites of **17α-hydroxylase** expression.
  b. ▼ **Excess ACTH** leads to hypercortisolism; examples include ACTH-secreting pituitary adenomas or a paraneoplastic syndrome associated with small cell lung carcinoma.
    i. ACTH is a trophic hormone and an excess causes growth of the adrenal glands.
    ii. Increased skin pigmentation may occur with ACTH excess since high doses of ACTH act at the MCR1 receptor.
    iii. **ACTH deficiency** causes secondary hypocortisolism and atrophy of the fasciculata and reticularis layers of the adrenal cortex. *The glomerulosa cells are spared because they are mainly supported by a trophic effect from angiotensin II.* ▼
11. Actions of aldosterone.
  a. The main effects of aldosterone are to conserve Na^+ in the extracellular fluid and promote K^+ excretion; *the absence of aldosterone is fatal.*
  b. The main site of action for the stimulation of Na^+ reabsorption and K^+ secretion is the renal collecting duct.
  c. Other aldosterone-sensitive epithelia include the distal colon, sweat glands, and salivary glands.
  d. The effects of aldosterone are mediated via the **mineralocorticoid receptor (MR).**
  e. Glucocorticoids can also act at the MR but is normally prevented by the enzyme **11β-hydroxysteroid dehydrogenase (11β-HSD),** which deactivates cortisol through its conversion to cortisone (Figure 8-23).
    i. ▼ *High levels of cortisol or synthetic glucocorticoids can overwhelm 11β-HSD.* **Licorice** *consumption also inhibits 11β-HSD activity and may lead to symptoms of mineralocorticoid excess.* ▼
12. Control of aldosterone secretion.
  a. *The renin-angiotensin system is the most important stimulus for aldosterone secretion.*
  b. Renin is secreted from the renal **juxtaglomerular (JG) apparatus** in response to low effective circulating blood volume.
  c. The stimulus for renin release is provided by three mechanisms acting together:
    i. Reduced renal perfusion through the afferent arteriole.
    ii. Reduced glomerular filtration rate signaled via tubuloglomerular feedback (see Chapter 6).

ALDOSTERONE TARGET CELL

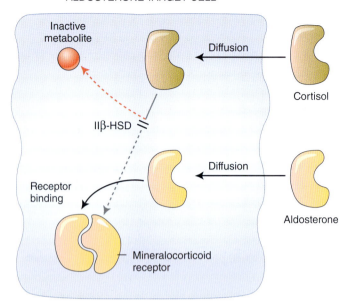

Figure 8-23. Metabolism of glucocorticoids by the enzyme 11 β-hydroxysteroid dehydrogenase (HSD) in the mineralocorticoid target cells.

  iii. Stimulation of the renal sympathetic nerves via β_1-**adrenergic receptors** on JG cells.
 d. The secretion of renin results in an increase in plasma angiotensin II and aldosterone concentrations as follows (Figure 8-24):

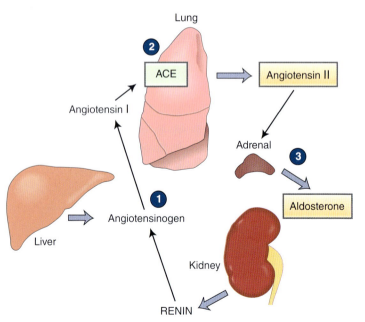

Figure 8-24. The renin-angiotensin-aldosterone system. Steps 1–3 are fully described in the text. **1,** Renin cleaves circulating angiotensinogen to produce angiotensin I; **2,** angiotensin-converting enzyme (ACE) converts angiotensin I to angiotensin II; **3,** angiotensin II stimulates aldosterone secretion from the adrenal cortex.

      i. **Renin** is an enzyme that cleaves **angiotensin I** from the circulating precursor protein **angiotensinogen.**

      ii. Angiotensin I is cleaved to produce the octapeptide **angiotensin II** by the action of **angiotensin-converting enzyme (ACE).** ACE is present on the vascular endothelial cells, with about 50% of ACE activity localized in the lung.

      iii. Angiotensin II binds to its AT_1 receptor in the adrenal cortical glomerulosa cells, which stimulates **aldosterone secretion.**

  e. *An increase in plasma $[K^+]$ is a secondary stimulus for aldosterone secretion* via direct depolarization of the glomerulosa cell membrane potential.

      i. Aldosterone increases K^+ excretion to restore normal plasma $[K^+]$.

  f. ACTH is a weak stimulus for aldosterone secretion; *aldosterone does not exert negative feedback control over ACTH secretion.*

13. Metabolism of aldosterone.

  a. Aldosterone is only approximately 60% protein bound in plasma.

  b. Aldosterone is mostly metabolized in the liver and conjugated with glucuronide prior to renal excretion.

14. ▼ Adrenocortical insufficiency.

  a. Most cases of adrenocortical insufficiency (**Addison's disease**) are due to primary failure of the entire adrenal cortex (e.g., autoimmune adrenalitis, tuberculosis).

  b. **Cortisol deficiency** results in fasting hypoglycemia due to low rates of hepatic gluconeogenesis; there is hypotension due to lack of vascular responsiveness to pressor action of catecholamines; patients commonly experience weakness and fatigue.

  c. **Aldosterone deficiency** further results in hypovolemia and hyponatremia as a result of urinary losses of NaCl and water; hyperkalemia and metabolic acidosis occur as a result of reduced urinary excretion of K^+ and H^+.

  d. Patients may become severely debilitated by the inability to mount a response to stress and are then described as being in **Addisonian crisis.**

  e. *In primary adrenal insufficiency, lack of negative feedback results in high levels of ACTH and a characteristic increase in skin pigmentation* (Figure 8-25).

  f. Deficiency of adrenal androgens in females may result in **reduced libido** and thinning of the public hair. These effects do not occur in males due to secretion of the gonadal androgens.

  g.

      i. Long-term **glucocorticoid therapy** (e.g., rheumatoid arthritis) can suppress the hypothalamic-pituitary-adrenal axis through feedback inhibition. *Adrenal insufficiency occurs if treatment is abruptly stopped.*

      ii. An **ACTH-stimulation test** is used to assess the adrenal cortex. After administration of an ACTH analogue (e.g., cosyntropin), the serum cortisol levels should increase appropriately; failure to do so indicates adrenocortical insufficiency. ▼

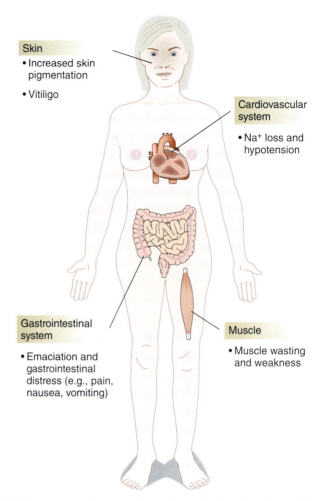

Figure 8-25. Characteristic features of a patient with chronic primary adrenocortical insufficiency (Addison's disease).

15. ▼ **Hypercortisolism (Cushing's syndrome)** is characterized by the following signs and symptoms (Figure 8-26):
    a. Hyperglycemia due to enhanced gluconeogenesis.
    b. Muscle wasting and weakness are due to protein catabolism.
    c. Truncal obesity and moon face caused by redistribution of body fat.
    d. Hypertension due to the mineralocorticoid effects of excess glucocorticoids.
    e. General causes of Cushing's syndrome include (Table 8-3):
        i. Primary hypercortisolism (e.g., adenoma of the adrenal cortex).
        ii. Secondary hypercortisolism (e.g., excess ACTH from a pituitary adenoma, specifically called **Cushing's disease**).
        iii. Tertiary hypercortisolism (excess CRH).
        iv. *Therapy with synthetic glucocorticoids* (e.g., for rheumatoid arthritis). ▼
16. ▼ Hyperaldosteronism.
    a. **Primary hyperaldosteronism** (Conn's syndrome) is the result of an aldosterone-producing adrenal adenoma. Symptoms include:
        i. **Hypertension** due to excessive retention of Na^+ and fluids by the kidney.
        ii. **Hypokalemia** due to increased urinary K^+ excretion.
        iii. **Metabolic alkalosis** due to increased urinary H^+ excretion.

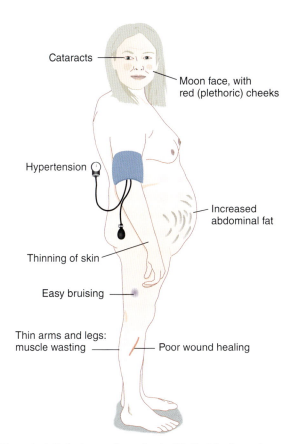

Cataracts

Moon face, with
red (plethoric) cheeks

Hypertension

Increased
abdominal fat

Thinning of skin

Easy bruising

Thin arms and legs:
muscle wasting

Poor wound healing

Figure 8-26. Characteristic features of a patient with Cushing's syndrome.

Table 8-3. Levels of Cortisol and Adrenocorticotrophic Hormone (ACTH) in Cushing's Syndrome

Disorder	Endogenous Cortisol Levels	ACTH Levels
Primary hypercortisolism (e.g., adrenal adenoma)	↑	↓
Secondary hypercortisolism (e.g., Cushing's disease)	↑	↑
Tertiary hypercortisolism	↑	↑
Exogenous glucocorticoid treatment	↓	↓

   b. **Secondary hyperaldosteronism** is chronic activation of the renin-angiotensin-aldosterone axis. Examples include:
      i. Renal artery stenosis.
      ii. Any condition producing a low effective circulating volume (e.g., congestive heart failure). *Note: Secondary hyperaldosteronism is common!* ▼
17. ▼ **Adrenogenital syndrome.**
   a. *The effects of adrenal androgen excess are more apparent in children and women since they do not secrete gonadal androgens.*
   b. Children and adult females develop male secondary sex characteristics, such as growth of facial and body hair and growth of the clitoris or the penis, called the **adrenogenital syndrome.**

  c. *The most common cause of androgen excess in females is **polycystic ovary***
   ***syndrome;** other causes include androgen-secreting adenoma of the ovary*
   or adrenal glands.

  d. *The most common congenital error in adrenal steroid metabolism is*
   ***21α-hydroxylase deficiency.** Complete enzyme loss simultaneously causes*
   deficiency of cortisol and aldosterone and an excess of androgens at birth
   (Figure 8-27).

    i. The clinical syndrome caused by 21α-hydroxylase deficiency is called
     virilizing congenital adrenal hyperplasia. *This congenital defect is most*
     readily apparent in female infants because the influence of androgens in
     utero produces ambiguous genitalia.

    ii. Adrenal hyperplasia is due to the trophic effect of high levels of ACTH,
     which is caused by loss of negative feedback inhibition from cortisol.

    iii. *Primary adrenal insufficiency due to loss of cortisol or aldosterone is the*
     most immediate life-threatening problem. ▼

18. Adrenal medulla.

  a. As part of the stress response, the adrenal medulla secretes epinephrine and
   norepinephrine into the blood in concert with activation of the sympathetic
   nervous system.

  b. Epinephrine and norepinephrine are made from the amino acid tyrosine via
   a series of enzymatically controlled reactions (Figure 8-28).

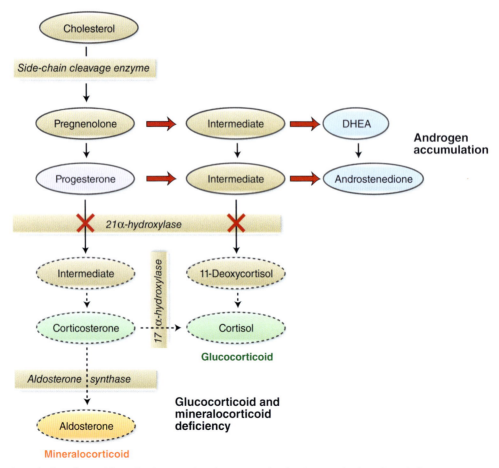

Figure 8-27. Shunting of adrenal steroid synthesis toward androgen production in 21 α-hydroxylase deficiency.

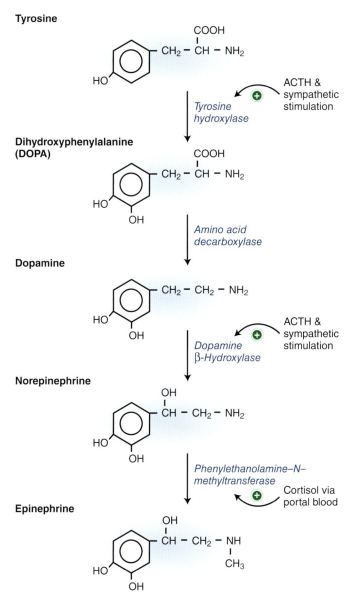

Tyrosine

Dihydroxyphenylalanine (DOPA)

Tyrosine hydroxylase — ACTH & sympathetic stimulation

Dopamine

Amino acid decarboxylase

Norepinephrine

Dopamine β-Hydroxylase — ACTH & sympathetic stimulation

Phenylethanolamine–N– methyltransferase — Cortisol via portal blood

Epinephrine

Figure 8-28. Catecholamine synthesis in the adrenal medulla. ACTH, adrenocorticotropic hormone.

i. *The rate limiting step is conversion of DOPA to dopamine by amino acid decarboxylase.*

ii. In sympathetic postganglionic neurons, the pathway ends with the production of norepinephrine.

iii. The final conversion from norepinephrine to epinephrine only occurs in the medullary chromaffin cells.

iv. Cortisol delivered via the portal blood vessels stimulates epinephrine synthesis.

c. *The release of catecholamines by the adrenal medulla is controlled by the central nervous system (CNS) via the preganglionic sympathetic neurons.*

i. The neurotransmitter acetylcholine is released and acts at the **nicotinic cholinergic receptors** on the chromaffin cells.

ii. *Chromaffin cells release 80% epinephrine and 20% norepinephrine.*

19. Actions of circulating catecholamines (Table 8-4).

   a. Responses in the target cells depend on the specific adrenergic receptor type that is expressed. There are five major receptor types:

      i. The α_1 **receptors** are coupled via $G_{\alpha q}$, which gives rise to increased intracellular $[Ca^{2+}]$ in the target cells.

      ii. The α_2 **receptors** suppress cAMP responses through coupling to $G_{\alpha i}$.

      iii. The β_1, β_2, **and** β_3 **receptors** all increase cAMP via $G_{\alpha s}$.

   b. Epinephrine has a similar binding affinity to norepinephrine at the α receptors but has greater affinity at the β_1 and β_2 receptors.

   c. Stress results in the enhanced secretion of catecholamines from the adrenal medulla and the secretion of cortisol from the adrenal cortex.

   d. Catecholamines coordinate a short-term stress response, which includes increased cardiac output, bronchodilation, and elevated blood glucose concentration.

   e. Cortisol initiates a more sustained stress response, which includes the mobilization of glucose, fatty acids, and amino acids, and suppression of the immune system.

Table 8-4. Selected Effector Organ Responses to Adrenal Medullary Hormones and Sympathetic Nerve Stimulation

Organ	Receptor Type	Response
Heart		
Sinoatrial node	β_1	Increased heart rate
Atrioventricular node and the His Purkinje system	β_1	Increased conduction speed
Myocardium	β_1	Increased contractility
Vascular smooth muscle	α_1	Constriction in skin, abdominal viscera, and kidney
	β_2	Dilation in skeletal muscle
Bronchiolar smooth muscle	β_2	Relaxation
Gastrointestinal tract		
Circular smooth muscle	α_2, β_2	Reduced motility
Sphincters	α_1	Constriction
Secretion	α_2	Inhibition
Liver	β_2	Glycogenolysis and gluconeogenesis
Adipose tissue	β_1, β_3	Lipolysis
Kidney	β_1	Renin secretion
Urinary bladder		
Detrusor	β_2	Relaxation of bladder wall
Sphincter	α_1	Constriction
Male sex organs	α_1	Ejaculation

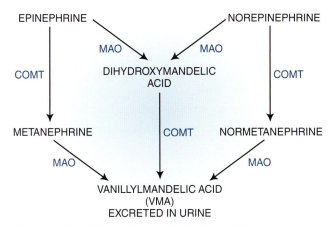

Figure 8-29. Degradation of circulating catecholamines. MAO, monoamine oxidase; COMT, catecholamine-O-methyltransferase.

20. Catecholamine metabolism.
    a. Circulating catecholamines are rapidly broken down by a series of enzymatic reactions, via **catecholamine-O-methyltransferase (COMT) and monoamine oxidase (MAO)** (Figure 8-29).
    b. The final product is **vanillylmandelic acid (VMA),** which is excreted in the urine.
       i. *Catecholamine production by the adrenal medulla is assessed by measuring the levels of catecholamines, metanephrines, and VMA in the urine.*
    c. ▼ Patients with **pheochromocytoma,** a secretory tumor of the adrenal medulla, hypersecrete catecholamines.
       i. Transient episodes of hypertension, palpitations, sweating, increased body temperature, and increased blood glucose concentration occur.
       ii. Diagnosis is aided by measuring the increased concentrations of catecholamines and their breakdown products in the urine. ▼

The Endocrine Pancreas

1. Endocrine cells in the pancreas form small aggregates called the **islets of Langerhans,** which have three major endocrine cell types (Figure 8-30):

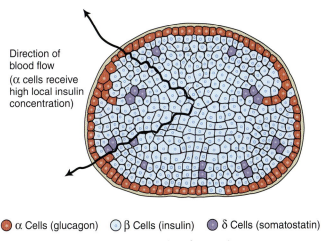

Direction of blood flow (α cells receive high local insulin concentration)

● α Cells (glucagon)   ○ β Cells (insulin)   ● δ Cells (somatostatin)

Figure 8-30. Endocrine cells in a pancreatic islet of Langerhans.

a. **α-cells** are mainly located at the periphery of the islets and secrete **glucagon.**

b. β-**cells** are mainly located toward the center of the islets and secrete **insulin, C peptide,** and **amylin.**

c. δ-**cells** secrete **somatostatin.**

d. Blood flows through the islets of Langerhans from the center toward the periphery so that the α-cells receive a high concentration of insulin; *insulin suppresses glucagon secretion.*

2. Insulin synthesis.

a. Insulin is cleaved from the precursor proinsulin (Figure 8-31).

b. Proinsulin has an A and a B domain joined by the connecting C-peptide.

c. The C domain is cleaved to yield insulin and a free C peptide.

d. ▼ *Urinary excretion of C peptide is a marker of insulin production because it is produced in a 1 to 1 ratio with insulin and is not degraded after secretion.*

   i. In endogenous hyperinsulinemia (e.g., insulinoma) both C peptide and insulin concentrations are elevated.

   ii. In exogenous hyperinsulinemia (e.g., insulin overdosing) C peptide will be absent. ▼

3. Effects of insulin.

a. The net effect of insulin on the plasma metabolite levels is a reduction in glucose, amino acids, fatty acids, and ketoacids.

b. *The three major effector organs for insulin are the liver, skeletal muscle, and adipose tissue.*

c. In the liver, insulin increases the following:

   i. Glycolysis and glycogen synthesis.

   ii. Conversion of glucose to triglycerides.

   iii. Net protein synthesis.

d. In skeletal muscle, insulin:

   i. Increases glucose uptake via **GLUT4.**

   ii. Increases glycolysis and glycogen synthesis.

   iii. Decreases metabolism of fatty acids, making more available for storage in the adipose tissue.

   iv. ▼ *Exercise improves control of blood glucose in patients with diabetes in part because GLUT4 is directly stimulated by increased muscle work via* **adenosine monophosphate (AMP) kinase.** ▼

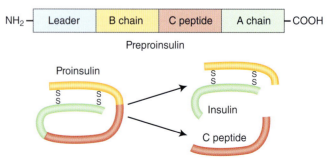

Figure 8-31. Processing of preproinsulin in the pancreatic β cells. Cleavage of C peptide from a region between the A and B chains of insulin produces equal amounts of C peptide and insulin. C peptide is stored in vesicles together with insulin, and both are secreted simultaneously during exocytosis.

   e. In adipose tissue, insulin increases:

      i. Glucose uptake via GLUT4.

      ii. Storage of circulating triglycerides via stimulation of the enzyme **endothelial lipoprotein lipase.**

   f. An independent rapid action of insulin is increased cellular uptake of K^+.

      i. Insulin secretion after a meal is important to quickly sequester ingested K^+.

      ii. ▼ *Insulin is used therapeutically to treat* **hyperkalemia;** *glucose is given at the same time to prevent hypoglycemia and Ca^{2+} is included to stabilize membrane potentials.* ▼

   g. ▼ *Insulin has long-term anabolic actions.* For example:

      i. **Insulin deficiency** in childhood impairs normal growth.

      ii. Chronic insulin excess in **type 2 diabetes mellitus** increases cancer risk and is associated with pathological growth of vascular smooth muscle. ▼

   h. The tissue effects of insulin are mediated via a **receptor tyrosine kinase.**

      i. Metabolic effects are mostly mediated via phosphoinositide signaling.

      ii. Growth promoting effects are mostly mediated via MAPK signaling.

      iii. ▼ *In type 2 diabetes mellitus the expression of insulin receptors and downstream signaling is impaired causing* **insulin insensitivity.** ▼

4. Control of insulin secretion.

   a. *The pancreatic β-cell is a fuel sensor that couples blood glucose concentration to insulin release* via the following four steps (Figure 8-32):

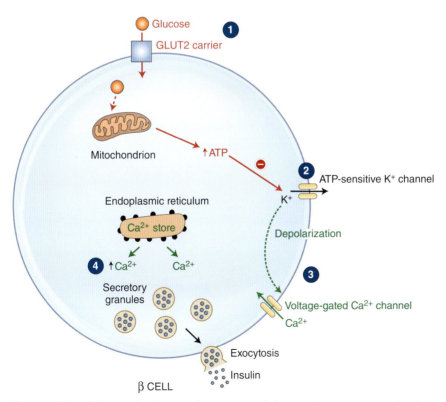

Figure 8-32. Cellular mechanism coupling increased plasma glucose concentration to insulin secretion from the pancreatic β cells. Steps 1–4 are fully described in the text. **1,** Uptake and oxidative metabolism of glucose; **2,** closure of adenosine triphosphate-sensitive K^+ channels; **3,** Ca^{2+} influx through voltage-operated Ca^{2+} channels following membrane depolarization; **4,** Ca^{2+}-induced Ca^{2+} release resulting in exocytosis of insulin and C peptide.

     i. Glucose is taken up via **GLUT2** and oxidized to produce ATP.

     ii. An increase in the ATP:ADP ratio inhibits **ATP-sensitive K⁺ channels,** resulting in depolarization of the β cell membrane potential.

     iii. Depolarization activates **voltage-sensitive Ca²⁺ channels,** causing influx of Ca²⁺.

     iv. Increased intracellular [Ca²⁺] triggers **exocytosis** of secretory granules containing insulin.

  b. Other factors that stimulate insulin release are:

     i. Amino acids and ketoacids (metabolized to increase ATP as above).

     ii. Parasympathetic simulation via acetylcholine.

     iii. **GLP-1** (incretin effect from gut).

     iv. Glucagon.

  c. Factors that inhibit insulin release are:

     i. Epinephrine and norepinephrine (via α_2 adrenergic receptors).

     ii. Somatostatin.

       • Physiological negative feedback operates in which somatostatin limits excess insulin secretion.

       • *Pharmacological doses of somatostatin can be used to treat insulin-secreting tumors.*

5. Glucagon.

  a. *Glucagon antagonizes the actions of insulin to increase the blood glucose concentration.*

  b. Several peptide hormones can be generated from the glucagon gene (Figure 8-33):

     i. α-cells in the pancreatic islets produce glucagon.

     ii. L cells in the intestine produce GLP-1.

6. Actions of glucagon.

  a. *The main target organ for glucagon is the liver.*

  b. The main effects of glucagon opposing insulin actions are to:

     i. Increase glucose production via glycogenolysis and gluconeogenesis.

     ii. Increase lipolysis in adipose tissue via stimulation of **hormone sensitive lipase.**

     iii. *Increase hepatic **ketone** (β hydroxybutyrate and acetoacetic acid) synthesis from fatty acids.*

       • Ketones provide an alternative energy source to glucose in many tissues, including the brain.

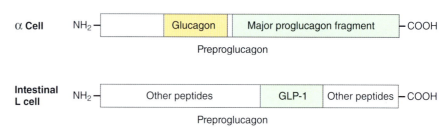

Figure 8-33. Products derived from the glucagon gene. Processing of preproglucagon produces glucagon in pancreatic α cells and glucagon-like peptide in intestinal L cells. GLP-1, glucagon-like peptide-1.

- Use of ketones for fuel conserves glucose and the cellular protein stores in prolonged fasting.

7. Control of glucagon secretion.
   a. *Secretion is stimulated by hypoglycemia, amino acids, vagal stimulation (acetylcholine), and by epinephrine (via β_2-adrenergic receptors).*
   b. Secretion is inhibited by hyperglycemia, insulin, and somatostatin.
   c. *Ingestion of a protein-rich meal stimulates both glucagon and insulin secretion.* Insulin increases amino acid uptake while glucagon prevents the development of hypoglycemia from increased insulin.

8. Integrated control of blood glucose concentration.
   a. Blood glucose concentration is determined by a balance between glucose input and output from the circulation (Figure 8-34).
      i. Glucose input to the circulation is dependent on the diet and on the production of glucose by the liver.
      ii. Glucose output from the circulation is a function of tissue metabolism.
   b. Insulin increases metabolic use and storage of glucose in response to hyperglycemia.
   c. Several counter-regulatory hormones decrease metabolic use of glucose and increase hepatic production of glucose in response to hypoglycemia, exercise, and stress:
      i. Glucagon and catecholamines are fast acting.
      ii. Cortisol and GH provide a sustained counter response to hypoglycemia.

9. Amylin:
   a. Is a peptide hormone stored in β-cell granules with insulin and C-peptide.
   b. Synthesis is stimulated by increased plasma glucose and fatty acids.
   c. Aids insulin action by decreasing spikes in blood glucose concentration by:
      i. Slowing gastric emptying.
      ii. Increasing satiety.
      iii. Inhibiting glucagon secretion.
   d. ▼ *Amylin is the main constituent of* **amyloid** *that accumulates and injures β-cells in type 2 diabetes.* ▼

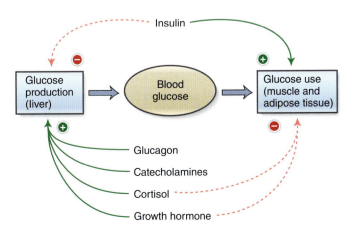

Figure 8-34. Integrated control of blood glucose concentration.

10. Somatostatin.
    a. Somatostatin is secreted by δ-cells in pancreatic islets in response to increased plasma nutrient levels.
    b. ▼ The physiological effect of pancreatic somatostatin is unclear but somatostatin agonists are used pharmacologically to:
        i. *Inhibit hormone secretion from **tumors** (e.g., insulinoma, glucagonoma, VIPoma, GH-secreting adenoma, etc.).*
        ii. *Manage **gastrointestinal bleeding** via vasoconstriction of splanchnic vessels.* ▼

11. Diabetes mellitus.
    a. *Diabetes mellitus causes hyperglycemia due either to inadequate insulin secretion or to insulin insensitivity.*
    b. ▼ **Hyperglycemia** causes widespread organ damage, and diabetes is the leading cause of blindness, nontraumatic lower extremity amputation, and end-stage renal disease. Diabetes-related abnormalities associated with lipid metabolism also result in the accelerated development of atherosclerosis. ▼
    c. *Type 1 diabetes results from β-cell destruction and is also referred to as insulin-dependent diabetes.* Type 1 diabetes:
        i. Only accounts for 5% of all diabetes cases.
        ii. Usually has an autoimmune cause.
        iii. *Is associated with ketoacidosis due to unopposed glucagon action.*
        iv. Results in a catabolic state.
    d. *Type 2 diabetes is caused by tissue insulin insensitivity and impaired β-cell response to glucose.*
        i. Insulin resistance parallels obesity in 90% of cases, especially **visceral obesity** (high waist circumference).
        ii. Inflammatory cytokines from adipose tissue induce insulin resistance.
        iii. Compensatory hyperinsulinemia is present in the early course of the disease.
        iv. *Type 2 diabetes is not usually associated with ketoacidosis* since there is some insulin action to oppose glucagon-stimulated hepatic ketogenesis.
        v. Progressive β-cell loss leads to insulin-dependence later in the disease.
    e. ▼ Type 2 diabetes is often associated with **metabolic syndrome,** defined as a cluster of three or more of the following objective findings:
        i. Abdominal obesity (waist circumference >40 inches in men, or >35 inches in women).
        ii. Plasma triglyceride >150 mg/dL.
        iii. HDL cholesterol <40 mg/dL in men or <50 mg/dL in women.
        iv. Systolic blood pressure >130 mm Hg or diastolic blood pressure >85 mm Hg.
        v. Fasting glucose >100 mg/dL. ▼
    f. Blood glucose testing.
        i. Normal fasting blood glucose concentration is 70–99 mg/dL.
        ii. 100–125 mg/dL alone indicates pre-diabetes.
        iii. *≥126 mg/dL is diagnostic for diabetes mellitus.*
        iv. *A random plasma glucose concentration ≥200 mg/dL indicates diabetes if the patient is experiencing the classic symptoms of diabetes:*
            • **Polyuria** and **polydipsia** due to osmotic diuresis from unreabsorbed glucose in the urine.

- Unintentional **weight loss** due to the catabolic state induced by the absence of insulin.

g. Glucose tolerance test (Figure 8-35).

  i. Serial blood samples are drawn before and after a fasting patient is given 75 g of an oral glucose solution.

  ii. *Diabetes is diagnosed if plasma glucose concentration ≥200 mg/dL after 2 hours.*

A. Normal

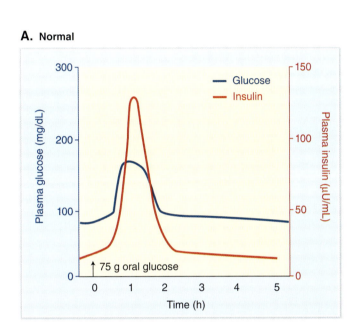

B. Type I diabetes mellitus

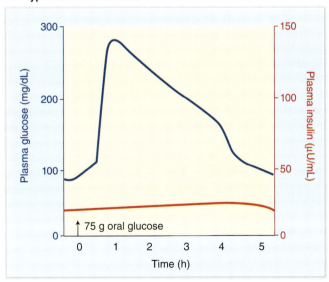

Figure 8-35. Glucose tolerance testing. **A.** In a normal fasting person, a 75-g oral glucose challenge produces an increase in the blood glucose concentration and an insulin secretion response during the first 2 hours after glucose ingestion. The resting blood glucose concentration is reestablished within 2 hours. **B.** Patients with type 1 diabetes mellitus do not secrete insulin in response to a glucose challenge. A plasma glucose concentration of ≥200 mg/dL more than 2 hours after glucose ingestion is diagnostic of diabetes mellitus. U, international insulin units.

   h. **Glycated hemoglobin A1C** is an indicator of glycemic control over the preceding 2–3 months.
      i. 4.0–5.6% = normal; 5.7–6.4% = pre-diabetes; >6.5% = diabetes.
      ii. *A treatment goal for patients with diabetes is maintaining HbA1C <7%.*

   i. ▼ Treatment of type 2 diabetes may include:
      i. Lifestyle change (exercise, diet, sleep, behavioral support, smoking cessation).
      ii. Insulin replacement as needed.
      iii. Biguanides (e.g., **metformin**) are first-line drugs and mainly act to decrease hepatic gluconeogenesis.
      iv. GLP-1 agonists or inhibitors of the enzyme **dipeptidyl peptidase 4 (DPP-4),** which degrades GLP-1. These agents promote physiologic incretin action to stimulate endogenous insulin secretion.
      v. Renal sodium-glucose cotransporter **(SGLT-2) inhibitors** to promote urinary glucose excretion.
      vi. **α-glucosidase inhibitors** of brush border enzymes in the small intestine to slow/decrease glucose digestion.
      vii. Thiazolidinediones activate the **nuclear peroxisome proliferator-activated receptor (PPAR)** to alter gene transcription of several targets that promote glucose disposal and improve lipid profile.
      viii. **Sulphonylureas** close K_{ATP} channels in β-cells and promote secretion of preformed insulin granules. ▼

Leptin

1. Leptin is a peptide hormone synthesized by adipocytes. Plasma levels vary in proportion to fat mass, giving rise to the concept of leptin as a "lipostat."
2. *Leptin functions as a long-term feedback control of body mass and acts on the hypothalamus to decrease appetite.*
3. ▼ Rare mutations in leptin or the leptin receptor cause severe obesity but *common obesity is a syndrome of **leptin resistance.*** ▼
4. Other effects of leptin include:
   a. Acting as a metabolic gate that signals adequate energy stores to **initiate puberty,** especially in females.
   b. Stimulating the sympathetic nervous system to increase energy expenditure. This is thought to contribute to **hypertension** in metabolic syndrome.

Hormones Regulating Calcium and Phosphate Balance

1. ***Parathyroid hormone (PTH)** and **vitamin D** are the main hormones that regulate Ca^{2+} and phosphate homeostasis.*
2. Ca^{2+} and phosphate balance are linked because they are both present in **hydroxyapatite** crystals in bone.
3. Ca^{2+} has many other critical functions, for example:
   a. Triggers muscle contraction.
   b. Triggers exocytosis.
   c. Is an intracellular second messenger.
   d. Modulates nerve excitability.
4. Key functions of phosphate are:
   a. Integral to DNA and RNA structure.

   b. Phosphate transfer reactions are the basis of cellular energy metabolism (e.g., ATP and ADP).

   c. Phosphorylation via kinases and dephosphorylation via phosphatases regulate protein function.

5. Ca^{2+} and phosphate balance (Figure 8-36).

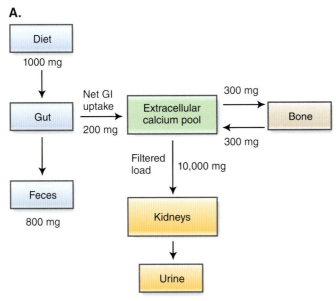

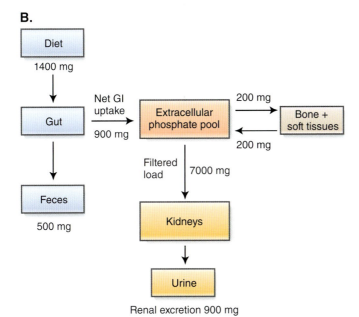

Figure 8-36. A. Normal daily Ca^{2+} balance. **B.** Normal daily phosphate balance. The normal Western diet includes a daily excess of Ca^{2+} and phosphate, which is only partially absorbed. Extracellular fluid contains a small proportion of total body Ca^{2+} and phosphate. In healthy adults, the net excretion of Ca^{2+} and phosphate by the renal system correlates with uptake from the diet. After growth has stopped, bone remodeling does not add or remove net Ca^{2+} or phosphate to or from the extracellular fluid. GI, gastrointestinal.

a. Inputs to and from the circulation must be balanced:

   i. *The inputs of Ca^{2+} and phosphate to the circulation are intestinal absorption plus resorption of bone.*

   ii. *Outputs of Ca^{2+} and phosphate from the circulation are renal excretion and bone formation.*

   iii. Bone is continuously remodeled with bone formation by **osteoblasts** and resorption by **osteoclasts.**

b. Ca^{2+} exists in three forms in plasma:

   i. Forty-five percent is **free ionized Ca^{2+}**. *The plasma concentration of free ionized Ca^{2+} is tightly regulated in the 1.0–1.3 mmol/L (4.0–5.2 mg/dL).*

   ii. Forty-five percent is **bound to plasma proteins,** particularly albumin.

   iii. Ten percent is **complexed with low-molecular-weight anions** such as citrate and oxalate.

   iv. ▼ *H^+ competes with Ca^{2+} for binding sites on albumin, resulting in increased free $[Ca^{2+}]$ in acidosis and decreased free $[Ca^{2+}]$ in alkalosis.* ▼

c. Phosphate occurs in two major forms in plasma: 80% is **alkaline phosphate (HPO_4^{2-})** and 20% is **acid phosphate ($H_2PO_4^-$).**

d. Plasma [phosphate] is less strictly regulated than Ca^{2+}, within the range of 0.8–1.5 mmol/L (2.5–4.5 mg/dL).

6. *PTH exerts dominant control of Ca^{2+} and phosphate homeostasis.* It is a peptide hormone that is:

a. Secreted from parathyroid gland **chief cells.**

b. Water soluble and circulates free in plasma.

c. Degraded by cleavage into smaller peptide fragments in the liver and by hydrolysis of the active N-terminal fragment in the kidney; its half-life is approximately 5 minutes.

7. Actions of PTH.

a. *PTH increases the free plasma Ca^{2+} concentration and decreases the plasma phosphate concentration.*

b. *PTH stimulates **bone resorption,*** which adds both Ca^{2+} and phosphate to plasma.

   i. PTH indirectly stimulates osteoclasts by stimulating osteoblasts to secrete a cytokine called the **RANK-ligand.**

   ii. ▼ Monoclonal antibodies against RANK-L are used to treat osteoporosis; the rate of organic bone matrix resorption can be assessed by measuring urinary excretion of **hydroxyproline.** ▼

c. *PTH decreases renal Ca^{2+} excretion,* due to stimulation of Ca^{2+} reabsorption in the thick ascending limb and the distal tubule of the nephron.

d. *PTH increases renal phosphate excretion,* due to the inhibition of phosphate reabsorption in the proximal renal tubule.

e. *The direct actions of PTH on Ca^{2+} cause an increase in the plasma $[Ca^{2+}]$.*

f. *The effect of PTH on phosphate is to cause movement of phosphate from bone to plasma and from plasma to urine, with the net effect of reducing the plasma [phosphate].*

g. PTH indirectly exerts more effects by also stimulating the final step in vitamin D synthesis (see Vitamin D).

8. The rate of PTH secretion is regulated by three factors (Figure 8-37):

a. *A decrease in the plasma free $[Ca^{2+}]$ is the most potent stimulus for PTH secretion.*

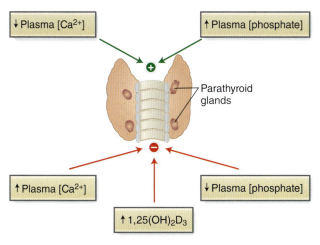

Figure 8-37. Regulation of parathyroid hormone secretion by plasma Ca^{2+} concentration, plasma phosphate concentration, and vitamin D. 1,25-$(OH)_2D_3$, 1,25 dihydroxycholecalciferol.

     i. Changes in plasma free $[Ca^{2+}]$ are detected by chief cells via the G-protein coupled **extracellular calcium-sensing receptor.**
  b. Increased plasma **phosphate concentration** stimulates PTH secretion.
  c. **Vitamin D** inhibits PTH secretion.
9. Vitamin D.
  a. Vitamin D is present in the body as **vitamin D$_2$ (ergocalciferol)** and **vitamin D$_3$ (cholecalciferol).**
  b. Cholecalciferol is a **fat-soluble vitamin** available from the diet or it may be synthesized from **7-dehydrocholesterol** in the skin in response to **ultraviolet light** exposure (Figure 8-38).
  c. Cholecalciferol is a precursor molecule that is modified to become the main active hormone **1,25-dihydroxycholecalciferol,** which is sometimes referred to as **1,25$(OH)_2D_3$,** or **calcitriol.**
    i. Hydroxylation of cholecalciferol at the 25 position occurs in the liver and is not regulated.
    ii. *Activation of vitamin D is completed by 1-hydroxylation in the kidney that is stimulated by PTH.*
    iii. ▼ Patients with **chronic renal failure** are often deficient in vitamin D because the diseased kidneys are unable to sufficiently convert inactive vitamin D to its active form. ▼
  d. *The major effect of vitamin D is stimulation of dietary Ca^{2+} and phosphate absorption in the small intestine (and to a lesser extent in the kidney).*
  e. The actions of vitamin D are mediated through an **intracellular receptor** and by alterations in gene transcription.
10. **Calcitonin.**
  a. Calcitonin is a peptide hormone secreted by the thyroid gland from parafollicular cells (thyroid C cells) in response to hypercalcemia.
  b. Calcitonin opposes the effects of PTH to reduce plasma Ca^{2+} by decreasing bone resorption by osteoclasts and increasing urinary Ca^{2+} excretion.
  c. ▼ *In humans, calcitonin has weak effects of Ca^{2+} homeostasis,* and neither the absence nor the excess of calcitonin causes a clinical defect in Ca^{2+} or phosphate homeostasis. However, it does have clinical applications:

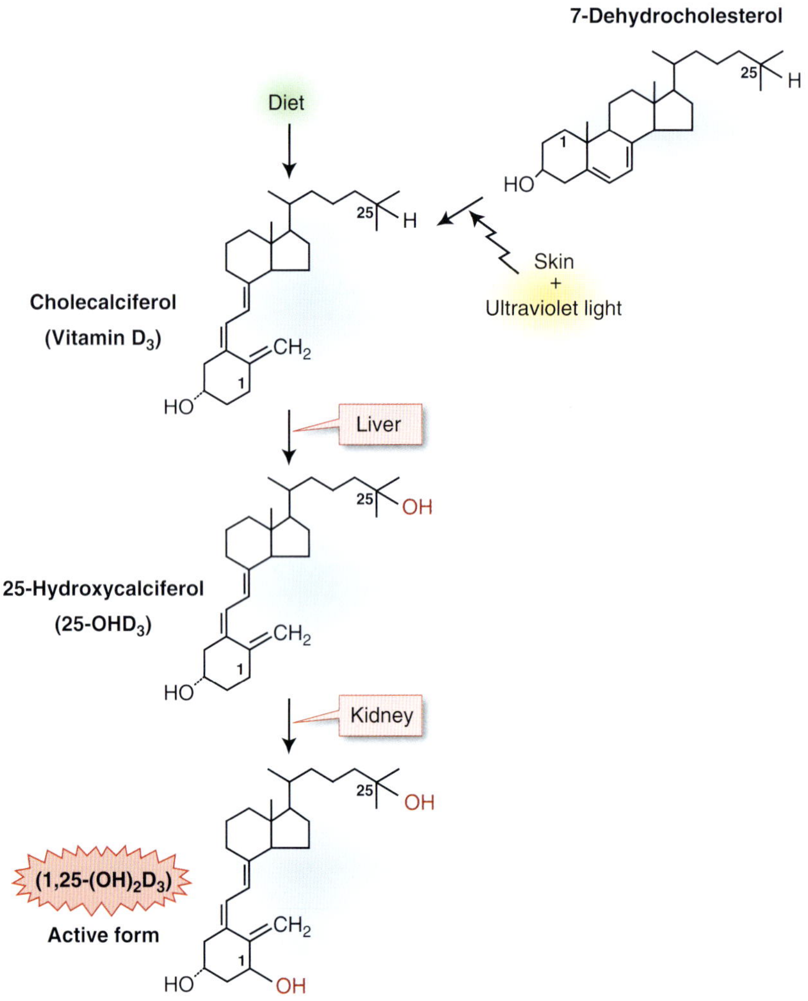

Figure 8-38. Synthesis and activation of vitamin D (cholecalciferol). Vitamin D is supplied from the diet and by synthesis from cholesterol-based precursors in the skin. Activation of vitamin D occurs in two stages: 25-hydroxylation in the liver (not regulated) and 1-hydroxylation in the kidney (stimulated by parathyroid hormone and hypophosphatemia).

   i. Calcitonin is a tumor marker for medullary thyroid cancer, which derives from thyroid C cells.
   ii. Calcitonin can be used as an adjunctive therapy in hypercalcemia and in **Paget's disease** of the bone. Additionally, the use of calcitonin as a therapy is a classic example of **tachyphylaxis,** the development of rapid tolerance to drugs following repeated administration. ▼

11. Phosphotonins.
   a. **Phosphotonins** are hormones released from bone in response to excess phosphate that in turn increase urinary phosphate excretion to create a **bone-renal axis** for phosphate regulation.
   b. *Fibroblast growth factor-23 (**FGF-23**) is the main phosphotonin.*
   c. FGF-23 decreases renal phosphate reabsorption and inhibits activation of vitamin D to suppress intestinal phosphate absorption.
   d. ▼ Genetic defects resulting in excess of FGF-23 cause phosphate wasting and bone deformities in children. An example is **autosomal-dominant**

hypophosphatemic rickets, which is caused by mutations in FGF-23 that make it resistant to breakdown. Other X-linked inheritance patterns occur for genes regulating FGF-23 expression. ▼

12. Integrated control of Ca^{2+} and phosphate balance.

   a. Ca^{2+} and phosphate are poorly soluble when they are present together in solution.

   b. The opposing actions of PTH to mobilize Ca^{2+} and increase phosphate excretion are important to prevent an excessive Ca^{2+} and phosphate ion product and precipitation of Ca^{2+}-phosphate crystals, known as **metastatic calcification.**

   c. *In general, the control of plasma $[Ca^{2+}]$ is dominant over the control of plasma [phosphate].*

13. Bone mineralization is a circumstance when both Ca^{2+} and phosphate are required together and is promoted by vitamin D:

   a. Vitamin D makes both ions available for bone formation through its actions on the gut and kidney.

   b. Vitamin D also suppresses PTH secretion, which would otherwise oppose bone formation.

   c. ▼ A **deficiency of vitamin D** during childhood causes a bone deformity called **rickets,** which is due to the poor mineralization of bone (Figure 8-39). **Osteomalacia** is the adult equivalent and increases risk of fractures. ▼

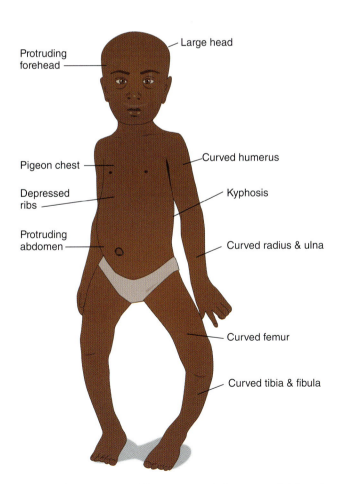

Figure 8-39. Bone deformities caused by vitamin D deficiency in childhood.

14. Vitamin D toxicity is caused by overdosing with supplements and causes hypercalcemia.

15. Response to hypocalcemia (Figure 8-40).

   a. **Hypocalcemia** stimulates PTH secretion, which in turn stimulates the production of $1,25\text{-}(OH)_2D_3$.

   b. To return the plasma Ca^{2+} concentration to normal, bone resorption and intestinal Ca^{2+} absorption increase and urinary Ca^{2+} excretion decreases.

   c. Bone resorption due to increased PTH concentration produces an unwanted phosphate input into the plasma; increased $1,25\text{-}(OH)_2D_3$ causes further addition of phosphate to plasma through increased intestinal absorption. *An increase in plasma phosphate concentration is prevented because PTH simultaneously increases urinary phosphate excretion.*

   d. ▼ *Hypocalcemia causes instability of membrane potentials, neuronal hyperexcitability, and muscle tetanus.*

      i. **Hypocalcemic tetany** can be assessed clinically by attempting to elicit either **Chvostek's sign** or **Trousseau's sign.**

      ii. Chvostek's sign is a facial spasm induced by tapping over the facial nerve just anterior to the ear.

      iii. Trousseau's sign is induction of carpal spasms by occluding the brachial artery for up to 3 minutes using a blood pressure cuff. ▼

16. Response to hypercalcemia.

   a. **Hypercalcemia** directly decreases PTH secretion and thereby decreases activation of vitamin D. As a result, plasma calcium is decreased by:

      i. Shifting the balance of bone turnover toward net bone formation.

      ii. Increasing urinary Ca^{2+} excretion.

      iii. Decreasing intestinal Ca^{2+} absorption.

   b. ▼ The phrase "bones, stones, moans, groans, and psychiatric overtones" indicates potential signs and symptoms of hypercalcemia: **bones**—bone pain; **stones**—kidney stones; **moans**—abdominal pains associated with

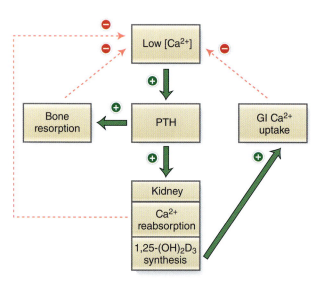

Figure 8-40. Integrated responses to hypocalcemia. PTH, parathyroid hormone; GI, gastrointestinal; $1,25\text{-}(OH)_2D_3$, 1,25 dihydroxycholecalciferol.

constipation or pancreatitis; **groans**—general malaise and weakness; **psychiatric overtones**—depression, delirium, and coma. ▼

17. Responses to hyperphosphatemia (Figure 8-41).

   a. **Hyperphosphatemia** directly stimulates PTH secretion, which together with phosphotonins increases urinary phosphate excretion.

   b. *Note: Hyperphosphatemia reduces the production of 1,25-(OH)$_2$D$_3$ independently of PTH. This is necessary to prevent increased PTH from activating vitamin D,* which would otherwise increase intestinal phosphate absorption.

18. Responses to hypophosphatemia.

   a. PTH secretion decreases and 1,25-(OH)$_2$D$_3$ production increases.

   b. As a result, the rate of urinary phosphate excretion decreases and dietary phosphate absorption increases until hypophosphatemia is corrected.

19. Disorders of PTH secretion and vitamin D production (Table 8-5).

   a. **Primary hyperparathyroidism** is an uncontrolled increase in PTH secretion that is most commonly caused by a solitary parathyroid adenoma.

      i. The clinical manifestations of primary hyperparathyroidism are due to the direct actions of PTH as well as to the high levels of 1,25-(OH)$_2$D$_3$, which are produced in response to PTH.

      ii. *Plasma [Ca^{2+}] is increased and plasma [phosphate] is reduced.*

      iii. Increased plasma [Ca^{2+}] is the result of increased bone resorption and increased intestinal Ca^{2+} absorption.

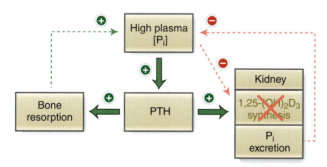

Figure 8-41. Integrated responses to hyperphosphatemia. PTH, parathyroid hormone; 1,25-(OH)$_2$D$_3$, 1,25 dihydroxycholecalciferol.

Table 8-5. Pathophysiology of Parathyroid Hormone (PTH)

Endocrine Disorder	PTH	1, 25-(OH)$_2$D$_3$	Plasma [Ca^{2+}]	Plasma [Phosphate]
Primary hyperparathyroidism	↑	↑	↑	↓
Humoral hypercalcemia of malignancy	↓	↑	↑	↓
Secondary hyperparathyroidism of chronic renal failure	↑	↓	↓	↑
Primary hypoparathyroidism	↓	↓	↓	↑
Pseudohypoparathyroidism	↑	↓	↓	↑

   iv. *Note: Despite the stimulation of renal tubular Ca^{2+} reabsorption by PTH, increased plasma $[Ca^{2+}]$ results in increased glomerular filtration of Ca^{2+} and often gives rise to the confusing finding of increased urinary calcium excretion (**hypercalciuria**) in hyperparathyroidism.*

   v. Decreased plasma [phosphate] is caused by increased urinary phosphate loss.

b. **Humoral hypercalcemia of malignancy** occurs in some cancers (e.g., squamous cell carcinoma of the lung) due to the secretion of **PTH-related peptide (PTH-rP)** by tumor cells.

   i. PTH-rP has the same actions as PTH; therefore, patients develop increased plasma $[Ca^{2+}]$ and decreased [phosphate].

   ii. *Note: PTH concentration is low because secretion is suppressed by negative feedback from the high plasma $[Ca^{2+}]$.*

c. **Secondary hyperparathyroidism** often complicates end-stage renal disease.

   i. Chronic renal failure causes inadequate renal phosphate excretion, which results in increased plasma [phosphate].

   ii. PTH secretion is stimulated by increased plasma [phosphate], accounting for secondary hyperparathyroidism.

   iii. *High PTH levels often result in bone demineralization in chronic renal disease, called **renal osteodystrophy.***

   iv. The levels of $1,25\text{-}(OH)_2D_3$ are low because of reduced functional renal mass.

d. **Primary hypoparathyroidism** is most commonly caused by surgical removal of the glands.

   i. The effects are the opposite of those described above for primary hyperparathyroidism; plasma $[Ca^{2+}]$ is decreased and [phosphate] is increased.

e. **Pseudohypoparathyroidism** is caused by a defective G protein in the kidney and bone that produces tissue resistance to PTH.

   i. Patients present with low plasma $[Ca^{2+}]$ and high [phosphate] because the normal tissue responses to PTH do not occur.

   ii. *PTH levels are high due to hypocalcemia but tissue resistance to PTH prevents a physiological response.*

20. Sex steroids and bone.

a. The sex steroids estradiol (in females) and testosterone (in males) are required for maintenance of normal bone mass.

b. *In postmenopausal women, there is a marked decline in estradiol levels, which is associated with a loss of bone mass, called **osteoporosis,** and a corresponding increase in bone fractures.*

c. Osteoporosis is less common in males due to a smaller and more gradual decline in testosterone levels with age.

d. ▼ *Fragility fractures associated with osteoporosis are a major cause of morbidity and mortality.* Characteristic fragility fractures occur in the vertebrae, hips, and distal radius (Colles' fracture). Hip fractures are associated with a 20% mortality rate, and about 50% of surviving patients have permanent disability. ▼

Introduction to the Hypothalamic-Pituitary-Gonadal Endocrine Axis

1. Sex steroids are essential for the differentiation and maintenance of the reproductive system (see Chapter 9).
2. There are three classes of sex steroids (Figure 8-42):
    a. **Progestins** are primarily female sex steroids. They prepare the uterine endometrium for implantation of a fertilized ovum and promote the development of the placenta and breasts during pregnancy. *The major progestin in the circulation is* **progesterone.**
    b. **Estrogens** play a major role in puberty in girls and in the menstrual (ovarian) cycle. Natural estrogens include **estrone (E$_1$), estradiol (E$_2$), and estriol (E$_3$).** *Estradiol is the major estrogen that is secreted from the ovaries during the ovarian cycle.*
    c. **Androgens** are the main sex steroids in males. *The major circulating androgen is testosterone, which is produced by the Leydig cells in the testes.*
        i. Testosterone is converted to **dihydrotestosterone** within target tissues, via the enzyme **5α-reductase.**
        ii. Adrenal androgens have weak direct effects but function as circulating precursors for conversion to active androgens in target tissues.
3. Production of sex steroids from the gonads is controlled by gonadotropins.
    a. Anterior pituitary gonadotrope cells secrete **LH** and **FSH.**
    b. In early pregnancy an LH-analog, **human chorionic gonadotropin (hCG),** is secreted by the developing placenta to maintain ovarian steroid production (see Chapter 9).
    c. LH and FSH secretion are under the control of the hypothalamic neurohormone **GnRH.**

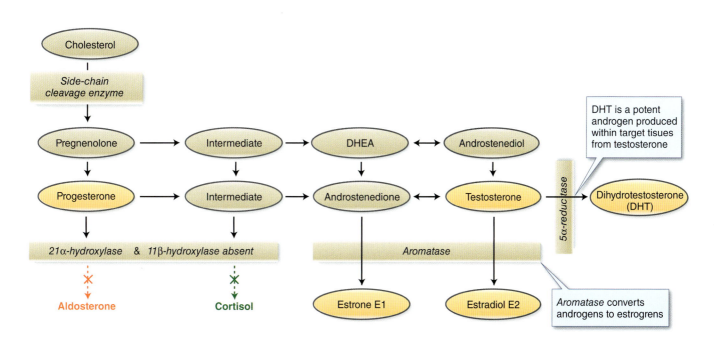

Figure 8-42. Gonadal synthesis of sex steroids. DHEA, dehydroepiandrosterone.

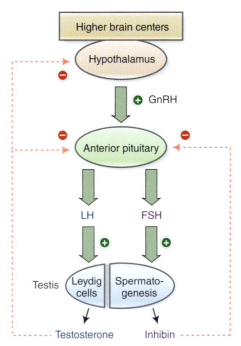

Figure 8-43. Hypothalamic-pituitary-gonadal axis in the male. LH, luteinizing hormone; FSH, follicle-stimulating hormone.

    d. *Pulsatile secretion of GnRH is necessary to maintain the stimulation of gonadotropes;* continuously applied GnRH downregulates LH and FSH secretion.

    e. Hierarchical negative feedback operates to control production of sex steroids. For example:

      i. In the mature male reproductive system, the effects of FSH and LH result in the secretion of testosterone and the production of sperm cells.

      ii. Testosterone feeds back to inhibit the secretion of FSH, LH, and GnRH.

      iii. FSH stimulates secretion of **inhibins** from Sertoli cells in the testis, which also exert negative feedback, specifically on FSH secretion (Figure 8-43).

      iv. See Chapter 9 for details of the hypothalamic-pituitary-gonadal axis in females.

Study Questions

Directions: Each numbered item is followed by lettered options. Some options may be partially correct, but there is only *ONE BEST* answer.

1. Analogues of guanosine triphosphate (GTP) such as GTP-γ-S can be used to activate G proteins in isolated cells. Which of the following signaling molecules would NOT be produced in response to GTP-γ-S?

    A. Arachidonic acid

    B. Cyclic adenosine monophosphate (cAMP)

    C. Diacylglycerol (DAG)

    D. Inositol 1,4,5-triphosphate (IP$_3$)

    E. Tyrosine kinase

2. A 28-year-old woman suffered severe trauma to the head in a horseback riding accident that resulted in the complete transection of the pituitary stalk. The plasma levels of which hormone would be expected to increase as a result of this accident?

   A. Adrenocorticotropic hormone
   B. Follicle-stimulating hormone
   C. Growth hormone
   D. Luteinizing hormone
   E. Oxytocin
   F. Prolactin
   G. Thyroid-stimulating hormone
   H. Vasopressin

3. A 4-year-old boy was diagnosed with visual disturbances due to a pituitary tumor secreting excess growth hormone. Which of the following conditions would this boy most likely develop without treatment?

   A. Acromegaly due directly to excess growth hormone
   B. Acromegaly due to excess insulin-like growth factor (IGF)-1 production
   C. Dwarfism due directly to excess growth hormone
   D. Dwarfism due to excess IGF-1 production
   E. Gigantism due directly to excess growth hormone
   F. Gigantism due to excess IGF-1 production

4. A 58-year-old woman complained of lethargy and weight gain over the ast year. Further investigation revealed a painless goiter, thick coarse skin, peripheral edema, and low iodine levels. Which of the following most likely describes this patient's diagnosis and plasma thyroid-stimulating hormone (TSH) level?

   A. Primary hyperthyroidism, high TSH
   B. Primary hyperthyroidism, normal TSH
   C. Primary hyperthyroidism, low TSH
   D. Primary hypothyroidism, high TSH
   E. Primary hypothyroidism, normal TSH
   F. Primary hypothyroidism, low TSH

5. A 42-year-old man visited his physician with a complaint that he was always tired. He described craving salty foods and feeling lightheaded after missing lunch. Physical examination shows a blood pressure of 100/70 mm Hg. Laboratory studies show a decreased plasma $[Na^+]$, increased plasma $[K^+]$, and decreased fasting plasma [glucose]. Over the past several months, he said that his skin had become tanned despite avoiding sun exposure. The physician suspected that the patient's adrenal gland was not functioning properly. Which profile of cortisol and adrenocorticotropic hormone (ACTH) levels are consistent with the symptoms described?

   A. High cortisol, high ACTH
   B. High cortisol, low ACTH
   C. Low cortisol, high ACTH
   D. Low cortisol, low ACTH

6. A genetically female infant was born with ambiguous genitalia. She remained in the hospital because of continual urinary salt and water losses during the first week of life. The differential diagnosis of 21α-hydroxylase deficiency would be supported by determining which of the following hormonal plasma profiles?

	Cortisol	Aldosterone	Adrenal Androgens	ACTH
A.	Low	Low	Low	Low
B.	Low	Low	High	High
C.	High	High	Low	Low
D.	High	High	High	High
E.	Low	Low	Low	High
F.	High	High	High	Low

7. A 22-year-old man was treated with a selective β_2-adrenoceptor agonist. Which of the following effects is expected to occur?

   A. Generalized vasoconstriction
   B. Increased gut motility
   C. Increased heart rate
   D. Reduced airway resistance
   E. Penile erection

8. A 28-year-old man with type 1 diabetes mellitus self-administered his routine insulin injection. Which of the following effects on plasma concentrations of glucose, fatty acids, and ketones would be expected 1 hour after insulin treatment compared with 1 hour before insulin treatment?

   A. ↑ glucose, ↑ fatty acids, ↑ ketones
   B. ↑ glucose, ↓ fatty acids, ↑ ketones
   C. ↑ glucose, ↓ fatty acids, ↓ ketones
   D. ↓ glucose, ↑ fatty acids, ↑ ketones
   E. ↓ glucose, ↓ fatty acids, ↑ increased ketones
   F. ↓ glucose, ↓ fatty acids, ↓ ketones

9. A 58-year-old man presented to his physician feeling generally unwell and complaining of excessive urination and thirst. He was morbidly obese. The urinalysis showed glycosuria and proteinuria but no ketonuria. Which of the following conditions is most consistent with these findings?

   A. Acromegaly
   B. Central diabetes insipidus
   C. Nephrogenic diabetes insipidus
   D. Primary hypothyroidism
   E. Type 1 diabetes mellitus
   F. Type 2 diabetes mellitus

10. A patient is found to have a rare genetic defect in a G protein that causes tissue resistance to parathyroid hormone (PTH) in kidney and bone. Which of the following profiles for plasma Ca^{2+}, phosphate (P), and PTH concentration would be expected in this patient?

	Plasma [Ca^{2+}]	Plasma [P]	Plasma PTH
A.	Low	Low	Low
B.	Low	Low	High
C.	Low	High	High
D.	High	High	High
E.	High	High	Low
F.	High	Low	Low

Reproductive Physiology

CHAPTER 9

Sexual Differentiation

1. Anatomic differentiation into male or female occurs in utero, but the final maturation of fully functional reproductive organs is not completed until puberty.
2. The complement of sex chromosomes determines sexual differentiation.
   a. Female gametes (**oocytes**) all have a 22X chromosomal makeup, whereas male gametes (**spermatozoa**) are either 22X or 22Y.
   b. *The **chromosomal sex** of the fetus is determined at fertilization when the male and female gametes combine; XX is female and XY is male.*
3. *The default **phenotypic sex** of the fetus is female if it does not have a Y chromosome.*
   a. The presence of a Y chromosome directs the undifferentiated gonad to become a testis rather than an ovary.
   b. A single gene (*SRY*), located in the **sex-determining region** of the Y chromosome, produces **testis-determining factor** that is required for male sexual differentiation.
4. Before sexual differentiation, the fetus has two parallel duct systems located near the undifferentiated gonads: the **mesonephric (Wolffian) duct** and the **paramesonephric (Müllerian) duct** (Figure 9-1).
   a. By week 10 of gestation, the fetal gonads can be distinguished as either **testes** or **ovaries.**
   b. In **males,** the primordial germ cells give rise to precursors of male gametes called **spermatogonia.**
      i. The germinal epithelium that will later produce male gametes is formed by spermatogonia plus support cells called **Sertoli cells.**
      ii. The surrounding mesenchyme becomes **Leydig cells,** which secrete testosterone.
   c. In **females,** the primordial germ cells give rise to precursors of female gametes called **oogonia.**
      i. The epithelium surrounding the oogonia differentiates into **granulosa cells,** and the surrounding ovarian mesenchyme becomes **thecal cells.**
      ii. In the sexually mature female, estrogens and progestins are secreted by the granulosa and theca cells.
5. *Differentiation of the genitalia depends only on the presence or absence of hormones secreted by the testes.*
   a. In the male fetus, the secretion of testosterone by Leydig cells directs each mesonephric duct to develop into an **epididymis,** a **vas deferens,** and a **seminal vesicle.**
   b. Leydig cells produce testosterone in response to the hormone human chorionic gonadotropin (hCG), which is secreted by the placenta.

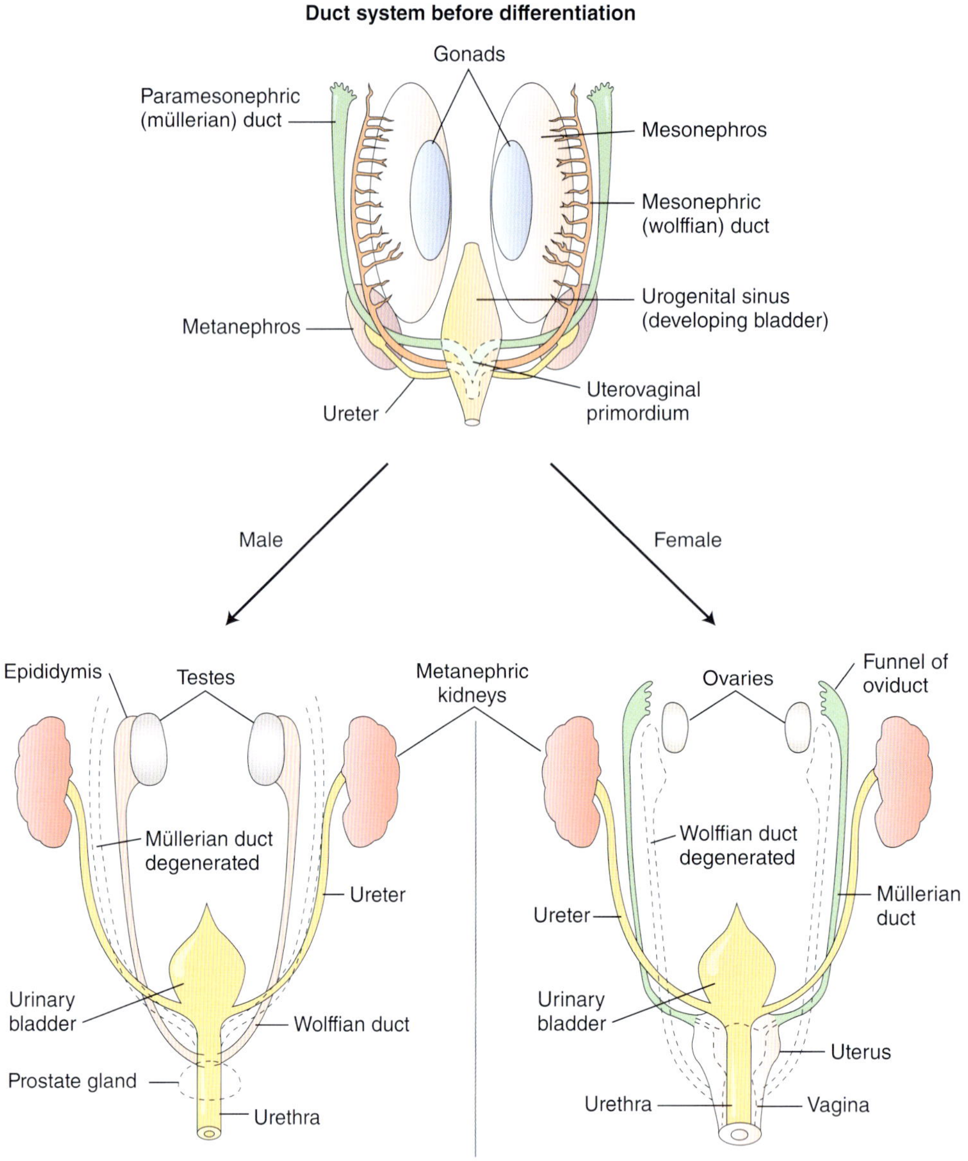

Duct system before differentiation

Figure 9-1. Differentiation of the internal reproductive organs. The mesonephric (Wolffian) and paramesonephric (Müllerian) duct systems of the early embryo run lateral to the undifferentiated fetal gonad. Secretion of testosterone in the male fetus results in the development of the mesonephric duct into the male reproductive organs; secretion of Müllerian-inhibiting substance by the Sertoli cells produces regression of the paramesonephric ducts. In the female fetus, the absence of testosterone allows the paramesonephric ducts to develop into the female reproductive organs and results in degeneration of the mesonephric ducts.

    c. The developing Sertoli cells are directed by *SRY* to secrete **Müllerian-inhibiting substance,** causing regression of the Müllerian duct system.

    d. The absence of the Müllerian-inhibiting substance in the female fetus allows the Müllerian duct system (instead of the Wolffian duct) to develop, leading to formation of the **fallopian tubes,** the **uterus,** and the **upper vagina.**

    e. *Fetal ovaries are not necessary for the development of the female genitalia* due to the high concentration of maternal estrogens that are present during pregnancy.

  6. Undifferentiated external genitalia consist of a genital tubercle and a urogenital slit, bounded by two lateral genital folds and two labioscrotal swellings (Figure 9-2).

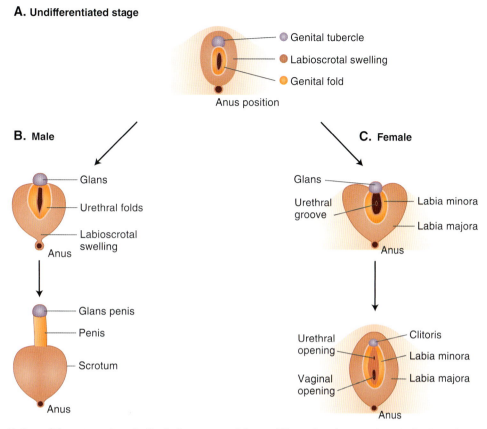

Figure 9-2. Differentiation of the external genitalia. **A.** Structures of the undifferentiated external genitalia. **B.** In the male fetus, fusion of the genital folds creates the penis, and fusion of the labioscrotal swellings forms the scrotum. **C.** In the female fetus, the genital folds do not fuse, allowing the vagina and urethra to open between the labia minora; the labia majora are formed from the labioscrotal swellings.

a. In males, the conversion of testosterone to **dihydrotestosterone,** via the enzyme **5α-reductase** within these target tissues, is necessary for formation of the **prostate gland** and the **male external genitalia.**

   i. The genital folds fuse to form the **penis;** the enlargement and fusion of the labioscrotal swellings form the **scrotum.**

   ii. *Descent of the fetal testes into the scrotum requires the secretion of the fetal gonadotropins and occurs during the last trimester of pregnancy.*

   iii. ▼ **Cryptorchidism** is the incomplete descent of the testis from the abdominal cavity to the scrotum and is associated with testicular malignancy and infertility. *In the setting of unilateral cryptorchidism, the fully descended testis may remain at risk of impaired sperm production or of becoming malignant.* ▼

b. In females, the urogenital slit remains open to form the **introitus** (vaginal opening).

   i. The **labia minora** are formed from the genital folds, and the **clitoris** forms anterior to the urethral opening.

   ii. The **labia majora** are formed from the labioscrotal swellings. *Exposure of the female fetus to androgens at this critical time of sexual differentiation can result in **masculinization** of the fetus, irrespective of the genetic or gonadal sex.*

      iii. ▼ **Virilization** of a fetus refers to a genetic female with normal ovaries and Müllerian duct structures (e.g., fallopian tubes, uterus, and upper vagina), but with masculinization of the external genitalia (e.g., clitoromegaly, fusion of the labioscrotal folds) due to excessive in utero exposure to androgens. ▼

7. Differences in sexual development (DSD).
   a. There are several conditions in which gonadal and phenotypic sex differ.
   b. **Complete androgen insensitivity syndrome (CAIS)** results from the lack of functional androgen receptors and illustrates the role of steroids in sexual differentiation, as follows:
      i. CAIS patients are 46 XY DSD. The gonads become testes since the Y chromosome is present; the testes remain undescended.
      ii. **Müllerian-inhibiting substance** continues to be secreted from the Sertoli cells, resulting in the absence of the female internal genitalia. Patients have a short, blind-ended vagina without a cervix, uterus, or ovaries.
      iii. **Dihydrotestosterone** is made but cannot direct the Wolffian duct to develop into male genitalia due to lack of androgen receptors; individuals have female external genitalia.
      iv. **Masculinization does not occur during puberty** because of the lack of testosterone action. Conversion of testosterone to estrogen causes breast development at puberty instead, but there is only a small amount of pubic hair. *Diagnosis is often determined following failure of the onset of the menstrual cycle.*
   c. **Deficiency of 5α-reductase** is another example of 46 XY DSD and causes ambiguous genitalia because it interferes with the conversion of testosterone to dihydrotestosterone.
      i. Testosterone is present but is a weaker androgen than DHT leading to varying degrees of failure of the genital and labioscrotal folds to close.
      ii. *Masculinization at puberty can occur because androgen receptors are present and respond to testosterone, distinguishing this condition from CAIS.*
   d. **Congenital adrenal hyperplasia (CAH)** is the most common reason for ambiguous genitalia in 46 XX DSD individuals.
      i. Deficiency of the enzyme **21-hydroxylase** in the steroid synthesis pathway is the most common cause of CAH and results in excessive production of adrenal androgens and virilization of a female fetus.
8. Puberty (Figure 9-3).
   a. Puberty is the final stage in the process of sexual differentiation and results in the mature individual, with the development of physical and behavioral attributes that allow reproduction.
   b. **Adrenarche** is the stage of maturation when the contribution of the adrenal glands occurs before the visible onset of puberty, with increased secretion of adrenal androgens in both males and females.
      i. *Adrenarche occurs at around 6–8 years of age and is independent of adrenocorticotropic hormone (ACTH) or gonadotropins.*
      ii. Increasing levels of the adrenal androgens initiate axillary and pubic hair growth.
   c. Puberty begins with activation of the gonadotropin-releasing hormone **(GnRH) pulse generator** within the hypothalamus.

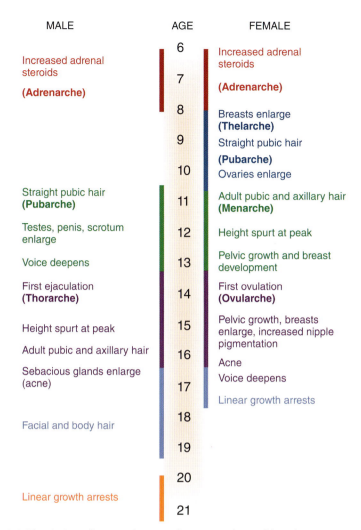

Figure 9-3. The timing of events during puberty in males and females.

i. The peptide neurotransmitter **Kisspeptin** stimulates GnRH neurons.

ii. **Leptin** is among the factors that stimulate Kisspeptin, especially in females, to signal adequate metabolic capacity for reproduction.

iii. The early stages of puberty are characterized by an increase in the pulsatile secretion of luteinizing hormone (LH) and follicle-stimulating hormone (FSH), which occurs during sleep.

d. In females, visible puberty begins between *8 and 10 years of age,* with breast enlargement (**thelarche**).

e. *The first menstrual cycle (**menarche**) usually occurs between the ages of 11 and 14 years (median age 12.4 years).*

f. **Female secondary sexual characteristics** develop over 2–3 years, mainly in response to increasing ovarian estrogen secretion, and include:

   i. **Breast development** characterized by growth of the lactiferous duct system and deposition of fat. *Final differentiation and development of the breast only occurs in pregnancy.*

   ii. Growth of pubic and axillary hair.

   iii. Enlargement of the uterus, the clitoris, and the labia, and keratinization of the vaginal mucosa.

   iv. Widening of the pelvis and deposition of fat on the hips and thighs.

g. Establishment of the monthly **ovarian cycle** requires progressive maturation of the hypothalamic-pituitary-ovarian axis:

   i. FSH and LH secretion increase.

   ii. Ovarian steroid secretion occurs in response to FSH and LH.

   iii. A midcycle positive feedback response to estrogen develops, causing an **LH surge** that initiates ovulation.

   iv. *Initial menstrual cycles may be anovulatory and are often irregular as the hormonal axis matures.*

h. Puberty visibly begins in **males** between *9 and 14 years of age,* with enlargement of the testes.

   i. The first ejaculation (**thorarche**) occurs between the ages of 12 and 14 years.

   ii. The testes increase in size and undergo maturation, involving secretion of testosterone by Leydig cells and **spermatogenesis** in the seminiferous tubules.

      • ▼ *Enlargement of the testes in puberty results from FSH secretion and can be used as a clinical indicator of normal function in the developing hypothalamic-pituitary axis.* ▼

   iii. The **scrotum** and **penis** enlarge.

   iv. **Secondary sexual characteristics** develop with increasing testosterone levels and include increases in:

      • Hair on the axilla, face, trunk, and pubis.

      • Bone mass.

      • Mass and strength of skeletal muscle.

      • Size of the larynx with associated deepening of the voice.

i. Pubertal growth spurt.

   i. Somatic growth is primarily controlled by the **growth hormone (GH)–insulin-like growth factor-1 (IGF-1) endocrine axis.**

   ii. Increased LH and FSH secretion at the beginning of puberty occurs together with increased GH secretion.

   iii. *The increase in GH secretion is caused by increasing estrogen levels in both sexes*; in males, estrogen is produced from testosterone via the enzyme **aromatase.**

   iv. The highest rates of GH secretion occur during puberty because the strength of negative feedback inhibition of GH secretion by IGF-1 is weak. *After puberty, the rate of GH production declines with age.*

j. Linear growth is completed in females by about age 17 and in males by about age 21. On average, men are 10–15 cm taller than women because:

   i. Growth during the pubertal growth spurt is more rapid in males than in females.

   ii. Puberty occurs later in males, allowing about 2 additional years of prepubertal growth before closure of the epiphyseal growth plates in long bones, *which occurs in response to sex steroids.*

k. ▼ **Precocious puberty** refers to early pubertal development, often before 8 years of age in girls and before 9 years of age in boys. In addition to early sexual maturation there is increased linear growth and skeletal maturation. *Children who experience precocious puberty are often tall for their age during childhood, but short for their age during adulthood.* ▼

l. ▼ Several genetic abnormalities cause delayed or absent puberty:

    i. Females with **Turner syndrome (45 XO)** lack one of their X-chromosomes and have rudimentary "streak" ovaries. There is phenotypic female sexual differentiation in utero but the inability to undergo puberty without hormone therapy.

    ii. Males with **Kleinfelter syndrome (47 XXY)** have an additional X chromosome, resulting in small testes and low testosterone levels. Puberty is often delayed or incomplete.

    iii. **Kallmann syndrome** is a gene (not chromosomal) defect, which leads to lack of GnRH neurons. The condition is more common in males due to X-linked inheritance of one of the causative genes. The syndrome causes **hypogonadotropic hypogonadism.** *Patients with Kallmann syndrome also have decreased or absent sense of smell (anosmia).* ▼

Male Reproductive Physiology

1. The male organs of reproduction include the paired testes, epididymis, vas deferens and seminal vesicles, and the prostate gland and penis (Figure 9-4A).

2. The paired **testes** are located outside the abdominal cavity, in the scrotum. The two major functions of the testes are:

    a. Testosterone secretion by Leydig cells.

    b. **Spermatogenesis** (production of spermatozoa), which occurs in numerous coiled tubes called seminiferous tubules.

        i. The testes are located outside the abdominal cavity within the scrotum and are maintained at a temperature about 2°C below normal body temperature, which is necessary for spermatogenesis to occur. *Spermatogenesis is strongly inhibited by heat.*

3. The epididymis and the vas deferens.

    a. The ducts of the seminiferous tubules exit the testis and converge to form a comma-shaped structure that lies behind the testis, called the **epididymis.**

    b. The duct of the epididymis is a single, highly coiled tube, about 6-m long. It is formed from the convergence of the seminiferous tubules at the upper pole of the testis.

    c. The tail of the epididymis is continuous with the **vas deferens** at the lower pole of the testis. *Final maturation of spermatozoa occurs during their storage in the epididymis.*

    d. The **vas deferens** is a muscular tube that expels spermatozoa to the urethra during **ejaculation.**

        i. The vas deferens passes up behind the testis, enters the abdomen via the inguinal canal, and follows a course around the abdominal and pelvic walls.

        ii. The vas deferens terminates by joining the duct of the seminal vesicle to form the **ejaculatory duct.**

        iii. The ejaculatory ducts on each side pierce the prostate gland and empty into the first portion of the urethra, just below the bladder.

        iv. *During ejaculation, spermatozoa combine with secretions from the seminal vesicles.*

    e. ▼ **Cystic fibrosis** affects the lungs and pancreas and also the genitourinary tract. *More than 95% of males diagnosed with cystic fibrosis have azoospermia*

A.

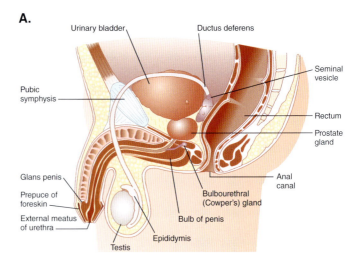

B.

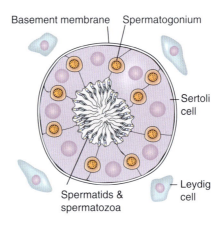

Figure 9-4. The anatomy of the male reproductive system. **A.** Midline vertical section showing the pathway taken by the vas deferens via the inguinal canal into the pelvis. Sperm from the testis and seminal plasma from the seminal vesicles and prostate gland are delivered into the prostatic part of the urethra during emission and are ejected from the penile urethra at ejaculation. **B.** Microscopic appearance of a single seminiferous tubule within the testis. Cells of the spermatogenic series, seen inside the tubule, are associated with the Sertoli cells. Steroid-secreting Leydig cells are located between the seminiferous tubules.

due to obliteration of the vas deferens by thick tenacious fluid secretions. Approximately 20% of women with cystic fibrosis are infertile due to abnormal fluid transport in the cervix and fallopian tubes. ▼

4. The seminal vesicles.

   a. The paired **seminal vesicles** are glandular outpouchings of the vas deferens, located behind the bladder.

   b. *Seminal vesicles secrete about 70% of semen by volume* and produce an electrolyte fluid rich in **fructose** for the nourishment of ejaculated spermatozoa within the female reproductive tract.

   c. Seminal vesicles secrete **semenogelins,** which are the main coagulant proteins responsible for coagulation of semen after ejaculation.

5. The prostate gland.

a. The **prostate gland** surrounds the first portion of the urethra and consists of lobules that drain directly into the urethra through small ducts.

b. Prostate secretion is an electrolyte fluid, rich in **acid phosphatase.** The prostate gland contains smooth muscle, which contracts to deliver secretions into the urethra during a phase called **emission,** just prior to ejaculation.

c. **Prostate-specific antigen (PSA)** is a protease that liquefies coagulated semen 15–30 minutes after ejaculation.

   i. ▼ *Increased serum PSA is used as a biochemical marker for prostate cancer in selected patients but is no longer used for population-based screening.* ▼

d. ▼ **Benign prostatic hyperplasia (BPH)** causes enlargement of the prostate, typically in the periurethral zone. Impedance of urinary flow is a common finding in BPH. *The pathophysiology of BPH involves increased levels of DHT in the prostate; inhibitors of 5α-reductase may be used for treatment of BPH.* ▼

6. The penis.

a. The functions of the penis are urination and (after puberty) intercourse.

b. The penis is composed of three columns of erectile tissue: two **corpora cavernosa** and the **corpus spongiosum.**

c. The **penile urethra** traverses the corpus spongiosum, which ends as the expanded **glans penis;** urine and semen exit via the **external urethral meatus** of the glans.

d. The prepuce, or **foreskin,** is a retractable fold of skin covering the glans penis, which is often surgically removed by **circumcision.**

e. ▼ Congenital anomalies of the penis include hypospadias and epispadias. **Hypospadias** is an abnormality in which the urethral opening is on the ventral surface of the penis and occurs when the urethral folds fail to fuse during development. **Epispadias** is a malformation in which the urethral opening is on the dorsal surface of the penis. ▼

7. Spermatogenesis.

a. The three phases of spermatogenesis are:

   i. **Proliferation of spermatogonia** to produce a large population of cells. Once a spermatogonium undergoes its final mitotic division, it becomes a **primary spermatocyte.**

   ii. **Generation of genetic diversity** by meiosis. After the first meiotic division, the developing gametes are called **secondary spermatocytes;** after the second (final) meiotic division, gametes are called **spermatids.**

   iii. **Maturation of sperm** with specializations that allow the journey to the oocyte within the female reproductive tract. Dramatic cellular remodeling of spermatids produces **spermatozoa** in a process called **spermiogenesis.**

b. The seminiferous epithelium consists of cells in the various stages of spermatogenesis (Figure 9-4B).

   i. Moving from the periphery of a seminiferous tubule toward the lumen, germinal cells are progressing in their development from spermatogonia to spermatozoa.

   ii. Developing spermatocytes are embedded in cytoplasmic extensions from the large nongerminal **Sertoli cells,** which provide support and nutrition as well as forming a **blood-testis barrier** to protect the microenvironment for spermatogenesis.

iii. The process of **spermiation** involves the release of spermatids from contact with Sertoli cells into the tubule lumen as spermatozoa.

c. Approximately 74 days are needed to produce mature spermatozoa from spermatogonia with approximately 60 days spent in the seminiferous tubules plus 14 days of final maturation of spermatozoa in the **epididymis.**

d. Mature spermatozoa have a **head region** containing the nucleus, which is surrounded by a large secretory vesicle, the **acrosome**; there is a **middle connecting section,** which is rich in mitochondria, and a **tail region,** which provides a swimming action (Figure 9-5).

e. *The **hypothalamic-pituitary-testis endocrine axis** controls spermatogenesis* (Figure 9-6):

   i. LH and FSH are secreted from the anterior pituitary under the control of GnRH from the hypothalamus.

   ii. *LH stimulates Leydig cells to produce testosterone,* which diffuses locally into the seminiferous tubules and also enters the systemic circulation.

   iii. *FSH stimulates the Sertoli cells,* resulting in the secretion of **androgen-binding protein** into the lumen of the seminiferous tubule.

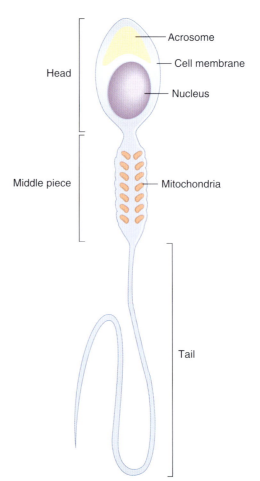

Figure 9-5. A spermatozoon. The head contains a large secretory vesicle, the acrosome, which releases hydrolytic enzymes on to the oocyte during fertilization. The middle section has many mitochondria, providing adenosine triphosphate (ATP) to power the swimming action of the tail.

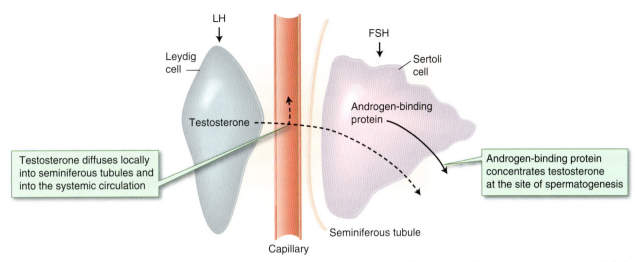

Figure 9-6. Effects of gonadotropins at the testis. Luteinizing hormone (LH) stimulates the Leydig cells to secrete testosterone. Follicle-stimulating hormone (FSH) stimulates the secretion of androgen-binding protein by the Sertoli cells into the lumen of the seminiferous tubules.

- *The function of androgen-binding protein is to increase the local concentration of testosterone at the site of spermatogenesis.*
- FSH also stimulates the secretion of **inhibin** from the Sertoli cells, which exerts negative feedback on FSH secretion by the anterior pituitary.

iv. Testosterone exerts negative feedback on the secretion of both FSH and LH.

8. Erection, emission, and ejaculation.
   a. *Penile erection is necessary for intercourse to occur and is controlled by the parasympathetic nervous system.*
   b. Erection can occur via a **spinal reflex,** by stimulation of the glans penis or the perineum. It can be induced (or suppressed) by **psychogenic stimuli** from higher centers at the level of the midbrain and amygdala.
      i. Erotic stimuli increase efferent parasympathetic activity, causing relaxation of vascular smooth muscle and vasodilation of penile blood vessels.
      ii. An erection results when vasodilation causes the sinusoidal spaces within erectile tissue to fill with blood.
      iii. Expansion of the corpora cavernosa compresses venous outflow, further increasing rigidity of the penis.
      iv. The corpus spongiosum does not contribute significantly to penile rigidity because the urethra must remain patent for passage of the ejaculate.
      v. *Nitric oxide is the most important transmitter causing vasodilation in erectile tissue through the second messenger cyclic guanosine monophosphate (cGMP).*
      vi. Nitric oxide may be released directly from parasympathetic nerve endings, or it may be produced in response to acetylcholine release.
   c. ▼ **Erectile dysfunction** can be related to many conditions, including endocrine disorders (e.g., diabetes mellitus or low testosterone levels due to

hypogonadism), drugs (e.g., antihypertensives or antidepressants), vascular disease, or psychogenic causes (e.g., stress).

   i. **Sildenafil** (Viagra) is a drug that is taken orally and can be used to treat some types of erectile dysfunction. Sildenafil inhibits **phosphodiesterase type V,** the enzyme responsible for breaking down cGMP. By inhibiting this key enzyme, *sildenafil potentiates the effects of cGMP, prolonging vasodilation of the erectile tissues.* ▼

  d. **Emission** occurs immediately prior to ejaculation:

    i. There is sequential contraction of smooth muscle in the vas deferens, the prostate, and the seminal vesicles, which results in spermatozoa and seminal plasma moving into the urethra.

    ii. *The emission phase is coordinated by* **sympathetic nerves.**

  e. **Ejaculation** is a spinal reflex that occurs after the entry of semen into the posterior urethra during emission.

    i. At ejaculation, semen is forcefully ejected from the urethra.

    ii. Contractions of the perineal musculature and pelvic floor are coordinated through somatic innervation via the **pudendal nerve.**

    iii. **Orgasm** is the pleasurable sensation, which, in males, accompanies ejaculation.

    iv. Contraction of the internal bladder sphincter (by α_1-adrenergic sympathetic stimulation) prevents the ejaculate from traveling up the urethra and into the bladder, known as **retrograde ejaculation.**

Female Reproductive Physiology

1. The female internal organs of reproduction are the ovaries, fallopian tubes, uterus, and vagina (Figure 9-7).

  a. The ovaries normally release a single **oocyte** (ovum or egg) into the reproductive tract, which occurs approximately once per month.

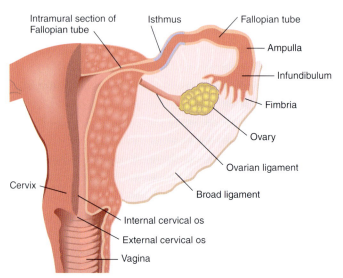

Figure 9-7. Female internal reproductive organs. The ovaries are placed laterally in the pelvis. Oocytes are released into the peritoneal cavity and caught by fimbria at the distal end of the fallopian tubes, which conduct the oocyte to the cavity of the uterus. The uterus communicates with the vagina via the cervix.

b. The oocyte travels along a **fallopian tube** to a hollow muscular organ, the **uterus.**

c. The fallopian tube is the normal site where **fertilization** of the ovum by a single sperm cell occurs; the uterus is the site of **implantation** and development of the embryo.

d. The lower reproductive tract consists of the **vagina** and the **vulva** (external genitalia). The functions of the vagina are to receive the penis during intercourse and to temporarily retain semen. The vagina and vulva also comprise the lowest part of the **birth canal.**

2. The ovaries and the fallopian tubes.

a. The paired **ovaries** are the female gonads; there is one ovary located laterally on each side of the pelvis.

b. *The ovary is the site of **gametogenesis (oogenesis)** and is the major source of the sex steroids.*

c. The microscopic appearance of the ovary varies throughout the ovarian cycle; oocytes in various stages of development within **follicles,** as well as a temporary endocrine gland, the **corpus luteum,** may be seen (Figure 9-8).

d. *The **fallopian tubes** transport the ovum and sperm to the site of **fertilization,** and transport the zygote to the site of **implantation** in the **uterus.***

e. There is one fallopian tube associated with each ovary and each one has four areas:

    i. The most distal part of a fallopian tube is funnel-shaped and bears finger-like projections called **fimbria,** which receive the ovum when it is released from the ovary at **ovulation.** A ciliated epithelial lining propels the ovum along the fallopian tube toward the uterus.

    ii. *The usual site of fertilization of the oocyte is a dilated area called the **ampulla.***

    iii. A narrow portion, called the **isthmus,** helps to retain the early embryo within the tube for 2–3 days after fertilization. During this time, there is final maturation of the **endometrium** (lining of the uterus) to facilitate implantation of the embryo.

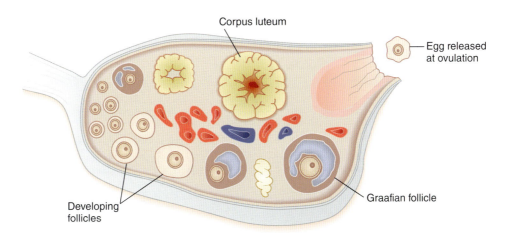

Figure 9-8. Microscopic appearance of the ovary. (*Note: The structures shown are not all present at the same time.*) In the first half of the menstrual cycle, several oocytes begin to develop as a cohort of follicles. A single dominant follicle is visible about midcycle, and has differentiated into a large Graafian follicle. Ovulation occurs by forceful rupture of the Graafian follicle. After ovulation, the Graafian follicle transforms into the corpus luteum.

iv. Each fallopian tube has an **intramural** portion, where it joins the hollow uterus. The point of entry of the fallopian tube is called the **cornua** of the uterus.

f. ▼ **Pelvic inflammatory disease (PID)** is caused by an ascending sexually transmitted disease.

i. PID is most commonly due to **chlamydia** or **gonorrhea,** and ascends from the cervix to the endometrium, to the fallopian tubes, and to the pelvic cavity.

ii. As a complication, the fallopian tubes can become scarred, increasing the risk of an **ectopic tubal pregnancy,** which is a potentially fatal condition! *The most common site of implantation of an ectopic pregnancy is the ampulla of the fallopian tube.* ▼

3. The uterus.

a. The uterus is a pear-shaped muscular organ within the pelvis, located between the bladder and rectum.

b. *The function of the uterus is to support the growing fetus during pregnancy.*

c. Growth of the uterus during pregnancy occurs by cell growth (hyperplasia) and production of new muscle cells from stem cells.

d. During **parturition** (childbirth), the uterine smooth muscle contracts powerfully to expel the fetus.

e. ▼ The uterus is supported in position by several connective tissue **ligaments.** *Damage to the uterine ligaments (e.g., during childbirth) may result in **prolapse** of the uterus downward into the vagina.* ▼

f. The structure of the uterus includes three areas:

i. The **fundus** is the area above the openings of the fallopian tubes.

ii. The **corpus** is the main body of the uterus. The lower third of the corpus is called the **lower uterine segment.** Contraction of this area draws the dilated cervix (lowest part of the uterus) upward during labor.

iii. The **cervix** is about 4-cm long and is mainly composed of connective tissue; this contrasts with the corpus, which is mainly composed of smooth muscle.

- Approximately half of the cervix protrudes into the upper vagina.
- The **cervical canal** joins the vaginal lumen and uterine cavity and is lined by a mucous-secreting epithelium.

g. The properties of **cervical mucus** change significantly during the **menstrual cycle.**

i. *About the time of ovulation at midcycle, under the influence of high estrogen and low progesterone, the mucus is thin and readily allows passage of sperm.*

- A sample of cervical mucus placed on a microscope slide at this time dries in a fern-like pattern, hence the term **ferning of cervical mucus.**

ii. *Later in the menstrual cycle, high concentrations of progesterone promote the secretion of thicker mucus, which resists the passage of sperm.*

h. ▼ **Cervical cancer** most commonly occurs at the squamocolumnar junction, which is the transition zone between vaginal epithelium and cervical epithelium.

i. An effective screening tool for the detection of cervical cancer was developed by George Papanicolaou and is known as the **Pap smear.**

ii. Cells collected from the cervical squamocolumnar junction are stained with the multichromatic Pap Stain and examined under the microscope for signs of dysplasia.

iii. Infection with **human papillomavirus (HPV) type 16 and 18,** among other types, plays an important etiologic role in the development of cervical cancer.

iv. HPV viral proteins have the capacity to inactivate tumor-suppressor genes, which may explain the carcinogenic effects of the virus.

v. *The development of an **HPV vaccine** (Gardasil) protects against infection with the virus and may significantly alter the epidemiology of cervical cancer in the future.*

vi. *HPV infection is also a leading risk factor for anal cancer. Vaccination of all children is now recommended between ages 11 and 12.* ▼

i. The endometrium.

   i. The **endometrium** is the epithelial lining of the uterus and undergoes dramatic changes during the monthly cycle. There are three phases of the monthly menstrual cycle:

- *The **proliferative phase** occurs in the first half of the cycle prior to ovulation and is under the influence of **high estrogen levels**. During* this time, there is marked thickening of the endometrium, growth of the **endometrial glands,** and the appearance of **spiral arteries.**

- *The **secretory phase** occurs after ovulation, during the second half of the monthly cycle when there is **progesterone dominance.*** There is copious secretion of a nutritive fluid from the endometrial glands in preparation for implantation of an embryo at this time.

- *The **menstrual phase** occurs if implantation of an embryo does not occur;* progesterone levels decrease toward the end of the cycle, causing the uterine spiral arteries to spasm. Tissue necrosis and bleeding (**menses**) occurs, usually over a period of 4–5 days, as the endometrial lining sloughs off.

4. The vagina and the vulva.

  a. The vagina is a tube that extends from the vaginal opening (**introitus**) to the cervix.

    i. Many mucous-secreting glands line the introitus and are stimulated during intercourse to provide lubrication.

    ii. The largest and most important of these glands is **Bartholin's gland,** which is located posterolaterally.

  b. The **vulva** is the collective name for the female external genitalia and comprises the **lower third of the vagina,** the **labia,** and the **clitoris** (Figure 9-9).

    i. The clitoris is the female homolog of the penis and consists of erectile tissue of the paired corpora cavernosa, ending in the sensitive **glans clitoris.**

    ii. The urethral opening lies between the clitoris and the introitus.

5. Oogenesis.

  a. **Oogenesis** is the process through which the mature female gamete is formed.

  b. Oogenesis begins in fetal life but is not completed until the time of fertilization.

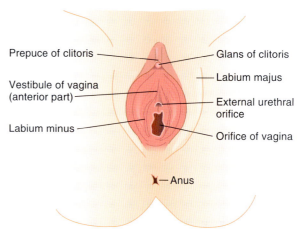

Figure 9-9. Female external genitalia.

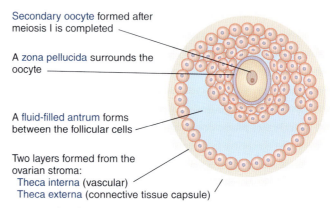

Figure 9-10. A Graafian follicle. The oocyte is surrounded by a gelatinous ring (the zona pellucida) by the granulosa cells of the cumulus oophorus and by the follicular fluid (the antrum). Thinning of the outer follicular wall of thecal cells occurs just prior to ovulation. Rupture of the follicle at ovulation ejects the oocyte-cumulus complex.

   c. The proliferation of oogonia by mitosis ends midway through fetal life, at which time oocytes are arrested in the first meiotic division.

   d. Thereafter, the number of oocytes gradually declines with age; there are about 1–2 million oocytes at birth and about 100,000 at puberty.

   e. Oocytes may be stimulated to develop for release at ovulation, or they will die through a process called **atresia.**

   f. Oogenesis occurs in the ovary within structures called **follicles.**

      i. Each unstimulated follicle contains a single **primary oocyte** surrounded by a single layer of **granulosa cells,** which in turn are associated with **thecal cells.**

   g. *With each monthly menstrual cycle, several follicles are stimulated to develop, but only one will become the dominant follicle that continues to ovulation:*

      i. The **oocyte** and granulosa cells in developing follicles enlarge.

      ii. A clear gelatinous ring of extracellular matrix appears around the oocyte, called the **zona pellucida.**

      iii. The dominant follicle becomes a **Graafian follicle** (Figure 9-10). After the LH surge, the oocyte within a Graafian follicle completes the first meiotic division to become a **secondary oocyte.**

    iv. Rupture of the Graafian follicle at **ovulation** expels the oocyte into the peritoneal space near the fimbria of the fallopian tube.

    v. The ruptured follicle collapses and granulosa cells proliferate to fill the space. *Under the influence of LH, structural transformation to the **corpus luteum** occurs.*

  h. ▼ *Trisomy 21, or **Down's syndrome,** is associated with increased maternal age.*

    i. The first meiotic division is arrested during fetal life and is not completed until years later at ovulation.

    ii. The mechanism that causes trisomy is thought to be related to **prolonged arrest of the first meiotic division** and age-dependent degradation of the meiotic proteins. ▼

6. The menstrual (ovarian) cycle (Figure 9-11).

  a. The cyclic activity of the hypothalamic-pituitary-ovarian axis results in ovulation and the simultaneous development of a uterine environment that is capable of supporting pregnancy.

  b. The terms menstrual cycle and ovarian cycle are both used to describe a sequence of events that recurs approximately every 28 days. *The first day of menstrual bleeding defines day 1 of a menstrual cycle.*

  c. From the perspective of events taking place in the ovary, the cycle is divided into **three phases:**

    i. **The follicular phase (days 1–14)** is the first half of the menstrual cycle.

- Toward the end of the previous cycle, the corpus luteum degenerates, resulting in a sharp decrease in the blood levels of progesterone, estrogen, and inhibin.
- The loss of negative feedback inhibition of FSH secretion allows plasma FSH concentration to increase.
- Under the influence of FSH, a cohort of primary follicles develops (a process that begins in the final 2–3 days of the previous cycle).
- **Granulosa cells** secrete estrogen and inhibin under the influence of FSH. *Note: Granulosa cells rely on a supply of androgens from thecal cells as a substrate for estrogen production.*
- By the midfollicular phase, FSH secretion is suppressed preventing the recruitment of more follicles.
- A **dominant follicle** emerges, which has *high sensitivity to FSH,* and continues to develop and to secrete estrogen, despite the now low levels of circulating FSH; the other follicles undergo **atresia** and die, leaving a single oocyte for release at ovulation.

    ii. **The ovulatory phase (days 13–15).**

- Ovulation occurs at the midpoint of a normal menstrual cycle, triggered by an **LH surge.**
- Ovulation occurs about 12 hours after the peak LH concentration.
- *The dominant follicle signals its maturity to the pituitary gland by a rapid increase in estrogen secretion, which exerts **positive feedback** on the anterior pituitary by sensitizing it to GnRH.*
- When the LH surge occurs, the primary oocyte completes the first meiotic division to form a larger **secondary oocyte,** which stops in the second meiotic division until fertilization.

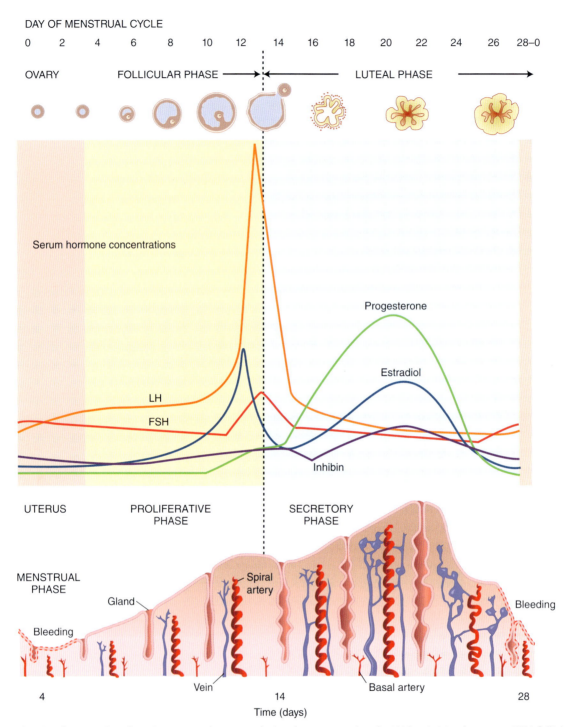

Figure 9-11. Ovarian, hormonal, and uterine events that occur during the menstrual cycle. LH, luteinizing hormone; FSH, follicle-stimulating hormone.

- **Ovulation** occurs due to thinning and rupture of the dominant follicle, under the influence of LH, progesterone, and locally released prostaglandins.
- The released oocyte is surrounded by the **zona pellucida** and granulosa cells.

iii. **The luteal phase (days 15–28).**

- After ovulation, the **corpus luteum** is formed, under the influence of LH, by differentiation of both theca and granulosa cells, into **theca-lutein** and **granulosa-lutein cells,** respectively.
- *Progesterone is the major secretory product of the corpus luteum,* although both estrogen and inhibin are also secreted.
- During the luteal phase, high levels of estrogen are unable to induce another LH surge due to the presence of high progesterone levels.
- If **pregnancy** does not occur, the corpus luteum spontaneously degenerates.

d. *Continued progesterone secretion by the corpus luteum is essential to early pregnancy.* If implantation of an embryo occurs, the trophoblast cells of the developing placenta secrete the LH analogue **human chorionic gonadotropin (hCG),** *which rescues the corpus luteum until the developing placenta assumes the production of progesterone.*

7. Menopause.

a. **Menopause** is a normal stage of life.

b. *The mean age of menopause is 51 years; 95% of women experience menopause between ages 45 and 55 years.*

c. The physiologic effects of menopause can be viewed as a syndrome of "ovarian failure." *Cessation of menstruation is a universal feature of menopause.*

d. **Withdrawal of estrogen** accounts for the symptoms of menopause, which include insomnia, hot flashes, variable degrees of vaginal atrophy, and decreased breast size.

e. *Estrogen deficiency causes bone loss and increases the risk of* **osteoporosis.**

f. The loss of ovarian function removes negative feedback on GnRH, producing high serum concentrations of FSH and LH.

   i. *FSH levels are particularly high in postmenopausal women* because inhibins, which exert selective negative feedback on FSH secretion, are no longer produced by the ovary.

g. ▼ **Menopausal hormone therapy (MHT)** involves use of either estrogen alone or in combination with progestins. Systemic estrogen is needed to treat hot flashes whereas topical estrogen can be used to treat vulvovaginal atrophy. *MHT should not be prescribed for disease prevention* because large-scale clinical trials in the Women's Health Initiative found an unfavorable risk-benefit profile (e.g., lower incidence of hip fracture but higher incidence of heart disease and breast cancer). ▼

h. ▼ **Endometrial cancer** is the most common malignant tumor of the female genital tract:

   i. It is primarily a disease of postmenopausal women and typically presents clinically as postmenopausal vaginal bleeding.

   ii. *Exposure to unopposed estrogen plays a critical etiologic role.* Risk factors include obesity, nulliparity (no pregnancies), late menopause, chronic anovulation (e.g., polycystic ovarian syndrome), and use of estrogen replacement therapy. ▼

i. **Andropause** occurs in men; *there is reduced testosterone secretion,* but the effects of andropause are usually mild compared to the effects of menopause in most women.

Human Sexual Responses

1. The physiology of human sexual responses is categorized in four phases as **excitement, plateau, orgasm,** and **resolution** (Figure 9-12). Physiologic changes during the human sexual response include vascular congestion, generalized muscle tension, and increased cardiorespiratory activity.

2. The four phases of the **male sexual response** proceed as follows:

    a. Penile erection is the first response to effective sexual arousal in the **excitement phase** and can occur through psychogenic or reflexogenic stimulation.

    b. During the **plateau phase,** there is a small increase in penile erection, the testes enlarge due to vascular congestion, and the scrotum contracts to draw the testes upward toward the perineum. Emission occurs shortly before ejaculation, depositing spermatozoa and seminal plasma into the posterior urethra.

    c. With adequate stimulation, **orgasm** and ejaculation occur simultaneously. There is an intense subjective sensation of pleasure and release of sexual tension.

A. Male sexual response

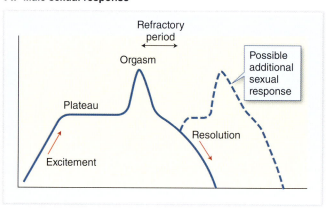

B. Female sexual responses

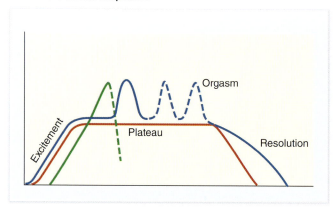

Figure 9-12. Phases of the human sexual response. **A.** The male sexual response involves penile erection in the excitement phase, emission of sperm and seminal plasma into the urethra in the plateau phase, a single orgasm associated with ejaculation, and a resolution phase with penile detumescence. **B.** The same phases are represented in the female sexual response, although the plateau and orgasm phases are more variable. There may be an extended plateau without orgasm, a short plateau with orgasm, or multiple orgasms due to the lack of a refractory period.

    d. During the **resolution phase,** penile **detumescence** (return to the flaccid state) typically occurs in two stages:

        i. In **stage 1,** the penis quickly returns to about half its erect size and is totally **refractory** to further stimulation.

        ii. In **stage 2,** the penis returns to its flaccid size over a longer period of time and is in a **relative refractory state,** when another full cycle of excitement through to orgasm may be possible.

3. The four phases of the **female sexual response** are as follows:

    a. Psychogenic and reflexogenic pathways function similarly in males and females during sexual arousal. The clitoris is the primary sensory sexual organ, though clitoral erection is a variable response in the **excitement phase;** vaginal lubrication is a more consistently observed response. There is expansion of the upper vagina, and the labia minora enlarge, moving outward away from the vaginal introitus.

    b. Engorgement and reddening of the labia minora are characteristics of the **plateau phase.**

    c. Female **orgasm** produces rhythmic contractions of the perineum and reproductive organs. Intense subjective sensations of pleasure are followed by release of general skeletal muscle tone.

        i. Female orgasm differs from male orgasm in that there is no ejaculation response; female orgasm can last longer and there is no refractory period before additional orgasms can occur.

    d. The **resolution phase** involves relaxation of the vagina and vascular decongestion of the reproductive organs.

4. ▼ **Dysfunction of the sexual response cycle** can occur at any stage; examples include desire disorders (more common in women), excitement disorders (e.g., erectile dysfunction in males or inadequate vaginal lubrication in females), anorgasmia (e.g., inadequate clitoral stimulation), dyspareunia (i.e., painful intercourse), or vaginismus (i.e., painful reflexive spasms of the paravaginal muscles, inhibiting any vaginal penetration). ▼

Fertilization and the Establishment of Pregnancy

1. At ejaculation, 100–600 million sperm are deposited into the vagina. After a few minutes, a small number of sperm have already reached the fallopian tube.

    a. **Sperm transport** results from the sperm's swimming motion and is assisted by contractions of the uterus and fallopian tubes (augmented during female orgasm, if it occurs).

    b. The oocyte is propelled along the fallopian tube by the action of cilia. The sperm and egg usually meet in the dilated ampulla of the fallopian tube.

2. *Successful fertilization occurs within a short time window, several hours after ovulation.*

    a. The fertilized egg is usually retained in the fallopian tube for about 3 days, where it divides into a solid mass of 12 or more cells called a **morula.**

    b. The morula develops into a **blastocyst** during the next 3 days as it floats freely in the uterine cavity.

    c. *Implantation of the blastocyst into the uterine endometrium occurs 6–7 days after ovulation.*

3. ▼ **Infertility** is defined as the inability to conceive after 12 months of unprotected sexual intercourse. Approximately 17% of infertility is

unexplainable, and 25% relates to male factors and about 58% relates to female factors.

4. Capacitation of spermatozoa:
   a. Is a final maturation event necessary for sperm to acquire the ability to penetrate the zona pellucida and fertilize the egg.
   b. Involves the removal of a protein coat that alters the membrane properties of the sperm.
   c. Occurs physiologically within the female reproductive tract, but it can also occur in vitro.

5. There are eight stages during fertilization of the egg by a sperm (Figure 9-13):
   a. The sperm head penetrates the layer of follicular cells surrounding the egg and binds to specific proteins in the zona pellucida.
   b. The sperm undergoes **the acrosome reaction.**
      i. The acrosome is a large secretory vesicle located in the head of the sperm, containing hydrolytic enzymes.
      ii. Binding of the sperm head to the zona pellucida produces an increase in intracellular $[Ca^{2+}]$ in the sperm, resulting in exocytosis of the contents of the acrosome on to the zona pellucida.
   c. The sperm **penetrates the zona pellucida** to reach the oocyte membrane.

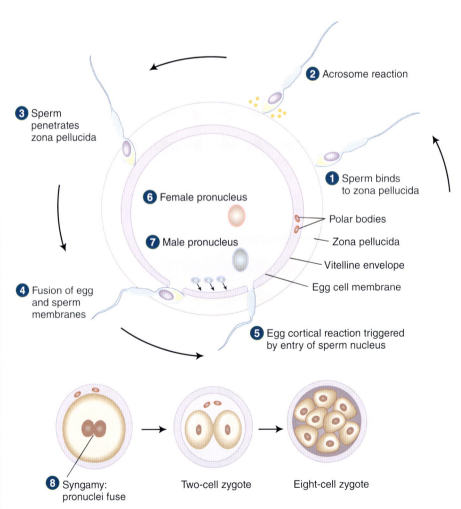

Figure 9-13. Stages of fertilization.

d. **The cell membranes of the sperm and egg fuse,** releasing the sperm nucleus and cytoplasm into the egg cytoplasm. This event causes depolarization of the egg cell membrane, which deters binding of other sperm heads to the egg.

e. The egg undergoes **the cortical reaction,** in which enzymes are released by the egg via exocytosis and results in hardening of the zona pellucida.

 i. The cortical reaction is caused by entry of the sperm nucleus, triggering a large inositol triphosphate-dependent increase in intracellular $[Ca^{2+}]$ in the egg.

 ii. *Together, with the egg cell membrane depolarization, hardening of the zona pellucida prevents entry of further sperm (**polyspermy**).*

f. The Ca^{2+} signal of the cortical reaction triggers **completion of the second meiotic division** by the secondary oocyte. Unfolding of chromosomes occurs to produce **the female pronucleus.**

g. Chromosomes in the sperm nucleus decondense, producing the **male pronucleus.**

h. **Male and female pronuclei fuse.** The union of chromosomes from the male and female, called **syngamy,** marks the end of fertilization. A **zygote** is formed with 23 chromosomes from each parent. *The chromosomal sex of the fetus has been determined, depending on whether the sperm is 22X or 22Y.*

i. ▼ **Hydatidiform mole** is a benign molar pregnancy that can be classified as either complete (most common) or incomplete.

 i. A complete hydatidiform mole results from fertilization of an empty egg with a single sperm, resulting in only paternally derived chromosomes.

 ii. An incomplete hydatidiform mole results from fertilization of a normal egg with two sperm, resulting in triploidy (three sets of chromosomes).

 iii. *Molar pregnancies are incompatible with life.* ▼

6. Implantation.

 a. The fertilized egg develops for 6–7 days before implantation.

 b. *Synchronized development of the fertilized egg and the endometrium are required for successful implantation.*

 i. The endometrium is in the secretory phase, under the influence of **progesterone** from the corpus luteum.

 ii. Endometrial secretions nourish the developing embryo within the lumen of the uterus prior to implantation.

 iii. Fluid within the uterine cavity is gradually absorbed via finger-like projections of the endometrium, called **pinopodes,** which appear only at this time.

 iv. Fluid absorption brings the embryo closer to the endometrium to facilitate contact and implantation.

 v. During the time when the developing embryo is floating in the uterine cavity, a process called "**hatching**" occurs, in which the zona pellucida and the follicular cells surrounding the blastocyst degenerate to expose the underlying embryonic cells.

 vi. *Once hatching is complete, the trophoblast cells of the developing embryo are able to come into direct contact with the endometrium.*

 c. **Implantation** can be described in the following **three stages**:

 i. **Apposition** is the formation of a loose connection between the trophoblast and the endometrium.

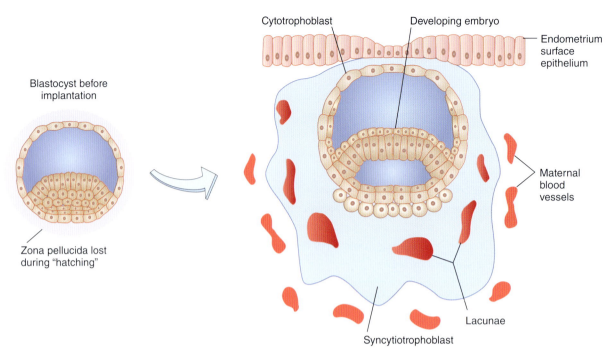

Figure 9-14. Embryo implantation. The embryo develops for approximately 1 week after fertilization of the egg, forming a blastocyst at the time of implantation. The endometrium is invaded by trophoblast cells that surround the blastocyst. Once implantation has occurred, the decidual reaction transforms the entire uterine endometrium into the decidual membranes of pregnancy.

ii. **Adhesion** occurs through specific ligand-receptor interactions when microvilli extend from the trophoblast cells. Adhesion is followed by rapid proliferation of trophoblast cells and differentiation into two layers: an inner **cytotrophoblast** cell layer and an outer multinucleated layer facing the endometrium, called the **syncytiotrophoblast.**

iii. **Invasion** of the endometrial stroma by the syncytiotrophoblast causes the embryo to become completely embedded in the endometrium (Figure 9-14).

d. After invasion by the syncytiotrophoblast, the entire endometrium undergoes further biochemical and morphologic change, called **decidualization (decidual reaction),** and forms the "membranes of pregnancy" called the **decidua.**

  i. *Decidualization begins at the site of implantation and spreads in a concentric wave around the entire endometrium.*

e. ▼ **Choriocarcinoma** is a malignant molar pregnancy that consists of both cytotrophoblasts and syncytiotrophoblasts. Due to the natural invasive nature of the syncytiotrophoblastic cells, this tumor is very invasive and hemorrhagic. The most common site of metastasis is hematogenous spread to the lung. ▼

7. The placenta.

a. The placenta is formed by elements from both the mother and the fetus. The two general functions of the placenta are:

  i. Transport of materials between the maternal and fetal circulations.

  ii. Secretion of hormones required for the maintenance of pregnancy.

b. The syncytiotrophoblast develops spaces within it called **lacunae,** as it invades deeper into the endometrium.

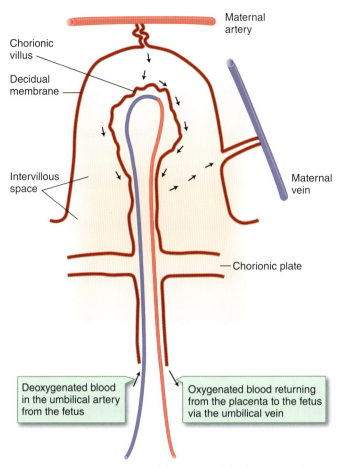

Figure 9-15. Schematic representation of the maternal-fetal exchange barrier.

  c. When maternal blood vessels in the endometrial wall are invaded, these spaces fill with maternal blood; lacunae coalesce into a single blood-filled space, called the **intervillous space.**

  d. **Chorionic villi** grow from the cytotrophoblast into the syncytiotrophoblast to make contact with lacunae.

  e. *The intervillous space behaves like a giant capillary, with fresh maternal arterial blood entering from the uterine spiral arteries and leaving via the placental veins* (Figure 9-15).

  f. Chorionic villi contain fetal blood capillaries. Numerous chorionic villi project into the intervillous space, resembling a forest of trees "rooted" to a discrete area called the **chorionic plate.**

    i. Fetal blood flowing through the chorionic villi arrives via **umbilical arteries.**

    ii. Blood returns from the chorionic villi to the fetus via the **umbilical veins.**

  g. The **maternal-fetal exchange barrier** between fetal and maternal blood consists of the following three components:

    i. The **fetal capillary endothelium.**

    ii. A layer of **cytotrophoblast** and **fetal mesenchymal cells.**

    iii. A layer of **syncytiotrophoblast** facing the maternal blood pool.

  h. ▼ The most common cause of bleeding during the third trimester is due to separation of the placenta from the uterine wall, a condition known as

placenta abruptio. *This potentially fatal condition classically presents as painful vaginal bleeding in the third trimester.* ▼

i. **Placental transport** occurs by a combination of active and passive mechanisms.

   i. Oxygen and carbon dioxide move by simple diffusion; glucose is transported to the fetus by facilitated diffusion; amino acids are mostly transported by secondary active transport.

   ii. Large molecules such as low-density lipoproteins (LDLs), antibodies, and other peptides (e.g., transferrin) are taken up by the syncytiotrophoblast via receptor-mediated endocytosis.

   iii. *Transport rates increase significantly in the final weeks of gestation, reflecting the accelerating growth rate of the fetus at this time.*

j. ▼ *Antibodies transported across the placenta augment the* **fetal immune system.** The immune system of a newborn predominately consists of maternal IgG. However, at approximately 6 months of age, the infant's immune system must begin to assume the major role in defense against infection, due to the degradation of the maternal IgG over time. Thus, **immunodeficiency disorders** (*e.g., severe combined immunodeficiency [SCID]*) *do not begin to present until after 6 months of age.* ▼

k. Gas exchange across the placenta.

   i. *Umbilical arteries carry deoxygenated blood* from the fetus to the placenta, and gas exchange with blood in the maternal intervillous space results in the *return of oxygenated blood to the fetus via the umbilical veins.*

   ii. The average P_{O_2} of blood in the intervillous space is about 30–35 mm Hg, which, in adults, would only produce about 60% saturation of hemoglobin and would result in hypoxemia.

   iii. **Fetal hemoglobin** *has a higher oxygen affinity than adult hemoglobin,* allowing 80–90% saturation of hemoglobin with a P_{O_2} of only about 30 mm Hg in the umbilical venous blood (Figure 9-16).

   iv. The P_{CO_2} of umbilical arterial blood is about 50 mm Hg, compared to the P_{CO_2} of about 42 mm Hg in the intervillous space. This diffusion gradient allows carbon dioxide excretion from the fetus to the mother; *the carbon dioxide produced by the fetus is excreted via the maternal lungs.*

The Endocrinology of Pregnancy

1. There are several hormones, including peptides, amines, and steroids, that are essential to the maintenance of pregnancy (Figure 9-17).
2. The placenta is a key endocrine organ, particularly after the first few weeks of gestation.
3. **Placental peptides.**
   a. The two major placental peptides, which are only secreted during pregnancy, are **human chorionic gonadotropin** (hCG) and **human chorionic somatomammotropin** (hCS).
   b. *hCG rescues the corpus luteum from degeneration* and allows continued progesterone secretion to support the early pregnancy.
      i. At about 8–9 weeks' gestation, the placenta will assume the production of progesterone. Thereafter, the plasma hCG concentrations decrease to

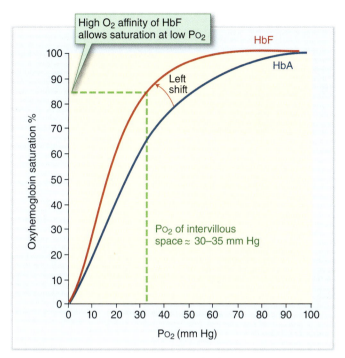

Figure 9-16. Oxyhemoglobin dissociation curves for fetal hemoglobin (HbF) and adult hemoglobin (HbA). The fetal curve shifts to the left, indicating the higher O_2 affinity of HbF that is necessary to ensure that O_2 is transferred in the direction from mother to fetus.

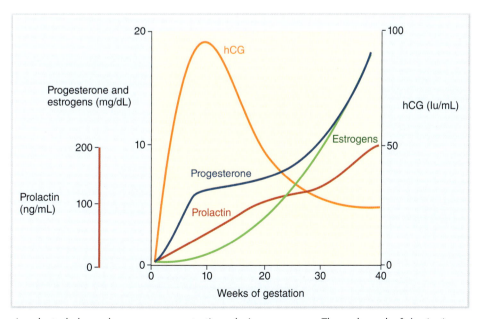

Figure 9-17. Changes in selected plasma hormone concentrations during pregnancy. The early peak of chorionic gonadotropin rescues the corpus luteum, which is responsible for the early rise in progesterone secretion. The placenta assumes production of progesterone by about gestation week 9. Estrogen secretion begins later because maturation of the fetal adrenal glands, which supplies androgen precursors to the placenta, is necessary for estrogen production.

lower levels but continue to be important for maintaining progesterone secretion by the syncytiotrophoblast.

ii. Placental hCG secretion is controlled in a paracrine manner, by locally produced GnRH.

iii. ▼ **Pregnancy tests** are able to detect the unique appearance of hCG in urine in early pregnancy. These tests are able to detect hCG in maternal urine 7–10 days after fertilization. *hCG is produced by the syncytiotrophoblast.* The plasma concentration of hCG normally doubles every 30–50 hours in the first 30 days of pregnancy. Levels of hCG are lower in ectopic pregnancy and will be elevated in cases of twin pregnancy, hydatidiform mole, and choriocarcinoma. ▼

c. Levels of **hCS** (also called **human placental lactogen**) are high during pregnancy; *hCS is structurally similar to GH and prolactin.*

i. The metabolic effects of hCS are similar to those of GH, with suppression of maternal glucose use and reduced maternal insulin responsiveness, which may preserve glucose for fetal use.

ii. *Fatty acids and ketones are important energy sources in the fetus and placenta,* and hCS stimulates production of these substrates.

iii. Higher concentrations of hCS found later in pregnancy also promote mammary gland development.

iv. ▼ hCS is the primary hormone in pregnancy that induces a state of insulin resistance in the mother to promote availability of glucose and fatty acids for the fetus but this increases the risk of developing **gestational diabetes mellitus** (i.e., the observation of hyperglycemia in a pregnant woman with no prior history of diabetes). ▼

4. Steroid hormone production by the maternal-placental-fetal unit (Figure 9-18).

a. Maternal levels of progesterone and estrogens are both much higher during pregnancy than at any time during the normal menstrual cycle.

b. High steroid levels are necessary to support pregnancy. For example, *progesterone is needed in the uterus to maintain the decidua and to relax the uterine smooth muscle to prevent early expulsion of the fetus.*

c. Beyond week 9 of gestation, most of the steroids present in the maternal circulation are secreted by the placenta.

d. **Maternally derived LDL cholesterol** is necessary for placental steroidogenesis because the placenta lacks enzymes needed to produce cholesterol from acetate. *The placenta can produce progesterone when provided with a supply of cholesterol.*

e. The placenta lacks enzymes needed to produce estrogens but has high **aromatase** activity to convert androgens to estrogens.

i. *The **fetal adrenal glands** supply the placenta with weak androgens for conversion to estrogens.*

ii. Fetal adrenals produce **dehydroepiandrosterone sulfate (DHEA-S),** most of which is converted to 16-hydroxy-DHEA-S by the fetal liver.

iii. **Estriol (E3)** is produced by the placenta from fetal 16-OH-DHEA-S. *Normally, estriol is not an important estrogen, but it is considered the major estrogen of pregnancy.*

iv. Estriol has weak estrogenic properties in most maternal organs but increases uteroplacental blood flow.

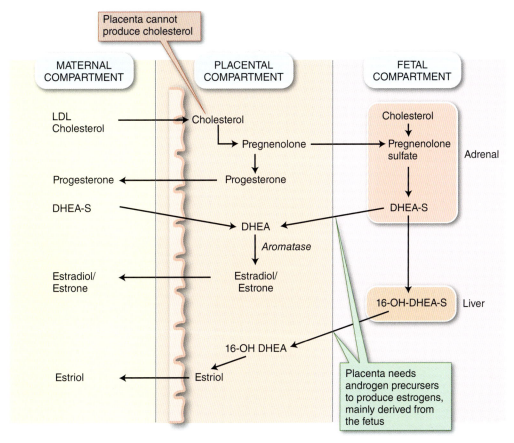

Figure 9-18. Steroid production by the maternal-placental-fetal unit. DHEA, dehydroepiandrosterone; DHEA-S, dehydroepiandrosterone sulfate; 16-OH-DHEA-S, 16-hydroxy-dehydroepiandrosterone sulfate; LDL, low-density lipoprotein.

    f. *The fetus does not produce progesterone or estrogens*, thereby avoiding exposure to high concentrations of these steroids. Although the fetus produces large amounts of weak adrenal androgens, *masculinization of the female fetus does not occur because the placenta acts as a large sink for fetal androgens.*

5. The level of activity in several **maternal endocrine axes** is altered during pregnancy:

    a. In pregnant women, *the total concentration of **thyroid hormones** (T_3 and T_4) is increased but the concentration of free T_3 and T_4 is normal.*

       i. Estrogens stimulate the maternal liver to increase the synthesis of thyroid hormone-binding globulin.

      ii. Increased levels of thyroid-binding globulin cause an initial decrease in free thyroid hormone concentration, which produces feedback stimulation of the hypothalamic-pituitary-thyroid axis to restore free T_3 and T_4.

    b. There is an increase in the maternal levels of **parathyroid hormone (PTH) and vitamin D,** which results in increased maternal Ca^{2+} uptake from the diet.

       i. The final activation of vitamin D_3 occurs in the placenta as well as in the kidney. *Changes in the PTH-vitamin D axis are necessary to support the high demand of fetal growth on the Ca^{2+} supply.*

c. The **renin-angiotensin-aldosterone axis** is upregulated in pregnancy, allowing the maternal blood volume to increase. Sensitivity to the pressor effects of angiotensin II is reduced to prevent high blood pressure.

d. ▼ *Preeclampsia (also known as **toxemia**) is defined by pregnancy-induced onset of hypertension, proteinuria, and edema.* Although the precise pathogenesis is unknown, preeclampsia results in systemic vasospasm and endothelial injury, causing multiorgan damage. If preeclampsia progresses to include seizure, the condition is referred to as **eclampsia.** ▼

Maternal Adaptations to Pregnancy

1. Numerous physiologic demands are placed on the mother by the fetus, which result in changes in virtually all of the maternal physiologic systems:

   a. **Blood volume** increases 40–50% during pregnancy. *The increase is necessary to provide a larger preload to meet the demands for increased cardiac output, to protect maternal venous return, and to provide a reserve against blood loss during childbirth.*

      i. The increased maternal cardiac output supplies the increased demand from the pregnant uterus, the placenta, the kidney (for excretion), the skin (to liberate additional heat), the breast (developing in readiness for lactation), and the heart (to support increased cardiac work).

      ii. The increase in maternal blood volume reflects an increase in both plasma volume and red cell mass.

      iii. *Plasma volume increases due to up-regulation of the renin-angiotensin-aldosterone axis in response to high levels of estrogen and progesterone.*

      iv. The increase in plasma volume is greater than the increase in red cell mass, producing a **dilutional anemia** during pregnancy.

   b. **Blood coagulability increases** to protect the mother from hemorrhage during childbirth.

      i. ▼ Pregnancy is a **hypercoagulable state** primarily because of increases in coagulation factors VII, VIII, and IX, and protein C.

      ii. The hypercoagulable state of pregnancy predisposes the mother to the development of **deep vein thrombosis** and **pulmonary embolism.** ▼

   c. **Alveolar ventilation** increases in pregnancy due to the action of progesterone on the medullary respiratory centers.

      i. Increased alveolar ventilation results from an increase in tidal volume rather than increased respiratory rate.

      ii. Maternal arterial P_{CO_2} decreases from about 40 mm Hg to about 30–34 mm Hg, facilitating CO_2 diffusion across the placenta from the fetus to the mother. The kidney compensates for this **mild respiratory alkalosis** and returns the plasma pH to normal by reducing the plasma bicarbonate concentration.

      iii. When compared to the nonpregnant state residual volume and functional residual capacity are decreased because the diaphragm is displaced upward by the enlarged uterus.

   d. The **glomerular filtration rate** increases by 40–50% by midpregnancy, with a consequent *decrease in the concentrations of plasma creatinine and urea.*

      i. *Glucose appears in the urine in 10–20% of pregnant women* because of increased filtered glucose load and relatively fixed tubular reabsorptive capacity for glucose.

e. **Nutritional demands** of pregnancy include notable increases in protein intake for growth of the fetus, placenta, uterus, and breasts.

   i. **Maternal iron deficiency** can develop due to the demands for production of fetal and maternal hemoglobin.

   ii. *Folate supplementation is also needed for increased hemoglobin synthesis as well as to reduce the risk of fetal* **neural tube defects.**

f. Suppression of cellular immunity is important to avoid fetal rejection. However, this causes pregnant women to become more susceptible to viral infections.

g. ▼ **Constipation** is a common problem during pregnancy because of the effects of progesterone on smooth muscle. Progesterone slows gastric and colonic motility, thereby increasing transit time and subsequent fluid absorption, which results in constipation. ▼

Parturition

1. *The human* **gestation period** *is approximately 40 weeks and is measured from the first day of the last menstrual period.*

2. Expulsion of the fetus, its placenta, and other membranes from the uterus occurs during **labor.** This process is characterized by thinning and dilation of the cervix and by strong regular contractions of the uterus.

3. Four phases of uterine activity can be described during pregnancy and labor:

   a. **Phase 0** is a long phase during which the uterus remains quiescent, under the influence of progesterone. The peptide **relaxin,** secreted by the corpus luteum, assists in maintaining the uterus in a relaxed state.

   b. **Phase 1** represents activation of the uterus when close to term.

      i. In the weeks preceding parturition (childbirth), there is weak low frequency myometrial activity called **contractures** (also known as **Braxton-Hicks** contractions or false labor).

      ii. In phase 1, there is increased myometrial expression of receptors for **oxytocin** and excitatory **prostaglandins (PGE$_2$, PGF$_{2\alpha}$).**

      iii. The appearance of many new **gap junctions** under the influence of rising estrogen levels promotes coordinated contraction of the myometrial smooth muscle cells. These changes are associated with a transition from contractures to true contractions.

   c. **Phase 2** is the dramatic stage of labor when there is stimulation of the uterus, with increasing oxytocin and prostaglandin levels inducing true **uterine contractions** and **dilation of the cervix.** *The products of conception are delivered at parturition, ending phase 2.*

   d. In **phase 3,** the uterus returns to its normal size with the assistance of sustained contraction of the myometrium, which also assists in **blood clotting.**

4. The **initiation of labor** is poorly understood. The **placental clock theory** proposes that the level of placental corticotropin-releasing hormone (CRH) controls the length of gestation, as follows:

   a. Placental CRH stimulates secretion of adrenocorticotropin (ACTH) from the fetal pituitary gland.

   b. Fetal ACTH stimulates the **fetal adrenal gland** to produce androgen.

   c. The placenta converts fetal androgens into estrogens for the maternal circulation.

d. The rising estrogen levels that stimulate uterine activity reflect maturity of the fetus and placental unit indicating readiness for parturition.

e. *A decrease in progesterone level just before term may also promote initiation of labor.*

5. Once labor is initiated, the local release of **prostaglandins** is important for ripening of the cervix and generating powerful uterine contractions.

6. **Oxytocin** is secreted in large amounts from the posterior pituitary during the expulsive stage of labor. The positive feedback stimulation of oxytocin secretion due to increasing cervical distension is known as the **Ferguson reflex.**

7. ▼ Prostaglandin and oxytocin analogues are used in the **induction of labor.** Cervical ripening is induced using vaginal prostaglandin suppositories and intravenous oxytocin is administered to induce uterine contractions. ▼

Lactation

1. Initial breast development at puberty produces a rudimentary system of ducts. During the first weeks of pregnancy, there is rapid growth and development to produce mammary alveoli and a differentiated system of ducts (Figure 9-19).

2. Breast differentiation in pregnancy is stimulated by ovarian and placental steroids with additional stimulation from insulin, cortisol, prolactin, and hCS.

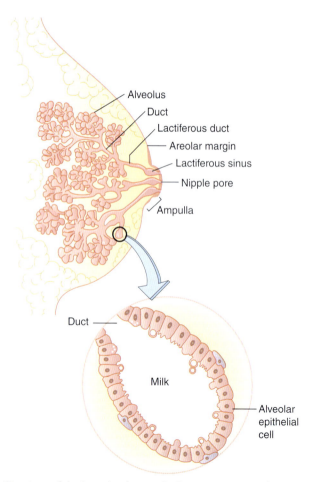

Alveolus
Duct
Lactiferous duct
Areolar margin
Lactiferous sinus
Nipple pore
Ampulla

Duct

Milk

Alveolar epithelial cell

Figure 9-19. Structure of the lactating breast. **A.** Gross anatomy. **B.** The mammary alveolus.

3. Each breast consists of 15–20 lobes and each lobe consists of 20–40 **terminal duct lobular units (TDLUs):**
   a. A TDLU consists of a cluster of mammary alveoli (acini) and their associated ducts.
   b. Alveolar epithelial cells are capable of transcellular fluid and electrolyte secretion as well as receptor-mediated transport of maternal immunoglobulins, and the synthesis and secretion of milk lipids and proteins.
4. **Breast milk** is a complex emulsion of lipids in an isotonic solution, which contains all the minerals founds in extracellular fluid.
   a. **Triglycerides,** constitute 3–5% of milk.
   b. Proteins make up about 1% of milk; the proteins **casein** and **lactalbumin** are only found in milk.
   c. The major sugar in milk is **lactose,** comprising about 7% of milk.
5. **Colostrum** is the thin, yellowish fluid produced within the first few days after parturition, before the main milk production begins. It contains more protein than milk, *including* **antibodies** *and immune cells, and provides the neonate with some immunologic protection.*
6. ▼ **Human breast milk** is the preferred food for full-term infants.
   a. Breast milk is rich in immunoglobulins (mainly IgA) and maternal macrophages, which are thought to protect the infant against upper respiratory tract and inner ear infections.
   b. In addition to reduced infections, breast-fed infants have a lower incidence of allergic diseases (e.g., food allergies and intolerances to foods).
   c. Breast-feeding also promotes bonding between the mother and the infant and hastens the return to prepregnancy weight for the mother. ▼
7. Endocrine control of lactation.
   a. **Prolactin** and **oxytocin** are the two key hormones involved in the control of lactation; *prolactin is required for milk production, and oxytocin stimulates milk ejection from the breast.*
      i. Prolactin is a peptide hormone secreted by the anterior pituitary lactotropes and is *essential for milk production by the lactating breast.*
      ii. Despite elevated prolactin levels during pregnancy, maternal milk production does not occur before the birth of the infant because high estrogen and progesterone levels inhibit the effects of prolactin at the breast.
      iii. There is a dramatic decline in sex steroid levels after expulsion of the placenta at birth, which removes their inhibitory effects on the actions of prolactin.
      iv. *Milk production in response to prolactin begins approximately 2 days after birth.* During the first few days postpartum, the breast secretes colostrum, before lactation begins.
   b. The neuroendocrine responses that occur when an infant suckles are known as **suckling reflexes.** *The afferent limb of the reflex is neuronal, and the efferent responses are hormonal.*
   c. Suckling stimulates **prolactin secretion,** acting via neural pathways to suppress the hypothalamic dopamine release.
      i. Elevated prolactin levels are sustained for as long as an infant breast feeds.

    ii. Peaks of prolactin concentration occur with each feeding session, so that *milk production meets the demands set by the infant.*

    iii. The prolactin released during a feed serves to stimulate milk production in readiness for the next feed.

  d. Suckling stimulates **oxytocin secretion** from neurons in the posterior pituitary.

    i. Oxytocin causes contraction of myoepithelial cells and **milk ejection** (let-down) from the breast.

    ii. The reflex can be conditioned, for example, by the sound of an infant crying.

  e. Suckling **inhibits the GnRH pulse generator,** which suppresses FSH and LH release and also *suppresses the menstrual cycle in most mothers who are breast-feeding.*

    i. The effectiveness of this suppression depends on feeding frequency and can result in the absence of menses for over 2 years.

    ii. Mothers who do not breast feed usually resume their menstrual cycles within 2–4 months after giving birth.

Contraception

1. Many **methods of contraception** have been developed that can interrupt the normal physiologic mechanisms of reproduction; for example:

  a. **Natural contraception** encourages the avoidance of coitus during the woman's midcycle fertile period, about the time of ovulation.

  b. **Barrier methods** such as condoms and the cap try to prevent the sperm from encountering the egg.

  c. **Intrauterine devices (IUDs)** disrupt implantation of the blastocyst.

  d. **Hormonal contraception** aims to disrupt the endocrinology of the menstrual cycle.

    i. **Combined oral contraceptives** contain both estrogen and progesterone and inhibit the increase of FSH that is needed to induce follicular development.

    ii. **Progestin-only pills** produce thick cervical mucus that inhibits sperm passage, and they also disrupt normal endometrial development and inhibit gonadotropin production.

    iii. ▼ Similar to pregnancy, **oral contraceptives** induce a hypercoagulable state and should be avoided in patients with a history of vascular disease (e.g., deep vein thrombosis or stroke). On the other hand, oral contraceptives have been associated with lower rates of ovarian and endometrial cancer. ▼

Study Questions

Directions: Each numbered item is followed by lettered options. Some options may be partially correct, but there is only *ONE BEST* answer.

1. A 34-year old-woman begins assisted fertility treatment to initiate ovulation. She is treated with an agent that acts via gonadotropin-releasing hormone (GnRH) receptors in the anterior pituitary. Which of the following treatments is most likely to be effective?

   A. GnRH agonist given in pulsatile doses

   B. GnRH agonist given continuously

   C. GnRH receptor blocker given in pulsatile doses

   D. GnRH receptor blocker given continuously

2. A 58-year-old man complained of loss of libido and reduced muscle strength. Serum analysis showed reduced levels of testosterone. Reduced activity in which of the following hormone-target cell axes could account for his symptoms?

   A. Luteinizing hormone (LH)—Leydig cell

   B. Follicle-stimulating hormone (FSH)—Leydig cell

   C. LH—Sertoli cell

   D. FSH—Sertoli cell

   E. LH—spermatogonium

   F. FSH—spermatogonium

3. A 17-year-old girl visited her physician because she had never had a menstrual period. Physical examination revealed a tall female with a short, blind-ended vagina and no palpable cervix. Ultrasound showed the absence of a uterus and no ovaries but the presence of undescended testes. Deficiency of which enzyme, hormone, or receptor is most likely to account for these findings?

   A. Androgen receptors

   B. Aromatase

   C. Estrogen receptors

   D. 21α-Hydroxylase

   E. Müllerian-inhibiting substance

   F. Progesterone

   G. 5α-Reductase

4. A 57-year-old man was prescribed the phosphodiesterase type 5 inhibitor sildenafil to enhance sexual function. Which of the following effects will most likely occur after he has taken sildenafil?

   A. Penile erection in the absence of erotic stimulation

   B. Enhanced penile erection following normal erotic stimulation

   C. Increased fluid release from seminal vesicles during emission

   D. Increased prostate secretion during emission

   E. Increased perineal muscle contractions during ejaculation

5. A blood sample is taken from a 27-year-old woman for hormone analysis. The sample contains low levels of follicle-stimulating hormone (FSH) and luteinizing hormone (LH) and high levels of estrogen, progesterone, and inhibin. Assuming a normal 28-day menstrual cycle, on which day of the woman's menstrual cycle was the blood sample taken?

   A. Day 1

   B. Day 7

   C. Day 14

   D. Day 21

   E. Day 28

6. A couple trying to conceive decided to use an ovulation predictor kit to indicate when intercourse should occur to maximize the probability of pregnancy. If ovulation occurs on day 15 of this woman's menstrual cycle, when would implantation of a successfully fertilized egg most likely occur in the uterus?

   A. Days 16–17
   B. Days 18–20
   C. Days 21–22
   D. Days 23–24
   E. Days 25–26

7. An experiment was performed in vitro in which motile sperm were placed in a dish with an egg that was released by natural ovulation. The sperm and egg were both loaded with fluorescent dyes that allowed intracellular $[Ca^{2+}]$ to be measured. A calcium signal was recorded in a single sperm, attached to the zona pellucida of the egg. This signal was most likely associated with which of the following events?

   A. Acrosome reaction
   B. Apoptosis
   C. Capacitation
   D. Cortical reaction
   E. Syngamy

8. Which of the following enzymes or substrates does the fetus provide for the placenta to produce estrogen?

   A. Aromatase
   B. Dehydroepiandrosterone sulfate (DHEA-S)
   C. 21α-Hydroxylase
   D. Pregnenolone
   E. Progesterone
   F. 5α-Reductase
   G. Testosterone

9. A 23-year-old woman consulted her midwife 1 day after the uncomplicated delivery of her first child. She was concerned about her lack of milk production and that she was only producing "a thin yellow fluid" at the breast. The midwife reassured her that this was normal and that milk production would begin within 1–2 days. Which hormone was suppressing her milk production?

   A. Estrogen
   B. Inhibin
   C. Oxytocin
   D. Prostaglandin E
   E. Prolactin

10. A 65-year-old woman was taken to the emergency department after fracturing her hip when stepping off a high curb. X-rays show a fracture at the head of the femur and also reveal very low bone density in general. Which of the following hormonal profiles for the pituitary-gonadal axis is predicted in this patient?

	FSH	LH	Estrogen
A.	Low	Low	Low
B.	Low	Low	High
C.	Low	High	High
D.	High	High	High
E.	High	High	Low
F.	High	Low	Low

Directions: Each numbered item is followed by lettered options. Select the best answer to each question. Some options may be partially correct, but there is only ONE BEST answer.

General Physiology and Neurophysiology

Questions 1–2

1. Nitrous oxide (N_2O) is a lipid soluble anesthetic gas. A 14-year-old girl was sedated with N_2O to relieve pain during an intra-articular injection. The N_2O concentration in her blood quickly equaled, but never exceeded, the alveolar N_2O concentration. What membrane transport mechanism is most likely to account for the uptake of N_2O from inspired air into her blood?

   A. Antiport with CO_2
   B. Cotransport with O_2
   C. Endocytosis
   D. Primary active transport
   E. Simple diffusion

2. The rate of N_2O uptake would increase if the:

   A. body temperature decreased
   B. diffusion distance from alveolus to blood increased
   C. inspired N_2O concentration increased
   D. rate of alveolar ventilation decreased
   E. rate of pulmonary blood flow decreased

Questions 3–5

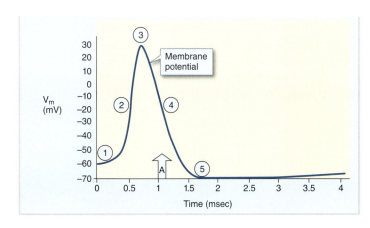

3. What change in ion channel activity is most responsible for the rapid depolarization of the neuronal membrane potential at position 2 (shown in the above figure)?

   A. Opening of K^+ channels
   B. Closure of K^+ channels
   C. Inactivation of K^+ channels
   D. Opening of Na^+ channels
   E. Closure of Na^+ channels
   F. Inactivation of Na^+ channels

4. During the repolarizing phase of the nerve action poten tial shown, which ionic currents are flowing when the membrane potential is 0 mV?

   A. Net current is zero at 0 mV
   B. Net inward K^+ current
   C. Net inward Na^+ current
   D. Net inward Cl^- current

5. If a second depolarizing stimulus of normal strength was applied at the arrow marked A on the figure, a second action potential

   A. has a lower peak voltage than normal
   B. has slower depolarization
   C. is additive with the first action potential
   D. is normal size but initiation is delayed
   E. would not be triggered

6.

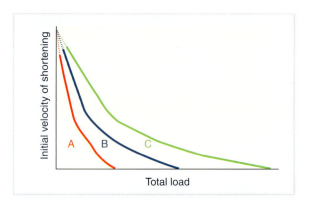

An isolated muscle was studied in the laboratory. The figure shows the relationship between shortening velocity and the total load placed on the skeletal muscle. A change in which of the following variables can explain the shift in this force-velocity relation from curve A to curve C?

   A. Increased preload
   B. Increased contractility
   C. Increased afterload
   D. Increased V_{max}

7. H$^+$ secretion was studied in selected cells taken from the human distal colon. H$^+$ secretion was found to be dependent on the presence of K$^+$ in the lumen of the colon, and was completely inhibited when the tissue was deprived of oxygen. Which mechanism of H$^+$ secretion is most consistent with the transport characteristics described?

   A. Exocytosis
   B. Facilitated diffusion
   C. H$^+$/K$^+$ cotransport
   D. H$^+$/Cl$^-$ antiport
   E. H$^+$ channels
   F. H$^+$/K$^+$-ATPase
   G. Simple diffusion through plasma membrane

8. A low serum K$^+$ concentration (hypokalemia) of 2.0 mM (normal range 3.5–5.5 mM) was measured in an 8-year-old boy after he experienced repeated episodes of diarrhea. K$^+$ was administered with intravenous fluids in an attempt to correct dehydration and hypokalemia. An excessive infusion of K$^+$ was given accidentally, which resulted in an acute increase in serum K$^+$ to 6.8 mM. What effect would this infusion have on the resting membrane potential (V_m) of most cells?

   A. No change in V_m because V_m is independent of E_K
   B. No change in V_m because E_K does not change
   C. Depolarization due to E_K becoming less negative
   D. Depolarization due to E_K becoming more negative
   E. Hyperpolarization due to E_K becoming less negative
   F. Hyperpolarization due to E_K becoming more negative

9. A skeletal muscle was stimulated with an increasing frequency of action potentials. The force of muscle contraction rose progressively to a plateau. The mechanism most likely to be responsible for this effect is

   A. increased Ca^{2+} entry from interstitial fluid
   B. increased amplitude of action potentials with increased stimulation frequency
   C. phosphorylation of myosin light chain kinase
   D. reduced sensitivity of troponin C to Ca^{2+}
   E. reduced time for Ca^{2+} reuptake into sarcoplasmic reticulum

10. As part of a physiology laboratory class, a two-point discrimination test is conducted on the tip of the left index finger of a healthy student volunteer. The axons of the primary sensory neurons that mediate these sensations can be found at which of the following locations?

   A. Left dorsal columns
   B. Right lateral spinothalamic pathway
   C. Left side of the thalamus
   D. Left internal capsule
   E. Left somatosensory cortex

11. A 52-year-old man developed a brain tumor that involved the suprachiasmatic nucleus. Which of the following functions or behaviors is likely to be abnormal as a result of this lesion?

    A. Feeding behavior
    B. Circadian rhythm generation
    C. Sexual behavior
    D. Short-term memory
    E. Temperature regulation
    F. Water balance

12. A 59-year-old woman was admitted to hospital with a 2-day history of altered mental status and headache. Her condition deteriorated, and she was transferred to the intensive care unit for airway protection. The woman was diagnosed with encephalitis due to herpes simplex virus infection. She remained hospitalized for 3 weeks and was treated with antiviral medication during this period. Upon recovery, she had aphasia, characterized by difficulty in comprehending written or spoken words. She mostly spoke in meaningless sentences and appeared to have memory loss. Which lobe of the brain was likely to have been most damaged as a result of the encephalitis?

    A. Frontal
    B. Insular
    C. Parietal
    D. Occipital
    E. Temporal

13. A 29-year-old man was stabbed in the back during a fight. The knife caused severe damage to the right half of the spinal cord at T11. Which of the following neurologic deficits would result from this injury?

    A. Loss of tactile sensation in the left leg
    B. Loss of positional sense from the left leg
    C. Paresis and spasticity of the left leg
    D. Loss of pain sensation in the right leg
    E. Loss of temperature sensation in the right leg
    F. Paresis and spasticity of the right leg

14. An 81-year-old woman suffers compression of the right optic nerve by a large aneurysm of her internal carotid artery. Which of the following visual field defects may occur as a result?

    A. Binasal hemianopia
    B. Bitemporal hemianopia
    C. Homonymous hemianopia
    D. Macula degeneration
    E. Monocular blindness

15. An 18-year-old man fails his driving test due to his inability to read the license plate on an automobile a few meters away. He visits an optometrist, who diagnoses nearsightedness. Which of the following lenses would correct this visual defect?

A. Concave

B. Convex

C. Cylindrical

D. Flat

16. A 17-year-old boy visited his physician because he had frequent headaches and because his academic performance at school was deteriorating despite his best efforts. He had also recently developed a slight tremor in his left hand. MRI scans revealed that both lateral ventricles and the third ventricle were enlarged; the fourth ventricle and subarachnoid space appeared normal. The physician determines that the boy has hydrocephalus. What is the most likely cause of hydrocephalus in this case?

A. Arachnoid granulation blockage

B. Cerebral aqueduct stenosis

C. Choroid plexus papilloma

D. Compression of the spinal canal

E. Ependymal cell dysfunction

17. Synaptic integration within a small neuronal network was studied in the laboratory. A recording electrode was placed in one output neuron, and stimulating electrodes were placed in several other input neurons. When weak stimulation was applied to any single input neuron, no action potentials were recorded in the output neuron. However, simultaneous stimulation of three or more input neurons consistently yielded action potentials in the output neuron. These results illustrate the phenomenon of

A. inhibitory postsynaptic potentials

B. quantal release

C. spatial summation

D. synaptic gating

E. temporal summation

18. A healthy 24-year-old woman runs 5 miles at a moderate pace. Her core body temperature increases to 40°C in the first 20 minutes of the run and remains stable at this value throughout the run (normal temperature = 36–38°C). Her sweating rate increases twofold during the run. Under these conditions, what is the most important mechanism through which sweating is stimulated?

A. Cholinergic parasympathetic neurons

B. Cholinergic sympathetic neurons

C. Circulating epinephrine

D. Norepinephrinergic parasympathetic neurons

E. Norepinephrinergic sympathetic neurons

19. A 68-year-old man was brought to the physician by his wife, who had noticed several changes in her husband over the past year. When greeting the patient, the physician noticed that the man had difficulty getting out of his chair and took a long time to begin walking toward her office. The man walked with a slow shuffling gait and had a characteristic tremor in both hands. He spoke slowly in a flat tone, without blinking. Physical examination revealed increased muscle tone in his arms and legs. What type of drug should this patient be prescribed to alleviate his symptoms?

A. Anticholinesterase
B. Barbiturate
C. Dopamine precursor
D. Sympathomimetic
E. Serotonin-reuptake inhibitor

20. A 59-year-old man is detained by police on suspicion of driving under the influence of alcohol after a minor automobile accident. The police officer assumed the man was severely impaired due to his very wide gait and inability to walk heel to toe in a straight line. However, a breath test revealed an alcohol level just below the legal limit. The man admitted being a heavy drinker for many years but insisted that he had not consumed any alcohol since the previous day. Neurologic examinations showed no sensory, cognitive, or memory deficits. Which of the following structures is most likely to be dysfunctional in this patient?

A. Amygdala
B. Basal ganglia
C. Cerebellum
D. Motor cortex
E. Vestibular labyrinth

21. A 35-year-old woman visited her physician because she had a severe throat infection for several days. She was prescribed an antibiotic but the infection was resistant to the drug and persisted for 5 weeks. After the inflammation had subsided, the woman complained of difficulty swallowing, loss of taste, and shooting pains in her throat. She had no speech problems. She also described frequent palpitations, which she had never felt before the throat infection. Which cranial nerve was most affected by this infection?

A. Abducens (CN VI)
B. Facial (CN VII)
C. Glossopharyngeal (CN IX)
D. Hypoglossal (CN XII)
E. Vagus (X)

22. A 44-year-old woman suffered a stroke that involved part of her midbrain. A hearing impairment resulted, which included a reduced ability to localize sound or to distinguish between sounds. Which structure in this area of the brain may have been damaged by the stroke and could account for these deficits?

A. Inferior colliculus
B. Medial lemniscus
C. Red nucleus
D. Reticular activating system
E. Substantia nigra

Blood and Cardiovascular Physiology

23.

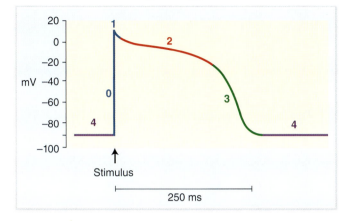

The above figure shows a single cardiac action potential measured in a normal ventricular myocyte. Which of the following stable ionic currents across the cell membrane is most responsible for phase 4?

A. Ca^{2+} current
B. Cl^- current
C. K^+ current
D. Na^+ current

24.

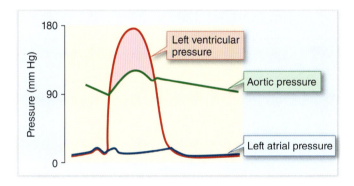

A 50-year-old man with a chronic heart valve abnormality is evaluated for valve replacement surgery. Cardiac catheterization produced the results shown in the figure above. Which of the following heart valve abnormalities does the patient have?

A. Aortic stenosis
B. Aortic insufficiency
C. Mitral stenosis
D. Mitral insufficiency

25.

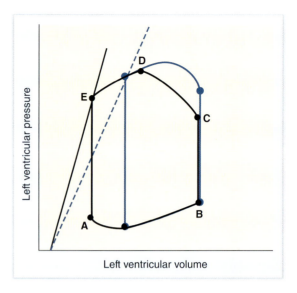

An 84-year-old woman visited her family physician complaining of severe shortness of breath at night and the need to urinate several times during the night. She said that she also became short of breath when lying down or during physical exertion. She was referred to a cardiologist for further investigation. Referring to the above figure, the patient's left ventricular pressure volume loop (*blue*) compared to the expected normal data (*black*). What changes would be expected in the left ventricular ejection fraction of this patient?

A. Decreased

B. Increased

C. No change

Questions 26–29

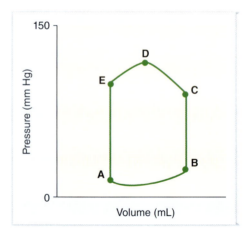

26. The above figure shows a schematic representation of a left ventricular pressure volume loop. During which interval are all the heart valves closed?

A. A–B

B. B–C

C. C–D

D. D–E

27. Which point in the above figure corresponds most closely with the aortic systolic blood pressure?

A. Point A
B. Point B
C. Point C
D. Point D
E. Point E

28. At which point in the above figure does the mitral valve close?

A. Point A
B. Point B
C. Point C
D. Point D
E. Point E

29. A heart murmur due to aortic stenosis would be heard throughout which of the following intervals?

A. A–C
B. B–D
C. C–E
D. D–A

30.

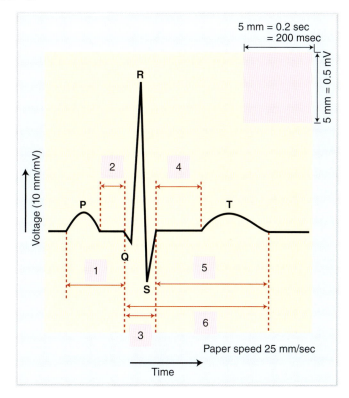

The above figure shows a single cardiac cycle measured in lead II of a normal electrocardiogram (ECG); segments and intervals are indicated by the numbers 1–6. Ventricular myocytes are in which phase of the action potential during period 4?

A. Phase 0
B. Phase 1
C. Phase 2
D. Phase 3
E. Phase 4

31. A 31-year-old woman fractured her pelvis in a skiing accident that resulted in a life-threatening hemorrhage. Because she was skiing in a remote area, 3 hours elapsed before the emergency services were able to administer a blood transfusion. When volume resuscitation was complete, her hematocrit was 40% but then decreased progressively to 24% after 30 days. Her plasma creatinine concentration increased from 1 mg/dL to 8 mg/dL over the same period. What is the most likely cause of this patient's anemia?

A. Decrease in glomerular filtration rate (GFR)
B. Decrease in erythropoietin (EPO) secretion
C. Bone marrow failure at the fracture site
D. Syndrome of inappropriate ADH secretion (SIADH)
E. The destruction of transfused blood

32.

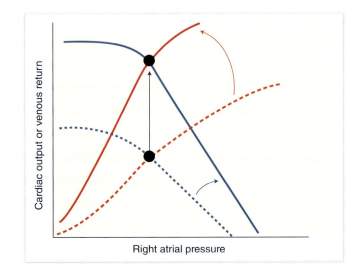

Solid lines in the above figure show changes in cardiac output and systemic vascular function caused by an unknown stressor; dashed lines indicate the normal resting state. The cardiovascular response depicted on the figure would occur in response to which of the following stressors?

A. Digestion of food
B. Dynamic exercise
C. Hypothermia
D. Severe hemorrhage

Respiratory, Renal, and Acid Base Physiology

33.

Patient A	Patient B	Patient C
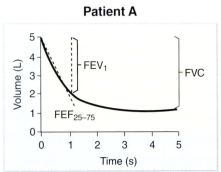	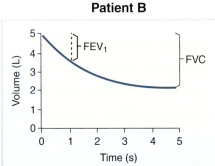	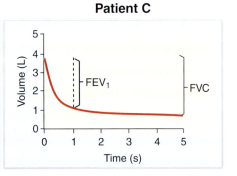

The above figure shows the results of a forced exhalation in three different male patients of similar age, height, and weight. Which one of the patients is most likely to have chronic bronchitis?

A. Patient A
B. Patient B
C. Patient C
D. No results are consistent with chronic bronchitis.

34.

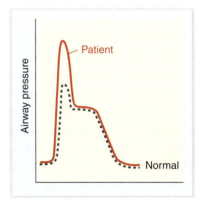

A 54-year-old woman with Guillain-Barré syndrome has received mechanical ventilation for the past 7 days. During the past 30 minutes, the amount of positive airway pressure required to deliver a tidal volume has increased. The above figure shows changes in airway pressure during a tidal breath in which a brief pause is applied just after the tidal volume is delivered. The red line shows the patient's current result; the dashed line shows the result of the same test applied 1 hour previously. What change in the patient's lung function can explain the present test result?

A. Decreased airway resistance
B. Increased airway resistance
C. Decreased static lung compliance
D. Increased static lung compliance

35.

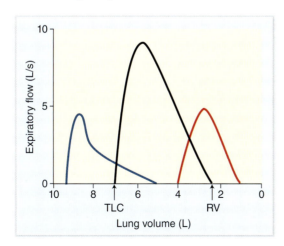

The above figure shows expiratory flow-volume curves for three female patients of similar age, height, and weight. Which diagnosis is consistent with the red curve?

A. Asthma

B. Chronic bronchitis

C. Emphysema

D. Pulmonary fibrosis

36.

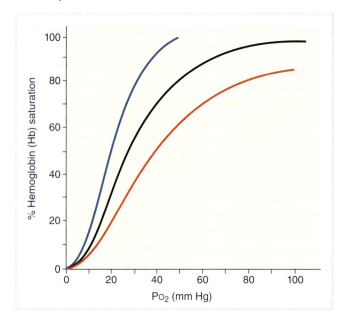

Which of the following changes in the properties of blood would result in a shift from the blue curve to the red curve shown in the above figure?

A. Decreased erythrocyte 2,3-bisphosphoglycerate (2,3-BPG) concentration

B. Decreased temperature

C. Decreased hematocrit

D. Increased partial pressure of CO_2

E. Increased pH

F. Increased plasma volume

37. A subject in a drug trial was infused with isotonic saline containing 200 mg inulin over a 1-hour period. At the end of the infusion period, plasma inulin concentration had stabilized at 1mg/dL. During the 1-hour infusion period, 100 mg of inulin was excreted in the urine. Use these data to approximate the subject's extracellular fluid volume.

A. 10 L

B. 20 L

C. 30 L

D. 40 L

E. 50 L

F. 60 L

38. A 24-year-old man entered a 5-mile road race on a hot day. Although in good health, he had not trained in preparation for the race, and he did not drink any replacement fluids during the race. What changes to his intracellular fluid (ICF) and extracellular fluid (ECF) volumes would be observed at the end of the race compared to just before the race?

A. ECF volume unchanged; ICF volume unchanged

B. ECF volume smaller; ICF volume smaller

C. ECF volume larger; ICF volume larger

D. ECF volume smaller; ICF volume larger

E. ECF volume larger; ICF volume smaller

39. A 52-year-old woman with a history of mitral valve disease developed acute low back pain while in the hospital awaiting heart valve surgery. A CT scan showed a single triangular area of infarction extending from the renal medulla to the outer cortex. Which feature of the renal blood supply accounts for this discrete pattern of infarction?

A. Countercurrent exchange in the vasa recta

B. Lack of anastomosis between the arcuate arteries

C. Low blood flow rate to the renal cortex

D. Low glomerular filtration of the cortical nephrons

E. Separate renal arteries to the upper and lower poles of the kidney

40. Cannulae were surgically implanted into the renal artery and vein of an experimental animal. The arterial-to-venous (a-v)O_2 content difference across the kidney was 1.5 mL (O_2) per 100 mL blood. Samples taken from the aorta and the inferior vena cava showed a systemic difference of 5 mL (O_2) per 100 mL of blood. Why was the renal a-v(O_2) difference smaller?

A. The renal O_2 consumption rate is low

B. The mixed venous O_2 content was pathologically low

C. The kidney has a high rate of blood perfusion

D. The cardiac output was pathologically low

41. A 56-year-old man visited his family physician for a routine health checkup. A urine test revealed significant excretion of albumin. Which cell type is most likely to be damaged or malfunctioning in this patient?

A. Glomerular endothelial cell

B. Juxtaglomerular cell

C. Mesangial cell

D. Podocyte

E. Vascular smooth muscle in afferent arteriole

42. Infusion of the α_1-adrenoceptor agonist phenylephrine into an experimental animal caused an increase in renal vascular resistance; there was greater constriction of the afferent arteriole than the efferent arteriole. What effect on renal blood flow, glomerular filtration, and filtration fraction would result from treatment with phenylephrine?

	Renal Blood Flow (RBF)	Glomerular Filtration Rate (GFR)	Filtration Fraction (FF)
A.	Decrease	Decrease	Decrease
B.	Decrease	Decrease	Unchanged
C.	Decrease	Unchanged	Decrease
D.	Unchanged	Decrease	Decrease
E.	Unchanged	Unchanged	Decrease
F.	Unchanged	Unchanged	Unchanged

43. A 48-year-old man who is 178 cm (5 ft 10 in) tall and weighs 75 kg (165 lb) was in the hospital for minor elective surgery, but laboratory studies showed that his plasma creatinine concentration was five times higher than normal. Which of the following is the most likely cause of this finding?

A. Acidosis
B. Dehydration
C. High plasma antidiuretic hormone (ADH) concentration
D. Large muscle mass
E. Low plasma Na^+ concentration
F. Low glomerular filtration rate (GFR)

44.

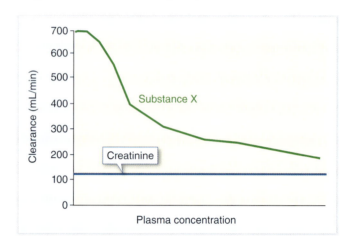

Based only on the information shown in the above figure, what can be deduced about the renal handling of substance X?

A. There is net tubular reabsorption of substance X
B. There is net tubular secretion of substance X
C. Substance X is freely filtered at the glomerulus but is not reabsorbed or secreted
D. Tubular transport of substance X occurs by simple diffusion

45. A 24-year-old man involved in an experiment is found to have a renal p-aminohippuric acid (PAH) clearance of 600 mL/min, a creatinine clearance of 100 mL/min, and a hematocrit of 50%. His rate of renal blood flow is calculated to be

A. 50 mL/min
B. 100 mL/min
C. 300 mL/min
D. 600 mL/min
E. 800 mL/min
F. 1000 mL/min
G. 1200 mL/min

46. A 24-hour urine sample is collected from a patient who was admitted to the hospital because of severe renal colic. Results of the urinalysis show urine creatinine concentration = 20 mg/mL and average urine flow rate = 1 mL/min. Plasma creatinine concentration was 0.2 mg/mL. What is the filtered load of creatinine?

A. 0.2 mg/min
B. 1.0 mg/min
C. 20 mg/min
D. 100 mg/min
E. 200 mg/min

47.

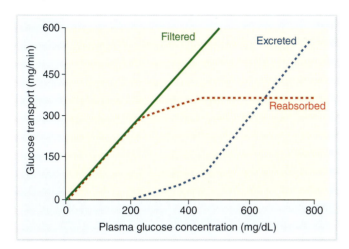

The above figure shows a renal titration curve for glucose. Use the figure to determine the renal threshold for glucose.

A. 0 mg/dL
B. 200 mg/dL
C. 600 mg/dL
D. 0 mg/min
E. 200 mg/min
F. 600 mg/min

48.

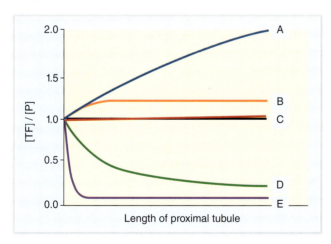

The figure shows tubular fluid-to-plasma (TF/P) concentration profiles for several solutes at increasing distance along the proximal tubule. Which solute would produce a profile similar to solute E?

A. Ca^{2+}
B. Creatinine
C. Glucose
D. K^+
E. Na^+

49. A 2-week-old infant was admitted to the hospital following a visit by the community nurse because he had not gained any weight since birth. On admission, he was found to be severely dehydrated and hypovolemic and was treated with intravenous fluids. Genetic tests were ordered because of the marked renal electrolyte wasting, which showed a mutation in the renal Na/2Cl/K cotransport system. Excessive renal loss of each of the following ions was measured EXCEPT

   A. Ca^{2+}
   B. Cl^-
   C. K^+
   D. Mg^{2+}
   E. Na^+
   F. phosphate

50. A 64-year-old woman with glaucoma is given the carbonic anhydrase inhibitor acetazolamide. Which ion would have the largest increase in its fractional excretion as a side effect of this drug?

   A. Ca^{2+}
   B. Cl^-
   C. HCO_3^-
   D. K^+
   E. Na^+

51. A healthy 59-year-old woman ingested 1 L of water over a 20-minute period. Her urine flow rate increased after 30 minutes and remained elevated for 3 hours. Which of the following changes in her renal function can account for increased water excretion?

   A. Aquaporin 2 expression in the collecting duct decreased
   B. End proximal tubule fluid became dilute
   C. Glomerular filtration rate (GFR) increased
   D. Na^+ reabsorption in the thin descending limb increased
   E. Renal urea production increased

52. A 15-year-old boy was busy with school activities and did not drink any liquids from 8 am to 5 pm. When he urinated late in the day, he noticed that his urine was dark yellow. All of the following events were occurring in his kidney during the day EXCEPT

   A. reduced fractional Na^+ excretion
   B. reduced fractional urea excretion
   C. increased plasma antidiuretic hormone (ADH) con centration
   D. increased Na^+ reabsorption in the thin descending limb
   E. increased aquaporin 2 expression in the collecting duct

53. The urine concentrating ability is evaluated in a 90-year-old woman who complained of polydipsia and polyuria. During the test period, urine flow rate = 2 mL/min, urine osmolarity = 295 mOsM, and plasma osmolarity = 295 mOsM. Free water clearance was calculated to be

A. 0 mL/min

B. 0.5 mL/min

C. 1.0 mL/min

D. 2.0 mL/min

54. A 19-year-old man involved in an automobile accident suffered internal bleeding that resulted in a significant decrease in effective circulating blood volume. The plasma concentration of each of the following hormones would be elevated EXCEPT

A. aldosterone

B. angiotensin II

C. antidiuretic hormone (ADH)

D. atrial natriuretic peptide (ANP)

E. epinephrine

55. A healthy 22-year-old man ate 200 g of salted peanuts. As a result, he became extremely thirsty and drank 1 L of water. What changes would occur to the physical forces acting at renal peritubular capillaries in response to this ingestion of salt and water?

A. Increased hydrostatic pressure and reduced oncotic pressure

B. Increased hydrostatic pressure and increased oncotic pressure

C. Reduced hydrostatic pressure and reduced oncotic pressure

D. Reduced hydrostatic pressure and increased oncotic pressure

56. A 29-year-old man had complained to his wife about bone pain, frequent headaches, and fatigue for over 1 year but had not visited his physician. After an episode of acute renal colic, he was evaluated in the hospital and found to have kidney stones. He was diagnosed with primary hyperparathyroidism. Compared to individuals with normal parathyroid function, his fractional renal Ca^{2+} excretion is expected to be

A. increased

B. decreased

C. unchanged

57. A 32-year-old man fell from a ladder and fractured his skull. On admission to the hospital, he was unconscious because of a closed head injury. Arterial blood gas analysis showed:

Po_2 = 106 mm Hg

Pco_2 = 25 mm Hg

pH = 7.52

$[HCO_3^-]$ = 21 mEq/L

Base excess = −1 mEq/L

Which of the following primary acid-base disturbances is present?

A. Respiratory alkalosis

B. Respiratory acidosis

C. Metabolic alkalosis

D. Metabolic acidosis

58. A 14-year-old girl with a history of poorly controlled type 1 diabetes mellitus is found unresponsive in her bed. Her parents call 911, and she is taken by ambulance to the emergency department. The arterial blood gas analysis at this time showed:

$Po_2 = 90$ mm Hg
$Pco_2 = 36$ mm Hg
$pH = 7.10$
$[HCO_3^-] = 7$ mEq/L
Base excess $= -20$ mEq/L

Which of the following primary acid-base disturbances is present in this patient?

A. Respiratory alkalosis
B. Respiratory acidosis
C. Metabolic alkalosis
D. Metabolic acidosis

59. A 27-year-old woman who weighs 60 kg was anesthetized using a drug that distributed equally throughout her total body water. Hepatic and renal function were both normal, and her body mass index was within the normal range. What is the approximate volume of distribution for the anesthetic in this patient?

A. 10 L
B. 20 L
C. 30 L
D. 40 L
E. 50 L
F. 60 L

60. A 64-year-old man was admitted to the hospital with evidence of low effective circulating blood volume. His past medical history includes a myocardial infarction 1 year ago but no previous kidney problems were noted. Clearance of PAH and creatinine are both reduced. Plasma creatinine is approximately three times higher than normal. Assuming normal diet and liver function, this patient's blood urea nitrogen (BUN) concentration would be expected to be

A. approximately the same as normal
B. approximately one third of normal
C. significantly less than one third of normal
D. approximately three times normal
E. significantly more than three times normal

61. A 21-year-old woman with a history of substance abuse was found unresponsive with a hypodermic needle in her arm. Arterial blood gas analysis showed:

$Po_2 = 68$ mm Hg
$Pco_2 = 84$ mm Hg
$pH = 7.02$
$[HCO_3^-] = 23$ mEq/L
Base excess $= -2$ mEq/L

Which of the following primary acid-base disturbances is present?

A. Respiratory alkalosis
B. Respiratory acidosis
C. Metabolic alkalosis
D. Metabolic acidosis

62. A 56-year-old man with chronic renal insufficiency was evaluated in the hospital in preparation for hemodialysis. Arterial blood gas analysis showed:

P_{O_2} = 90 mm Hg
P_{CO_2} = 28 mm Hg
pH = 7.32
$[HCO_3^-]$ = 15 mEq/L
Base excess = -10mEq/L

The patient was diagnosed with partially compensated

A. respiratory alkalosis
B. respiratory acidosis
C. metabolic alkalosis
D. metabolic acidosis

Gastrointestinal Physiology

63. During surgery to remove a tumor, an area of normal small intestine was removed and placed in a tissue bath for study. A peptide with endocrine activity was added to the bathing solution. The peptide caused secretion of fluid from surface epithelium and simultaneous relaxation of smooth muscle. The peptide was most likely to be

A. cholecystokinin
B. gastrin
C. glucose-dependent insulinotropic polypeptide
D. motilin
E. vasoactive intestinal polypeptide

64. A novel antibiotic drug was tested in animals. Side-effects of the drug included increased intestinal motility, which was characterized by waves of peristaltic contractions approximately every 90 minutes. Which hormone is the antibiotic most likely to mimic?

A. Cholecystokinin
B. Gastrin
C. Glucagon-like peptide-1
D. Motilin
E. Secretin

65. A 62-year-old man was admitted to the hospital with low blood pressure and evidence of active bleeding from the upper gastrointestinal tract. He was administered fluid intravenously and a drug that vasoconstricts splanchnic blood vessels. The drug also reduces gastric acid production and pancreatic secretion. Which hormone does the drug mimic?

A. Acetylcholine
B. Cholecystokinin
C. Gastrin
D. Secretin
E. Somatostatin

66.

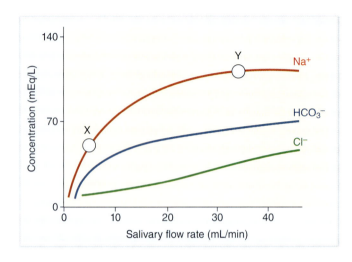

Which one of the following interventions would result in the sample taken at point Y in the figure compared to a control sample obtained at point X?

A. Dehydration of the subject
B. Exposure of the subject to low ambient temperature
C. Induction of sleep by meditation
D. Infusion of aldosterone
E. Stimulation of parasympathetic nerves to the salivary gland

67. A 3-year-old boy swallowed a steel ball bearing 1 cm in diameter. An x-ray taken 6 hours later showed that the object was located in his distal ileum. Which pattern of gastric motility allowed the ball bearing to pass through the pyloric sphincter?

A. Antral systole
B. Migrating motor complex
C. Phasic contractions of the fundus
D. Tonic contraction of proximal stomach

68. A preparation of normal pancreatic acinar cells obtained from a surgical sample was studied in vitro. Fluorescent imaging was used to measure changes in intracellular Ca^{2+} concentration in response to a series of agonists. Which of the following hormones would produce the largest increase in intracellular $[Ca^{2+}]$?

A. Cholecystokinin
B. Gastrin
C. Glucagon
D. Secretin
E. Vasoactive intestinal polypeptide

69. A 39-year-old woman is treated for pancreatic cancer by complete surgical removal of the pancreas and duodenum. Without supplemental treatment, which of the following mineral deficiencies would most likely develop in this patient in the following weeks and months?

   A. Iron and Ca^{2+}
   B. K^+ and Ca^{2+}
   C. K^+ and iron
   D. Na^+ and K^+
   E. Na^+ and Ca^{2+}

70. A 40-year-old man with hereditary hemochromatosis visited his physician because he was concerned about a recent darkening of his skin. A program of controlled blood removal by venipuncture was begun to reduce body iron levels. What process is responsible for iron overload in this patient?

   A. Excess production of transferrin
   B. Excess intestinal absorption of iron
   C. Excess hepatic secretion of hepcidin
   D. Failure of tissue ferritin production
   E. Inadequate renal iron excretion

71. Sugar absorption was studied in a segment of jejunum perfused in vitro. What is the most likely effect on glucose absorption of adding equimolar galactose to the luminal solution?

   A. Glucose absorption is abolished
   B. Glucose absorption continues at a reduced rate
   C. Glucose absorption is unaffected
   D. Glucose absorption continues at an increased rate

72. A 28-year-old man visited his physician because of diarrhea and bloating, which has been an increasing problem for the past 6 months. Fecal analysis showed that fecal osmolarity was not accounted for by the electrolytes present in the sample. Which condition could account for the presence of this "fecal osmolar gap"?

   A. Achalasia
   B. Diabetes mellitus
   C. Lactase deficiency
   D. Secretory diarrhea
   E. Xerostomia

73. A patient with chronic steatorrhea is most likely to develop deficiency of which of the following vitamins?

   A. Vitamins A and B_1
   B. Vitamins A and C
   C. Vitamins A and D
   D. Vitamins B_1 and C
   E. Vitamins B_1 and D
   F. Vitamins C and D

74. A 3-month-old infant was being breast-fed in the physician's reception room. Just before entering the physician's office for her examination, the child defecated into her diaper. Which of the following gastrointestinal reflexes is most likely to account for this untimely defecation?

    A. Enterogastrone reflex
    B. Gastroileal reflex
    C. Gastrocolic reflex
    D. Ileal brake
    E. Rectosphincteric reflex

75. A group of normal subjects was given a range of test meals, each of the same volume. The rate of gastric emptying was determined using noninvasive imaging procedures. Which of the following meals would take the longest time to empty from the stomach?

    A. Pure water, pH = 7.0
    B. 1% glucose solution, pH = 7.0
    C. 1% glucose + 0.1% oleic acid, pH = 7.2
    D. 1% glucose + 0.1% oleic acid + 0.9% saline, pH = 7.2
    E. 1% glucose + 0.1% oleic acid + 0.9% saline + HCl, pH = 6.2

Endocrinology and Reproductive Physiology

76. A stable derivative of cholesterol was synthesized as part of a drug discovery program. Which of the following properties is this new molecule most likely to have when injected into test subjects?

    A. Binds mostly to surface membrane receptors on target cells
    B. Circulates bound to plasma proteins
    C. Enters target cells by carrier-mediated transport
    D. Has effects lasting a few minutes
    E. Induces an increase in intracellular cAMP in target cells

77.

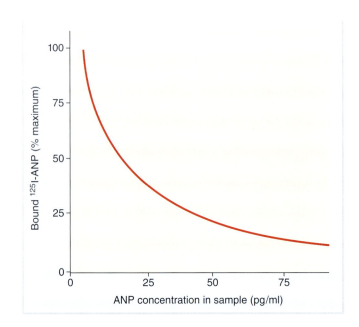

Plasma atrial natriuretic peptide (ANP) concentration was measured by radio-immunoassay in a healthy 31-year-old man. The standard curve shown in the figure above was obtained by displacing radioactive ^{125}I-ANP from anti-ANP antibodies with ANP standards. A sample of a patient's serum caused 50% of ^{125}I-ANP to remain bound to the antibody. What was the patient's approximate plasma ANP concentration?

A. 0 pg/mL
B. 20 pg/mL
C. 40 pg/mL
D. 60 pg/mL
E. 80 pg/mL

78. A 54-year-old woman visited her physician because of persistent headaches and blurred vision. The physician noted that the woman has very large hands and feet, a wide jaw, a large tongue, and a prominent forehead. Which of the following metabolic abnormalities would most likely be present in this patient?

A. Decreased blood fatty acid concentration
B. Decreased hepatic gluconeogenesis
C. Decreased protein synthesis
D. Increased blood glucose concentration
E. Increased uptake of glucose in skeletal muscle

79. A 19-year-old patient produced a copious amount of dilute urine following a head injury sustained in a motor vehicle accident. Damage to which of the following sites could account for these symptoms in this patient?

A. Anterior pituitary
B. Mamillary body
C. Median eminence
D. Superior hypophyseal artery
E. Supraoptic nucleus

80. A healthy 29-year-old man was injected with thyroid-stimulating-hormone (TSH) as part of a clinical research study. Increased levels of serum thyroid hormones were detected within a few minutes. Which major form of thyroid hormone was detected in this subject?

A. Monoiodothyronine
B. Diiodothyronine
C. Triiodothyronine
D. Reverse triiodothyronine
E. Thyroxine

81. A 28-year-old woman visited her physician because of anxiety. She was perspiring heavily and complained about the high temperature of the waiting room. Physical examination showed a thin patient with notable tremor, muscle weakness, tachycardia, and an ophthalmopathy with a staring gaze. What is the most likely profile of serum thyroxine (T_4) and thyroid-stimulating hormone (TSH) concentrations in this patient?

A. Low T_4, high TSH

B. Low T_4, low TSH

C. High T_4, low TSH

D. High T_4, high TSH

82. A fine needle adrenal biopsy was performed in a 71-year-old man who had an unidentified adrenal mass. Tests performed on the sample included the expression of the enzyme aldosterone synthase. Which area of the adrenal gland would show positive staining for this enzyme?

A. Zona glomerulosa

B. Zona fasciculata

C. Zona reticularis

D. Medullary chromaffin cells.

83. A 2-year-old boy is brought to a pediatrician because he has acute viral laryngitis and has developed difficulty breathing. He was previously treated for 3 days with a large dose of oral glucocorticoids to reduce inflammation of his larynx. The effects of this treatment on the child's fasting plasma glucose and fatty acids levels would most likely be

A. increased glucose and increased fatty acids

B. increased glucose and decreased fatty acids

C. decreased glucose and increased fatty acids

D. decreased glucose and decreased fatty acids

84. Excessive licorice consumption may result in secondary hypertension due to inhibition of the enzyme 11β-hydroxysteroid dehydrogenase in renal epithelial cells. The Na^+ retention that follows is due to interaction between which agonist–receptor pair?

A. Glucocorticoids—glucocorticoid receptors

B. Mineralocorticoids—mineralocorticoid receptors

C. Mineralocorticoids—glucocorticoid receptors

D. Glucocorticoids—mineralocorticoid receptors

85. A 68-year-old woman became acutely ill while on holiday. She was confused and unable to give the attending physician her medical history. The physician noticed the patient had a moon face, truncal obesity, and bruising on large areas of skin on both legs. Laboratory studies showed fasting hyperglycemia and low levels of both cortisol and adrenocorticotropic hormone (ACTH). Which of the following conditions is consistent with the physical examination and laboratory data?

A. ACTH-secreting tumor

B. Chronic glucocorticoid medication

C. Cortisol-secreting tumor

D. Destructive tumor of the anterior pituitary

E. Primary adrenocortical insufficiency

86. A 45-year-old woman suffered episodes of headache, nausea, sweating, and palpitations that were becoming more frequent and severe. One such episode occurred while she was visiting a friend in the hospital. A nurse measured her heart rate and blood pressure during the episode, which were 142 beats/min

and 180/145 mm Hg, respectively. A resident suggested the differential diagnosis of pheochromocytoma. Which of the following profiles of catecholamine excretion in the urine would support this diagnosis?

	Vanillylmandelic acid (VMA)	Metanephrine	Epinephrine
A.	Low	Low	Low
B.	Low	Low	High
C.	Low	High	High
D.	High	High	High
E.	High	High	Low
F.	High	Low	Low

87. A 28-year-old medical resident who was accustomed to eating regular meals was forced to skip breakfast and lunch one day because of a heavy work schedule. By midafternoon, he was feeling lightheaded and very hungry. Compared to his typical day, the plasma concentration of which of the following hormones would be decreased at this time?

    A. Cortisol
    B. Epinephrine
    C. Glucagon
    D. Growth hormone
    E. Insulin

88. A healthy 21-year-old man was intravenously infused with a saline solution containing a mixture of amino acids, including arginine and leucine. Which pair of secretory responses in insulin and glucagon would occur in response to this challenge?

    A. Increased insulin and increased glucagon
    B. Increased insulin and decreased glucagon
    C. Decreased insulin and decreased glucagon
    D. Decreased insulin and increased glucagon

89. A healthy 12-year-old girl consumed a 100-g bar of chocolate. Her plasma insulin concentration increased significantly soon after eating, with only a modest increase in plasma glucose concentration. Which hormone is released by mucosal endocrine cells of the gastrointestinal tract that could help to account for these observations?

    A. Enterogastrone
    B. Gastrin
    C. Glucagon
    D. Glucagon-like peptide-1
    E. Insulin

90. A 19-year-old woman visited her physician complaining of frequent urination and of being thirsty all the time. On physical examination, the woman appeared extremely malnourished. Plasma analysis showed high concentrations of both glucose and ketones. Which hormone is most responsible for the presence of high ketone concentrations in this patient?

A. Cortisol
B. Epinephrine
C. Glucagon
D. Growth hormone
E. Insulin

91. A healthy 34-year-old woman runs 5 miles at a fast pace, resulting in a large increase in the rate of glucose oxidation in her muscles. Which pair of hormones is most important to minimize the decrease in plasma glucose concentration during her run?

A. Cortisol and growth hormone
B. Cortisol and insulin
C. Epinephrine and insulin
D. Glucagon and epinephrine
E. Glucagon and thyroxine
F. Growth hormone and thyroxine

92. A 23-year-old medical student ingests several liters of cola in an effort to stay awake over a 24-hour period of studying. This ingestion of cola represents a large intake of phosphate ions, which results in increased urinary phosphate excretion. Which hormone is most responsible for stimulating phosphate excretion in this case?

A. Calcitonin
B. Ergocalciferol
C. Parathyroid hormone
D. 1,25-$(OH)_2$ Vitamin D_3

93. A 46-year-old man with bone cancer is found to have high plasma levels of parathyroid hormone-related peptide (PTH-rp). Which of the following profiles for plasma Ca^{2+}, phosphate (P), and parathyroid hormone (PTH) concentration would be expected in this patient?

	Plasma [Ca²⁺]	Plasma [P]	Plasma [PTH]
A.	Low	Low	Low
B.	Low	Low	High
C.	Low	High	High
D.	High	High	High
E.	High	High	Low
F.	High	Low	Low

94. A 17-year-old girl visited her physician because she had never had a menstrual period. Physical examination revealed a tall female with a short, blind-ended vagina and no palpable cervix. Ultrasound showed the absence of a uterus and no ovaries and the presence of undescended testes. Deficiency of which enzyme, hormone, or receptor is most likely to account for these findings?

A. Androgen receptors
B. Aromatase
C. Estrogen receptors

D. 21α-Hydroxylase

E. Müllerian-inhibiting substance

F. Progesterone

G. 5α-Reductase

95. A blood sample is taken from a 27-year-old woman for hormone analysis. The sample contains low levels of follicle-stimulating hormone (FSH) and luteinizing hormone (LH) and high levels of estrogen, progesterone, and inhibin. Assuming a normal 28-day menstrual cycle, on which day of this woman's menstrual cycle was the blood sample taken?

A. Day 1

B. Day 7

C. Day 14

D. Day 21

E. Day 28

96. An indicator dilution technique was used to estimate plasma volume in a pregnant woman at the beginning of her third trimester. Plasma volume was found to be about 30% higher than that expected for a nonpregnant woman of similar height and weight. Increased secretion of which hormone accounts directly for this large increase in plasma volume?

A. Aldosterone

B. Atrial natriuretic peptide

C. Chorionic gonadotropin

D. Cortisol

E. Estrogen

F. Oxytocin

G. Progesterone

97. An arterial blood sample was taken from a 28-year-old pregnant woman. Blood gas analysis showed:

$Po_2 = 91$ mm Hg

$So_2 = 97\%$

$Pco_2 = 31$ mm Hg

$pH = 7.42$

$HCO_3^- = 21$ mEq/L

Which primary physiologic adaptation to pregnancy is responsible for changes in acid-base status compared to normal nonpregnant women?

A. Increased alveolar ventilation

B. Decreased alveolar ventilation

C. Increased insulin responsiveness

D. Decreased insulin responsiveness

E. Increased glomerular filtration rate

F. Decreased glomerular filtration rate

98. A 37-year old-woman who is breast-feeding her 4-month-old son is taking the train to see her mother who lives several hours away. When the woman hears the cry of another infant, she notices that milk has been expressed from both her breasts. The release of which hormone can account for this response?

A. Estrogen

B. Inhibin

C. Oxytocin

D. Progesterone

E. Prolactin

99. A 36-year-old woman who is pregnant with her third child is in labor. Her serum oxytocin levels were measured at regular intervals over a 24-hour period. Measurements were taken at the onset when the woman began having low back pains 1 day before delivery and ended 3 hours after delivery of the infant, just before the woman was to begin breast-feeding the infant. A normal vaginal delivery was completed without medical intervention. At what time was the oxytocin concentration in maternal blood most likely to be highest?

A. Before labor

B. At the onset of back pain

C. Uterine contractions 20 minutes apart

D. During the expulsive stages of labor

E. Three hours after delivery

100. A 32-year-old woman and her partner were trying to conceive a child. The woman had regular menstrual cycles of about 30 days in length. Four days after missing her menstrual period, she bought a commercial pregnancy testing kit. The couple was excited to discover that her urine sample indicated a positive result for pregnancy. Which of the following hormones was detected in her urine?

A. Human chorionic gonadotropin

B. Estrogen

C. Follicle-stimulating hormone

D. Gonadotropin-releasing hormone

E. Inhibin

F. Luteinizing hormone

G. Progesterone

101. Fetal acquisition of glucose occurs by placental glucose transport. What is the first cell layer within the placenta that glucose must cross during transport from maternal to fetal blood?

A. Cytotrophoblast

B. Decidua

C. Inner cell mass

D. Mesenchyme

E. Syncytiotrophoblast

102. The luteinizing hormone surge measured during the ovulatory phase of the menstrual cycle results from positive feedback exerted by which of the following hormones?

A. Estrogen

B. Follicle-stimulating hormone

C. Gonadotropin-releasing hormone

D. Inhibin

E. Progesterone

103. A 36-year-old woman visited her gynecologist to have a routine annual examination. A cervical Pap smear was performed to check for abnormal cells. The mucus sample was thin and produced a fern-like pattern when it dried on a microscope slide. Assuming a normal 28-day menstrual cycle, on which day of this woman's menstrual cycle was the smear taken?

    A. Day 1
    B. Day 7
    C. Day 14
    D. Day 21
    E. Day 28

104. A 37-year-old man with four children elected to have a vasectomy. This procedure prevents conception because

    A. no sperm is ejaculated
    B. secretion from seminal vesicles is not ejaculated
    C. secretion from the prostate gland is not ejaculated
    D. no semen is ejaculated

105. A child born with ambiguous genitalia was found to have a 46XY karyotype. Testes were present at birth, and there was a small phallus with a urethral opening at its mid point. The child entered puberty late, but masculinization was evident. Which deficiency could account for these findings?

    A. Aromatase
    B. 21α-Hydroxylase
    C. Luteinizing hormone receptor
    D. 5α-Reductase
    E. Testosterone

106. Ovarian granulosa cells were grown in primary cell culture in vitro. The cells failed to secrete significant amounts of estrogen when exposed to follicle-stimulating hormone (FSH) and luteinizing hormone (LH) until they were cultured together with ovarian thecal cells. A likely explanation for the failure of granulosa cells to produce estrogens when cultured alone is

    A. inability of granulosa cells to synthesize cholesterol
    B. lack of androgen precursors from which to produce estrogens
    C. lack of aromatase activity
    D. lack of 5α-reductase activity
    E. lack of progesterone precursor from which to produce estrogens

107. When the gas composition of umbilical arterial blood is compared to umbilical venous blood, the arterial blood has

    A. lower P_{O_2} and higher P_{CO_2}
    B. lower P_{O_2} and lower P_{CO_2}
    C. higher P_{O_2} and lower P_{CO_2}
    D. higher P_{O_2} and higher P_{CO_2}
    E. the same P_{O_2} and P_{CO_2}

108. An 18-year-old man visited his physician because he was concerned about his height. He is 152 cm tall (5 ft). He described himself when he was in elementary school as being self-conscious because he was taller than his peers. He also recalled developing pubic and axillary hair at about age 7 or 8. Physical examination showed a healthy male of short stature with normal genitalia and male secondary sexual development. Which endocrine abnormality best explains the findings in this patient?

    A. Early maturation of the hypothalamic-pituitary-gonadal axis
    B. Failure of pulsatile gonadotrophin-releasing hormone secretion at puberty
    C. Growth hormone excess in early childhood
    D. Insulin-like growth factor-1 deficiency
    E. Panhypopituitarism

Answers

Chapter 1

1. **(C) Facilitated diffusion**

   Facilitated diffusion only occurs passively down the solute electrochemical gradient; it occurs via uniporters, with no dependence on other solutes and is saturable.

2. **(A) Isosmotic**

   Lumen osmolarity = $2 \times 150 = 300$ mOsm/L; bathing solution osmolarity = $1 \times 300 = 300$ mOsm/L. The solutions are therefore isosmotic.

3. **(B) Water moves out of the intestine**

   Effective osmolarity (tonicity) = osmolarity $\times$ reflection coefficient. Lumen tonicity = $300 \times 0.9 = 270$ mOsm/L; bath tonicity = 300×1.0 = 300 mOsm/L. The luminal solution is hypotonic with respect to the bathing solution; water therefore moves out of the intestine by osmosis.

4. **(F) −90 mV**

   When the cell membrane is selectively permeable for one ion (in this case K^+), an electrochemical equilibrium for that ion is established. Membrane potential is therefore equal to E_K (−88 mV).

5. **(A) Depolarization**

   Opening Cl^- channels results in total membrane conductance being shared between K^+ and Cl^-. V_m is the weighted average of E_K and E_{Cl}. No fractional conductances are given, but V_m lies between E_K (−88 mV) and E_{Cl} (−46 mV) and is thus depolarized compared to the control condition.

6. **(A) Cl^- moves out of the cell**

   The electrochemical gradient ($V_m - E_{Cl}$) is the driving force for Cl^- flux. Under the initial conditions $V_m - E_{Cl} = -88 - (-46) = -42$ mV. By convention, a negative electrochemical gradient directs outward anion flux. Opening Cl channels would shift V_m (−88 mV) toward E_{Cl} (−46 mV), such that V_m would become less negative; negatively charged Cl^- ions must move out of the cell to make the cell interior less negative.

7. **(C) Failure of acetylcholine release from the motor nerve terminal**

   Voltage-operated calcium channels in the presynaptic membrane open in response to action potentials in the motor nerve. Calcium entry triggers the release of acetylcholine by exocytosis. The neurotoxic peptide ω-conotoxin causes this to fail.

8. **(C) Decreased acetylcholine breakdown at the neuromuscular junctions**

Acetylcholinesterase breaks down acetylcholine to choline and acetic acid within the synaptic cleft. In myasthenia gravis, there is reduced nicotinic acetylcholine receptor availability in the skeletal muscle membrane. Blocking acetylcholinesterase increases the amount and duration of acetylcholine presence in the synaptic cleft, increasing the probability of muscle stimulation.

9. **(A) A band**

The A bands are composed of thick filaments and have a fixed length. Contraction with muscle shortening causes Z disks to approach each other and the I band to shorten, as thin filaments are drawn over thick filaments.

10. **(E) Decreased myosin light chain phosphatase activity**

Excitation contraction coupling in smooth muscle involves activation of thick filaments by phosphorylation. Myosin phosphorylation is determined by a balance between myosin light chain kinase and myosin light chain phosphatase enzymes. A decrease in myosin light chain phosphatase activity favors myosin phosphorylation and greater smooth muscle tone.

Chapter 2

1. **(B) Brain capillary endothelium**

The blood-brain barrier prevents the free access of most solutes from plasma to the brain extracellular fluid. The blood-brain barrier is formed by the capillary endothelial cells and supporting glial cells. The choroid plexus also contributes, to a lesser extent, by actively regulating cerebrospinal fluid composition.

2. **(B) Demyelination of central nervous system (CNS) neurons**

The involvement of somatic sensory and motor functions, as well as autonomic functions such as urinary continence, indicates the involvement of many parts of the nervous system. This presentation in a young woman is consistent with a diagnosis of multiple sclerosis, which is caused by the autoimmune destruction of myelin sheaths around neurons in the brain and spinal cord.

3. **(B) Glutamate**

The neurotransmitter produces an excitatory postsynaptic potential in this case. Glutamate is the most common excitatory neurotransmitter in the central nervous system; the others are all inhibitory transmitters. Enkephalin and somatostatin are large molecule transmitters present in lower abundance than the other examples given.

4. **(F) Left dorsal column**

   Touch (as well as vibration and proprioception) sensations are conveyed via the dorsal column white matter to the brain. This pathway crosses over at the level of the caudal medulla, so that touch sensation from the left leg is represented in left side of the spinal cord.

5. **(B) Bitemporal hemianopia**

   A tumor pressing on the optic chiasm disrupts optic fibers crossing from one side to the other, from the nasal half of each retina. These neurons are excited by light from the temporal parts of the visual field.

6. **(B) Left optic nerve**

   The absence of both the direct and consensual light reflex response when light is shone in the left eye indicates a problem with the afferent part of the pupillary light reflex pathway on the left. A normal response on both sides when light is shone in the right eye demonstrates that the efferent parts of the reflex pathway, including the Edinger Westphal nucleus and cranial nerve III, are unaffected. The superior colliculus and visual cortex are not involved in the pupillary light reflex.

7. **(A) Weber test lateralizes to the left; Rinne test shows air conduction > bone conduction**

   The patient is most likely to have damaged hair cells in her right ear by listening to loud music selectively in this ear for a prolonged period of time. This produces a sensorineural hearing loss due to failure of the hair cell transduction mechanism (rather than a failure of sound conduction through the middle ear). In unilateral sensorineural hearing loss, the Weber test lateralizes to the unaffected side and air conduction of sound is better than bone conduction.

8. **(D) Olfaction**

   The sensory pathway for olfaction does not involve the thalamus and would therefore result in the least thalamic neuronal activity. The olfactory pathway involves the nasal mucosa, olfactory bulb, and olfactory tract, leading to the olfactory cortex in the temporal lobe. The pathways of all the other sensory modalities listed involve the thalamus.

9. **(B) Cerebellum**

   The presence of an intention tremor, and the lack of coordination during complex movements, indicates dysfunction in the cerebellar hemispheres. The gait abnormality described is consistent with dysfunction in the circuits of the spinocerebellum.

10. **(H) Raphe**

    The loss of serotonergic neurons in the raphe nucleus is the most consistent with development of mood and sleep problems. Loss of the amygdaloid nuclei reduces aggressiveness. The arcuate, paraventricular, suprachiasmatic, and supraoptic nuclei are all hypothalamic nuclei; the caudate, dentate, and fastigial nuclei are associated with the motor system; and the Edinger–Westphal nucleus is a parasympathetic nucleus.

Chapter 3

1. **(C) Normocytic, hypoproliferative anemia**

   Low hemoglobin concentration and hematocrit demonstrate the presence of anemia. Mean cell volume is normal because the red blood cell count is reduced in proportion to the reduced hematocrit; therefore a normocytic anemia is present. The reticulocyte count is not increased, as would occur, for example, in hemorrhage or hemolytic disease, indicating that the anemia is hypoproliferative (low red cell production).

2. **(A) Antithrombin III defect**

   The patient is likely to be in a hypercoagulable state, predisposing her to deep vein thrombosis. Defects in anticoagulants, such as antithrombin III, produce a hypercoagulable state. Decreased platelets, fibrinogen, or factor VIII all oppose coagulation; hematocrit is not directly relevant.

3. **(E) Chelates Ca^{2+} ions**

   Citrate ions chelate Ca^{2+}, which is required as a cofactor for several steps in the coagulation cascades.

4. **(C) Inhibition of platelet function**

   Aspirin and other NSAIDs inhibit the production of *thromboxane A_2* by blocking the key enzyme cyclooxygenase (COX). These agents therefore inhibit platelet activation.

5. **(D) Prolonged prothrombin time (PT)**

   Vitamin K deficiency reduces the production of prothrombin (and other clotting factors) in the liver. In mild vitamin K deficiency, the prothrombin time is therefore prolonged. Platelet production is not dependent on vitamin K; bleeding time is an indicator of platelet function and is not affected. The INR provides a normalized value of the prothrombin time and would therefore also be increased. Prolonged partial prothromboplastin time reflects function of the intrinsic clotting pathway and does not become affected until vitamin K deficiency is severe.

Chapter 4

1. **(D) Decreased contractility and decreased TPR**

   The baroreceptor reflex would cause a decrease in sympathetic nervous tone as a result of this sudden blood volume expansion. The intrinsic contractility of the heart would decrease due to less norepinephrinergic stimulation (*Note: "contractility" refers to intrinsic contraction strength for a given preload; in this case, SV may be increased due to high preload but contractility is reduced.*) Reduced vasoconstrictor tone causes decreased TPR.

2. **(F) Increased vagal tone**

   A decrease in resting HR and an increase in SV is a characteristic of endurance training that allows a greater increase in cardiac output during exercise. This adaptation of training results from increased vagal tone to the SA node.

3. **(E) Purkinje fibers**

The results of this patient's ECG are consistent with complete heart block. In the normal hierarchy of pacemakers, the AV node would be next to initiate ventricular beating at about 40 beats/min, when the SA node is unable to excite the ventricles. A pacemaker originating in the AV node or bundle of His would produce normally shaped QRS complexes. Excitation that spreads from a bundle branch or Purkinje fiber takes longer to reach all parts of the ventricles, producing wide QRS complexes. Purkinje fibers have a slow rate of spontaneous depolarization, consistent with a HR of 25 beats/min.

4. **(C) Mitral stenosis**

Diastolic murmurs include mitral stenosis and aortic insufficiency; an opening snap is characteristic of mitral stenosis. Dyspnea on exertion and paroxysmal nocturnal dyspnea suggest pulmonary edema. Pulmonary edema is consistent with increased left atrial (and therefore pulmonary capillary) pressure, which results from impedance of blood flow through the mitral valve.

5. **(A) Decreased aortic compliance**

The patient has isolated systolic hypertension. Vascular tone appears to be normal because diastolic pressure is most affected by changes in peripheral resistance. Sympathetic stimulation would cause increases in both systolic pressure and diastolic pressure; parasympathetic tone has little impact on blood pressure. In any case, the patient's HR is normal, indicating that there is no abnormal autonomic nervous system activity. Low aortic compliance produces high systolic pressure in response to the ejection of a normal SV.

6. **(C) inadequate blood flow autoregulation**

Autoregulation is the dominant mechanism of blood flow control in the cerebral circulation. Autoregulation is reset in chronic hypertension to regulate cerebral blood flow around higher than normal blood pressures. In this case, treatment of hypertension reduces blood pressure to a value below the autoregulatory range, causing cerebral blood flow to decrease.

7. **(B) diastolic blood pressure**

Systolic pressure is primarily determined by SV, aortic compliance, and the diastolic pressure. In this case, diastolic pressure is increased, causing systolic pressure to be higher; pulse pressure is normal (40 mm Hg), suggesting that SV and aortic compliance are normal.

8. **(E) Increased capillary hydrostatic pressure**

Mitral stenosis causes increased left atrial pressure, which results in increased pulmonary capillary pressure, thereby accounting for the signs of pulmonary edema. Systemic edema is present, most likely resulting from failure of the right ventricle, which developed over time due to high pulmonary vascular resistance; right ventricular failure increases venous and capillary pressures in the systemic circulation. Increased capillary hydrostatic pressure increases the formation of interstitial fluid.

9. **(B) Decreased capillary oncotic pressure**

The patient has liver failure and is therefore unlikely to synthesize enough albumin to maintain a normal plasma oncotic pressure. Capillary oncotic pressure is the major force opposing filtration of plasma out of capillaries; low capillary oncotic pressure therefore results in edema.

10. **(E) Patent ductus arteriosus**

A patent ductus arteriosus is a communication between the aorta and the pulmonary artery, which normally closes shortly after birth. In most cases, this disorder becomes apparent in infants. A continuous murmur is produced because turbulent blood flow occurs along the ductus throughout the cardiac cycle (because pressure is always higher in the aorta than in the pulmonary artery). Increased pulmonary blood flow and venous filling to the left side of the heart have, over time, resulted in left ventricular hypertrophy. Low diastolic blood pressure results from pathologic runoff of blood along the patent ductus. The increased pulse pressure reflects the large left ventricular SV, which is the result of increased venous filling on the left side.

Chapter 5

1. **(D) Pulmonary fibrosis**

FVC and FEV_1 are expected to be reduced in all these conditions. The coexistence of low FRC indicates reduced resting lung volume and is consistent with the low static lung compliance found in patients with pulmonary fibrosis.

2. **(C) The thoracic volume on the right would be larger**

A pneumothorax interrupts the pleural fluid between the lung and chest wall, allowing each structure to assume its equilibrium position. Therefore, the lung collapses to a small volume and the chest wall expands; the diaphragm is part of the chest wall and also moves outward (i.e., flattens to a lower position compared to the unaffected side).

3. **(D) Intrapulmonary shunt**

Severe O_2 refractory hypoxemia results from right-to-left intrapulmonary shunting of blood. This patient is hyperventilating, indicated by his low arterial Pco_2. A high respiratory rate results from pain and splinting as a result of rib fractures. A severe reduction in pulse pressure suggests low cardiac output. The source of intrapulmonary shunt in this case is a tension pneumothorax, with a collapsed lung that is perfused but not ventilated.

4. **(A) Alveolar hypoventilation**

The patient is hypoventilating, causing CO_2 retention and hypercapnia. As a result, alveolar CO_2 is increased and O_2 is decreased.

5. **(B) dead space ventilation is increased**

The patient has a decreased alveolar ventilation rate, evidenced by the increased arterial Pco_2. Decreased alveolar ventilation in the presence of increased total exhaled minute ventilation can only be explained if dead space ventilation is increased.

6. **(C) Increased Pco_2 and decreased Po_2**

Pulmonary emboli create areas of the lung that are ventilated but not perfused, thereby increasing dead space, reducing alveolar ventilation, and decreasing CO_2 excretion. Blood is forced to flow to other areas of the lung, some of which are not ventilated, creating a degree of intrapulmonary shunt, which decreases oxygenation.

7. **(D) Increased Pco_2**

Breathing into and out of a paper bag will result in accumulation of CO_2 and depletion of O_2 in the bag. The same changes will, therefore, be reflected in alveolar air and in arterial blood. Accumulation of CO_2 will also result in a decrease in the blood pH. However, in normal subjects, the most potent drive to breathe is the arterial Pco_2, acting through central chemoreceptors.

8. **(A) Decreased alveolar Po_2**

Chronic pulmonary hypertension is caused by a sustained increase in pulmonary vascular resistance. In patients with alveolar hypoxia, active vasoconstriction increases the vascular resistance. High lung volume contributes to the increased vascular resistance to a lesser degree. Vascular resistance is at a minimum at the FRC. Patients with emphysema have an increased resting lung volume, which causes compression of pulmonary capillaries and therefore increases vascular resistance. Pulmonary vascular resistance is not significantly affected by autonomic nerves.

9. **(D) Rectus abdominus**

The abdominal muscles are the most powerful expiratory muscles; the internal intercostal muscles are weak expiratory muscles. The diaphragm is the primary inspiratory muscle, supported by the external intercostal muscles; the sternocleido-mastoid is an accessory muscle of inspiration.

10. **(A) Bicarbonate ions**

Even in the presence of elevated Pco_2 levels, bicarbonate ions convey the majority (approximately 90%) of the CO_2 in blood.

Chapter 6

1. **(A) ECF volume smaller; ICF volume unchanged**

Acute blood loss is an example of isosmotic volume contraction. Volume loss is from the ECF. No change in ECF osmolarity occurs; therefore no fluid movement between the ECF and ICF occurs.

2. **(A) +16 mm Hg**

Using Equation 6-3 (in the text): $P_{UF} = P_{GC} - (\pi_{GC} + P_{GC})$. $P_{UF} = 50 - (26 + 8) = +16$ mm Hg (favoring filtration).

3. **(D) Efferent arteriole dilation**

An increase in RBF without an increase in blood pressure indicates a decrease in renal vascular resistance. Dilation of the efferent arteriole increases glomerular capillary outflow and reduces P_{GC}, causing GFR to decrease. Filtration fraction decreases because GFR is smaller and RBF is larger.

4. **(C) 48 mL/min**

Clearance is the ratio of excretion rate to plasma concentration. In this case, excretion rate is provided (often it must be calculated from the product of urine concentration and urine flow rate): C_{urea} = 12 mg/min / 0.25 mg/mL = 48 mL/min.

5. **(A) Proximal tubule**

The patient has a condition called acquired Fanconi syndrome. The presence of high levels of glucose, HCO_3^-, and phosphate together in the urine suggest proximal tubule dysfunction because this is their main site of reabsorption.

6. **(B) Loop diuretic**

A powerful diuretic is needed to remove fluids and reduce pulmonary edema. Inhibition of the thick ascending limb by loop diuretics provides the largest natriuresis and diuresis.

7. **(A) Central diabetes insipidus**

Removal of drinking water for 6 hours would increase urine osmolarity in cases of compulsive water drinking or in patients with diabetes mellitus. Restoration of urine concentration with exogenous ADH demonstrates a failure of endogenous ADH secretion and a diagnosis of central diabetes insipidus.

8. **(D) Insulin/glucose**

Acid infusion or aldosterone blockade would elevate serum potassium further. Insulin activates Na/K/ATPase and causes uptake of potassium by cells to alleviate the problem. α-Adrenoceptor agonists and PTH have no effect.

9. **(C) Metabolic alkalosis**

Plasma [HCO_3^-] is high and base excess is elevated, defining metabolic alkalosis. There is alkalemia but no respiratory compensation.

10. **(B) respiratory acidosis**

The patient has high $Paco_2$ (respiratory acidosis) and high plasma HCO_3^- (metabolic alkalosis). The pH remains acidic, indicating that the primary disorder is the acidosis, which has been partially compensated. This is a chronic condition. The expected compensation for this condition is an increase of 0.4 mEq/L HCO_3^- for every 1 mm Hg increase in $Paco_2$.

Chapter 7

1. **(D) Ileum**

   The microspheres travel with the meal and reflect the transit time of the meal. After 8 hours, the meal would typically progress to the distal small intestine. The beads are small enough not to be arrested by sphincters.

2. **(C) Splanchnic sympathetic nerves**

   Most afferent nerves conveying pain in the gastrointestinal tract travel in the sympathetic division of the autonomic nervous system.

3. **(A) Upper esophageal sphincter**

   High resting pressure indicates the sensor was located in a sphincter. The pattern of pressure changes upon swallowing describes the action of upper esophageal sphincter.

4. **(A) Relaxation of the upper esophageal sphincter**

   Achalasia is a condition that affects the intrinsic nerves of the ENS in the esophagus. Relaxation of the lower sphincter and the organization of peristalsis are particularly affected. The upper esophageal sphincter is controlled by extrinsic nerves and is minimally affected by achalasia.

5. **(G) Histamine + gastrin + acetylcholine**

   There is potentiation between histamine, gastrin, and acetylcholine so that the combined response is greater than the sum of individual responses.

6. **(D) Reduced volume of pancreatic juice**

   Cystic fibrosis Cl^- channels are required for fluid secretion by pancreatic ducts, which secrete most of the volume of pancreatic juice. Cl^- channels supply Cl^- from the cell to drive HCO_3^- secretion into the duct lumen. The secretion of HCO_3^- drives Na^+ secretion and fluid secretion. Without a functional Cl^- channel, fluid secretion is reduced very significantly.

7. **(C)**

   The clinical signs and symptoms suggest blockage of the lower biliary tract with a gallstone. Obstructive jaundice develops, in which the liver conjugates bilirubin, which leaks into the systemic circulation. The capacity of hepatocytes to continue conjugating bilirubin decreases when the outflow pathway into the biliary tract is blocked. Therefore, serum free bilirubin levels increase. The lack of conjugated bilirubin entering the intestines prevents formation of urobilinogen; therefore the levels of urobilinogen are low.

8. **(A) Anemia**

   The distal ileum is a specific site for absorption of vitamin B_{12}. Deficiency of this vitamin leads to pernicious anemia.

9. **(E) All of the above**

   The patient has fat malabsorption. Hyperacidity can denature pancreatic lipase. Pancreatic insufficiency results in inadequate pancreatic lipase secretion. Obstructive gallstone disease limits bile delivery and reduces fat assimilation. Inflammatory bowel disease may prevent adequate absorption of dietary fat even when digestion is normal.

10. **(B) Excess secretion of potassium in the large intestine**

    Potassium secretion in the distal large intestine occurs through luminal membrane potassium channels. The delivery of increased amounts of sodium and fluid to the large intestine in diarrhea drives excess potassium secretion.

Chapter 8

1. **(E) Tyrosine kinase**

   Tyrosine kinases do not couple to G proteins; all other choices are second messengers that are produced through activation of G-protein–coupled receptors.

2. **(F) Prolactin**

   Prolactin is the only hormone under primarily negative control from the hypothalamus, via dopamine release. Sectioning of the pituitary stalk therefore increases prolactin secretion, due to loss of dopamine action on lactotrope cells of the anterior pituitary.

3. **(F) Gigantism due to excess IGF-1 production**

   Excess growth hormone produces gigantism in prepubertal children because the epiphyseal growth plates in long bones have not closed. The effects of growth hormone on linear growth are mediated via IGF-1.

4. **(D) Primary hypothyroidism, high TSH**

   Iodine deficiency prevents normal production of thyroid hormone by the thyroid gland, producing primary hypothy-roidism. Lack of negative feedback inhibition by thyroid hormone on the hypothalamus and pituitary results in high TSH levels.

5. **(C) Low cortisol, high ACTH**

   The symptoms describe adrenal insufficiency, with Na wasting, volume depletion, and K retention due to low aldosterone levels. Fasting hypoglycemia and fatigue are due to low cortisol levels. Increased pigmentation suggests high levels of ACTH. High ACTH would occur in primary adrenal insufficiency due to a lack of negative feedback from cortisol.

6. **(B)**

   The enzyme 21-hydroxylase is required for cortisol and aldosterone synthesis (Figure 8-11). Low levels of cortisol result in high levels of ACTH due to loss of negative feedback. Build up of steroid precursors in adrenal cortex is shunted toward the formation of excess adrenal androgens, which causes virilization.

7. **(D) Reduced airway resistance**

   β_2 receptors mediate relaxation of bronchioles to reduce airway resistance. Vasodilation of skeletal muscle arterioles and mobilization of glucose and fatty acids in the liver also occur through activation of β_2 receptors.

8. **(F) ↓ glucose, ↓ fatty acids, ↓ ketones**

   Insulin directs increased uptake, use, and storage glucose, and increased storage of fatty acids as triglycerides. Ketone production in the liver is increased by glucagon and suppressed by insulin.

9. **(F) Type 2 diabetes mellitus**

   Glycosuria indicates diabetes mellitus. Mature onset and obesity are most likely to be associated with type 2 diabetes mellitus; the absence of ketonuria suggests type 2 rather than type 1 diabetes. Polyuria is due to osmotic diuresis from hyperglycemia. Proteinuria may indicate renal damage as a result of diabetes mellitus.

10. **(C)**

    If PTH is ineffective due to tissue resistance, there is inadequate renal Ca^{2+} retention and failure to produce enough $1,25\text{-}(OH_2) D_3$, in turn resulting in low dietary Ca^{2+} uptake. With ineffective PTH, there is low Ca^{2+} mobilization from bone. Urine phosphate excretion is inadequate. Low Ca^{2+} and high phosphate stimulate PTH secretion.

Chapter 9

1. **(A) GnRH agonist given in pulsatile doses**

   Pulsatile GnRH mimics the physiologic release pattern. Continuous dosing is ineffective because it downregulates pituitary gonadotropes.

2. **(A) Luteinizing hormone (LH)—Leydig cell**

   Leydig cells produce testosterone in response to LH.

3. **(A) Androgen receptors**

   The patient has complete androgen insensitivity (testicular feminization) in which androgen-induced development of the mesonephric duct fails. Sertoli cells continue to secrete müllerian-inhibiting substance, so female internal reproductive organs also fail to develop.

4. **(B) Enhanced penile erection following normal erotic stimulation**

   Sildenafil decreases the clearance of cyclic guanine monophosphate (cGMP), which mediates vasodilation in erectile tissues following NO release. NO is not produced or released unless parasympathetic nerves are activated by normal erotic stimulation. Emission and ejaculation are mediated via sympathetic nerves, independent of NO-cGMP.

5. **(D) Day 21**

   A high concentration of estrogen, progesterone, and inhibin, all at the same time, indicates peak secretion from the corpus luteum about days 18–24. Negative feedback produces low LH and FSH.

6. **(C) Days 21–22**

   Implantation normally occurs 6–7 days after ovulation.

7. (A) Acrosome reaction

Binding of the sperm head to specific proteins of the zona pellucida causes a calcium signal in the sperm, resulting in the acrosome reaction.

8. (B) Dehydroepiandrosterone sulfate (DHEA-S)

Human placenta has a very high aromatase enzyme activity that converts androgens to estrogens but lacks the ability to produce the androgen substrate. DHEA-S and its 16-hydroxylated derivative are produced by fetal adrenal for this purpose.

9. (A) Estrogen

Estrogens suppress the milk-producing effects of prolactin during pregnancy to prevent milk production before birth. Expulsion of the placenta at birth removes the source of estrogen. At about day 2 postpartum, milk production in response to prolactin begins.

10. (E)

Ovarian failure after menopause causes estrogen, progesterone, and inhibin levels to decrease to very low levels. The loss of negative feedback results in high levels of gonadotropin secretion by the anterior pituitary. This patient has osteoporosis, a common complication of sustained low estrogen.

Chapter 10

1. (E) Simple diffusion

Small lipid soluble gas molecules such as N_2O readily diffuse through biological membranes. The inability to increase blood N_2O concentration above that in the lung alveolus is consistent with simple diffusion and the absence of any primary or secondary active transport process.

2. (C) inspired N_2O concentration increased

According to Fick's law of diffusion, the rate of simple diffusion of N_2O is proportional to its membrane permeability and to its concentration gradient. The N_2O concentration gradient is increased if the inspired N_2O concentration is increased, but is decreased if alveolar ventilation or pulmonary blood flow are decreased. The rate of simple diffusion is slower at colder temperatures or if the diffusion distance is increased.

3. (D) Opening of Na^+ channels

When a depolarizing stimulus causes the threshold membrane potential (of about -55 mV) to be exceeded, voltage sensitive Na^+ channels rapidly open, resulting in fast depolarization.

4. (C) Net inward Na^+ current

At 0 mV during repolarization, Na^+ channels are inactivating but many remain open. K^+ channels are opening rapidly at this time. The electrochemical driving force is inward for Na^+ and outward for K^+. Therefore, there is net outward K^+ flow and net inward Na^+ flow at this time. A significant Na^+ conductance must still be present to account for a membrane potential of 0 mV.

5. **(E) would not be triggered**

    The stimulus is applied during the absolute refractory period. No second action potential is possible because too many Na^+ channels are now inactivated.

6. **(A) Increased preload**

    Curves intersect the x-axis when there is zero shortening ("isometric" contraction). The total force on the muscle at this point is indicative of preload; therefore curve C has the largest preload. If a total load is selected on the x-axis and a vertical line is drawn, the curves may be compared; increased preload results in faster muscle shortening.

7. **(F) H $^+$/K$^+$-ATPase**

    Primary active transport has a direct dependence on adenosine triphosphate hydrolysis and would be inhibited under anaerobic conditions. Secretion moves H^+ out of the cell; dependence on external K^+ suggests an exchange with H^+.

8. **(C) Depolarization due to E_K becoming less negative**

    In most cells, V_m is a function of $[K^+]_o$ because K^+ channels provide the dominant membrane conductance at rest. Acutely increasing $[K^+]_o$ results in a less negative value for E_K, according to the Nernst equation. V_m becomes less negative, or depolarize as a result.

9. **(E) reduced time for Ca^{2+} reuptake into sarcoplasmic reticulum**

    The question describes temporal summation, in which the muscle is tetanized. The basis of this effect is accumulation of Ca^{2+} in the sarcoplasm with repeated stimulation due to insufficient time for Ca^{2+} reuptake by sarcoplasmic reticulum. A plateau is reached when maximal cross-bridge cycling has occurred.

10. **(A) Left dorsal columns**

    The primary sensory neurons for touch, vibration, and proprioception are conveyed by the ipsilateral dorsal columns. Second-order neurons cross over in the medulla and ascend to the thalamus; third-order neurons are conveyed via the internal capsule to the somatosensory cortex.

11. **(B) Circadian rhythm generation**

    The suprachiasmatic nucleus is a key site for the "body clock" and therefore the generation and maintenance of circadian rhythms.

12. **(E) Temporal**

    The patient has aphasia consistent with damage to Wernicke's area, which is at the junction of the temporal and parietal lobes. The presence of memory loss is consistent with damage to the hippocampal formation, which is in the medial temporal lobe.

13. **(F) Paresis and spasticity of the right leg**

    Transection of the right lateral corticospinal tracts (which have already crossed over) causes loss of upper motor neurons controlling movement of the right leg. Therefore, there is right leg paresis and spasticity. Transection of the right dorsal columns causes loss of touch, vibration, and proprioception from the right leg because these neurons cross over in the medulla. Transection of the anterolateral spinothalamic tracts results in loss of contralateral (left in this case) pain and temperature sensation; these modalities are absent in two to three spinal segments below the lesion due to the path of sensory neurons via Lissauer's tract.

14. **(E) Monocular blindness**

Loss of an optic nerve involves only the affected eye. Bitemporal hemianopia is caused by damage to fibers crossing at the optic chiasm; homonymous hemianopia (loss of one half of the visual field) is caused by lesions beyond the optic chiasm. Binasal hemianopia would require selective damage at the lateral aspect of the optic chiasm on both sides. Macular degeneration is loss of the central vision due to damage to the macula area of the retina.

15. **(A) Concave**

Nearsightedness (myopia) is usually the result of eyeballs that are too long, causing light to be focused in front of the retina. A concave lens corrects this problem by causing light to diverge before it enters the eye. A convex lens would worsen the problem by converging light rays further; a cylindrical lens is used to correct for astigmatism.

16. **(B) Cerebral aqueduct stenosis**

Expansion of the ventricular system is isolated to areas upstream of the cerebral aqueduct, suggesting this is a site of obstruction that results in hydrocephalus.

17. **(C) spatial summation**

Since only action potentials were being recorded in an output neuron, no synaptic events were measured directly. Simultaneous stimulation from several input neurons demonstrates spatial summation of inputs to reach threshold for action potential in the output neuron. If increased intensity of stimulation in a single input neuron produces action potentials in the output neuron, this would demonstrate temporal summation.

18. **(B) Cholinergic sympathetic neurons**

Physiologic sweating in response to increased body temperature is mediated by cholinergic sympathetic nerves, which are activated by the hypothalamic temperature controller. Adrenergic sweating can also occur to a lesser degree and may contribute, for example, to the presentation of sweating and vasoconstriction in patients with shock.

19. **(C) Dopamine precursor**

The patient has the classic clinical findings of Parkinson's disease. The paucity of movement reflects loss of dopaminergic input to the basal ganglia from the substantia nigra pars compacta. Exogenous administration of a dopamine precursor capable of entering the brain, such as levodopa, will alleviate symptoms.

20. **(C) Cerebellum**

The wide ataxic gait and inability to walk heel to toe without falling suggest a cerebellar problem; chronic alcohol abuse is a common cause of cerebellar damage. Loss of proprioception via the dorsal column pathways would also cause a similar pattern of symptoms.

21. **(C) Glossopharyngeal (CN IX)**

The glossopharyngeal nerve is sensory to the pharynx and motor to several striated muscles involved in the pharyngeal component of swallowing. It conveys taste from the posterior third of the tongue. The sinus nerve joins the glossopharyngeal nerve; dysfunction in the baroreceptor reflex may, therefore, play a role in the appearance of palpitations. The facial nerve is secretomotor to salivary glands and serves taste to the anterior two thirds of the tongue; it may be affected, but it is not involved with swallowing or mediating sensations from the pharynx. The vagus nerve is important for modulation of gastrointestinal and cardiac function, but it is not necessary for swallowing or involved in oral sensations. The hypoglossal and abducens are only motor nerves to the tongue and extraocular muscles, respectively.

22. **(A) Inferior colliculus**

The inferior colliculus is a key relay in the auditory pathway. The medial lemniscus is a sensory fiber tract; the red nucleus and substantia nigra are part of the motor system. The reticular activating system is part of the diffuse modulatory systems and is not directly related to the auditory system.

23. **(C) K^+ current**

Phase 4 is the resting membrane potential, which is most dependent on the presence of open K^+ channels that mediate an outward K^+ current.

24. **(A) Aortic stenosis**

High left ventricular pressure is developed by the left ventricle to overcome the impedance to ejection of blood through a narrowed aortic valve. In severe valve disease such as this, the aortic systolic pressure is reduced due to low stroke volume.

25. **(A) Decreased**

The patient has a clinical history consistent with systolic heart failure. The pressure-volume relation confirms reduced ventricular contractility. The ejection fraction is reduced systolic heart failure. In contrast, ventricular contractility and ejection fraction would be preserved in diastolic heart failure, but cardiac filling would be reduced and diastolic heart pressures increased.

26. **(B) B–C**

During isovolumic contraction, the atrioventricular valves close because of increasing ventricular pressure, but the semilunar valves are not yet open because ventricular pressure has not exceeded the pressure in the aorta (or the pulmonary artery).

27. (D) Point D

The aortic valve opens at point C and ventricular ejection occurs from C–E; the peak left ventricular pressure is almost equal to the peak aortic (systolic) pressure.

28. (B) Point B

Diastolic filling is completed from A–B; isovolumic contraction begins at B, causing the mitral valve to close.

29. (C) C–E

Narrowing of the aortic valve causes turbulent blood flow during ventricular ejection. Therefore, the murmur is heard from the opening of the aortic valve at point C to its closure at point E.

30. (C) Phase 2

Period 4 is the ST segment in which the ECG recording is on the isoelectric baseline, indicating that all ventricular cells are at the same potential (no electrical dipole is measured). In this period, ventricular cells are between depolarization (QRS complex) and repolarization (T wave) and are therefore in the plateau (phase 2) of the action potential.

31. (B) Decrease in erythropoietin (EPO) secretion

Hematocrit is the percentage of whole blood contributed by red blood cells. Destruction of transfused blood is unlikely, assuming blood type is correctly matched. Dilution of red cells by water retention in SIADH is possible, but a decrease to 24% hematocrit represents massive water retention. GFR has decreased, as shown by the high plasma creatinine concentration, but GFR is not a direct determinant of the hematocrit. Low GFR indicates renal insufficiency, which will be accompanied by failure to secrete EPO, thereby causing anemia. There are many sites of active bone marrow away from the fracture site for erythrocyte production.

32. (B) Dynamic exercise

The stressor results in an increase in cardiac output and venous return associated with increased cardiac contractility (increased cardiac output for the same atrial pressure). Systemic vascular resistance is reduced, evidenced by the increased slope of the vascular function curve. During exercise, the activation of the sympathetic nervous system provides positive inotropic stimulation to the heart, thereby increasing cardiac output. Dilation of muscle blood vessels is responsible for reducing systemic vascular resistance. During digestion, blood would be redistributed to the gastrointestinal organs but without a change in cardiac output. In hypothermia, cardiac output would decrease because cooling inhibits heart rate and contractility. In severe hemorrhage, cardiac output would decrease due to decreased venous return.

33. (B) Patient B

Chronic bronchitis is an obstructive lung disorder, characterized by reduced FVC, FEV_1, and a reduced ratio of FVC to FEV_1.

34. **(B) Increased airway resistance**

The peak inspiratory pressure is increased, showing that dynamic compliance is reduced. However, the plateau pressure, which is measured in the absence of airflow, is unchanged compared to the previous test, indicating that the increased peak airway pressure is associated with air flow. Increased airway resistance therefore accounts for the high airway pressure needed to ventilate the patient. If the plateau of pressure had increased, this would indicate that the lung and chest compliance were low.

35. **(D) Pulmonary fibrosis**

The red curve depicts a patient breathing from a reduced resting lung volume. This occurs in pulmonary fibrosis due to low lung compliance. The blue curve depicts a patient with emphysema who breathes from an increased resting lung volume due to highly compliant lungs.

36. **(D) Increased partial pressure of CO_2**

The red oxyhemoglobin dissociation curve is right-shifted, which may be caused by increased temperature, increased P_{CO_2}, or increased erythrocyte 2,3-BPG concentration, or by decreased pH.

37. **(A) 10 L**

Inulin is a marker for ECF volume. Using Equation 1-1 (see Chapter 1), $V = (Q - q)/C$: $V = (200 \text{ mg} - 100 \text{ mg})/1 \text{ mg/dL} = 100 \text{ dL} = 10 \text{ L}$.

38. **(B) ECF volume smaller; ICF volume smaller**

Sweat is a hypotonic saline solution. Sweating reduces ECF volume and raises ECF osmolarity, causing water to flow from ICF to ECF. Both ICF and ECF have a reduced final volume and higher osmolarity (hyperosmotic volume contraction).

39. **(B) Lack of anastomosis between the arcuate arteries**

Lobar branching of a single renal artery reflects the embryologic development of the kidney in lobes. The arcuate arteries arising from the lobar arteries appear to meet and anastomose along the corticomedullary boundary, but there is little functional anastomosis.

40. **(C) The kidney has a high rate of blood perfusion**

The A-V(O_2) differences given in the question are normal, suggesting no pathologic problems. Renal a-v(O_2) is low because renal blood flow is normally very high, providing an excess of O_2 delivery despite high renal O_2 demand.

41. **(D) Podocyte**

The glomerular barrier restricting protein filtration is located partly in the glomerular basement membrane and partly by filtration slits between foot processes of podocytes.

42. **(B)**

Constriction of afferent arteriole increases vascular resistance and reduces RBF. Blood flow into the glomerulus decreases, resulting in a decrease in

P_{GC} and, therefore, a decrease in GFR. RBF and GFR both decrease, leaving the filtration fraction unchanged.

43. (F) Low glomerular filtration rate (GFR)

High plasma creatinine is most likely to indicate a decrease in GFR. Dehydration can also cause a decrease in GFR, but not so much as to cause a fivefold increase in P_{cr}. Creatinine levels are not affected by ADH or acid-base status. Increased creatinine is observed in body builders due to high muscle mass, but this patient has a low body weight that is not consistent with this explanation.

44. (B) There is net tubular secretion of substance X

Clearance of substance X is larger than that of creatinine at all plasma concentrations. When clearance of a solute exceeds glomerular filtration, the solute must be secreted in addition to filtration. The decline in the clearance of substance X with increased plasma concentration indicates a saturable carrier-mediated transport process rather than simple diffusion.

45. (G) 1200 mL/min

C_{PAH} is the effective renal plasma flow rate. Applying Equation 6-6 (see Chapter 6), renal blood flow (RBF) = renal plasma flow (RPF)/(1-Hct): RBF = 600 (mL/min)/0.5 = 1200 mL/min.

46. (C) 20 mg/min

In the case of creatinine, a marker for the glomerular filtration rate, the excretion rate equals the filtered load. Excretion rate is the product of urine concentration and urine flow rate: FL_{cr} = 20 mg/mL × 1 mL/min = 20 mg/min.

47. (B) 200 mg/dL

Renal threshold is defined as the plasma concentration at which a solute first appears in the urine. The blue curve indicates glucose excretion, which begins at a plasma glucose concentration of about 200 mg/mL.

48. (C) Glucose

The rapid decline in tubular solute concentration at the start of the proximal tubule indicates a preferentially absorbed solute. Nutrients and $HCO_3\sim$ have this pattern of proximal tubule absorption.

49. (F) phosphate

The infant has Bartter's syndrome. Loss of function in the thick ascending limb causes dramatic urinary electrolyte losses, reflecting what is normally reabsorbed in this segment. Phosphate is the only electrolyte listed that does not have a high rate of transport in the thick ascending limb; phosphate is mainly reabsorbed in the proximal tubule.

50. (C) HCO_3^-

Carbonic anhydrase is required to recover filtered $HCO_3\sim$ in the proximal tubule. Inhibition by acetazolamide results in a large urinary loss of $HCO_3\sim$. *Note: in this case, acetazolamide was used for its effect on the eye to reduce the rate of aqueous humor secretion by the ciliary epithelium.*

51. (A) Aquaporin 2 expression in the collecting duct decreased

Ingestion of a large volume of water causes hypotonic plasma and suppresses antidiuretic hormone (ADH) secretion. Low ADH levels inactivate the countercurrent system. Water reabsorption is inhibited in the collecting duct because aquaporin 2 water channels are internalized by principal cells. Changes in free water excretion are not mediated by changes in GFR or proximal tubule absorption.

52. (D) increased Na$^+$ reabsorption in the thin descending limb

Dehydration increases plasma osmolarity and stimulates ADH secretion. ADH stimulates Na$^+$ and urea reabsorption as part of the countercurrent mechanism. Na$^+$ reabsorption is stimulated in the ascending limb, not the descending limb of the loop of Henle. Aquaporin 2 expression increases to allow water retention by the collecting duct.

53. (A) 0 mL/min

Equations 6-7 and 6-8 (see Chapter 6) could be applied, but in this case urine is exactly isosmotic with respect to plasma, so no free water can have been added or removed in the formation of urine.

54. (D) atrial natriuretic peptide (ANP)

ANP causes excretion of more Na$^+$. This endocrine axis is suppressed in response to hemorrhage because blood volume and atrial stretch are reduced.

55. (A) Increased hydrostatic pressure and reduced oncotic pressure

Increasing extracellular fluid (ECF) volume with salt and water ingestion dilutes plasma proteins and reduces plasma oncotic pressure generally. Increased ECF volume includes increased plasma volume, the largest fraction of which is in the systemic veins. Increased systemic venous pressure increases capillary pressures, including the peritubular capillary hydrostatic pressure. These changes to Starling's forces suppress tubular fluid reabsorption and therefore promote renal Na$^+$ and water excretion.

56. (B) decreased

Parathyroid hormone stimulates renal Ca^{2+} reabsorption by the distal tubule, causing a decrease in fractional excretion.

57. (A) Respiratory alkalosis

Pco$_2$ is depressed. The patient is hyperventilating and has respiratory alkalosis. There is alkalemia with no metabolic compensation.

58. (D) Metabolic acidosis

Plasma [HCO$_3^-$] is very low and there is a large base deficit, defining metabolic acidosis. The pH is acidic, and there is no respiratory compensation present.

59. (C) 30 L

Total body water can be estimated as 50% of body weight in women of normal body mass index (and 60% of body weight in men). Therefore, a female patient weighing 60 kg would have approximately 30 L of body water.

60. **(E) significantly more than three times normal**

The patient has low effective circulating volume and reduction in renal blood flow and filtration (C_{PAH} and C_{CR}). BUN will be elevated due to the low glomerular filtration rate and further increased due to the high antidiuretic hormone levels in this low volume state. The ratio of BUN to creatinine is expected to be high; because P_{CR} is three times normal, BUN will be significantly more elevated than this.

61. **(B) Respiratory acidosis**

P_{CO_2} is very elevated, defining respiratory acidosis. pH is acidic. No metabolic compensation is present.

62. **(D) metabolic acidosis**

The patient has low plasma [HCO_3^-] (metabolic acidosis) and low P_{CO_2} (respiratory alkalosis). The pH is acidic, indicating primary metabolic acidosis. The expected compensation is a 1.3 mm Hg decrease in P_{CO_2} for every 1 mEq/L decrease in plasma HCO_3^-.

63. **(E) vasoactive intestinal polypeptide**

VIP is a potent secretagogue in small intestine. The other choices (i.e., gastrin, cholecystokinin, motilin, and glucose-dependent insulinotropic polypeptide) have little effect on fluid secretion.

64. **(D) Motilin**

The contractions described are the migrating motor complex. Motilin stimulates this pattern of motility, under the direction of the enteric nervous system.

65. **(E) Somatostatin**

Somatostatin is a potent inhibitor in the gastrointestinal system. Other substances listed are either stimulatory for secretion in the stomach (acetylcholine and gastrin) or pancreas (secretin and cholecystokinin).

66. **(E) Stimulation of parasympathetic nerves to the salivary gland**

At point Y, salivation has been stimulated. The primary control of salivation is via parasympathetic tone. Sleep and dehydration reduce salivation. Sympathetic tone has minor effects on salivation. Aldosterone slightly increases Na^+ absorption from saliva.

67. **(B) Migrating motor complex**

The pyloric sphincter only allows small particles to pass during the fed state. It is only during the fasting state that the migrating motor complex flushes residual stomach contents into the duodenum.

68. **(A) Cholecystokinin**

Cholecystokinin is the most important agonist that stimulates pancreatic acinar cells to release zymogen granules by exocytosis. Acetylcholine is a weak agonist (not listed here).

69. **(A) Iron and Ca^{2+}**

The duodenum is the main site of iron and Ca^{2+} uptake, particularly iron uptake. Other ions are extensively reabsorbed along the small intestine; Na^+ is also reabsorbed in large intestine.

70. **(B) Excess intestinal absorption of iron**

Iron overload is caused by excessive intestinal uptake because no regulated excretion pathway exists for iron. In hereditary hemochromatosis, there is a failure of negative feedback control of intestinal uptake through the hepcidin pathway.

71. **(B) Glucose absorption continues at a reduced rate**

Galactose and glucose have equal affinity at the same Na-linked cotransport protein (SGLT1). Equimolar galactose would compete for binding to the transporter, reducing the rate of glucose uptake.

72. **(C) Lactase deficiency**

A fecal osmolar gap indicates the presence of organic molecules that are measured as part of the total osmolarity but are present in addition to electrolytes such as Na^+ and K^+. Lactase deficiency would cause undigested lactose in the feces, resulting in osmotic diarrhea.

73. **(C) Vitamins A and D**

Fat-soluble vitamins rely on normal fat reabsorption for their assimilation. A high proportion of dietary fat-soluble vitamins remain in fecal fat in patients with steatorrhea (excess fecal fat excretion). Vitamins A and D are fat soluble; vitamins B_1 and C are water soluble.

74. **(C) Gastrocolic reflex**

The presence of food in the stomach and duodenum stimulates the gastrocolic reflex. This is a feed-forward reflex in which mass movement contractions occur in the colon to propel feces into the rectum. The response is particularly well developed in young children in whom reflex defecation follows.

75. **(E) 1% glucose + 0.1% oleic acid + 0.9% saline + HCl, pH = 6.2**

Enterogastrones cause feedback inhibition of gastric emptying. Low pH, high osmolarity, and high nutrient content of chyme all stimulate enterogastrones.

76. **(B) Circulates bound to plasma proteins**

A cholesterol derivative is most likely to behave like a steroid hormone. Steroids are usually bound to carrier proteins in blood. Classic steroid effects are long lasting; they are mediated by diffusion into cells, binding to intracellular receptors and changes in gene transcription.

77. **(B) 20 pg/mL**

Reading the standard curve across from the y-axis, a value of 50% ^{125}I-ANP displacement corresponds to a serum ANP concentration of about 25 pg/mL.

78. **(D) Increased blood glucose concentration**

The signs and symptoms noted in this patient are classic manifestations of growth hormone excess after puberty (acromegaly). Growth hormone has diabetogenic actions that result in an increase in blood glucose concentration, including increased gluconeogenesis in the liver and inhibition of glucose uptake by muscle.

79. **(E) Supraoptic nucleus**

Symptoms suggest loss of antidiuretic hormone (ADH) action (diabetes insipidus). Acquired central diabetes insipidus may be caused by a head injury. ADH is produced mainly in the supraoptic nucleus so damage here would compromise ADH secretion.

80. **(E) Thyroxine**

Ninety percent of secreted thyroid hormone is T_4. T_3 is the most potent form, but is produced in the tissues by the action of $5'/3'$ deiodinase.

81. **(C) High T_4, low TSH**

The symptoms describing this patient indicate hyperthyroidism. Ophthalmopathy suggests Graves' disease, in which thyroid-stimulating immunoglobulins (TSI) act as TSH agonists, driving high levels of T_4 secretion. Negative feedback suppresses endogenous TSH secretion to produce low TSH levels.

82. **(A) Zona glomerulosa**

The zona glomerulosa is the sole source of aldosterone because it is the only region of gland to express aldosterone synthase.

83. **(A) increased glucose and increased fatty acids**

Glucocorticoids mobilize glucose, amino acids, and fatty acids.

84. **(D) Glucocorticoids—mineralocorticoid receptors**

11β-Hydroxysteroid dehydrogenase modifies cortisol to prevent it from acting at the mineralocorticoid receptor. This is necessary because it is an agonist at the receptor, and it circulates at much higher concentration than aldosterone. Inhibition of 11β-hydroxysteroid dehydrogenase by licorice allows cortisol to activate the mineralocorticoid receptor, causing salt retention.

85. **(B) Chronic glucocorticoid medication**

The patient's clinical signs are characteristic of glucocorticoid excess. However, there is low cortisol and low ACTH, so physical signs can only be explained by exogenous glucocorticoid medication.

86. **(D)**

Pheochromocytoma is a secretory tumor of adrenal medullary chromaffin cells. High levels of the catecholamines epinephrine and norepinephrine are excreted in the urine. Metabolism of catecholamines via catechol-*O*-methyltrans-ferase (COMT) and monoamine oxidase (MAO) enzymes produce high levels of metanephrine and VMA, which are excreted in urine.

87. (E) Insulin

The resident is likely to be hypoglycemic due to prolonged fasting. Insulin secretion is stimulated by hyperglycemia and suppressed by hypoglycemia. All the other listed hormones are stimulated by hypoglycemia.

88. (A) Increased insulin and increased glucagon

Insulin increases net protein synthesis, and insulin secretion is stimulated by increased plasma amino acid concentration. To prevent hypoglycemia from developing, glucagon secretion is also stimulated by increased plasma amino acid concentration.

89. (D) Glucagon-like peptide-1

Enteroendocrine cells release glucose-dependent insulinotropic polypeptide (GIP) and glucagon-like peptide-1 in response to a carbohydrate-rich meal. These incretins stimulate insulin release by pancreatic **P** cells as an "anticipatory" response to an impending glucose load.

90. (C) Glucagon

The patient has type 1 diabetes mellitus. Lack of insulin prevents proper oxidation of fatty acids. High levels of glucagon direct hepatic formation of ketones from acetyl CoA instead.

91. (D) Glucagon and epinephrine

Glucagon and epinephrine stimulate gluconeogenesis by the liver and increase the supply of glucose precursors from muscle to the liver. Other effects include increased release of fatty acids from adipose tissue and the increased rate of glycogen breakdown in liver and muscle.

92. (C) Parathyroid hormone

Urine phosphate excretion is controlled by parathyroid hormone, which inhibits tubular phosphate reabsorption.

93. (F)

The patient has humoral hypocalcemia of malignancy due to PTH-rp secretion, whose action is similar to endogenous PTH. Ca^{2+} retention and phosphate excretion occur. Hypercalcemia suppresses PTH secretion.

94. (A) Androgen receptors

The patient has complete androgen insensitivity (testicular feminization). Androgen-induced development of the mesonephric duct fails. Sertoli cells continue to secrete müllerian-inhibiting substance, so female internal reproductive organs also fail to develop.

95. (D) Day 21

High concentrations of estrogen, progesterone, and inhibin, all at the same time, indicate peak secretion from the corpus luteum around days 18–24. Negative feedback produces low LH and FSH.

96. **(A) Aldosterone**

Changes in renal function that increase plasma volume in pregnancy are due to up-regulation of the renin-angiotensin II-aldosterone axis. High levels of progesterone and estrogen bring about this up-regulation, but do not act directly themselves to increase plasma volume.

97. **(A) Increased alveolar ventilation**

Alveolar ventilation increases in pregnancy due to higher tidal volumes. CO_2 levels decrease as a primary result. Renal compensation brings about a decrease in $[HCO_3\sim]$ to compensate the pH.

98. **(C) Oxytocin**

The lactation reflex occurs in response to a baby suckling, which produces a surge of oxytocin secretion and milk ejection. This reflex can be conditioned by stimuli such as the sound of a baby crying.

99. **(D) During the expulsive stages of labor**

Oxytocin secretion increases in a positive feedback fashion as the cervix dilates, resulting in high concentrations about the time of birth, which produce powerful uterine contractions.

100. **(A) Human chorionic gonadotropin**

Human chorionic gonadotropin is a pregnancy-specific hormone secreted by the early embryonic trophoblast. Trace amounts can be detected in urine as early as 7–10 days after ovulation.

101. **(E) Syncytiotrophoblast**

The syncytiotrophoblast persists in the mature placenta as a multinucleated cell layer outermost in chorionic villi, and is bathed in maternal blood within the intervillous space.

102. **(A) Estrogen**

A sustained high estrogen concentration produces positive feedback stimulation of luteinizing hormone secretion by sensitizing gonadotropes to gonadotropin-releasing hormone.

103. **(C) Day 14**

Ferning of cervical mucus indicates the most receptive time for passage of sperm. This thinner mucus is produced during estrogen dominance about midcycle.

104. **(A) no sperm is ejaculated**

The vas deferens carries sperm from the epididymis to the ejaculatory duct. Severing the vas prevents sperm from being added to seminal plasma.

105. **(D) 5α-Reductase**

In this child, there is failure of male external genitalia to develop correctly with a normal XY karyotype. External genitalia require dihydrotestosterone for development, which is synthesized in the tissues from testosterone via the enzyme 5α-reductase. Testosterone is produced normally by the testes, allowing masculinization at puberty.

106. (B) lack of androgen precursors from which to produce estrogens

Estrogens are produced in a two-cell system of granulosa and theca cells. Theca cells provide androgen precursors under the influence of LH. Granulosa cells use androgens to synthesize estrogens, which is accomplished via FSH-stimulated aromatase activity.

107. (A) lower P_{O_2} and higher P_{CO_2}

Blood in the umbilical artery is returning from fetal tissues to the placenta for oxygenation and removal of CO_2.

108. (A) Early maturation of the hypothalamic-pituitary-gonadal axis

This is a case of true precocious puberty in which normal puberty has occurred, but too early. A pubertal growth spurt caused the patient to be tall as a child. Early production of sex steroids caused early closure of epiphyseal growth plates, resulting in short adult height.

Index

Page numbers followed by f and t indicate figures and tables respectively.